Computational Models of Visual Processing

edited by Michael S. Landy and
J. Anthony Movshon

Computational Models of Visual Processing

A Bradford Book
The MIT Press
Cambridge, Massachusetts
London, England

This book was set in Palatino by Asco Trade Typesetting Ltd., Hong Kong,
and was printed and bound in the United States of America.

Library of Congress Cataloging-in-Publication Data

Computational models of visual processing / edited by Michael S. Landy and
J. Anthony Movshon.
    p. cm.
  Based on a workshop held at the Cold Spring Harbor Laboratory's Banbury
Center in June 1989.
  "A Bradford book."
  Includes bibliographical references and index.
  ISBN 0-262-12155-7 (hc)
  1. Visual pathways—Computer simulation—Congresses. I. Landy,
Michael S. II. Movshon, J. Anthony.
  [DNLM: 1. Computer Simulation—congresses. 2. Models,
Neurological—congresses. 3. Visual Perception—physiology—congresses.
WW 105 C7385 1989]
QP475.C62   1991
599'.01823'0113—dc20
DNLM/DLC
for Library of Congress   90-13590
                                           CIP

Contents

Preface   ix

Contributors   xi

Part I   **The Task of Vision**   1

1   **The Plenoptic Function and the Elements of Early Vision**   3

Edward H. Adelson and James R. Bergen

Part II   **Receptors and Sampling**   21

2   **Learning Receptor Positions**   23

Albert J. Ahumada, Jr.

3   **A Model of Aliasing in Extrafoveal Human Vision**   35

Carlo L. M. Tiana, David R. Williams, Nancy J. Coletta, and P. William Haake

4   **Models of Human Rod Receptors and the ERG**   57

Donald C. Hood and David G. Birch

Part III   **Models of Neural Function**   69

5   **The Design of Chromatically Opponent Receptive Fields**   71

Peter Lennie, P. William Haake, and David R. Williams

6   **Spatial Receptive Field Organization in Monkey V1 and its Relationship to the Cone Mosaic**   83
Michael J. Hawken and Andrew J. Parker

7   **Neural Contrast Sensitivity**   95
Andrew B. Watson

8   **Spatiotemporal Receptive Fields and Direction Selectivity**   109
Robert Shapley, R. Clay Reid, and Robert Soodak

9   **Nonlinear Model of Neural Responses in Cat Visual Cortex**   119
David J. Heeger

Part IV   **Detection and Discrimination**   135

10   **A Template Matching Model of Subthreshold Summation**   137
Jacob Nachmias

11   **Noise in the Visual System May Be Early**   147
Denis G. Pelli

12   **Pattern Discrimination, Visual Filters, and Spatial Sampling Irregularity**   153
Hugh R. Wilson

Part V   **Color and Shading**   169

13   **A Bilinear Model of the Illuminant's Effect on Color Appearance**   171
David H. Brainard and Brian A. Wandell

14   **Shading Ambiguity: Reflectance and Illumination**   187
Michael D'Zmura

15   **Transparency and the Cooperative Computation of Scene Attributes**   209
Daniel Kersten

Part VI   **Motion and Texture**   229

16   **Theories for the Visual Perception of Local Velocity and Coherent Motion**   231
Norberto M. Grzywacz and Alan L. Yuille

17   **Computational Modeling of Visual Texture Segregation**   253
James R. Bergen and Michael S. Landy

18   **Complex Channels, Early Local Nonlinearities, and Normalization in Texture Segregation**   273
Norma Graham

19   **Orthogonal Distribution Analysis: A New Approach to the Study of Texture Perception**   291
Charles Chubb and Michael S. Landy

Part VII   **3D Shape**   303

20   **Shape from X: Psychophysics and Computation**   305
Heinrich H. Bülthoff

21   **Computational Issues in Solving the Stereo Correspondence Problem**   331
John P. Frisby and Stephen B. Pollard

22   Stereo, Surfaces, and Shape   359
Andrew J. Parker, Elizabeth B. Johnston,
J. Stephen Mansfield, and Yuede Yang

Author Index   383
Subject Index   391

Preface

The task of understanding vision is a formidable one and has commanded the attention of biologists, psychologists, physicists, and philosophers for many centuries. The past three decades have seen an extraordinary explosion in our empirical knowledge of the psychophysical and neurobiological basis of visual function, so that accurate and detailed information is now available about many stages of the process by which light in the world gives rise to the sensations of vision. As in all maturing fields of science, the growth of empirical knowledge has led to the development of new theories and models. In the case of vision, the shape of recent theories has been strongly influenced by the concurrent development of the digital computer and the accompanying challenge of building machines that see. Thus many models of visual function are now built not only as abstract formal models, but also as computational theories instantiated as computer programs that simulate the operation of the parts of the system under study.

The advent of computational models of visual processing has brought theory and experiment together in many new and exciting ways. This volume is intended to provide a snapshot (circa 1990) of contemporary research on modeling the visual system. Our emphasis is on the "early" processes of vision—the translation of retinal images into neural representations of the visual world—rather than on the more cognitive problems of perceiving and identifying objects, although computational approaches are beginning to make their influence felt there also (Richards, 1990). The contributions span the range from neurophysiology to psychophysics, and from retinal function to the analysis of visual cues to motion, color, texture, and depth. After an introductory chapter by Edward Adelson and James Bergen that provides a new and elegant formalization of the elements of early vision, the book treats six areas: (1) receptors and sampling; (2) models of neural function; (3) detection and discrimination; (4) color and shading; (5) motion and texture; and (6) three-dimensional shape.

This book grew out of a workshop held at the Cold Spring Harbor Laboratory's Banbury Center in June, 1989. The workshop immediately preceded the Cold Spring Harbor Laboratory summer course in Computational Neuroscience, and the participants were able to make use of the computer laboratory assembled for that course. In combination with the very special setting, the availability of machines for hands-on modeling transformed the workshop into a uniquely interactive experience. We have tried to reflect the particular character of the workshop in this volume.

The workshop and this volume would not have been possible without the efforts of many individuals. At Cold Spring Harbor, we owe special thanks to Susan Hockfield, tireless organizer of the summer courses and promoter and securer of funding for the workshop. The staff of the Laboratory and of the Banbury Center, especially Jan Witkowski, Bea Tolliver, and Herb Parsons, were unfailingly helpful and tolerant of having their beautiful conference center littered with machines and draped with cables. We also owe special thanks to Ellen Hildreth, co-organizer of the Computational Neuroscience course, for her help in securing and setting up the computer laboratory, and to Karl Gegenfurtner and Ian Horswill, the student assistants both for the workshop and for the course.

After the participants dispersed the real work began, and we owe special thanks to Fiona Stevens at The MIT Press for the continued support and encouragement that helped keep this project in motion.

The workshop was supported by the Office of Naval Research. Funding for the computer laboratory was provided by the Alfred P. Sloan Foundation, supplemented by the loan of equipment by the Massachusetts Institute of Technology.

Reference

Richards, W. S. (1990). *Natural Computation*. Cambridge, MA: MIT Press.

Contributors

Edward H. Adelson
Media Laboratory, Massachusetts Institute of
Technology, Cambridge, MA

Albert J. Ahumada, Jr.
NASA Ames Research Center, Moffett Field, CA

James R. Bergen
SRI/David Sarnoff Research Center, Princeton, NJ

David G. Birch
Retina Foundation of the Southwest, Dallas, TX

David H. Brainard
Department of Psychology, University of California,
Santa Barbara, CA

Heinrich H. Bülthoff
Department of Cognitive and Linguistic Sciences,
Brown University, Providence, RI

Charles Chubb
Department of Psychology, Rutgers University,
New Brunswick, NJ

Nancy J. Coletta
College of Optometry, University of Houston,
Houston, TX

Michael D'Zmura
Department of Cognitive Sciences, University of
California, Irvine, CA

John P. Frisby
University of Sheffield, Sheffield, England

Norma Graham
Department of Psychology, Columbia University,
New York, NY

Norberto M. Grzywacz
The Smith-Kettlewell Eye Research Institute,
San Francisco, CA

P. William Haake
Center for Visual Science, University of Rochester,
Rochester, NY

Michael J. Hawken
Center for Neural Science, New York University,
New York, NY

David J. Heeger
NASA Ames Research Center, Moffett Field, CA

Donald C. Hood
Department of Psychology, Columbia University,
New York, NY

Elizabeth B. Johnston
University Laboratory of Physiology, Oxford, England

Daniel Kersten
Department of Psychology, University of Minnesota,
Minneapolis, MN

Michael S. Landy
Department of Psychology, New York University,
New York, NY

Peter Lennie
Center for Visual Science, University of Rochester,
Rochester, NY

J. Stephen Mansfield
University Laboratory of Physiology, Oxford, England

J. Anthony Movshon
Center for Neural Science, New York University,
New York, NY

Jacob Nachmias
Department of Psychology, University of Pennsylvania,
Philadelphia, PA

Andrew J. Parker
University Laboratory of Physiology, Oxford, England

Denis G. Pelli
Institute for Sensory Research, Syracuse University,
Syracuse, NY

Stephen B. Pollard
AI Vision Research Unit, University of Sheffield,
Sheffield, England

R. Clay Reid
Center for Neural Science, New York University,
New York, NY

Robert Shapley
Center for Neural Science, New York University,
New York, NY

Robert Soodak
The Rockefeller University, New York, NY

Carlo L. M. Tiana
The Institute for Optics, University of Rochester,
Rochester, NY

Brian A. Wandell
Department of Psychology, Stanford University,
Stanford, CA

Andrew B. Watson
NASA Ames Research Center, Moffett Field, CA

David R. Williams
Center for Visual Science, University of Rochester,
Rochester, NY

Hugh R. Wilson
Visual Sciences Center, University of Chicago,
Chicago, IL

Yuede Yang
University Laboratory of Physiology, Oxford, England

Alan L. Yuille
Division of Applied Sciences, Harvard University,
Cambridge, MA

Part I

The Task of Vision

To model the visual system, one must begin with an analysis of the problem. What precisely is the visual stimulus, and what features of the stimulus carry the most information about the visual world? In this first chapter, Adelson and Bergen approach these questions from a general viewpoint. By defining a multidimensioned "plenoptic function" that captures all the information potentially available in the image, and by considering the utility of simple analyses in the various subdimensions of this function, they show that structures already known to be helpful in detecting simple visual forms can almost effortlessly be translated into other dimensions, where they have clear and useful properties in analyzing such other elements as motion, color structure, depth, and motion parallax. This chapter offers a new, unified, and appealing description of visual processing as the search for basic structures in the plenoptic view.

The Plenoptic Function and the Elements of Early Vision

Edward H. Adelson and James R. Bergen

What are the elements of early vision? This question might be taken to mean, What are the fundamental atoms of vision?—and might be variously answered in terms of such candidate structures as edges, peaks, corners, and so on. In this chapter we adopt a rather different point of view and ask the question, What are the fundamental *substances* of vision? This distinction is important because we wish to focus on the first steps in extraction of visual information. At this level it is premature to talk about discrete objects, even such simple ones as edges and corners.

There is general agreement that early vision involves measurements of a number of basic image properties including orientation, color, motion, and so on. Figure 1.1 shows a caricature (in the style of Neisser, 1976), of the sort of architecture that has become quite popular as a model for both human and machine vision. The first stage of processing involves a set of parallel pathways, each devoted to one particular visual property. We propose that the measurements of these basic properties be considered as the elements of early vision. We think of early vision as measuring the amounts of various kinds of visual "substances" present in the image (e.g., redness or rightward motion energy). In other words, we are interested in how early vision measures "stuff" rather than in how it labels "things."

What, then, are these elementary visual substances? Various lists have been compiled using a mixture of intuition and experiment. Electrophysiologists have described neurons in striate cortex that are selectively sensitive to certain visual properties; for reviews, see Hubel (1988) and DeValois and DeValois (1988). Psychophysicists have inferred the existence of channels that are tuned for certain visual properties; for reviews, see Graham (1989), Olzak and Thomas (1986), Pokorny and Smith (1986), and Watson (1986). Researchers in perception have found aspects of visual stimuli that are processed pre-attentively (Beck, 1966; Bergen & Julesz, 1983; Julesz & Bergen,

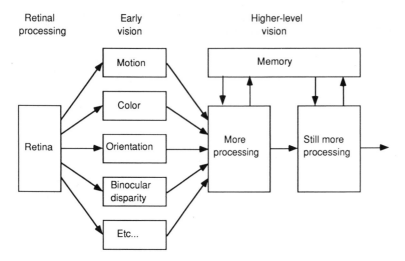

Retinal processing   Early vision   Higher-level vision

Fig. 1.1
A generic diagram for visual processing. In this approach, early vision consists of a set of parallel pathways, each analysing some particular aspect of the visual stimulus.

1983; Treisman, 1986; Treisman & Gelade, 1980). And in computational vision, investigators have found that certain low-level measurements are useful for accomplishing vision tasks; for examples, see Horn (1986), Levine (1985), and Marr (1982).

These various approaches have converged on a set of superficially similar lists, but there is little sense of structure. Why do the lists contain certain elements and not others? Or, indeed, are there other unknown visual elements waiting to be discovered?

Our interest here is to derive the visual elements in a systematic way and to show how they are related to the structure of visual information in the world. We will show that all the basic visual measurements can be considered to characterize local change along one or more dimensions of a single function that describes the structure of the information in the light impinging on an observer. Since this function describes everything that can be seen, we call it the *plenoptic function* (from *plenus*, complete or full, and *optic*). Once we have defined this function, the measurement of various underlying visual properties such as motion, color, and orientation fall out of the analysis automatically.

Our approach generates a list of the possible visual elements, which we think of as somewhat analogous to Mendeleev's periodic table in the sense that it displays systematically all the elemental substances upon which

vision can be based. This table catalogues the basic visual substances and clarifies their relationships.

This cataloging process makes no assumptions about the statistics of the world and no assumptions about the needs of the observing organism. The periodic table lists every simple visual measurement that an observer could potentially make, given the structure of the ambient light expressed in the plenoptic function. A given organism will probably not measure all of the elements, and of those that it measures it will devote more resources to some than to others.

In what follows we will make reference to some of the relevant psychophysical and physiological literature on early vision. Our topic is quite broad, however, and if we were to cite all of the relevant sources we would end up listing hundreds of papers. Therefore our references will be sparse, and readers are encouraged to consult the various books and review articles cited above.

The Plenoptic Function

We begin by asking what can potentially be seen. What information about the world is contained in the light filling a region of space? Space is filled with a dense array of light rays of various intensities. The set of rays passing through any point in space is mathematically termed a *pencil*. Leonardo da Vinci refers to this set of rays as a "radiant pyramid":

The body of the air is full of an infinite number of radiant pyramids caused by the objects located in it. These pyramids intersect and interweave without interfering with each other during their independent passage throughout the air in which they are infused. (Kemp, 1989)

If a pinhole camera happens to positioned at a given point, it will select the pencil of rays at that point and will reveal that they form an image. An observer's eye acts in the same way (neglecting the finite aperture of the pupil for now): It reveals the structure of the pencil of light at the pupil's location. The fact that image information fills space is expressed by Leonardo in his notebooks; he invites the reader to perform a thought experiment:

I say that if the front of a building—or any open piazza or field—which is illuminated by the sun has a dwelling opposite to it, and if, in the front which does not face that sun, you make a small round hole, all the illuminated objects will project their images through that hole and be visible inside the dwelling on the opposite wall which may be made white; and there, in fact, they will be upside down, and if you make similar openings in several places in the same wall you will have the same result from each. Hence the images of the illuminated objects are all everywhere on this wall and all in each minutest part of it. (Richter, 1970)

J. J. Gibson referred to a similar notion when he spoke of the structure of ambient light (Gibson, 1966): "The complete set of all convergence points ... constitutes the permanent possibilities of vision, that is, the set of all points where a mobile individual might be."

Let us follow this line of thought a bit further and consider the parameters necessary to describe this luminous environment. Consider, first, a black and white photograph taken by a pinhole camera. It tells us the intensity of light seen from a single viewpoint, at a single time, averaged over the wavelengths of the visible spectrum. That is to say, it records the intensity distribution P within the pencil of light rays passing through the lens. This distribution may be parameterized by the spherical coordinates, $P(\theta, \phi)$, or by the Cartesian coordinates of a picture plane, $P(x, y)$ (figure 1.2; see discussion below). A color photograph adds some information about how the intensity varies with wavelength λ, thus: $P(\theta, \phi, \lambda)$. A color movie further extends the information to include the time dimension t: $P(\theta, \phi, \lambda, t)$. A color holographic movie, finally, indicates the observable light intensity at every viewing position, V_x, V_y, and V_z: $P(\theta, \phi, \lambda, t, V_x, V_y, V_z)$. A true holographic movie would allow reconstruction of every possible view, at every moment, from every position, at

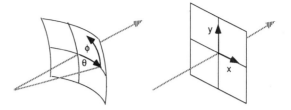

Fig. 1.2
The image information available from a single viewing position is defined by the pencil of light rays passing through the pupil. The rays may be parameterized in angular coordinates or in Cartesian coordinates. The Cartesian approach is commonly used in machine vision and computer graphics, but the angular approach can more easily represent the full sphere of optical information impinging on a point in space.

every wavelength, within the bounds of the space-time-wavelength region under consideration. The plenoptic functions is equivalent to this complete holographic representation of the visual world.

Such a complete representation would contain, implicitly, a description of every possible photograph that could be taken of a particular space-time chunk of the world (neglecting the polarization and instantaneous phase of the incoming light). Note that the plenoptic function need not contain any parameters specifying the three viewing angles describing the direction of gaze and orientation of the eye, since rotating the eye without displacing it does not affect the distribution of light in the bundle of rays impinging on the pupil, but merely changes the relative positions at which they happen to strike the retina. The fact that some rays are behind the eye and are therefore blocked is irrelevant to the present discussion, which is intended to characterize the optical information potentially available at each point in space, as if the hypothetical eye had a 360° field of view. Figure 1.3 shows a pair of samples from this function, with the eye placed at different positions in a natural scene.

To measure the plenoptic function one can imagine placing an idealized eye at every possible (V_x, V_y, V_z) location and recording the intensity of the light rays passing through the center of the pupil at every possible angle (θ, ϕ), for every wavelength, λ, at every time t. It is simplest to have the eye always look in the same direction, so that the angles (θ, ϕ) are always computed with respect to an optic axis that is parallel to the V_z axis. The resulting function takes the form:

$$P = P(\theta, \phi, \lambda, t, V_x, V_y, V_z). \tag{1}$$

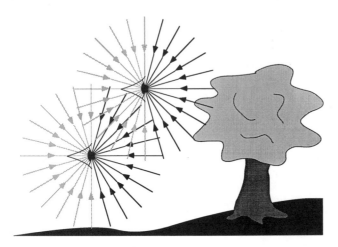

Fig. 1.3
The plenoptic function describes the information available to an observer at any point in space and time. Shown here are two schematic eyes—which one should consider to have punctate pupils—gathering pencils of light rays. A real observer cannot see the light rays coming from behind, but the plenoptic function does include these rays.

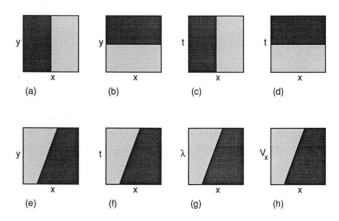

Fig. 1.4
Some edgelike structures that might be found along particular planes within the plenoptic function (note the various axes, as labeled on each figure): (a) a vertical edge; (b) a horizontal edge; (c) a stationary edge; (d) a full-field brightening; (e) a tilting edge; (f) a moving edge; (g) a color sweep; (h) an edge with horizontal binocular parallax.

Alternatively, one may choose to parameterize the rays entering the eye in terms of (x, y) coordinates, where x and y are the spatial coordinates of an imaginary picture plane erected at a unit distance from the pupil. This is the approach commonly adopted in computer graphics and machine vision. The parameterization then becomes:

$$P = P(x, y, \lambda, t, V_x, V_y, V_z). \tag{2}$$

The spherical parameterization more easily suggests the fact that the light impinges on a given point in space from all directions and that no direction has special status. However, the Cartesian parameterization is more familiar, and we will use it in the discussion that follows.

The plenoptic function is an idealized concept, and one does not expect to completely specify it for a natural scene. Obviously one cannot simultaneously look at a scene from every possible point of view, for every wavelength, at every moment of time. But, by describing the plenoptic function, one can examine the structure of the information that is potentially available to an observer by visual means.

The significance of the plenoptic function is this: The world is made of three-dimensional objects, but these objects do not communicate their properties directly to an observer. Rather, the objects fill the space around them with the pattern of light rays that constitutes the plenop-

tic function, and the observer takes samples from this function. The plenoptic function serves as the sole communication link between physical objects and their corresponding retinal images. It is the intermediary between the world and the eye.

Plenoptic Structures

It may initially appear that the plenoptic function is extremely complicated. Since it has seven dimensions, it is difficult to visualize. However, much of the information that the plenoptic function contains describes familiar structures of the visual world. One can develop a sense of the structure of the plenoptic function as a whole by considering some planar slices.

Figure 1.4 shows a variety of slices along various planes passing through the x-axis. The figure illustrates a number of edgelike structures that might occur within a given plenoptic function. Part A, in the (x, y) plane, shows a vertical edge. Part B, also in the (x, y) plane, shows a horizontal edge. Part C, in the (x, t) plane, shows a stationary edge. Part D, also in the (x, t) plane, shows a temporal edge—a sudden increase in intensity. Part E, in the (x, y) plane, shows a tilted edge. Part F, in the (x, t) plane, shows a moving edge. Part G, in the (x, λ) plane, shows a patch that changes color across space. Part H, in the (x, V_x) plane, shows an edge that projects a changing

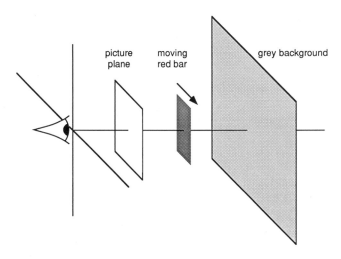

picture plane   moving red bar   grey background

Fig. 1.5
A hypothetical scene that produces a variety of simple plenoptic structures. See figure 1.6.

retinal image as the eye is translated in the V_x direction—that is, an edge with horizontal parallax.

Figure 1.5 shows a concrete example of a particular simple scene. The eye views a red bar at a certain distance, moving against a grey background at a larger distance. The figure also shows the imaginary picture plane at a unit distance from the eye.

Figure 1.6 shows a variety of slices through the plenoptic function for this scene. All the slices shown pass through the x-axis; thus all of the parameters other than the two diagrammed in the slice are taken to be zero if not otherwise specified. The only exception is wavelength, λ, which we will let default to 550 nm, which is the approximate center of the human visible spectrum.

Part B of figure 1.6 shows an (x, y) slice, which is simply the view at 550 nm, at the moment $t = 0$, given the eye is in position $(0, 0, 0)$. It consists of a darker bar against a lighter background. Part C shows an (x, t) slice, which can be thought of as the temporal record of horizontal raster lines appearing at height $y = 0$; wavelength is 550 nm, and the eye is at $(0, 0, 0)$. This image consists of a spatiotemporally "tilted" bar, the tilt corresponding to the changing position over time. Part D shows an (x, λ) slice, which one might call a "spatiospectral" or "spatiochromatic" slice, taken at height $y = 0$, time $t = 0$, and viewing position $(0, 0, 0)$. The fact that the bar is red leads to the variation in intensity along the wavelength dimension in the middle region of the slice: Long wavelengths have high intensities while short wavelengths have low in-

tensities. Part E shows an (x, V_x) slice, representing the series of views obtained as the eye position shifts from left to right. Part F shows a similar slice for (x, V_y), as the eye position shifts up and down. Finally, part G shows an (x, V_z) slice, representing the changing image as the eye moves backward or forward.

It is clear from examining these slices that similar structures are to be found along various planes in the plenoptic function. In the case of the example shown, extended edgelike features appear in all planes, with different tilts and curvatures. Each plane offers useful information about different aspects of the stimulus. The (x, y) plane contains information about instantaneous form; the (x, λ) plane contains information about chromatic variation in the x direction; the (x, V_x) plane contains information about horizontal parallax—information that could be gathered either through head motion or through stereo vision; the (x, V_z) plane contains information about the looming that occurs when the eye advances along the z-axis, and so on. All of the information in the plenoptic function is potentially useful.

The Plenoptic Function and Elemental Measurements in Early Vision

The Task of Early Vision

We suggest that the first problem of early vision is to extract as much informaton as possible about the structure of the plenoptic function. The first task of any visual system is to measure the state of the luminous environment. As pointed out by Koenderink and van Doorn (1987), only by representing this information internally can all potential visual information be made available for subsequent analysis. By definition, the state of the luminous environment is described by the plenoptic function. Clearly, only a small portion of the potential information present in this environment can be extracted.

As noted above, much of the structure of the plenoptic function describing simple stimulus configurations may take the form of oriented patterns at various angles within plenoptic space. An oriented pattern is one that changes in one direction more rapidly than in another direction; characterizing this anisotropy is a useful first step in analyzing the local structure of a signal. We therefore offer the following propositions:

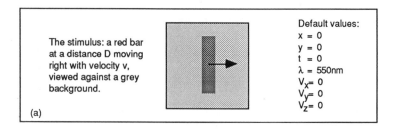

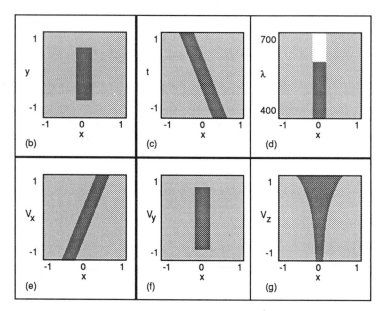

Fig. 1.6
The plenoptic strcutures found along various planes for the scene illustrated in figure 1.5. Each picture represents a slice through the plenoptic function, where all the unspecified parameters take on their default values.

• *Proposition 1.* The primary task of early vision is to deliver a small set of useful measurements about each observable location in the plenoptic function.

• *Proposition 2.* The elemental operations of early vision involve the measurement of local change along various directions within the plenoptic function.

These two propositions establish a useful "null hypothesis" regarding the existence of early visual mechanisms. If some local descriptor of the plenoptic function exists, then we may (in general) expect a visual system to compute this descriptor. If the system does not do this, we have reason to ask why this particular aspect of visual information is not being extracted. By comparing what is extracted by a visual system (as specified by the basic measurements that it makes) with what might be ex-

tracted (specified by the structure of the plenoptic function), we can learn something about the nature of the system's visual process. What exactly are the fundamental measurements implied by these propositions?

Extraction of Information from the Plenoptic Function

Efficient extraction of information from the plenoptic function requires that each sample contain as much information as possible about the most important aspects of the function. An additional desideratum is that the information represented by each sample be simply interpretable without reference to many other samples. Representations motivated by these requirements can take many forms. Since local change defined in arithmetic terms is equivalent to a derivative, a reasonable choice for conceptual purposes consists of the low order directional derivatives of the plenoptic function at the sample points. This set of measures fits well with the goal of capturing the simple structure of the plenoptic function since it consists of oriented linear filters in the plenoptic hyperplanes. In this sense, these derivatives may be thought of as "feature detectors," corresponding to the structures shown in figure 1.6. However, since these are linear filters they are not really detecting features; rather they are measuring the amount of a particular type of local structure.

Another way to think about this type of representation is as a truncated Taylor series expansion around each sample point. Koenderink and van Doorn (1987) have developed a theory of early representation based on *local jets* which pursues such an interpretation. If we compute all of the derivatives at each point, each set of derivatives contains the information present in all of the samples (assuming that the function is smooth). By computing only the low order derivatives, we construct a synopsis of the local structure of the function at each point. This explicit representation of local structure allows analysis of salient local characteristics without repeated examination of multiple samples. The appropriateness of this representation depends on the plenoptic function having the kind of locally correlated structure described in the previous section. It would not make sense if the plenoptic function looked like uncorrelated random noise or were otherwise chaotic in structure.

Mathematically, a derivative is taken at a point, but for characterizing a function within a neighborhood it is more useful to work with the local average derivative of the function, or the derivative of the local average of the function, which is the same thing. The equivalence of these alternate processes follows trivially from the commutativity of linear systems, but it is worth emphasizing, as illustrated in figure 1.7. Let the original function $f(s)$, where s is the variable of interest, have the form of a trapezoid for purposes of illustration. The figure shows three paths to the same result. In one path, a local average is taken by convolving $f(s)$ with a smoothing function, $g(s)$; then this smoothed function is differentiated to produce the final result, $f(s) * g'(s)$. In a second path, the derivative is taken, and then this function is smoothed by local averaging. In the third path, shown on the diagonal, the two steps are combined into one: A single linear filter (the derivative of the smoothing function) is used to produce the final output.

Along with the three paths are three verbal descriptions: taking a derivative of an averaged signal; taking an average of a differentiated signal; and convolving the

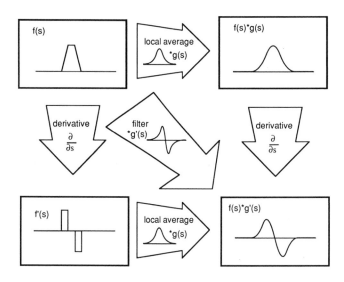

Fig. 1.7
The local average of a derivative is the same as the derivative of a local average.

signal with a single filter. The result is the same in each case.

We can use the standard notation of vector calculus to describe the first few directional derivatives of the plenoptic function. By convention, we assume that any dimensions not mentioned are averaged over. In other words, D_x denotes a filter that averages locally (say, with a Gaussian weighting function) in all directions, and then differentiates in the x direction. Similarly, D_{xy} means differentiation in x and in y (the sequence is irrelevant). For second derivatives we write D_{xx} (for example) or $D_{\lambda\lambda}$. For derivatives in directions other than along coordinate axes, such as "up and to the right," we can write D_{x+y} (a diagonal derivative) or D_{x+t} (a horizontally moving one). These latter are in fact equal to $D_x + D_y$ and $D_x + D_t$, respectively, but it is useful to use the other notation sometimes to emphasize the fact that these are no more complicated than D_x or D_y, just taken in a different direction.

Examples of these operators are shown in figure 1.8. If we designate the axes shown as u and v, the operator in the upper left corner is D_v. To the right of that are D_{vv} and D_{uv}. The lower row consists of D_{u+v}, $D_{(u+v)(u+v)}$, D_{uvv}, and D_{uuvv}.

The only slightly more complicated case that we need to consider is the Laplacian operator, shown in the upper right corner. This is not a directional derivative per se, but it is the sum of second directional derivatives: $L_{uv} =$

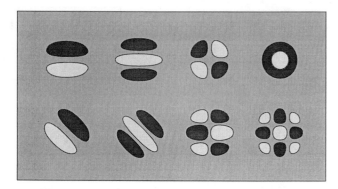

Fig. 1.8
The low order derivative operators lead to a small number to
two-dimensional receptive field types.

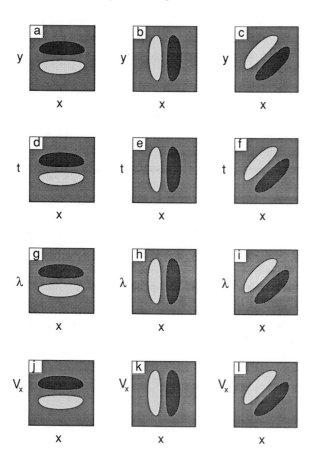

Fig. 1.9
The same receptive field structures produce different visual
measurements when placed along different planes in plenoptic space.

$D_{uu} + D_{vv}$. We do not wish to suggest that center-surround structures in biological visual systems are necessarily constructed in this way; we are simply describing the formal relationships among the various types of operators.)

Visual Mechanisms for Extracting Plenoptic Structure

The visual mechanisms suggested by this approach include some familiar receptive field structures, as well as some that are more novel (cf. Young, 1989). Figure 1.9 shows some examples of idealized receptive fields that one could construct to analyze change in various directions in plenoptic space—ignoring implementational constraints for the moment. These particular receptive fields represent only two dimensions of information, and one of the dimensions shown is always the spatial dimension x. All receptive fields have an implicit shape in the full set of plenoptic dimensions; they are assumed to be bloblike in all of the dimensions not shown.

Although these measurements do not precisely correspond to properties that are described by ordinary language, it is possible to assign approximate labels for them: (a) horizontally oriented structure (edgelike); (b) vertically oriented structure (edgelike); (c) diagonally oriented structure (edgelike); (d) full-field brightening; (e) static spatial structure; (f) moving edgelike structure; (g) full-field bluish color; (h) achromatic edgelike structure; (i) spatiochromatic variation; (j) full-field intensity change with eye position; (k) absence of horizontal parallax (edgelike structure); (l) horizontal parallax (edgelike structure).

Plenoptic Measurements in the Human Visual System

We have presented an idealized view of the basic structure available in the plenoptic function, and of the measurements that early vision could employ to characterize that structure. We now ask how these measurements, or closely related measurements, might be implemented in the human visual system. (While we refer to the "human" visual system, much of the evidence upon which our analysis is based comes from physiological studies of other mammals. We will assume without arguing the point that the early stages of processing are similar across species.)

At any given moment, a human observer has access to samples along five of the seven axes of the plenoptic function. A range of the x and y axes are captured on the surface of the retina; a range of the λ-axis is sampled by the three cone types; a range of the t-axis is captured and processed by temporal filters; and two samples from the V_x-axis are taken by the two eyes. In order to sample the V_y-axis at an instant, we would need to have a third eye, vertically displaced, and in order to sample the V_z-axis, we would need an extra eye displaced forward or backward. It is possible to accumulate information about V_y and V_z over time by moving the head—that is, using ego-motion—but the information is not available to a static observer at a given moment, and therefore we exclude any detailed consideration of this information from our discussion here.

For human observers then, the available plenoptic function involves the five parameters, x, y, t, λ, and V_x, and may be parameterized:

$$P = P(x, y, t, \lambda, V_x). \tag{3}$$

Each dimension is analyzed by the human visual system with a limited resolution and a limited number of samples. Given that the visual system can only extract a finite number of samples, it is quite interesting to observe where the sampling is dense and where it is sparse. The sampling in x and y (or visual angle, if one prefers), is by far the densest, corresponding to hundreds of thousands of distint values. The sampling in wavelength is much cruder: The cones extract only three samples along the wavelength dimension. The sampling in horizontal viewing position is cruder still, with only two samples. Time is represented continuously, but the dimensionality of the representation at any given instant is probably quite low.

The fact that different dimensions are sampled with different densities may reflect a number of factors, such as: (1) some dimensions have greater physical variance than others and thus simply contain more information (Maloney, 1986), (2) some dimensions contain information that is more important for survival than other dimensions, and (3) some dimensions are easier to sample than others, given biological constraints. It is worth noting that the eyes of certain mantis shrimps have been reported to analyze the spectrum with as many as ten distinct photoreceptor types (Cronin & Marshall, 1989); these organisms can presumably make much finer chromatic distinc-tions than humans can, although their spatial resolution is much poorer than that of humans. Denser sampling in one domain requires sparser sampling in another, and so the tradeoffs chosen in a given organism reflect the way in which visual information is weighted in that organism's niche. It is also significant that in the human visual system the sampling is not uniform across space, being far denser in the fovea than in the periphery. Thus the direction of gaze has a major impact on the actual information available to the observer, even though it does not affect the information potentially available in the pencil of rays entering the pupil.

We now consider the way that human (and other mammalian) visual systems analyze the various dimensions of the plenoptic function. Both the commonalities and the variations are quite interesting.

Space

The two spatial dimensions (or visual angle dimensions), which we will consider together, are analyzed in far more detail than any other dimensions. Spatial receptive fields may have more lobes than the two or three expected from the lowest order derivative operators: indeed, neurons with six or more lobes have been reported in visual cortex (De Valois, Thorell & Albrecht, 1985; Young, 1985), which would suggest derivative orders of 5 or more. In addition, the spatial analysis is performed at many positions and at many scales, and the analysis is more detailed in the fovea than in the periphery. The extensive and diverse analysis that is devoted to the spatial domain indicates that it is far more important than any other sampled dimension for primate (and presumably for human) vision.

Spatial receptive fields at the level of the retina and the lateral geniculate nucleus (LGN) tend to be circular or slightly elliptical. But the receptive fields of cells devoted to spatial analysis in primary visual cortex are almost invariably oriented, except for the cells in layer 4, which receive direct input from LGN. As far as we know, cells with "crisscross" receptive fields, such as would result from separable analysis of two spatial directions, are not found.

Time

The time dimension is unusual in two ways. First, all filtering must be causal, which is to say that the impulse

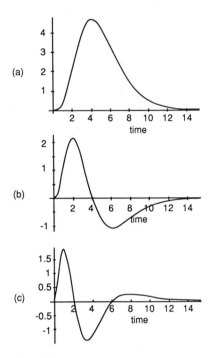

Fig. 1.10
Since temporal impulse responses must be causal, they do not have the same form as the weighting functions observed along other axes. Shown here are the zeroth, first, and second derivatives of a fourth-order Butterworth filter. The amplitude spectra of these filters are similar to those of the corresponding Gaussian and Gaussian derivative filters, although the phase spectra are quite different.

response can only include events in the past and not in the future. This means that (unless unreasonable amounts of delay are introduced) the temporal weighting functions cannot have the symmetrical form found in the space domain. Rather, they tend to look more like those shown in figure 1.10, which shows impulse responses corresponding to a lowpass filter of the form $t^4 e^{-t}$, along with its first and second derivatives.

A second peculiarity of the time dimension is that it is not discretely sampled. All other dimensions are sampled by a finite number of neurons, but since these neurons produce continuously varying outputs (neglecting the fact that they must convey this output via a spike train) there seems to be no equivalent sampling in time. The amount of information conveyed in the cell responses is, of course, limited by the stochastic character of the spike train; moreover, there is a temporal frequency bandlimit on the cell's response, and this can be used to compute an effective temporal sampling rate.

One can also ask about the dimensionality of the temporal analysis that is available at a given retinal position at a given time. If only a single cell were responding the dimensionality would be unity, but if several cells are responding simultaneously to different temporal epochs (as with lagged cells) or to different temporal frequency bands (as with flicker and motion cells), then it becomes reasonable to speak of the dimensionality of the temporal representation at an instant. This dimensionality is likely to be small, as there seem to be only two or three broadly tuned temporal channels at a given location (Graham, 1989).

It is worth noting that, from the standpoint of the plenoptic function, simple temporal change (brightening, dimming, and flicker) is at least as fundamental as is motion, which involves correlated change across space and time.

Wavelength

In humans the wavelength axis is sampled at only three points, by three cone types (neglecting the rods). The broad cone action spectra can be thought of as prefilters required by this sparse sampling that prevent high frequency aliasing in the wavelength domain (cf. Barlow, 1982). An averaging across wavelength, without any derivatives, leads to an achromatic signal, as shown in figure 1.11A. A first derivative operator in wavelength corresponds to a blue-yellow opponent signal, as shown in figure 1.11B. A second derivative operator corresponds to a red-green opponent signal, as shown in figure 1.11C. Note that this red-green signal receives positive input from both the short-wave and long-wave cones, which is consistent with many results in psychophysics and physiology. These three idealized weighting functions are qualitatively similar to the ones that are actually found experimentally, although they differ in detail.

It is also interesting to characterize common chromatic neurons with spatiochromatic receptive fields. Color opponent "blob" cells (those without spatial structure) correspond to derivatives in wavelength without any derivatives in space (D_λ); figure 1.12A illustrates an (x, λ) slice of an idealized cell. Double opponent cells correspond to derivatives in wavelength and circular (Laplacian) derivatives in space (in one dimension $D_{xx\lambda}$); a slice is shown in figure 1.12B. Single opponent cells, as in figure 1.12C, do

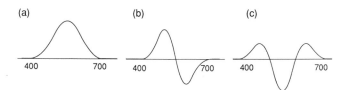

Fig. 1.11
The zeroth, first, and second derivatives of a Gaussian weighting function along the wavelength axis are similar to the luminance, blue-yellow, and red-green weighting functions found in the human visual system.

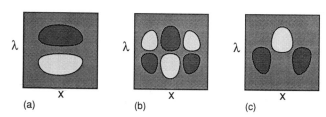

Fig. 1.12
Spatiochromatic receptive fields may be used to characterize various color selective neurons: (a) an opponent color cell with no spatial structure; (b) a double opponent cell; (c) a single opponent cell. Note that this cell type does not correspond to a standard derivative type, although it may be constructed by taking sums of derivatives.

not have any simple interpretation in terms of derivatives, although one can synthesize them as sums of derivatives (in fact $D_\lambda + D_{xx} + D_{yy}$). Cells that are spatiochromatically oriented (not illustrated here) would respond to chromatic ramps or edges.

Horizontal Parallax (Binocular)

The axis corresponding to horizontal eye position (V_x) is sampled at only two discrete positions by the two eyes. This creates potential ambiguities in the interpretation of this dimension by the visual system. The finite size of the pupil offers a very small amount of spatial prefiltering, which is entirely inadequate to prevent the aliasing introduced by such sparse sampling. Aliasing in the V_x-axis is the source of the "correspondence problem" in stereo vision (also known as the problem of ghosts). If the eyes were somehow able to prefilter properly along the V_x-axis, the correspondence problem would vanish. However, this would be optically impossible, and even if it were possible it would greatly reduce the accuracy with which stereo disparity could be measured.

Figure 1.13 shows examples of how the (x, V_x) plane can be analyzed with simple derivative operators. We

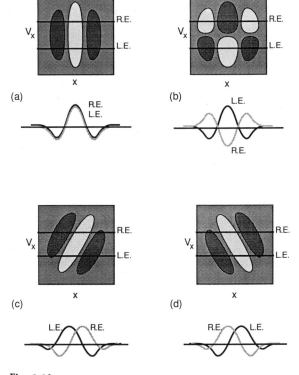

Fig. 1.13
Four examples of binocular receptive fields. Humans only take two samples from the V_x axis, as shown by the two lines labeled R.E. and L.E. for right eye and left eye). The curves beneath each receptive field indicate the individual weighting functions for each eye alone. The four receptive field types shown here correspond to: (a) binocular correlation; (b) binocular anticorrelation; (c) uncrossed disparity; (d) crossed disparity. These could be used to produce cells that would be categorized as "tuned excitatory," "tuned inhibitory," "far," and "near."

show the plane itself, along with the two linear samples that correspond to the images acquired by the left eye (L.E.) and right eye (R.E). For these examples we assume that the two eyes are fixating a common point at a finite distance; note that this condition differs from our earlier convention that the eye's axis is always parallel to the z-axis. When the eyes are fixating a point at an intermediate distance, then near points and far points exhibit parallax of different signs. Below each of the receptive fields is a diagram showing the individual responses of the right eye and left eye alone; these individual responses would be linearly summed to produce sampled versions of the underlying receptive fields.

Part A of figure 1.13 shows a receptive field for zero disparity, which will respond well when an object lies in the plane of fixation. Part B shows a receptive field for binocular anticorrelation, which will respond well to an object that is giving different or opposite contrasts to the two eyes (leading to the percept known as "luster"). Part C shows a receptive field sensitive to objects beyond the plane of fixation (i.e., uncrossed disparity); part D shows a receptive field sensitive to objects before the plane of fixation (i.e., crossed disparity). Poggio and Poggio (1984) describe "tuned excitatory," "tuned inhibitory," "near," and "far" cells, which might correspond to the receptive field types shown here.

Parallax in V_x, V_y, and V_z

A free observer can gather information about parallax along arbitrary directions in space by actively translating the eye through a range of viewing positions. The information is known as motion parallax, and it includes horizontal and vertical parallax for the V_x and V_y direction as well as the looming effects of the V_z direction. To produce a receptive field for motion parallax, one must combine information about the observer's motion with information about the changing retinal image; such mechanisms are more complex than the ones we have chosen to discuss under the heading of early vision, but in principle they could be analyzed in similar terms.

Periodic Tables for Early Vision

We have considered the structure of information in the luminous environment and how this information appears to be sampled in mammalian visual systems. We are now in a position to list systematically the possible elements of early vision, i.e. to build our periodic table of visual elements. Figure 1.14 shows a set of measurements that can be made by taking derivatives along single axes of the plenoptic function (D_u and D_{uu}). Since there are five axes, there are five entries for each. For the first derivative we find measurements as follows: x-axis: vertical "edge"; y-axis: horizontal "edge"; t-axis: flicker (brightening); λ-axis: blue-yellow opponency; V_x-axis: binocular anticorrelation (luster). For the second derivative, which we have shown with on-center polarity, we find: x-axis: vertical "bar"; y-axis: horizontal "bar"; t-axis: flicker (pulse); λ-axis: green-red opponency. There is no meaningful measurement for the V_x-axis given only the samples from two eyes.

The range of possible measurements becomes richer when we allow variation in two dimensions instead of just one. A given receptive field type now may occur with any pair of different axes. Thus we arrive at a 5 by 5 matrix of possible measurements for a given receptive field type. An example is shown in figure 1.15. The receptive field consists of a diagonal second derivative ($D_{(u+v)(u+v)}$). The possible axes are listed along the sides of the matrix; each pair of axes leads to a preferred stimulus, which is listed in the matrix. The diagonal entries are meaningless, and the upper triangle is identical to the lower triangle in this particular case by symmetry. Thus only the lower triangle is filled.

Each entry has four descriptors, corresponding to the spatial, temporal, chromatic, and binocular aspects of the preferred stimulus. The default values for the descriptors are: full-field (no spatial variation); static (no temporal variation); achromatic (no wavelength variation), and no binocular disparity. For each entry, the "interesting values" are shown in boldface, while the default values remain in plain text.

Some of the entries correspond to well-known cell types that respond to common experimental stimuli, such as tilted or moving bars. Both horizontal and vertical disparity also appear in the matrix. Some of the chromatic measurements are unexpected: wavelength variation correlated with space, time, and eye position lead to measurements of what we call spatial and temporal hue-sweeps, and to chromatic luster. Although these chromatic properties may sound obscure, they correspond to properties that an observer can encounter in the world. For example, a spatial hue-sweep can occur when an object's color varies across space; a temporal hue-sweep can occur when an object changes color over time; and a binocular hue difference can occur with certain kinds of lustrous objects, especially iridescent ones. Interestingly, Livingstone and Hubel (1984) reported a cell in the striate cortex of a monkey that was chromatically double opponent in both eyes but with opposite sign; that is, in the right eye it was $R^+ G^-$ center, $R^- G^+$ surround, while in the left eye it was $R^- G^+$ center, $R^+ G^-$ surround.

Another example is shown in figure 1.16. In this case, the measurement consists of a pair of single derivatives taken separably along two dimensions (D_{uv}). Once again the upper and lower triangles are identical symmetry, and the diagonal entries are not meaningful. This leaves us with the ten measurements listed in the matrix. Some

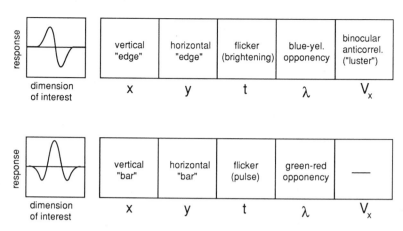

Fig. 1.14 (first derivative)

	x	y	t	λ	Vx
response / dimension of interest	vertical "edge"	horizontal "edge"	flicker (brightening)	blue-yel. opponency	binocular anticorrel. ("luster")

Fig. 1.14 (second derivative)

	x	y	t	λ	Vx
response / dimension of interest	vertical "bar"	horizontal "bar"	flicker (pulse)	green-red opponency	—

Fig. 1.14
Derivatives along single dimensions lead to a number of basic visual measurements.

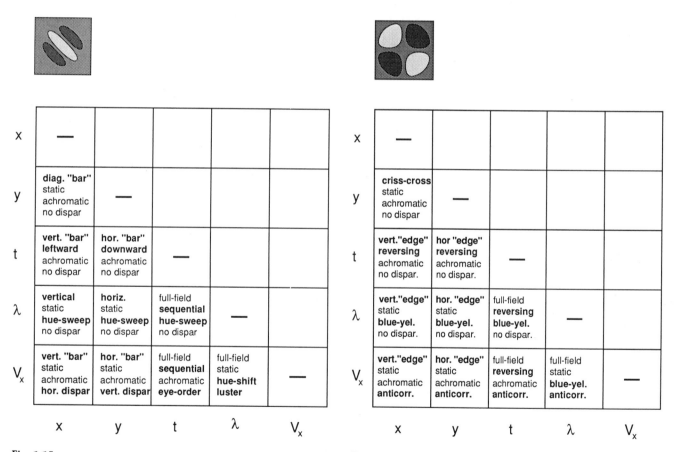

Fig. 1.15

	x	y	t	λ	Vx
x	—				
y	diag. "bar" static achromatic no dispar	—			
t	vert. "bar" leftward achromatic no dispar	hor. "bar" downward achromatic no dispar	—		
λ	vertical static hue-sweep no dispar	horiz. static hue-sweep no dispar	full-field sequential hue-sweep no dispar	—	
Vx	vert. "bar" static achromatic hor. dispar	hor. "bar" static achromatic vert. dispar	full-field sequential achromatic eye-order	full-field static hue-shift luster	—

Fig. 1.16

	x	y	t	λ	Vx
x	—				
y	criss-cross static achromatic no dispar	—			
t	vert."edge" reversing achromatic no dispar.	hor "edge" reversing achromatic no dispar.	—		
λ	vert."edge" static blue-yel. no dispar.	hor. "edge" static blue-yel. no dispar.	full-field reversing blue-yel. no dispar.	—	
Vx	vert."edge" static achromatic anticorr.	hor. "edge" static achromatic anticorr.	full-field reversing achromatic anticorr.	full-field static blue-yel. anticorr.	—

Fig. 1.15
The ten entries in the section of the periodic table corresponding to a tilted second derivative. The entries on the diagonal are meaningless, and the entries in the upper triangle are the same as those in the lower triangle by symmetry.

Fig. 1.16
The entries in the periodic table corresponding to separable first derivatives along both axes. There are ten elementary measurements of this type.

of the measurements are familiar, such as reversing (i.e., counterphase flickering) edges. The spatial "crisscross" measurement would seem to be straightforward enough, but cells showing this receptive field are rarely if ever found in cortex. Chromatic flicker and binocular luster (anticorrelation) are among the other measurements appearing in the table.

For each receptive field type one can construct a similar table. For a given shape of two-dimensional receptive field, there correspond twenty basic measurements, or ten when there is symmetry about the diagonal. Consider the receptive fields (RF) shown in figure 1.8. The seven oriented and separable RF types will lead to a total of some 100 distinct elemental measurements. (The exact number depends on how one chooses to treat symmetries.)

These 100 measurements can be considered to be the first stage of a periodic table of visual elements. Note that these measurements only include derivatives of order one and two, and that they do not include measurements involving derivatives along three or more dimensions of the plenoptic function. Thus, for example, a moving chromatic bar would not be properly analyzed at this level.

Several points emerge from this exercise. First, the plenoptic function is quite rich in information: At every point within it there are some 100 distinct and independent local measurements that can be used to characterize is structure, even when the measurements are restricted to the simplest sort. Second, it would be an enormous burden for the human visual system to sample and represent all of these measurements at high density, and so it is necessary that only the more important ones be analyzed in detail. Third, as one allows higher derivatives and more plenoptic dimensions, the number of potential elements grows through a combinatorial explosion.

Psychophysical experiments can be performed to determine human sensitivity to change along various axes in plenoptic space. Indeed, many psychophysical tasks can be shown to have unexpected relationships through such an analysis. Some interesting examples are discussed in the appendix.

Further Computations

The linear derivative-like computations we have discussed offer a starting point for early vision. Later stages

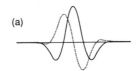

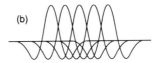

Fig. 1.17
Energy computation: (A) a pair of receptive fields that are in quadrature phase can be used to compute a local energy measure; (B) complex cells in striate cortex may compute local energy measures by combining the rectified outputs of several adjacent receptive fields.

in vision can make use of these initial measurements by combining them in various ways.

In some cases one may wish to measure the magnitude of local change within the plenoptic function in a region of the visual field, without specifying the exact location or spatial structure within that region. One may wish to know, for example, that there exists an oriented contour without specifying whether it is an edge, a dark line, or a light line. In this case a "local energy measure" can be computed that pools similar derivative-like signals within a spatial region. The term "local energy" is motivated by the fact that this pooling can be accomplished by summing the squared outputs of two linear receptive fields differing in phase by 90°. This arrangements is shown in figure 1.17A. This nonlinear combination gives a single-peaked positive response to edges and lines, regardless of sign (Adelson & Bergen, 1985; Granlund, 1978; Knutsson & Granlund, 1983; Ross, Morrone & Burr, 1989); the response extends smoothly over a patch centered on the feature of interest. Similar properties are obtained in general if an array of related linear subunits, as shown in figure 1.17B, are passed through a rectifying nonlinearity and then summed over some region. Complex cells in striate cortex seem to be performing a computation similar to this (Movshon, Thompson & Tolhurst, 1978; Spitzer & Hochstein, 1985). In addition, motion-selective complex cells may compute spatiotemporal energy measures by pooling the outputs of receptive fields that are oriented in space-time (Adelson & Bergen, 1985; Emerson,

Bergen & Adelson, 1987, 1991). By performing similar operations along other axes in the plenoptic function one can compute local energy measures for binocular disparity (Jacobson & Gaska, 1990; Ohzawa, DeAngelis & Freeman, 1990; cf. Sanger, 1988), flicker, chromatic saturation, and so on.

Energy measures can also be combined and cascaded to form more complex measurements (Granlund, 1978). Such an approach may be used to form cells that are end-stopped or side-stopped, or which are selective for more complex properties such as curvature. There is abundant evidence for this sort of complexity in striate cortex and beyond, but a discussion is outside our present scope (cf. Dobbins, Zucker & Cynader, 1987; Koenderink & van Doorn, 1987).

Conclusion

The world is filled with light, and the structure of this light is determined by the physical arrangement of the materials that fill the world. An observer can learn about the world by making measurements of the structure of the light passing through a given point.

We introduce the plenoptic function to specify formally the way that light is structured. For a given wavelength, a given time, and a given viewing position in space, there exists a pencil of light rays passing through the viewing point. Each ray has an intensity, and the collection of rays constitutes a panoramic image. This panoramic image will vary with time, viewing position, and wavelength. The plenoptic function thus has seven dimensions and may be parameterized as $P(x, y, t, \lambda, V_x, V_y, V_z)$.

One of the tasks of early vision is to extract a compact and useful description of the plenoptic function's local properties; the low order derivatives offer such a description under reasonable assumptions about world statistics. If one takes locally weighted first and second derivatives along various axes in plenoptic space, a full range of elemental visual measurements emerges, including all of the familiar measurements of early vision.

The actual information extracted by the human visual system is a small subset of the information that is physically available in the plenoptic function. Humans gather information from only two viewing positions at a time, obtaining two samples along the V_x axis, both taken at a single value of V_y and V_z. Humans sample the wavelength axis with only three cone types. The most densely sampled axes are those corresponding to visual angle, namely, the spatial axes of the retinal image. Time is the only axis that is represented continuously.

One can develop a taxonomy of derivative types, and for each type one can construct a table of visual measurements corresponding to different choices of axes. In this way one can construct a kind of periodic table of the visual elements. A basic table (constructed with the simple derivative types applied to one or two axes at a time) contains 100 elementary measurements.

The periodic table is constructed from first principles, using only the constraints imposed by the available optical information. It is not dependent on the statistics of the world or on the needs of any particular organism. Thus the periodic table offers a null hypothesis about the measurements that an organism could make, with no further assumptions about the environment or the organism's place in it. It then becomes interesting to compare the list of potential measurements with the list of actual measurements that a given organism makes.

The entries in the periodic table include all of the basic visual properties that are commonly considered to constitute early vision, such as orientation, color, motion, and binocular disparity. Other less popular properties also appear in the list, including flicker, binocular correlation and anticorrelation, and hue-shift in space and time. Finally, there are some unexpected properties, such as binocular chromatic anticorrelation.

Many psychophysical and physiological experiments can be considered as explorations of sensitivity to the elemental measurements listed in the periodic table. Over the years, experimenters have filled in the entries of the table in a somewhat random fashion; but it is possible to approach the problem systematically. Physiologists can look for neurons that fall into the various elemental categories, and psychophysicists can look for channels selective for the various elemental properties.

Appendix

Psychophysical Experiments in Plenoptic Space

A variety of paradigms have been developed over the years to assess the limits of human visual performance.

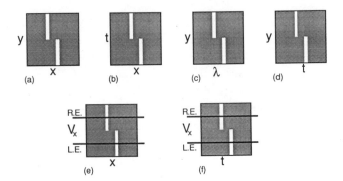

Fig. 1.18
A variety of psychophysical stimuli that seem unrelated turn out to have the same plenoptic structure. The basic spatial vernier task (a) transforms into: (b) temporal displacement discrimination; (c) spatial (top–bottom bipartite field) wavelength discrimination; (d) biparite simultaneity or temporal order judgement; (e) stereoacuity; (f) dichoptic simultaneity or eye-order judgement.

When these experiments are depicted in plenoptic space, a number of unexpected parallels emerge. As an example, the stimuli shown in figure 1.18 correspond to a variety of tasks involving spatial acuity, motion thresholds, wavelength discrimination, and so on. The tasks seem diverse but their structure in plenoptic space is quite similar, as we will now describe.

Part A of figure 1.18 shows the case in which the axes are (x, y); this is just the classic vernier offset task, in which one vertical line is displaced with respect to another. Part B shows the (x, t) case. This corresponds to a vertical line undergoing a jump in position; in other words, it measures sensitivity to small sudden displacements. Part C shows the (λ, y) case. This is a bipartite field, split into top and bottom halves, in which the top half has a different wavelength than the bottom half. In other words, this is a wavelength discrimination task. Part D shows the (t, y) case. This is a bipartite field in which the top half is briefly pulsed and then the bottom half is briefly pulsed. The task is to determine the temporal order in which the two half-fields are pulsed.

Parts E and F of figure 1.18 involve the eye position axis, V_x. Since humans have only two eyes, they take only two samples from this axis, and the locations of these samples are indicated by the horizontal lines marked R.E. and L.E. Part E depicts a stimulus of two vertical lines, one in each eye, with a horizontal displacement—in other words, a test for the detection of stereoscopic disparity. Part F depicts a stimulus in which a full-field flash is presented first to one eye and then to the other.

Figure 1.19 enumerates all the variants of such a stimulus, using pairwise combinations of the five dimensions of x, y, t, λ, and V_x. Every stimulus makes sense, although some of them seem a bit odd at first. For example, the (λ, V_x) stimulus represents a static field of one wavelength in the left eye and a different wavelength in the other eye; the task is to detect the wavelength difference.

Other stimulus classes are shown in figures 1.20 and 1.21. Figure 1.20 shows a stimulus that looks like a piece of a checkerboard in (x, y). but which takes on various sorts of chromaticity, temporal steps, and binocular anti-correlation when the different axes are used. The cells in the upper right triangle are left blank, as they are identical to the lower left triangle by symmetry. Figure 1.21 shows a stimulus that is a diagonal bar in the (x, y) plane, but can become a rainbow, a moving bar, or other stimuli in other planes.

The stimuli we have depicted in the tables above can

	x	y	t	λ	V_x
x	—	**hor. vernier** static achromatic no dispar.	**vert. bipart. pulse order** achromatic no dispar.	**vert. edge** static λ **diff.** no dispar.	—
y	**vert. vernier** static achromatic no dispar.	—	**hor. bipart. pulse order** achromatic no dispar.	**hor. edge** static λ **diff.** no dispar.	—
t	**vert. line jump left** achromatic no dispar.	**horiz. line jump down** achromatic no dispar.	—	**full-field sequential** λ **change** no dispar.	—
λ	**2 vert. lines** static λ **change** no dispar.	**2 hor. lines** static λ **change** no dispar.	**full-field pulse order blue-yel.** no dispar.	—	—
V_x	**vert. line** static achromatic **h disp.**	**horiz. line** static achromatic **v disp.**	**full-field pulse order** achromatic **anticorr.**	**full-field static** λ **diff.** **anticorr.**	—

Fig. 1.19
A table of the psychophysical stimuli corresponding to the basic vernier structure.

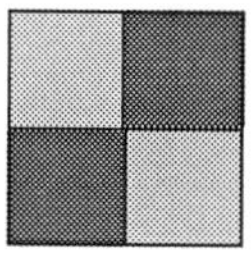

	x	y	t	λ	Vx
x	—				
y	**checker** static achromatic no dispar	—			
t	**vert. edge reversing** achromatic no dispar.	**horiz. edge reversing** achromatic no dispar.	—		
λ	**vert. edge** static **blue-yel.** no dispar.	**horiz. edge** static **blue-yel.** no dispar.	full-field **exchange blue-yel.** no dispar.	—	
Vx	**vert. edge** static achromatic **anticorr.**	**horiz. edge** static achromatic **anticorr.**	full-field **exchange** achromatic **anticorr.**	full-field static **blue-yel. anticorr.**	—

Fig. 1.20
A table of the psychophysical stimuli corresponding to the checkerboard structure.

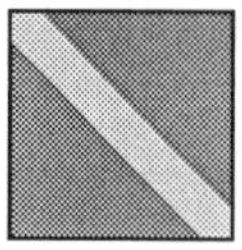

	x	y	t	λ	Vx
x	—				
y	**diag. bar** static achromatic no dispar	—			
t	**vert. bar leftward** achromatic no dispar	**horiz. bar downward** achromatic no dispar	—		
λ	**vertical** static **rainbow** no dispar	**horiz.** static **rainbow** no dispar	full-field **sequential rainbow** no dispar	—	
Vx	**vert. bar** static achromatic hor. dispar	**horiz. bar** static achromatic vert. dispar	full-field **sequential** achromatic eye-order	full-field static **hue-shift luster**	—

Fig. 1.21
A table of psychophysical stimuli corresponding to a tilted bar structure.

be described with only two axes, but many psychophysical stimuli require more. For example, a diagonal chromatic moving bar in depth would require a full five-dimensional description.

References

Adelson, E. H. & Bergen, J. R. (1985). Spatiotemporal energy models for the perception of motion. *Journal of the Optical Society of America A, 2*, 284–299.

Barlow, H. B. (1982). What causes trichromacy? a theoretical analysis using comb-filtered spectra. *Vision Research, 22*, 635–643.

Beck, J. (1966). Perceptual grouping produced by changes in orientation and shape. *Science, 154*, 538–540.

Bergen, J. R. & Julesz, B. (1983). Rapid discrimination of visual patterns. *IEEE Transactions on Systems, Man and Cybernetics, 13*, 857–863.

Cronin, T. W. & Marshall, N. J. (1989). A retina with at least ten spectral types of photoreceptors in a mantis shrimp. *Nature, 339*, 137–140.

De Valois, R. L. & De Valois, K. K. (1988). *Spatial Vision*. New York: Oxford University Press.

De Valois, R. L., Thorell, L. G., & Albrecht, D. G. (1985). Periodicity of striate-cortex-cell receptive fields. *Journal of the Optical Society of America A, 2*, 1115–1123.

Dobbins, A., Zucker, S. W., & Cynader, M. (1987). Endstopped neurons in the visual cortex as a substrate for calculating curvature. *Nature, 329*, 438–441.

Emerson, R. C., Bergen, J. R., & Adelson, E. H. (1987) Movement models and directionally selective neurons in the cat's visual cortex. *Society for Neuroscience Abstracts, 13*, 1623.

Emerson, R. C., Bergen, J. R., & Adelson, E. H. (1991). Directionally selective complex cells and the calculation of motion energy in cat visual cortex. *Vision Research*, in press.

Gibson, J. J. (1966). *The senses considered as perceptual systems*. Boston: Houghton Mifflin.

Graham, N. V. S. (1989). *Visual pattern analysers*. New York: Oxford University Press.

Granlund, G. (1978). In search of a general picture processing operator. *Computer Graphics and Image Processing, 8*, 155–173.

Horn, B. K. P. (1986). *Robot vision*. Cambridge, MA: The MIT Press.

Hubel, D. H. (1988). *Eye, brain and vision*. San Francisco: Freeman.

Jacobson, L. D. & Gaska, J. P. (1990). A s/sf energy model for estimating binocular disparity. *Investigative Ophthalmology and Visual Science (Suppl.), 31*, 91.

Julesz, B. & Bergen, J. R. (1983). Textons, the fundamental elements in preattentive vision and perception of textures. *Bell Systems Technical Journal, 62*, 1619–1645.

Kemp, M. (1989). *Leonardo on painting*. New Haven: Yale University Press.

Knutsson, H. & Granlund, G. H. (1983). Texture analysis using two dimensional quadrature filters. In *IEEE CAPAIDM*, p. 206–213, Silver Spring, MD.

Koenderink, J. J. & van Doorn, A. J. (1987). Representation of local geometry in the visual system. *Biological Cybernetics, 55*, 367–375.

Levine, M. D. (1985). *Vision in man and machine*. New York: McGraw-Hill.

Livingstone, M. S. & Hubel, D. H. (1984). Anatomy and physiology of a color system in the primate visual cortex. *Journal of Neuroscience, 4*, 309–356.

Maloney, L. T. (1986). Evaluation of linear models of surface spectral reflectance with small numbers of parameters. *Journal of the Optical Society of America A, 3*, 1673–1683.

Marr, D. (1982). *Vision*. San Francisco: Freeman.

Movshon, J. A., Thompson, I. D., & Tolhurst, D. J. (1978). Receptive field organization of complex cells in the cat's striate cortex. *Journal of Physiology, 283*, 79–99.

Neisser, U. (1976). *Cognition and reality*. San Francisco: Freeman.

Ohzawa, I., DeAngelis, G., & Freeman, R. (1990). Stereoscopic depth discrimination in the visual cortex: neurons ideally suited as disparity detectors. *Science, 249*, 1037–1041.

Olzak, L. & Thomas, J. P. (1986). Seeing spatial patterns. In K. R. Boff, L. Kaufman, & J. P. Thomas. (Eds.), *Handbook of perception and human performance*: Vol. (pp. 7-1–7-56). New York: Wiley.

Poggio, G. F. & Poggio, T. (1984). The analysis of stereopsis. *Annual Review of Neuroscience, 7*, 397–412.

Pokorny, J. & Smith, V. C. (1986). Colorimetry and color discrimination. In K. R. Boff, L. Kaufman, & J. P. Thomas (Eds.), *Handbook of perception and human performance*: Vol. 1 (pp. 8-1–8-51). New York: Wiley.

Richter, J. P. (1970). *The notebooks of Leonardo da Vinci*: Vol. 1. New York: Dover.

Ross, J., Morrone, M. C., & Burr, D. C. (1989). The conditions under which mach bands are visible. *Vision Research, 29*, 699–715.

Sanger, T. D. (1988). Stereo disparity computation using Gabor filters. *Biological Cybernetics, 59*, 405–418.

Spitzer, H. & Hochstein, S. (1985). A complex cell receptive field model. *Journal of Neurophysiology, 53*, 1266–1286.

Treisman, A. (1986). Properties, parts and objects. In K. R. Boff, L. Kaufman, & J. P. Thomas, (Eds.), *Handbook of perception and human performance*: Vol. 2 (pp. 35-1–35-70). New York: Wiley.

Treisman, A. and Gelade, G. (1980). A feature integration theory of attention. *Cognitive Psychology, 12*, 97–137.

Watson, A. B. (1986). Temporal sensitivity. In K. R. Boff, L. Kaufman, & J. P. Thomas, (Eds.), *Handbook of perception and human performance*: Vol. 1 (pp. 6-1–6-43). New York: Wiley.

Young, R. A. (1985). *The gaussian derivative theory of spatial vision: Analysis of cortical cell receptive field line-weighting profiles* (Tech. Rep. GMR-4920). General Motors Research Publication.

Young, R. A. (1989). Quantitative tests of visual cortical receptive field models. In *OSA Annual Meeting, 1989, Technical Digest*, p. 93, Washington, DC.

Part II

Receptors and Sampling

Before visual signals enter the brain, they are captured by the photoreceptors and processed by the neural elements of the retina. Aspects of retinal function, especially the sensitivity, size, number, and distribution of the photoreceptors, impose fundamental limits on visual capacity that have recently received substantial attention. Of particular interest is the sampling array provided by the cones, the photoreceptor type that subserves high resolution vision under most usual conditions of illumination.

The cone mosaic resembles a tightly packed hexagonal array near the center of gaze, but cone positions become less and less orderly in the peripheral retina. It may be that this disorder has adaptive value (Yellott, 1982). In the fovea, the Nyquist limit (the most finely resolved pattern that can be accurately represented by the cone sampling) is near 60 cycles/degree of visual angle, a value agreeably close to the finest pattern that can be imaged under optimal conditions by the optical apparatus of the eye. Thus in the center of the retinal image, the optics filter the input to eliminate those patterns that would exceed the capacity of the receptor array. In the periphery this is not the case: The optics resolve fine patterns beyond the sampling limit imposed by the cones. An undesirable consequence of undersampling is "aliasing," in which the sampled signal contains spurious components not present in the original image. When sampling is regular, regular patterns produce an alias that is another regular pattern; importantly, this aliased pattern cannot be distinguished from a real pattern quite different from the one actually present in the image. Disorder in the sampling array does not remove aliasing, but it has the effect of making regular patterns produce irregular aliases that resemble spatial "noise" like that seen on a television tuned between channels. If we make the reasonable assumption that the visual system is more interested in things that have regular images than in things that resemble noise, it can be argued that the aliasing produced by irregular arrays might be less disruptive than that produced by regular ones.

Alternatively, it might be possible to trade temporal resolution for spatial resolution by taking multiple samples separated by small eye movements and comparing the resulting images; this effectively increases the sampling resolution at the expense of not being able to process rapidly changing images (Maloney, 1989).

An assumption of these models of cone sampling and aliasing is that the visual system can reconstruct the full two-dimensional visual stimulus from the discrete spatial samples. To do this correctly, the system must not only know the values of the image at each sample point, but also the positions of those sample points. The chapter by Ahumada describes three learning algorithms that a visual system could use to learn the positions of the input samples, to learn the appropriate interpolation weights, and to refine the estimates of cone positions as they change over time (with development, disease, or minor changes in the optics).

Williams and his colleagues have done a great deal of work on the consequences of the cone sampling properties on the appearance of static and moving spatial patterns (Coletta & Williams, 1987; Williams, 1985a,b, 1986, 1988; Williams & Coletta, 1987). His chapter, coauthored by Tiana, Coletta, and Haake, provides a computational model that predicts the appearance of spatiotemporal patterns both within and outside the resolution limits imposed by sampling. This model deals in turn with the optical imaging apparatus, the spatial structure of the sampling mosaic, and the central nervous system's processing of the resulting signal. The model nicely predicts the results of a variety of perceptual experiments in which special optical methods are used to probe visual processing of stimuli that exceed the normal resolution limits of the eye.

In addition to its role in sampling the image, the retina has a major role in the transformation of visual signals from a representation based on the local absolute luminance of the image to a representation based on image contrast (Shapley & Enroth-Cugell, 1984). This transformation is accomplished partly by neural hardware that compares nearby image values, but the most important retinal component concerns light adaptation. Photoreceptors change their gain in response to changes in the prevailing illumination, so that they are most sensitive to variations about that prevailing level. Hood and Birch's chapter describes data obtained from electroretinographic recordings of the activity of human photoreceptors, and a model that accounts for the changes in their response pattern with illumination. The structure of this model draws from a body of earlier work incorporating several putative mechanisms for modifying receptor gain and provides a satisfactory and comprehensive account that has implications both for processing images and for further studies of the underlying neuronal mechanisms.

References

Coletta, N. J. & Williams, D. R. (1987). Psychophysical estimate of extrafoveal cone spacing. *Journal of the Optical Society of America A*, 4, 1503−1513.

Maloney, L. T. (1989). Combining information across multiple sampling arrays. *Investigative Ophthalmology and Visual Science (Suppl.)*, 30, 54.

Shapley, R. M. & Enroth-Cugell, C. (1984). Visual adaptation and retinal gain controls. *Progress in Retinal Research*, 3, 263−353.

Williams, D. R. (1985a). Aliasing in human foveal vision. *Vision Research*, 25, 195−205.

Williams, D. R. (1985b). Visibility of interference fringes near the resolution limit. *Journal of the Optical Society of America A*, 2, 1087−1093.

Williams, D. R. (1986). Seeing through the photoreceptor mosaic. *Trends in Neurosciences*, 9, 193−198.

Williams, D. R. (1988). Topography of the foveal cone mosaic in the living human eye. *Vision Research*, 28, 433−454.

Williams, D. R. & Coletta, N. J. (1987). Cone spacing and the visual resolution limit. *Journal of the Optical Society of America A*, 4, 1514−1523.

Yellott, J. I., Jr. (1982). Spectral analysis of spatial sampling by photoreceptors: Topological disorder prevents aliasing. *Vision Research*, 22, 1205−1210.

Learning Receptor Positions

Albert J. Ahumada, Jr.

The human retinal cones are not arrayed in regular rows and columns like the elements of current solid-state video sensors. The cone density drops surprisingly steeply as one moves away from the center of the fovea (Østerberg, 1935). Even in the fovea, where the cone array is most regular, there is significant variation in density and packing orientation (Ahnelt, Kolb & Pflug, 1987; Curcio, Sloan, Packer, Hendrickson & Kalina, 1987): Psychophysics and visual experience suggest that somehow this array of sensors leads to an extremely accurately reconstructed image in terms of geometric position. Theories explaining the ability to make fine geometric judgments typically assume knowledge of cone position either implicitly or explicitly (Geisler, 1984; Geisler & Davila, 1985). The goal here is to introduce some computational theories that provide plausible solutions to the problem of how the brain knows the positions of the photoreceptors. These theories have been developed in collaboration with others and have been described previously (Ahumada & Mulligan, 1989,1990; Ahumada & Pavel, 1989; Ahumada & Yellott, 1989; Maloney, 1988a,b, 1989; Maloney & Ahumada, 1989).

Three separate models will be described. In models 1 and 2, spontaneous activity generates calibration signals inside the visual system. These can be thought of as pre-experiential models. Model 1 performs the task of copying the configuration of receptor positions from the retinal level to a higher level. Model 2 performs the task of interpolating the image between these positions, allowing other visual processes to sample the reconstructed image at arbitrary positions. External visual images form the input for model 3. This model refines the image reconstruction on the basis of experience, allowing compensation for optical distortions, imperfections in the prior mechanisms, and new errors that may develop as the retina continues to develop after birth.

Although each model performs a useful task on its own and need not be associated with the others, the second two use results of their predecessors. The interpolation function construction process of model 2 assumes that certain points in the reconstructed image correspond to the receptor positions, presumably as copied by model 1. Model 3 uses an interpolated image to evaluate its measure of quality, the difference between its current samples and the samples from an interpolated image at a previous position. All three models are self-organizing, in that they do not depend on feedback from external systems. Mathematically, however, they have the character of feedback processes rather than competitive processes. They use locally derived error signals to guide the calibration process.

Methods

Model 1: Copying Receptor Positions

The goal of this process is to position units in a plane at a higher neural level so they have the same configuration as that of the retinal receptors. The process adjusts the unit positions at the higher level so that the distances between units are proportional to the distances between their corresponding receptors. Figure 2.1 illustrates the process. Each receptor has the capability to send one of two messages to its corresponding unit, depending on the state of activity of the receptor. If the receptor is active, it signals this fact to its unit. If the receptor is inactive, it reports the level of local activity to its unit. One at a time, receptors become spontaneously active and generate activity at all higher units through two pathways. In the first pathway, activity spreads laterally in the retina from the active receptor to the others. The local level of this activity is passed from each inactive receptor to its unit. The activity is assumed to decrease with distance and represents the retinal distance from the active receptor to each of the other receptors. In the second pathway, the active receptor signals its corresponding unit to initiate a similar spread of activity in the higher neural plane. This activity represents the distance between the active unit and the others. The difference between the two levels of activity is then used as an error signal to move the units corresponding to the inactive receptors to positions at the correct distance from the active unit. Although these adjustments may be detrimental to the distances among the inactive units, these distances get corrected later. When

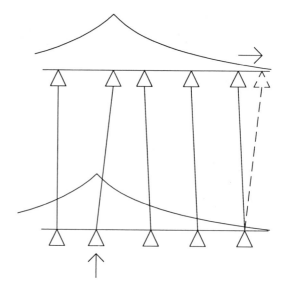

Fig. 2.1
A diagram of the position learning process of model 1. A retinal unit (*upward arrow*) is spontaneously active and generates an activity gradient in the retina. Its corresponding unit at the higher level also generates a gradient, and the difference between these two gradients causes the higher level unit on the far right, for example, to move to the right where the gradients are equal. For positions along a single dimension, as illustrated here, all the units would move to correct relative positions with a single activation. In two dimensions, more activations are generally required, as illustrated in figure 2.2

units become spontaneously active in a random sequence, the configuration converges towards the correct one.

Let i be the index of the currently active receptor, with retinal coordinates x_i and y_i. Let $d_{i,j}$ be the distance from the ith receptor to the jth receptor,

$$d_{i,j} = \sqrt{(x_i - x_j)^2 + (y_i - y_j)^2}. \tag{1.1}$$

The activation at the jth receptor is given by

$$s_{i,j} = f(d_{i,j}), \tag{1.2}$$

where f is a monotonically decreasing function, representing decremental spread of activity with distance. Using the prime symbol (') to indicate the corresponding quantities for the higher level units, the activity at the jth unit from activity spreading at this level is given by

$$s'_{i,j} = f(md'_{i,j}), \tag{1.3}$$

where m is the magnification factor relating the activity spread functions at the two levels. A nonzero difference between these two activity levels,

$$e_{i,j} = s_{i,j} - s'_{i,j}, \tag{1.4}$$

indicates an error in the distance $d'_{i,j}$. Since f decreases with distance, a positive error indicates that $d'_{i,j}$ is too large, so point j is moved toward point i by adding increments to the coordinate of point j,

$$\Delta x'_j = r(x'_i - x'_j)e'_{i,j}$$

$$\Delta y'_j = r(y'_i - y'_j)e'_{i,j} \qquad (1.5)$$

where r is a small positive fraction, the learning rate. These increments move the point (x'_j, y'_j) toward or away from (x'_i, y'_i) along the line connecting them. Since the idea of the method is to move the point using physiologically plausible information, it may seem inappropriate that the actual coordinates appear in the formula. They only play the role of determining the direction of point i from point j at the higher level. An equivalent, locally determined formula could be constructed using the gradient of the spread function at the higher level.

If the retinal receptor remains active and the adjustments are repeated, the inactive unit positions will converge to a point which is the correct distance away, where

$$md'_{i,j} = d_{i,j}. \qquad (1.6)$$

The physiologically plausible process can thus be simulated by using increments that move directly to this point,

$$\Delta x'_j = k(x'_i - x'_j),$$

$$\Delta y'_j = k(y'_i - y'_j). \qquad (1.7)$$

where

$$k = 1 - \frac{d_{i,j}}{md'_{i,j}}. \qquad (1.8)$$

This adjustment rule is conveniently independent of f and r.

Even if only one point is out of position, a single adjustment will not usually be in the correct direction, as illustrated in figure 2.2. But as different points are activated at random, simulations have always managed to untangle completely random initial configurations as illustrated in figure 2.3. Mathematical analyses of similar processes have been described by Kohonen (1989, chapter 5), but actual convergence proofs are not known to me. Simulations of the process have been done serially, which could take a long time for millions of receptors. Multiple units could be spontaneously active, so long as their activity regions do not overlap, This could be ensured by

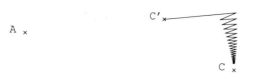

Fig. 2.2
Path of a point C′ when points A and B are alternately activated. Points A′ and B′ are assumed to be correctly positioned at points A and B, respectively, and C is the correct position for C′.

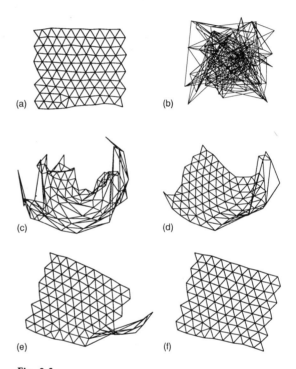

Fig. 2.3
An example of position learning using the fovea cone position data of Hirsch and Hylton (1984). (a) The retinal configuration. (b) The randomized positions. (c) The configuration after 1 cycle (102 activations with 101 adjustments each). (d) After 2 cycles. (e) After 6 cycles. (f) After 10 cycles.

the spreading activity of one receptor inhibiting the spontaneous activation of the others.

Model 2: Constructing the Interpolation Functions

Once the positions have been copied to the higher level, the way is paved for the construction of a network that can compute a continuous interpolation of the sampled image. This network, which will compensate for the uneven spacing of the receptors, will be formed by a learning process that also depends on spontaneous activity.

Before describing this process, we review some concepts in reconstructing images from samples.

Interpolation of Regularly Spaced Samples

It is somewhat counter to intuition that if a continuous image has no contrast at spatial frequencies above the Nyquist frequency of a discrete rectangular sampling grid, it can be reconstructed perfectly from the discrete sample values by sinc interpolation (Jerri, 1977). A two-dimensional spatial frequency component is below the Nyquist frequency if the spatial frequencies in both sampling directions are less than half the sampling rate. The reconstruction process, illustrated for one dimension and one sample point in figure 2.4, is additive. At each sample point, a sinc function image, with a peak contrast equal to that of the sample, is added into the reconstructed image. Since the sinc function is unity at the sample point and zero at the others, the reconstructed image will be correct at the sample points; and the reconstruction thus interpolates between them (correctly if the image is appropriately limited in spatial frequency). The general equation for a linear reconstruction $a'(x, y)$ of an image $a(x, y)$ from discrete samples,

$$a_i = a(x_i, y_i),\qquad(2.1)$$

is given by

$$a'(x, y) = \sum_i a_i s_i(x, y).\qquad(2.2)$$

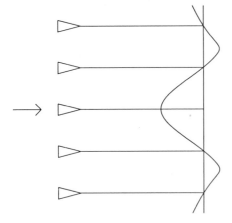

Fig. 2.4
Sinc interpolation. The waveform illustrates the interpolated image generated by the activation of a single receptor (*arrow*). The response to a general input would be a weighted sum of such waves from each input.

It is a sinc interpolation if $s_i(x, y)$ is the two-dimensional sinc function centered at (x_i, y_i),

$$s_i(x, y) = \text{sinc}\left(\frac{x - x_i}{d}\right)\text{sinc}\left(\frac{y - y_i}{d}\right).\qquad(2.3)$$

The one-dimensional sinc function is given by

$$\text{sinc}(x) = \frac{\sin \pi x}{\pi x},\qquad(2.4)$$

and d is the constant spacing between the rectangularly arrayed samples.

Uneven Samples

When the sample position (x_i, y_i) are not evenly spaced, this formula can lead to very poor reconstructions. If points are close, the image will "pile up" and large spaces between samples will result in "holes" in the image. Clearly we could improve the reconstruction by boosting the gains of the reconstruction functions in the neighborhood of gaps and dropping the gains for closely spaced positions. If we introduce weights, not only from sample to reconstruction function, but from all samples to each reconstruction function, it is possible to correct for all the errors at the sample points and obtain an interpolation (a reconstruction that is correct at the sample points), as illustrated in figure 2.5. Let us call the $s_i(x, y)$ spread functions and reserve the term reconstruction function for the functions that result from a unit input to a single receptor. The ith reconstruction function is now

$$r_i(x, y) = \sum_j w_{i,j} s_j(x, y),\qquad(2.5)$$

where the $w_{i,j}$ are the network gains or weights. The image is now reconstructed as

$$a'(x, y) = \sum_i a_i r_i(x, y).\qquad(2.6)$$

If the spread functions are the sinc functions and the weights are chosen so that the reconstruction functions are interpolators, the reconstruction is called least squares interpolation (Chen & Allebach, 1987).

The condition that our reconstruction be an interpolation, i.e., be correct at the sample points, is that

$$r_i(x_k, y_k) = \delta'_{i,k}\qquad(2.7)$$

where the Kronecker delta, $(\delta_{i,k})$ equals one if $i = k$, and zero otherwise. From equation 2.5 we see that we are

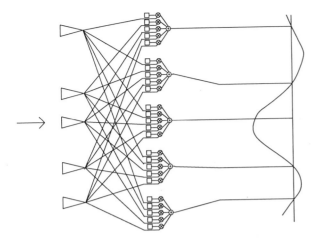

Fig. 2.5

Least squares interpolation. The weights of the network form a combined interpolation from a weighted sum of sinc functions centered at the receptor positions. The weights are selected so that the output from a single input has unity gain at its own position and is zero at all the other receptor positions.

seeking $w_{i,j}$ that satisfy

$$\sum_j w_{i,j} s_{j,k} = \delta'_{i,k} \qquad (2.8)$$

where $s_{j,k}$ is $s_j(x_k, y_k)$, the jth spread function evaluated at the kth receptor position. In matrix language, the matrix of $w_{i,j}$ is the inverse of the matrix of $s_{j,k}$.

Interpolation Weight Learning

Is there a physiologically plausible mechanism for setting the $w_{i,j}$ to be the matrix inverse of the $s_{j,k}$? The matrix inverse relation is symmetric, so equation 2.8 can be rewritten as

$$\sum_i s_{k,i} w_{i,j} = \delta_{k,j}. \qquad (2.9)$$

This equation implies that when the kth spread function is input into the network in place of an image, the network output should be unity at position k and zero at the other positions. That is, the spread functions are network inputs for which the outputs are known (and simple). The delta rule of neural network learning theory (Stone, 1986; Widrow & Hoff, 1960) was developed to solve this problem—the calculation of weights that transform known inputs into known outputs. In the delta rule, inputs are selected one at a time and fed into the network. The difference between the output and the desired output is computed to form an error term. The network weights are

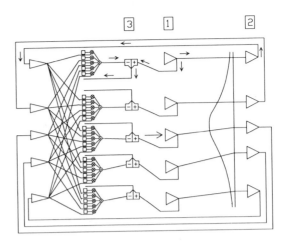

Fig. 2.6

The weighted interpolation network of figure 2.5 modified for weight calibration by model 2. Layer 1 has spontaneously active units that activate the spread functions formerly activated by the network output. An active unit (*large arrow*) generates a spread function signal (the Gaussian curve) in the reconstructed image plane (*vertical line*). Layer 2 has units positioned according to the receptor spacing in this plane. They sample this image and feed it back into the network. Layer 3 computes an error signal as the difference between the activity in layer 1 and the network output. The error signal (*unterminated lines*) is used to adjust the weights as shown in figure 2.7. Small arrows indicate the direction of signal flow.

then adjusted with a combination (the outer product) of the input and the error.

Figures 2.6 and 2.7 show a network that can implement the delta rule process for this application. Figure 2.6 shows the network of figure 2.5 reconfigured for weight learning. Three new layers appear in the figure. The first new layer is a layer of spontaneously active units, placed intermediate between the network and the spread functions. It replaces the weight network outputs as the activators of the spread functions. When one unit is active, its spread function becomes the interpolated image, as illustrated. The second new layer in figure 2.6 samples the interpolated image at positions corresponding to the receptor positions (furnished by model 1) and feeds these values back to provide the weight network input. If the kth spontaneous unit is active, the ith input to the weight network will be $s_{k,i}$ and the jth output from the network will be given by the left-hand side of equation 2.9. The third new layer is a layer of subtracting units. They compute the error, the difference between the desired output and the network output. The desired output, $\delta_{k,j}$, is conveniently available as the state of the spontaneously active units. The error at the jth network output when the

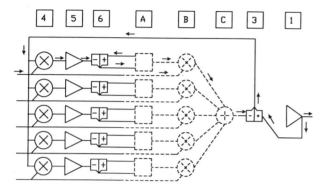

Fig. 2.7

The weight adjustment network of model 2. The dotted lines show the original signal weighting network. Layer A shows the weights, which are multiplied by the input values in layer B and summed at layer C. Layer 1 has a spontaneous unit which has generated the signal in layer 2 (not shown here) that is entering on the input lines (*unterminated*) on the far left. Layer 3 sends the error signal back to layer 4, which computes the product of the error and the input. Layer 5 adjusts the gain by the learning rate. Layer 6 subtracts the modified error signal from the weight and returns the new value. Small arrows indicate the direction of signal flow.

kth spread function is activated is given by

$$e_{k,j} = \delta_{k,j} - \sum_i s_{k,i} w_{i,j}. \qquad (2.10)$$

In figure 2.6 the lines carrying the error are shown going back toward the weights they will help adjust.

Figure 2.7 shows the additional circuitry needed at each weighting unit to adjust the weights. A fourth new layer, a layer of multipliers compute the product of the ith input, $s_{k,i}$ and the jth error, $e_{k,j}$. A fifth new layer multiplies this product by a constant gain factor r, the learning rate. The sixth and last new layer subtracts the weighted error from the old value of the weight and returns the difference as the new weight. The network weights are thus adjusted by the delta rule increments

$$\Delta w_{i,j} = r s_{k,i} e_{k,j}. \qquad (2.11)$$

As in model 1, the actual value of the learning rate r plays no role if the same input is repeated until the error for that input goes to zero. The effect is the same as using the learning rate which does zero the error in one step,

$$r = \frac{1}{\sum_i s_{k,i}^2}. \qquad (2.12)$$

As illustrated in figure 2.6, spread functions are not required to be sinc functions. Other functions can be used

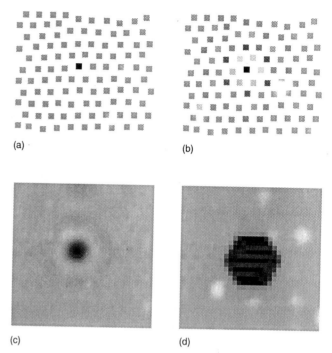

Fig. 2.8

An interpolation example. An interpolation for the Hirsch and Hylton (1984) foveal receptor positions based on Gaussian spread functions. Gray scale representations in which black is positive and white is negative. (A) A sampled input which is unity at one receptor (black) and zero at the others (gray). (B) The interpolation weights from that receptor position to the others. The immediately surrounding weights are negative (light gray). (C) The interpolation function from that receptor position. (D) The Fourier amplitude transform of that interpolation function.

for s and the corresponding w will generate an interpolation. Figure 2.8 shows an example interpolation using Gaussian spread functions for a nearly hexagonal sampling array. For rectangular sampling, the sinc interpolation function is the Fourier transform of a rectangular box function. For hexagonal (triangular) sampling, the corresponding interpolator is the Fourier transform of a hexagon. The interpolation for the selected input point in figure 2.8 is seen to have a fairly hexagonal transform. Gaussian spread functions were selected originally just to see how they would work, but they could be a good choice since the optical spread function of the eye is approximately Gaussian (Campbell & Gubisch, 1966). Oakley and Cunningham (1990) have shown that for regularly sampled signals that are not strictly band-limited but have been filtered with a Gaussian optical point spread, the interpolator constructed by model 2 is "ideal" if its spread function is the Gaussian whose standard deviation is root two times that of the optical spread.

Unlike the case of model 1, where the process requires that spontaneously active units not have active neighbors, the process of model 2 does not. Any pattern of activity in the spontaneously active layer is the desired network output for the network input that it generates. The case of single active units is just simpler to describe (and simulate).

Model 3: Experiential Refinement

In principle, the above system could create a fairly accurate copy of the retinal image, but in practice it would be dependent on the accuracy of the positions provided by model 1, which depend on activity spread functions being only a function of retinal distance. It could do nothing about optical distortions. If there were known calibration images, the delta rule could be used to train the weights to compensate for optical as well as sampling effects. For example, if we knew that we were looking straight at a lone star, we could try to minimize the outputs at all other places. Maloney (1988a,b; 1989) proposed that the image translations generated by eye movements could be used to compute an error term for training the weights. Following this suggestion we have written computer programs that use the delta rule algorithm with internally generated error. They successfully train weights without knowledge of the input images. These weights linearly transform input samples into estimates of samples from image positions assumed by the visual system.

External Translation

Again we assume an image $a(x, y)$ sampled at a number of points giving a list of input values,

$$a_i = a(x_i, y_i). \tag{3.1}$$

These are transformed by a network of weights $w_{i,j}$ into estimates a'_j of samples at positions (x_j, y_j),

$$a'_j = \sum_i a_i w_{i,j}. \tag{3.2}$$

We next assume that there is a new image b generated by translating a by the amount t_x in the x direction and t_y in the y direction,

$$b(x, y) = a(x - t_x, y - t_y). \tag{3.3}$$

The internal representation of this image is given by

$$b'_j = \sum_i b_i w_{i,j}. \tag{3.4}$$

Internal Translation

Next we assume that the internal signal a' is interpolated into a continuous function $a'(x, y)$ from the $a'(j)$ such that

$$a'(x_j, y_j) = a'_j. \tag{3.5}$$

This reconstructed image is translated internally by (t_x, t_y) and sampled at the points (x_j, y_j), forming a list of sample points,

$$b''_j = a'(x_j - t_x, y_j - t_y). \tag{3.6}$$

Weight Adjustment

If the weights were correct, the internally translated values b''_j would match the externally translated values b'_j, so we use the b''_j as the desired output for the b'_j in the delta rule process. The error for the process becomes

$$e_j = b''_j - b'_j, \tag{3.7}$$

and the adjustment rule becomes

$$\Delta w_{i,j} = r b_i e'_j \tag{3.8}$$

where r is again a learning rate.

Additional Complexities

If feedback were correct, this would be the delta rule and, as in delta rule learning, to ensure that the process will converge to the correct weights, the dimensionality of the input image space must not exceed the number of input and output units; and the sequence of input images must include all stimulus subspaces infinitely often (Bitmead, 1984). The translation adds additional restrictions. The input space now includes translations of the original space and these translations must not unduly increase the dimensionality of the space. The translations must occur in two independent directions (Raugh, 1985), and all stimulus subspaces have to be moved in both directions infinitely often.

The interpolation function used was not the sinc function, which is appropriate for stimuli which are specified by their continuous Fourier transform, but was the Fourier series equivalent, the sum of cosines (Green & Swets, 1966, Section 6.3.2),

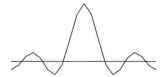

Fig. 2.9
The sum of cosines interpolation function for 7 equidistant samples.

$$\Psi(x) = \frac{\frac{1}{2} + \sum_{f=1}^{f_{max}} \cos(2\pi f x)}{\frac{1}{2} + f_{max}}. \tag{3.9}$$

Figure 2.9 illustrates this periodic equivalent of the sinc function.

Translation invariance does not force a unique solution like correct feedback does. Any translation-invariant filtering by the weight matrix goes undetected by the error computation. A unique solution is determined if either the receptive field of an output unit or the projective field of an input unit is fixed. However, while all projective fields depend on the positions of other units, the correct receptive field for an output at the same position as an input is simple: a weight of unity for that input and a weight of zero for all others. We thus arbitrarily select one input k to correspond to one output, j, and fix the receptive field of that output accordingly.

$$w_{i,j} = \delta_{i,k}. \tag{3.10}$$

The delta rule with correct feedback converges if

$$0 < r \sum_i b_i^2 < 2, \tag{3.11}$$

and it zeros the error for this input if

$$r = 1 / \sum_i b_i^2. \tag{3.12}$$

We have had better learning from a learning rate half this size, presumably because it does not pay to take such large steps if you are not going in the right direction. Actually, the direction in our simulations is a little worse than the above equations suggest. They represent the sequence "look, move, look, and learn." It seems more plausible that a biological system would repeat the sequence "move, look, and learn." The image being translated internally to form b_j'' is then based on one earlier $w_{i,j}$.

An Example Simulation

Figure 2.10 shows a 5 by 5 jittered lattice of input sample points and regular lattice corresponding to the internal representation. The translation-invariant learning rule and the delta rule with correct feedback were both tried on a white noise input image. Figure 2.11 shows three error curves as a function of iterations, one for the delta rule and two for the translation-invariance rule. The error for the delta rule (labeled "delta") and the external-internal error for translation invariance (labeled "ext-int") are the root-mean-square differences between the external image and the internal image at the rectangular grid points. The internal-internal error is the root-mean-square of the internally measured errors of equation 3.7, which the learning process seeks to minimize. The figure illustrates correct feedback training the weight matrix to correct for random errors in receptor positions ("delta"). It also illustrates that translation-invariance errors ("int-int") are corrected almost as fast as the delta rule corrects its errors. The actual errors for the translation invariance rule ("ext-int") are lagging behind, but are also converging towards zero, essentially because correctly fixing the receptive field of one unit has made the correct solution the only translation-invariant one.

Some Intuitions from a Special Case

To gain some insight into how the process works, suppose that the input samples and the output samples are in the same regular positions, but are not correctly connected. Assume the sampled input image is unity at the ith receptor and zero at the others,

$$a_j = \delta_{i,j}. \tag{3.13}$$

If the translation is a step from position i to position k,

$$b_j = \delta_{k,j}. \tag{3.14}$$

Putting these images through the weight matrix gives the projective fields of the ith and kth inputs,

$$a_j' = w_{i,j}' \tag{3.15}$$

$$b_j' = w_{k,j}. \tag{3.16}$$

The internal translation of a_j' to create b_j'' is then the projective field of the ith receptor moved to the position of the kth receptor. If $r = 1$ we find that

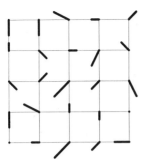

Fig. 2.10
A 5 by 5 rectangular lattice (the internal representation) and a jittered version (the external sample points). The jitter is uniform in x and y with a width equal to the sample spacing.

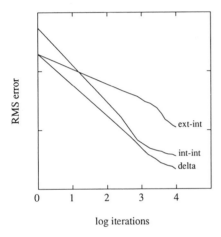

Fig. 2.11
Learning curves for translation-invariance learning of interpolation weights for the jitter in figure 2.10, using model 3. The actual interpolation error is labeled "ext-int" and is the average root-mean-square difference between the external image and the internal image, both sampled at the rectangular positions. The curve labeled "int-int" is the average root-mean-square value of the translational errors used to adjust the weights. The bottom curve labeled "delta" shows the actual interpolation error when the delta rule (correct feedback from the external image) was used.

$$\Delta w_{i,j} = \delta_{i,k}(b_j'' - w_{k,j}). \qquad (3.17)$$

Only the kth projective field is changed and it is replaced by the ith projective field appropriately translated. If one projective field is fixed, it is copied to all the others. If one receptive field is fixed, one element of each projective field is fixed. Once all positions have been reached, the correct projective field is formed and is then dragged around to the other positions. When the learning rate is less than unity, the process does not copy from one place to another; it replaces the new one with a weighted average of the old and the new, asymptotically giving the same result.

In this special case, when a projective field is fixed, starting at the position of the fixed field and moving the point image to each position in turn finishes learning in n steps if there are n receptors. In the general delta rule case (with correct feedback), only n steps are needed if each sampled input is orthogonal to all the previous ones. In the general translation case, faster learning occurs if the translations move over an input image in a systematic way, with steps large enough so that successive images are relatively independent.

Discussion

Previous Work

The Present Models

The first two models have been previously described by Ahumada and Yellott (1989). That presentation also describes ways of speeding up the convergence of the matrix inversion calculation, while still maintaining one computational advantage of the method described here, its ability to take advantage of locality in the spread functions. Initial convergence considerations for all three models appear in Ahumada and Mulligan (1989). Ahumada and Pavel (1989) explored alternative adjustment algorithms, such as gradient descent, using the second position as the correct feedback for the first, and the look-twice method mentioned above. No appreciable differences were found in the performance of these algorithms, which all seem more difficult to implement physiologically.

Maloney (1988a,b; 1989) developed the idea of using translation invariance to calibrate a visual system. The theory is presented in Maloney and Ahumada (1989), along with a brief description of the simulation algorithm of model 3. The paper also proposes an alternative way of making the translation-invariant weights unique. In model 3, uniqueness was forced by fixing one receptive or projective field. Maloney also realized that if the weights were made invariant for rotation and zoom transformations, uniqueness would result. Rotation invariance corrects the phases of all the frequency components of the projective fields and zoom invariance corrects their relative amplitudes.

A serious plausibility problem with model 3 is that the visual system is assumed to know the exact amount of translation. Ahumada and Mulligan (1990) demonstrate that if the system is only slightly miscalibrated, the estimation of the translation can be done by the visual system from the incorrectly calibrated internal images. This also supports the need for other mechanisms, such as the first two models, for bringing the system into good initial calibration.

Related Computational Models

Sperry (1956) pioneered experimental work on the general problem of how the visual pathways might maintain topological (neighbor to neighbor) order during development, and proposed a two-gradient model for the reconstruction of retinal maps. Model 1 can be thought of as a gradient model in which each receptor has its own gradient. A more general model that allows an arbitrary number of gradients was developed by von der Malsburg and Willshaw (1977). Competitive learning algorithms that develop topologically correct (neighbor-relation preserving) maps have been frequently described (Amari, 1988; Kohonen, 1989). These maps are not geometrically precise, because the area associated with an input increases monotonically with the frequency of activity of the input (Ritter & Schulten, 1986). Correlational approaches have also been proposed to develop maps. Toet, Blom, and Koenderink (1988) use response overlap to recover receptor configurations, while Linsker (1989) proposes recreating maps by maximizing information transmission.

Banks (1987, 1988) has reviewed the developmental changes in the visual system that require recalibration and proposed methods by which the adjustments might be made, including the use of scale invariance (zoom) to calibrate gain at different spatial frequencies. While most artificial visual systems are calibrated with known test images, electron beam lithography presented a case where the calibration image could not be constructed or positioned as accurately as the desired calibration (Raugh, 1985). Raugh showed that two different translations are enough to determine a calibration transformation under the assumption that it is possible to exactly determine the coordinates of corresponding points in the output images.

Why Construct a Geometrically Correct Interpolated Image?

It is often pointed out that the goal of vision science is not to generate an image in the head where there is no one to look at it, the goal is to analyze the image. Unlike the wholistic view of the Gestaltists (Köhler, 1947), modern vision theory stresses the multiplicity of computational problems that the vision system must solve (Marr, 1982) and the physiology seems to support the notion that independent processing streams solve these problems in parallel (DeYoe & Van Essen, 1988). Barlow (1979) appealed to the ability to make hyperacuity judgments when he proposed that a visual image is interpolated in the cortex. But Snyder (1982), in a paper claiming that hyperacuity "demands some form of neural interpolation," also admits, "With prior knowledge of the task, some measure of hyperacuity is theoretically possible even without interpolation." Obviously if the hyperacuity stimulus is placed in one retinal position, the system could learn the pattern without learning the receptor positions. It is the success of fine position discriminations despite their varying retinal position that suggests that translation invariant measures must be used. Model 3 does not care what kind of receptive field it is constructing; if one receptive field is fixed to be an oriented bandpass filter or spatial frequency channel (Watson & Ahumada, 1989), the model will construct a set of translation invariant filters that can represent the image as well as a single spatial image. However, the interpolation of the image is still required during the learning process to represent translations of the image at a scale finer than the cone representation, unless the motions are integral multiples of internal lattice spacings.

An early goal of this work was to provide a way for artificial vision systems to take advantage of the benefits of variable resolution and irregular spacing. Our visual system has the striking characteristic of providing what appears to be a very high-resolution view of the world despite having very few cones. This is accomplished with a variable resolution design. Yellott (1984) has argued that the increased irregularity of the extrafoveal cone array serves the purpose of reducing structured aliasing from this region but has also shown that this benefit can not be realized unless the actual positions are known (Yellott, 1987). For artificial vision systems to take advantage of variable density, irregular sampling and still use algorithms for image processing that are based on regular arrays, an interpolation system is required, and a self-calibrating one is an extra bonus. Computational models of visual system channels are a special case of artificial vision systems and are also usually implemented to process regularly sampled images. Interpolation process models allow them to include visual effects of retinal sampling in their image processing.

Other Applications

The ability to geometrically recalibrate a sensor array without known calibration images would be a valuable ability for remote systems whose optical and sensor properties might alter or degrade over time. As long as the average density of sensors remains above the Nyquist limit of the optical system, images could in principle be perfectly reconstructed despite random sensor loss. One could also imagine processes that could generate extremely high-density sensor arrays with noisy positions like that of film, for which this kind of recalibration would be more appropriate than the usual optical calibration based on a small number of polynomial coefficients. Finally, the translation-invariance calibration can be used to postprocess images from sensors that may have lost calibration during use. All that is required is that images partially overlap. Although the stress here has been on geometric calibration, the diagonal elements of the weight array alone provide a photometric calibration, which can be performed alone at great savings in computation.

Acknowledgments

I gratefully acknowledge the helpful suggestions of Misha Pavel, Jeff Mulligan, Dave Williams, Mike Landy, Lee Stone, and Kathy Turano.

References

Ahnelt, P. K., Kolb, H. & Pflug, R. (1987). Identification of a subtype of cone photoreceptor, likely to be blue sensitive, in the human retina. *Journal of Comparative Neurology, 225,* 18–34.

Ahumada, A. J., Jr. & Mulligan, J. B. (1989). Learning in interpolation networks for irregular sampling: Some convergence properties. *Applied Vision: Optical Society of America Technical Digest Series, 16,* 24–27.

Ahumada, A. J., Jr. & Mulligan, J. B. (1990). Learning receptor positions from imperfectly known motions. *Proceedings of the SPIE conference on Human vision, visual processing & digital display, 1249,* Paper 10.

Ahumada, A. J., Jr. & Pavel, M. (1989). Receptor position learning from known motions. *Optical Society of America Technical Digest Series 18,* 142 (Abs.).

Ahumada, A. J., Jr & Yellott, J. I. Jr. (1989). Reconstructing irregularly sampled images by neural networks. *Proceedings of the SPIE conference on Human vision, visual processing & digital display, 1077,* 228–235.

Amari, S. (1988). Dynamical stability of formation of cortical maps. In M. A. Arbib & S. Amari (Eds.), *Dynamic interactions in neural networks: Models and data* (pp. 15–34). New York: Springer-Verlag.

Barlow, H. B. (1979). Reconstructing the visual image in space and time. *Nature, 279,* 189–190.

Banks, M. S. (1987). Mechanisms of visual development: An example of computational models. In J. Bisanz, C. J. Brainerd & R. Kail (Eds.), *Formal models in developmental psychology: Progress in cognitive development research.* New York: Springer-Verlag.

Banks, M. S. (1988). Visual recalibration and the development of contrast and optical flow perception. In A. Yonas (Ed.), *Perceptual development in infancy: The Minnesota symposia on child psychology: Vol. 20.* Hillsdale, NJ: Erlbaum.

Bitmead, R. R. (1984). Persistence of excitation conditions and the convergence of adaptive schemes. *IEEE Transactions in Information Theory, 30,* 183–191.

Campbell, F. W. & Gubisch, R. W. (1966). Optical quality of the human eye. *Journal of Physiology, London, 186,* 558–578.

Chen, D. S. & Allebach, J. P. (1987). Analysis of error in reconstruction of two-dimensional signals from irregularly spaced samples. *IEEE Transactions in Acoustic, Speech & Signal Processing, 35,* 173–180.

Curcio, C. A., Sloan, K. R., Packer, O., Hendrickson, A. E. & Kalina, R. E. (1987). Distribution of cones in human and monkey retina: Individual variability and radial asymmetry. *Science, 236,* 579–582.

DeYoe, E. A. & Van Essen, D. C. (1988). Concurrent processing streams in monkey visual cortex. *Trends in Neuroscience, 11,* 219–226.

Geisler, W. S. (1984). Physical limits of acuity and hyperacuity. *Journal of the Optical Society of America A, 1,* 775–782.

Geisler, W. S. & Davila, K. D. (1985). Ideal discriminators in spatial vision: two-point stimuli. *Journal of the Optical Society of America A, 2,* 1483–1497.

Green, D. M. & Swets, J. A. (1966). *Signal detection theory.* New York: Wiley.

Hirsch, J. & Hylton, R. (1984). Quality of the primate photoreceptor lattice and limits of spatial vision. *Vision Research, 24,* 347–356.

Jerri, A. J. (1977). The Shannon sampling theorem—Its various extensions and applications: A tutorial review. *Proceedings of the IEEE, 65*, 1565–1597.

Köhler, W. (1947). *Gestalt psychology*. New York: Mentor.

Kohonen, T. (1989). *Self-organization and associative memory*. New York: Springer.

Linsker, R. (1989). *How to generate ordered maps by maximizing the mutual information between input and output signals* (IBM Research Report RC 14264 No. 65530). Yorktown Heights, NY.

Maloney, L. T. (1988a). Spatially irregular sampling in combination with rigid movements of the sampling array. *Investigative Ophthalmology & Visual Science, 29*, (ARVO Suppl.), 58 (Abs.).

Maloney, L. T. (1988b). Learning algorithm that calibrates a simple visual system. *Optical Society of America Technical Digest Series, 11*, 133 (Abs.).

Maloney, L. T. (1989). Calibrating a linear visual system by comparison of inputs across camera/eye movements. *Applied Vision: Optical Society of America Technical Digest Series, 16*, 28–31.

Maloney, L. T. & Ahumada, A. J., Jr. (1989) Learning by assertion: Two methods for calibrating a linear visual system. *Neural Computation, 1*, 392–401.

von der Malsburg, C. & Willshaw, D. J. (1977). How to label nerve cells so that they can interconncet in an ordered fashion. *Proceedings of the National Academy of Science, 74*, 5176–5178.

Marr, D. (1982). *Vision*. San Francisco: Freeman.

Oakley, J. P. & Cunningham, M. J. (1990). A function space model for digital image sampling and its application in image reconstruction. *Computer Vision, Graphics, and Image Processing, 49*, 171–197.

Østerberg, G. (1935). Topology of the layer of rods and cones in the human retina. *Acta Ophthalmologica (Suppl.), 6*, 1–103.

Raugh, M. R. (1985). Absolute two-dimensional sub-micron metrology for electron beam lithography: A calibration theory with applications. *Precision Engineering*, 3–13.

Ritter, H. & Schulten, K. (1986). On the stationary state of Kohonen's self-organizing sensory mapping. *Biological Cybernetics, 54*, 99–106.

Snyder, A. W. (1982). Hyperacuity and interpolation by the visual pathways. *Vision Research, 22*, 1219–1220.

Sperry, R. W. (1956). The eye and the brain. *Scientific American, 194*, 48–52.

Stone, G. O. (1986). An analysis of the delta rule and the learning of statistical association. In D. E. Rumelhart & J. L. McClelland (Eds.), *Parallel distributed processing:* Vol. I. (pp. 444–459). Cambridge, MA: The MIT Press.

Toet, A., Blom, J. & Koenderink, J. J. (1988). The construction of a simultaneous functional order in nervous systems. IV. The influence of physical constraints on the resulting functional order. *Biological Cybernetics, 57*, 275–286.

Watson, A. B. & Ahumada, A. J., Jr. (1989). A hexagonal orthogonal-oriented pyramid as a model of image representation in visual cortex. *IEEE Transactions in Biomedical Engineering, 36*, 97–106.

Widrow, B. & Hoff, M. E. (1960). Adaptive switching circuits. *Institute of Radio Engineers WESCON Record*, Part 4, 96–104.

Yellott, J. I. Jr. (1984). Image sampling properties of photoreceptors: A reply to Miller and Bernard. *Vision Research, 24*, 281–282.

Yellott, J. I. Jr. (1987). Consequences of spatially irregular sampling for reconstruction of photon noisy images. *Investigative Ophthalmology & Visual Science, 28*, (ARVO Suppl.), 137 (Abs.).

3

A Model of Aliasing in Extrafoveal Human Vision

Carlo L. M. Tiana,
David R. Williams,
Nancy J. Coletta,
and P. William Haake

When interference fringes are used to avoid blurring by the optics of the eye, spatial aliasing by the cone mosaic can be observed with the fovea (Byram, 1944; Campbell & Green, 1965; Williams, 1985b, 1986, 1988). In the range of spatial frequencies from roughly 60 to 150 cycles/degree, most observers see a distorted pattern of wavy lines or "zebra stripes" that corresponds to a moiré pattern formed between the interference fringe and the cone mosaic. Williams (1985a, 1988) has described a model of foveal cone sampling that accurately predicts the effect of spatial frequency and orientation of the interference fringe on these zebra stripes, allowing the spacing and packing arrangement of foveal cones to be estimated in the living eye.

Aliasing phenomena have also been reported in the extrafoveal retina (Coletta & Williams, 1987; Smith & Cass, 1987a,b; Thibos, Cheney & Walsh, 1987; Thibos, Walsh & Cheney, 1987; Williams & Coletta, 1987), in which case interference fringes take on the appearance of two-dimensional spatial noise. The percept of two-dimensional noise is thought to arise from undersampling by a disordered array of sampling elements corresponding to cones at moderate retinal eccentricities, with a possible contribution from later sampling stages in the far periphery. Though the percept of noise associated with these high-frequency stimuli is consistent with an explanation in terms of disordered sampling by the visual system, it is not particularly compelling evidence by itself. One of the motivations of this chapter is to evaluate the psychophysical evidence on this noisy percept in order to provide a strong quantitative link to the sampling properties of the visual system, so that a theory of the appearance of fine interference fringes can be constructed from the morphology of the retina. This chapter describes a model of the early stages of the human visual system that accurately simulates two peculiar aspects of the appearance of this spatial noise, which we will refer to as the *motion reversal* and the *orientation reversal* phenomena, to be described shortly. The model incorporates the sampling properties of the cone mosaic and implicates aliasing by the mosaic as the cause of these psychophysical phenomena, at least for retinal eccentricities within about 20° of the fovea.

Perhaps the most compelling early evidence for spatial aliasing in vision comes from observations of insects viewing moving gratings. In this situation, flies typically exhibit an optomotor response: They rotate their bodies in order to stabilize the grating drifting with respect to the arrays of photoreceptors that constitute their compound eyes. A fly is attached to a torque meter centered on the axis of a rotating cylinder, on the inside of which are painted vertical black and white stripes. At low spatial frequencies, the fly attempts to rotate its body in the direction of the bars. When the spatial frequency of the bars is higher, however, the fly rotates in the direction opposite to that of the cylinder (von Gavel, 1939; Goetz, 1965). This is what one would expect from spatial aliasing because the (lower frequency) moiré pattern formed between the grating and the photoreceptor array moves in the opposite direction from that of the grating.

Coletta, Williams, and Tiana (1990) have demonstrated a similar motion reversal phenomenon in human vision. Their psychophysical results provide the primary data for the development of the model described in this chapter, so we briefly review these results below. Interference fringes of various spatial frequencies were drifted at a fixed temporal frequency in either a leftward or rightward direction, randomly determined, during each stimulus presentation. The observer's task was to indicate the direction of motion of the stimulus on each trial, without feedback. The solid line in figure 3.1 shows a psychometric function obtained from a single observer at a single retinal eccentricity (3.8° in the horizontal meridian). Chance performance is 50 percent correct. Observers could correctly identify the direction of fringe motion as long as the spatial frequency remained below a certain critical frequency, which we will refer to as the *first motion null*. At this frequency, the direction of motion was ambiguous. At higher frequencies the stimulus resembled two-dimensional spatial noise with a perceived direction of motion in the direction *opposite* to that of the stimulus. In this range of frequencies, percent correct on the motion discrimination task fell reliably below chance performance. At a still higher frequency, the direction of motion is ambiguous again and performance rises to the chance

level a second time. We will refer to this spatial frequency as the *second motion null*. At even higher frequencies, there is a tendency to report the correct direction of motion (performance rises slightly above chance). Finally, at the very highest frequencies, performance goes to chance and the stimulus presentation itself goes undetected.

Note that the first motion null (indicated in figure 3.1 as the first spatial frequency at which the data cross chance performance) corresponds roughly to the Nyquist frequency of the human cone mosaic calculated from the data of Curcio, Sloan, Pacter, Hendrickson and Kalina (1987) and the second motion null corresponds roughly to the cone sampling frequency (or twice the Nyquist frequency). Figure 3.2 shows that this correspondence is preserved over a large range of Nyquist frequencies, corresponding to retinal eccentricities from 0° to 30°. The left panel shows the first motion nulls for five observers collected at a number of retinal eccentricities plotted as a function of anatomical Nyquist frequency; the right panel shows the corresponding data for the second motion null. The line at 45° indicates perfect agreement between the motion null and the Nyquist frequency. The first motion nulls fall below the line at large retinal eccentricities, where the Nyquist frequency is low, a point we will return to later. The second motion null, on the other hand, agrees reasonably well with the sampling frequency over the entire range, though there may be a slight tendency to lower values at the very lowest Nyquist frequencies (largest eccentricities). The model developed in this paper will establish a plausible basis for this agreement.

Coletta and Williams (1987) described a second phenomenon involving the appearance of high-frequency interference fringes viewed extrafoveally. They showed that there is a range of spatial frequencies, roughly centered on the cone sampling frequency, for which the noise appears anisotropic. Specifically, it has a predominant orientation that is perpendicular to the true orientation of the interference fringe. The dotted line in figure 3.1 shows a psychometric function for an orientation discrimination task, which reveals the orientation reversal phenomenon. The observer was shown either a vertical or a horizontal stationary interference fringe on each trial and was asked to identify its orientation. There is a range of spatial frequencies in which observers reliably report the *wrong* orientation for the stimulus presented. Note that the minimum of this psychometric function lies near the cone

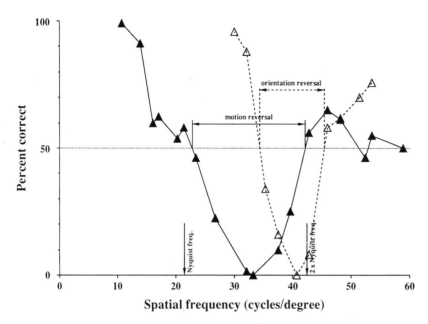

Fig. 3.1
Psychometric functions for orientation discrimination (*open symbols*) and direction of motion discrimination (*filled symbols*). The anatomical values for the Nyquist frequency and twice the Nyquist frequency from Curcio et al. (1987) are marked by the vertical arrows on the x-axis. The orientation curve represents the average for vertical and horizontal grating presentations at 3.8° eccentricity in the nasal retina. The orientation data are from Coletta and Williams (1987) and the motion data are from Coletta, Williams and Tiana (1990).

sampling frequency. Coletta and Williams showed that this correspondence held across the central retina and attributed this orientation reversal to aliasing by the cone mosaic. They simulated the phenomenon with an optical model. In this chapter, we simulate it with a computational model as a test of the theory of fringe appearance described here. That is, if the theory is correct, a single set of parameters for the model should be able to generate both the motion reversal and the orientation reversal effects with the proper quantitative relationship to each other and to the known sampling properties of the retina.

Figure 3.1 and 3.2 contain the empirical results that our model will describe and explain. One goal is to simulate these results with a visual system model incorporating a small number of stages, where each stage is plausible and is defined as much as possible by parameters taken from independent anatomical and psychophysical experiments. A second goal is to determine to what extent these perceptual phenomena reflect the effect of sampling alone. Specifically, we ask how spatial filtering in the visual

system either prior to or following the sampling operation might influence the psychophysical effects, to determine whether they can be expected to provide reliable measures of the spacing between sampling elements.

One-dimensional Model of the Motion Reversal Effect

Figure 3.3 illustrates a simple one-dimensional model of sampling that provides an intuitive justification for looking for the source of the motion reversal phenomenon in a sampling stage of the system. In this figure a regular array of photoreceptors of spacing s is depicted sampling a sinusoidal grating drifting rightward (as can be seen by following one of its peaks through the three different time "frames"). A lower frequency alias of this grating is shown as the dashed line in the figure. Given the information available at the sample points, this alias is one of many alternative interpretations of the actual stimulus. Note that the alias moves in the opposite direction to that of the actual stimulus. Thus spatial aliasing can produce motion reversals as can temporal aliasing, which is perhaps more familiar. For example, temporal aliasing is responsible for the familiar reversal in the rotation of wagon wheels in films due to the inadequate frame rate in the motion picture camera.

This simple model, while intuitively appealing, suffers from a number of shortcomings that led us to the development of the more elaborate model described in the

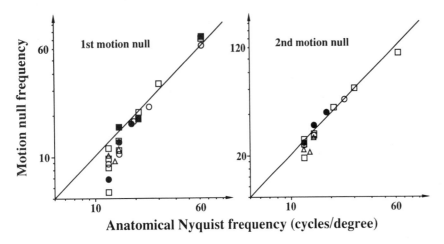

Fig. 3.2

Left, Spatial frequencies corresponding to the first motion null for five observes as a function of anatomical Nyquist frequency. Motion nulls were estimated from psychometric functions like those shown in figure 3.1. *Right,* Spatial frequencies corresponding to the second motion null versus anatomical Nyquist frequency. Note the difference in the ordinates of the two panels, indicating the two-fold difference between first and second motion nulls. Estimates of the anatomical Nyquist frequency in the human are from Curcio et al. (1987). (Reprinted with permission from *Vision Research,* Coletta, N. J., Williams, D. R., and Tiana, C. L. M., Consequences of spatial sampling for human motion perception. Copyright 1990, Pergamon Press.)

next section. These shortcomings include:

• The simple model above has a one-dimensional sampling array rather than a two-dimensional array like the human retina.

• The simple model employs a regular sampling array rather than the disordered one like the actual cone mosaic.

• The simple model does not address the impact of spatial filtering prior to the sampling operation, such as would result from the finite aperture of cones.

• The model above can indicate what stimuli imaged on a sampling array will be confused by the visual system, but it does not offer a mechanism by which the visual system adopts one particular interpretation or another. For example, there is nothing in the model to determine which of the two interpretations illustrated in figure 3.3 will actually be perceived. That is, the simple model is a theory of the discrimination of spatiotemporal stimuli, but it is not a theory of their appearance. This is quite analogous to the fact that trichromacy (which refers to sampling along the dimension of wavelength) places con-

straints on the range of spectral distributions that can be discriminated by the eye, but it does not tell us how they will appear. A proper theory of color appearance requires a postreceptoral stage that specifies how cone signals are combined and then related to appearance. The model described below incorporates mechanisms following the sampling operation to meet this need.

The Model

Overview

Figure 3.4 shows a diagram of the proposed model, indicating cascaded stages in visual processing that would be relevant for the psychophysical tasks of orientation and motion discrimination. The model was implemented in the spatiotemporal frequency domain for computational efficiency and because intuitions about the effects of sampling are more easily grasped in frequency terms rather than in space-time. The model is initially described primarily in the context of the motion reversal phenomenon, and its application to the orientation reversal effect is addressed later.

The input to the model was restricted to analytic descriptions of sinusoidal gratings that had the same characteristics as those used in the psychophysical experiments reviewed earlier. The main independent variable in both the simulation and the psychophysical experiments was spatial frequency. Grating contrast was always unity, and because the psychophysical experiments were performed with interference fringes that avoid diffraction and aberrations by the dioptrics of the eye (Campbell &

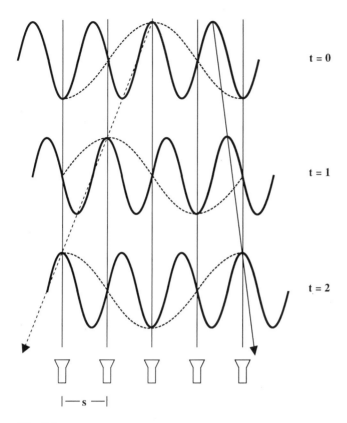

Fig. 3.3
A one-dimensional model of sampling that illustrates the origin of the motion reversal phenomenon. Photoreceptors (*bottom*) of constant spacing s sample a sinusoidal grating (*solid line*) drifting past them. The grating has a spatial frequency higher than the Nyquist frequency of the sampling array, so that the dashed grating is a lower frequency alias of the solid grating consistent with the sampling information. Thus, whereas the solid grating is drifting rightward (as shown by the arrow connecting its rightmost peak through the different points in time), the lower frequency alias is seen to drift leftward (*dashed arrow*).

Green, 1965; Saleh, 1982), the optical quality of the eye is not included as a stage in the model.

First, we provide a brief overview of the model with detailed descriptions of each stage to follow. The model has three stages, the first of which involves the optical properties of the cone mosaic. The model incorporates two effects of the cone mosaic: (1) spatial filtering that results from the finite apertures of individual cone photoreceptors, and (2) the spatial sampling properties that depend on the locations of receptors in the mosaic. The effect of the cone aperture can be computed by the convolution of the input stimulus with the cone aperture function. In the spatiotemporal frequency domain imple-

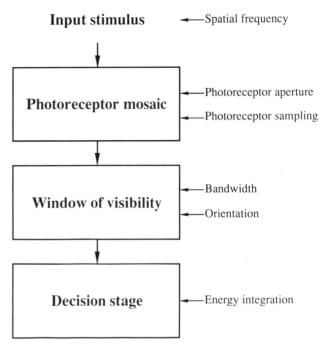

Fig. 3.4
Block diagram of the model. To the right of each box we have shown the main parameters.

mented in the model, the effect of the aperture is computed by multiplying the Fourier spectrum of the input stimulus, $S(f_x, f_y, f_t)$ by the Fourier transform of the cone aperture, $A(f_x, f_y)$. The effects of spatial sampling are described by the product of the input stimulus, filtered by the cone aperture, and the array of cone locations, whose Fourier transform is $M(f_x, f_y)$. In the spatiotemporal frequency domain, this multiplication corresponds to a convolution. Therefore, the spectrum of the output of the photoreceptor mosaic is:

$$O'(f_x, f_y, f_t) = \{[S(f_x, f_y, f_t) \times A(f_x, f_y)] \otimes M(f_x, f_y)\}, \quad (1)$$

where $\otimes$ denotes convolution.

The sampling operation produces aliases of the input stimulus with a variety of different frequency components. The second stage of the model is a spatial filter, $W(f_x, f_y)$, or window of visibility that represents postreceptoral information loss in the visual system. It specifies which frequency components are available to the decision stage, the final stage in the model. Thus, the output of the second stage of the model is:

$$O''(f_x, f_y, f_t) = O'(f_x, f_y, f_t) \times W(f_x, f_y). \quad (2)$$

The decision stage uses the information available from the postreceptoral filter to compute whether the stimulus moved to the left or right in the case of the motion discrimination task, or whether the orientation was horizontal or vertical in the case of the orientation discrimination task. The model does not incorporate an *ideal* decision rule, that is, the model is not an ideal observer (e.g., Geisler, 1989). Rather, the model has been tailored to mimic the performance of real human observers.

Initially, we set the parameters of the model with anatomical and psychophysical data obtained at an eccentricity of $3.8°$ in the nasal retina, since the most extensive independent evidence about the values of these parameters was available there. Then we investigated the effects of each stage by varying each of their defining parameters over a wide range. This allowed us to generalize the performance of the model to see how it would perform with parameter values from other retinal eccentricities.

We next examine each stage of the model in detail.

The Input Stimulus

As we mentioned above, the stimuli we used were sinusoidal luminance gratings. For the motion discrimination simulations, we used analytic descriptions of the stimuli employed in the psychophysical experiments: unity contrast vertical gratings of variable spatial frequency and drifting either leftward or rightward at 10 Hz (the use of a constant 10 Hz temporal modulation means that the grating velocity is inversely proportional to its spatial frequency). For the orientation discrimination simulations, we used analytic descriptions of vertical and horizontal gratings. The general form for the input to the model is:

$$s(x, y, t) = L_0\{1 + \cos[2\pi(f_{0x}x + f_{0y}y - f_{0t}t)]\}, \quad (3)$$

where L_0 is the mean luminance of the stimulus, f_{0x} and f_{0y} are the spatial frequency components along the x- and y-axes, and f_{0t} is the temporal frequency.

The Fourier transform of this expression is given by:

$$S(f_x, f_y, f_t) = \begin{cases} L_0\{\delta(f_x, f_y, f_t) + \\ \frac{1}{2}\delta(f_x - f_{0x}, f_y - f_{0y}, f_t - f_{0t}) + \\ \frac{1}{2}\delta(f_x + f_{0x}, f_y + f_{0y}, f_t + f_{0t})\} \end{cases} \quad (4)$$

which consists of a δ function at the origin, with two flanking δ functions. Figure 3.5 illustrates the space in which we choose to represent our stimuli. The vertical axes (labeled f_t) in each panel represent temporal frequen-

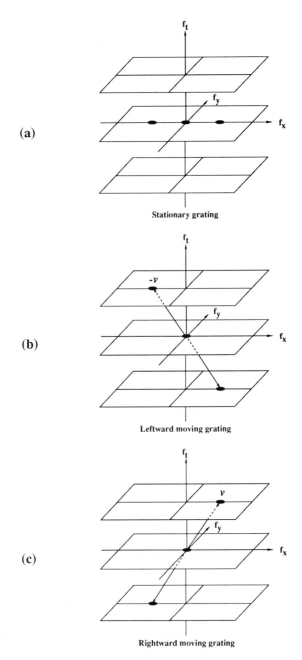

(a)

Stationary grating

(b)

Leftward moving grating

(c)

Rightward moving grating

Fig. 3.5
The spatiotemporal frequency domain showing the Fourier spectra of stationary and drifting gratings. f_x and f_y are the spatial frequency coordinates, f_t is the temporal frequency coordinate. The solid discs represent δ functions. (A) The transform of a vertical stationary grating lies on the plane at the origin of the temporal frequency axis, oriented along the f_x-axis. (B) The case of a leftward moving grating. Its velocity is given by the ratio of its temporal frequency and its spatial frequency. In this case the velocity is oriented towards the negative f_x-axis and is denoted as $-v$. (C) The case of a rightward moving grating. In this case the velocity is oriented toward the positive f_x-axis and is denoted as v.

cy. The axes labeled f_x and f_y define the spatial frequency plane at a temporal frequency of 0. Part A shows the case for a stationary vertical grating: its transform (the three δ functions represented by black ovals in the diagram) lies along the f_x-axis, wholly in the plane at 0 temporal frequency. The transform of a horizontal grating (not shown) would lie entirely along the f_y-axis. Part B shows the transform of a vertical grating drifting *leftward*. It contributes a δ function at the origin of the spatiotemporal frequency space (the first term in equation 4), a δ function in the plane at temporal frequency f_{0t} (the second term in equation 4), and one at $-f_{0t}$ (the third term in equation 4). We refer to these three δ functions respectively as residing in the 0 Hz, 10 Hz, and -10 Hz spatial frequency planes, respectively. In this space, the slope of the vectors joining the origin and the δ functions in the 10 Hz spatial frequency plane represent the speed of the grating. Part C shows the transform of a grating drifting *rightward* (with velocity v).

The Photoreceptor Mosaic

The two optical properties of the cone mosaic that we consider are the effect of the cone aperture and the effect of cone locations. These are discussed in turn below.

Spatial Filtering by the Cone Aperture

The finite aperture of the elements of a sampling array has the effect of demodulating the image. The precise shape of the cone aperture is not known, nor is enough known about the waveguide properties of receptors to calculate the aperture function from anatomical estimates of cone morphology. However, MacLeod, Williams and Makous (in press) have developed a psychophysical technique that has provided estimates of the size of the aperture at various retinal eccentricities. We assume here for convenience that the aperture function $a(x, y)$ is Gaussian, where the standard deviation, σ_a is a measure of aperture size:

$$a(x, y) = e^{-(x^2 + y^2)/2\sigma_a^2} \tag{5}$$

For example, figure 3.6 shows adjacent cones taken from the 3.8° mosaic, the inner segments of which are delimited by circles. The Gaussian intensity distribution within each cone corresponds to the aperture estimate of MacLeod et al. (1985). At 3.8° eccentricity, $\sigma_a = 17.6$ sec arc.

The Fourier transform of the Gaussian aperture func-

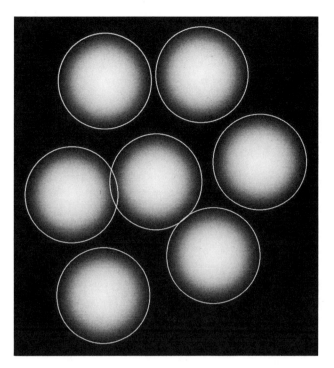

Fig. 3.6
The cone aperture. A cluster of cones from the primate cone mosaic at 3.8° eccentricity where the anatomical inner segments are represented by circles. The cone aperture has an isotropic Gaussian sensitivity profile with a standard deviation taken from the psychophysical data of MacLeod, Williams, and Makous (in press). The overlap between some of the cones is not meant to suggest that cones do overlap in any physical way, but rather reflects the fact that the measures for cone size are an average over a number of cones at a given eccentricity. The inner segment diameter at this eccentricity in the human is about 6.5 μm or 81 sec arc. The standard deviation of the Gaussian aperture in the spatial domain is $\sigma_a = 17.6$ sec arc, which is equivalent to a standard deviation in the Fourier domain of 32.5 cycles/degree.

tion specifies the spatial filtering properties of each cone. This modulation transfer function, $A(f_x, f_y)$, is also Gaussian:

$$A(f_x, f_y) = e^{-2\pi^2\sigma_a^2(f_x^2 + f_y^2)}. \tag{6}$$

In this domain, the bandwidth of the cone aperture (defined as the standard deviation of the Gaussian modeling it) is 32.5 cycles/degree.

Cone Locations in the Mosaic

We implemented two different types of photoreceptor mosaic in the model. The first was a regular, triangular packed mosaic, described by (e.g., Williams, 1988):

$$m_{reg}(x, y) = \frac{r^2}{\sqrt{3}} \sum_{m=-\infty}^{\infty} \sum_{n=-\infty}^{\infty}$$
$$\times \delta\left[x - r(m+n), y - \frac{r}{\sqrt{3}}(m-n)\right], \quad (7)$$

where r is the spacing between sensors along a row. This spacing is $\sqrt{3}/2$ times the center-to-center spacing. Its Fourier transform is:

$$M_{reg}(f_x, f_y) = \sum_{m=-\infty}^{\infty} \sum_{n=-\infty}^{\infty}$$
$$\times \delta\left[f_x - \frac{(m+n)}{2r}, f_y - \frac{\sqrt{3}(m-n)}{2r}\right] \quad (8)$$

The Nyquist frequency of this array is defined as the inverse of twice the row spacing: $f_{N_{reg}} = 1/2r$. Though this crystalline mosaic is not biologically plausible, it approaches the more regular packing of cones found in the fovea (Williams, 1988). This mosaic is useful in the present model to contrast with the disordered mosaics described below.

The disordered mosaics were taken from photographs of actual cone distributions in retinal whole mounts (from a *Macaca mulatta*) provided by Perry (see Perry & Cowey, 1985). These photographs were scanned into our computer with an image digitizer. The locations of the cone centers were then picked out by hand using a pointing device and stored as a set of coordinates. Mosaics were collected from four different eccentricities in the nasal retina (fovea, 3.8°, 10°, and 30°). Figure 3.7 shows subsets of the mosaics at each of these eccentricities, rescaled to display a constant number of cones in each image. The reason for this rescaling was to evaluate the impact of disorder in the packing arrangement with retinal eccentricity uncontaminated by changes in cone density. We assume that the disorder that characterizes the monkey cone mosaic is comparable to that in man. Estimates of cone spacing at various eccentricities were taken from human anatomical data (Østerberg, 1935; Curcio et al., 1987).

The numerical Fourier transforms of the mosaics in figure 3.7 are shown in figure 3.8. Consider first the transforms of the three extrafoveal mosaics, which are similar in appearance. This transform was first described by Yellott (1982, 1983). It consists of a noisy annulus of energy surrounding a central peak of energy, with rela-

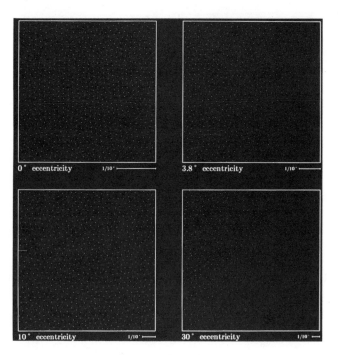

Fig. 3.7
Photoreceptor mosaics at various eccentricities across the retina. All photoreceptor locations were digitized from photomicrographs of retinal whole mounts, as described in the text, but only a region from the whole mosaic is shown here: All regions have the same number of cones, to allow a comparison of irregularity among the different eccentricities.

tively little energy in between. Outside of this ring lies energy with a lower average magnitude than that of the ring, and extending out to the highest spatial frequencies. In some cases, a second and even a third ring can be discerned in the midst of this energy, concentric with the first.

The foveal transform preserves some of the triangular structure present in the transform of a crystalline array with triangular packing. This is consistent with the results of Hirsch and Miller (1987), who showed an abrupt increase in regularity toward the foveal center. As can be seen in figure 3.8, extrafoveal cone mosaics at all eccentricities have similar sampling characteristics once they are appropriately scaled. This will allow us to consider only one mosaic in what follows and scale its average spacing appropriately for various eccentricities. We use the packing arrangement of the mosaic at 3.8° eccentricity because that is the eccentricity at which most of the psychophysical data were collected. Model results at other extrafoveal eccentricities did not differ in any important

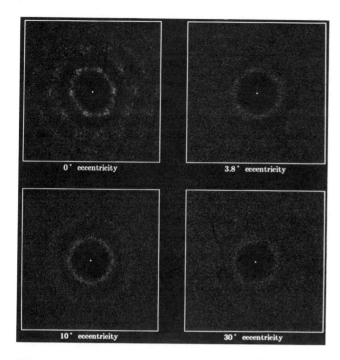

Fig. 3.8
The numerical Fourier transforms of the photoreceptor mosaics shown in figure 3.7. Lightness is proportional to the intensity in the transform. Each transform is centered on the origin of the spatial frequency plane. Only spatial frequencies·below 6 f_N in the f_x (horizontal) and f_y (vertical) directions are shown.

manner once the change in absolute cone spacing was accounted for.

Figure 3.9 allows us to compare the features of these transforms of actual mosaics with that of a crystalline triangular mosaic of the same cone density. We have plotted the radial energy density distribution for the transforms shown in the previous figures. This distribution consists of the average energy per unit radial spatial frequency interval, plotted against spatial frequency.[1] Note that the spatial frequency corresponding to the radius of the ring, defined by the peak in the radial energy distribution, is not affected by the amount of disorder in the mosaic and corresponds closely in every case to the fundamental frequency of the crystalline array (shown as the

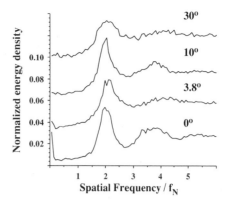

Fig. 3.9
Superimposed radial energy density plots for all mosaic transforms shown in figure 3.8. The vertical axis applies to the 0° transform, whereas all other eccentricities have been shifted vertically upwards by 0.03 units each, for clarity. The peak of each function occurs at a spatial frequency corresponding to the radius of the annulus of noise shown in figure 3.8. The point corresponding to $f/f_N = 0$ has been omitted for each transform. The value at this point is 1 in each case. The dashed vertical lines shown represent the radial energy density plot for the transform of a crystalline triangular mosaic.

dashed line at a value of 2 on the normalized spatial frequency axis). Consequently, we define the sampling frequency of these disordered lattices as the radius of the ring, and we define the Nyquist frequency f_N as half the radius of the ring.

Effects of Cone Sampling of Gratings

Before considering later stages in the model, it will be useful to illustrate how sampling affects the Fourier spectrum of drifting gratings. Since the sampling operation in space can be represented by the product of the array of sampling elements and the grating intensity distribution (recalling that these gratings have already been demodulated by the cone aperture), in Fourier space this translates to a *convolution* of the transforms of the mosaic and of the grating. The mosaic's transform is replicated at each δ function location, appropriately weighted (Yellott, 1982, 1983).

---

1. It is obtained by integrating energy at a given distance from the origin of the spatial frequency plane, over an annulus centered on the origin and of preset width Δ and normalizing by the annulus' area, thus:

$$D(r) = \frac{\sum_r M(f_x, f_y)}{2\pi r\Delta + \pi\Delta^2} \qquad (9)$$

where $\forall r \in [0, 6f_N]$, $r \leqslant \sqrt{f_x^2 + f_y^2} < r + \Delta$. $M(f_x, f_y)$ is the Fourier transform of a photoreceptor mosaic. The numerator is the integral (on a discrete space) of the transform over an annulus of spatial frequencies contained in the interval $[r, r + \Delta]$. The denominator is the area of this annulus. The distribution is calculated for all frequencies between 0 and 6 times the Nyquist frequency and is plotted in figure 3.9 for $\Delta = 1$ pixel.

In figure 3.10 we show the spatiotemporal representation of the spectrum of a sampled grating *drifting rightward* at 10 Hz. The rightmost replica in the spectrum of the stationary sampled grating is now displaced out of the 0 Hz spatial frequency plane into a positive spatial frequency plane at 10 Hz, while the leftmost replica is displaced to the negative spatial frequency plane at −10 Hz. The vectors drawn in figure 3.10 from the origin of the space show that the spectrum of the sampled stimulus contains components of different spatial frequency, orientation, and velocity, all temporally modulated at 10 Hz. These additional components that result from disordered sampling do not drift in a coherent fashion. Some of this energy even moves in the direction *opposite* to that of the stimulus, as represented by the leftmost vector in the diagram. This raises the question of how the postreceptoral visual system will interpret this rather complex distribution of spatiotemporal frequency components and reach a decision about the predominant direction of motion. The remaining two stages in the model propose one algorithm that the visual system could use.

Window of visibility

The second stage in our model, following the sampling operation, is a postreceptoral spatial filter, or "window of visibility." This stage is required because the postreceptoral visual system must have some limitation on its spatial frequency bandwidth. This concept, introduced by Pearson (1975), has been successfully applied before to the study of apparent motion (Watson, Ahumada & Farrell, 1986) as well as photoreceptor sampling (Coletta & Williams, 1987; Williams 1988; Williams & Coletta, 1987; Williams, Collier & Thompson, 1983). The postreceptoral filter behaves like a window in the postreceptoral frequency domain that is transparent for some spatial frequency components in the spectrum of the sampled grating, but not others.

We adopt a similar approach, but to more easily explain it we first offer a simplification of the complex picture presented in figure 3.10. Note that all information about the speed, direction, and spatial frequency of energy components produced by the sampled stimulus can be gleaned from an examination of the 10 Hz spatial frequency plane alone. Changing the spatial frequency of the input stimulus produces symmetric changes in the 10 Hz and −10 Hz spatial frequency planes and no change in the 0 Hz spatial frequency plane, so we can investigate the effect of this key parameter by looking at only one plane. Fixing the temporal frequency of the stimulus allows us to treat our window of visibility as being dependent on spatial frequency only.

We now explore the effect of grating spatial frequency on the spatial frequency components that pass through a very simple window of visibility, as illustrated in figure 3.11. This exercise provides critical insight into our explanation for the origin of the motion reversal and orientation reversal phenomena and shows how the window of visibility provides a theory of appearance of these grating stimuli. The figure shows five spatial frequency planes (each at 10 Hz), where each plane contains the spectrum of a sampled rightward moving grating of a different spatial frequency. (Recall that this spectrum consists of the replica of the transform of the mosaic centered on a δ function corresponding to the input stimulus). The f_t-axis passes through the center of each plane perpendicular to

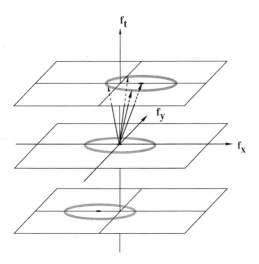

Fig. 3.10
The spatiotemporal Fourier transform of a sampled moving grating. As depicted, the grating is drifting rightward parallel to the x-axis, its spatial frequency given by the distance of the positive temporal frequency δ function to the temporal frequency axis, on the f_x-axis. Its temporal frequency is given by the height of the positive temporal frequency plane. The circles represent the replicas of the transform of the cone mosaic. Nonrigidity in the sampled stimulus motion is demonstrated by the vectors pointing to energy that is associated with motion in directions and speeds different from that of the grating. The visual system adopts the lower spatial frequency, nonrigid interpretation of the motion of the stimulus, even though there exists a rigid motion interpretation possible (the veridical one).

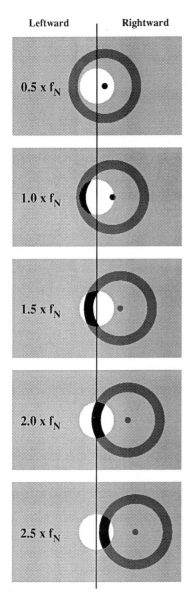

Leftward | **Rightward**

$0.5 \times f_N$

$1.0 \times f_N$

$1.5 \times f_N$

$2.0 \times f_N$

$2.5 \times f_N$

Fig. 3.11
Effect of spatial frequency on the energy passed by the postreceptoral spatial filter.

those falling to the right correspond to rightward motion. We do not define any temporal frequency bandwidth for the window of visibility because all the temporal frequency components are confined to 10 Hz, which is in the range of temporal frequencies to which the visual system is most sensitive.

Recall that the psychophysical results (see figure 3.1) that this model should simulate show that observers can correctly discriminate the direction of motion up to roughly the Nyquist frequency, perceive a reversed direction between f_N and twice f_N, and again perceive the correct direction just above twice f_N. Consider the first panel, in which the spatial frequency of the stimulus is one-half f_N. Only the grating delta function passes through the window and the model faithfully reproduces the grating moving in the correct direction, without aliasing distortion. In the second panel, however, when the stimulus spatial frequency is the same as the mosaic's f_N, there is some rightward energy associated with the original stimulus but also leftward energy associated with the mosaic replica, namely, aliasing. So the overall direction of motion is ambiguous in this case, leading to the first "motion null." Note, however, that the leftward energy is dispersed in spatial frequency and orientation, which is consistent with the noisy percepts that are first described near this spatial frequency.

For frequencies between f_N and twice f_N (such as illustrated in the third panel) the leftward energy predominates, despite the fact that the grating is actually moving rightward. This is the case of "motion reversal." The fourth panel presents the case of the mosaic sampling a grating of frequency twice f_N. Near this spatial frequency the ring of energy straddles the center of the window, making roughly equal contributions to the leftward and rightward motion. This corresponds to the model's explanation for the second motion null observed psychophysically. Finally, consider the case (bottom panel) where the spatial frequency of the stimulus rises beyond twice the array's f_N. Now the rightward energy should exceed the leftward energy again, and the stimulus is again perceived to be moving in the correct direction. This perception of movement in the correct direction will persist until either the annulus is completely outside the window, or the grating is completely demodulated by the cone aperture.

This analysis can also explain the orientation reversal phenomenon (Coletta & Williams, 1987) discussed in the introduction to this chapter. Consider the panel showing

the page. The input spatial frequency increases from top to bottom in the five panels. The window we have chosen is simply a cylinder function in the plane with a radius corresponding to the Nyquist frequency, f_N. In the figure, this window is illustrated as a light hole in an otherwise translucent gray screen. This window is centered on zero spatial frequency. Frequency components falling to the left of the vertical line down the center of the figure (the f_y-axis) are drifting in a generally leftward direction, while

a grating frequency of twice the Nyquist frequency. The energy passed through the window is dispersed vertically, as is characteristic of *horizontal* stimuli, even though the original stimulus was vertical. The model incorporating this simple window of visibility captures the essential qualitative features of the psychophysical results on motion and orientation discrimination.

To compute the spatial frequencies that produce both the motion nulls and the orientation reversal with a single model, we chose a somewhat different window of visibility. We expect the filter to have a high-frequency rolloff, from fundamental physical considerations: The information channels in the system must have finite bandwidth. Indeed, the contrast sensitivity function demonstrates a high-frequency rolloff even when blurring by the optics of the eye is avoided by interferometry (Campbell & Green, 1965; Williams, 1985b). This spatial bandwidth limitation would be the kind imposed by the centers of ganglion cell or lateral geniculate nucleus receptive fields (Derrington & Lennie, 1984), and it is tempting to identify the window with these physiological sites. However, the locus of the window is irrelevant to the functioning of the model. We assumed that the window of visibility had the same shape as the neural contrast sensitivity function. Williams and Coletta (1987, figure 1) measured contrast sensitivity for two observers with interference fringe stimuli at 3.8° in the nasal retina. Both sets of data were well fit by a Gaussian with a standard deviation $\sigma_{c.s.f.} = 9.5$ cycles/degree. This standard deviation includes the effect of the cone aperture, which has already been accounted for in the mosaic stage of the model, so we made a small correction in the window bandwidth to take this into account. The window standard deviation then became 10 cycles/degree.

The Decision Stage

The final stage in the model is the decision stage, the function of which is to use that information passed by the window of visibility to determine motion direction or orientation of the grating. We describe below two different decision stages, one tailored for the motion discrimination experiment and one for the orientation discrimination experiment. All the versions of these stages that we have tried are essentially *opponent* in nature (e.g., Adelson & Bergen, 1985) in that they compare energy in different regions of the spatial frequency plane.

Motion discrimination schemes

A variety of strategies could be employed to weight the energy on either side of the origin of the frequency plane in the stimulus transform. We tried a technique that allowed us to vary the spatial frequency resolution of the filter by averaging the spatiotemporal energy distribution in the stimulus over patches of variable size.

Consider first two decision rules that are extreme cases on a continuum of possible rules. Because we have no psychophysical data describing the decision rule actually employed in the visual system, we chose these two extremes to cover the widest range of possibilities. In the case that we shall refer to as *full integration,* all energy passing through the right-hand half of the window of visibility (associated, as we have seen, with rightward moving components of the stimulus) is integrated, then all energy passing through the left-hand half of the window of visibility (associated with leftward moving components of the stimulus) is integrated, and the difference between these energies is computed. This difference, as a function of the stimulus spatial frequency, is the output of the opponent energy model; we call it an energy function (E.F.). Specifically:

$$E.F._{\cdot in}(f_{0x}, f_t) = \left\{ \int_0^\infty df_x \int_{-\infty}^\infty df_y \| O''(f_x - f_{0x}, f_y, f_t) \| \right\}$$
$$- \left\{ \int_{-\infty}^0 df_x \int_{-\infty}^\infty df_y \| O''(f_x - f_{0x}, f_y, f_t) \| \right\} \quad (10)$$

where the symbol $\|(expr)\|$ denotes complex magnitude.

At the other extreme is the case of *peak detection*: the maximum of the energy distribution passing through the right-hand side of the window is compared in opponent fashion to the *maximum* passing through the left-hand side. Since the energy distribution is a discrete two-dimensional pixel map, the maximum of the energy distribution is simply the maximum pixel value; each pixel represents a small two-dimensional bin of size determined by the resolution of our image in Fourier space.

Between these two approaches lies a generalized integration strategy which we call the *patch integration scheme*: The spatial frequency plane can be thought of as tiled by a lattice (in our case, square) of two-dimensional frequency patches. The energy in each of the patches is weighted by the postreceptoral filter on a point-to-point basis and integrated over each patch. The greatest of the integrals over all patches under the right-hand half of the filter is then compared in opponent fashion, to the greatest under the left-hand side. The patch size can, in theory, be varied at will, from the smallest possible patches encompassing a single-pixel in the spatial frequency plane (recovering the case of peak detection) to just two large patches encompassing the right and left half-planes (recovering the full integration case). The mathematical description for the patch integration scheme is given by:

$$E.F._{pa}(f_{0x}, f_t)$$

$$= MAX\left\{\int_{n\Delta}^{(n+1)\Delta} df_x \int_{m\Delta}^{(m+1)\Delta} df_y \|O''(f_x - f_{0x}, f_y, f_t)\|\right\}$$

$$- MAX\left\{\int_{(-n-1)\Delta}^{-n\Delta} df_x \int_{(-m-1)\Delta}^{-m\Delta} df_y \|O''(f_x - f_{0x}, f_y, f_t)\|\right\}$$

$$\text{for } n = 0, \ldots, +\infty \text{ and } m = -\infty, \ldots, +\infty, \quad (11)$$

where Δ denotes the patch size.

Implicit in all of these approaches, which are implemented in the frequency domain, is the notion that motion information is perfectly integrated in space. That is, the amplitudes of the spatial frequency components that are weighed to reach a decision are computed from the entire stimulus field. A second class of decision rules (which we did not try) could be based on the outputs of many spatially localized motion detectors within the stimulus field. The psychophysical experiments typically employed relatively small fields at each eccentricity, which helps to justify the assumption of perfect spatial integration. However, the two classes of decision rules would be strictly equivalent only if the outputs of such spatially localized filters were combined *linearly* prior to the nonlinear decision-making process.

Orientation Discrimination Schemes

The same opponent decision rule, based on an integration, peak detection, or patch integration scheme, can be used to discriminate between vertical and horizontal energy, associated respectively with a horizontal or vertical input stimulus. To apply the model to this task, we used the same Gaussian window of visibility as we had used for the motion direction discrimination task, except that we now think of this as the sum of two components, one tuned in the horizontal direction, one in the vertical direc-

tion. The decision on the grating orientation then occurs based on the opponent difference between the amount of energy passed by each of the windows.

We adopted the following functional form for the sub-window tuned to detect horizontally oriented energy (shown in figure 3.12):

$$W(f_x, f_y) = e^{-(f_x^2 + f_y^2)/2\sigma_w^2} \times \frac{f_x^2}{f_x^2 + f_y^2} \quad (12)$$

(where we have to take care to define $W(0, 0) \equiv 1$; this discontinuity at the origin is not important for practical purposes, since energy that falls exactly at the origin does not have any horizontal or vertical component). The first term is an isotropic Gaussian, while the second term is a weighting term equal to 1 along the f_x-axis and 0 along the f_y-axis, thus weighting energy moving in a horizontal direction more strongly. Changing the numerator of the second term to f_y^2 rotates the filter by 90°, which is what we need for the purposes of detecting vertically oriented

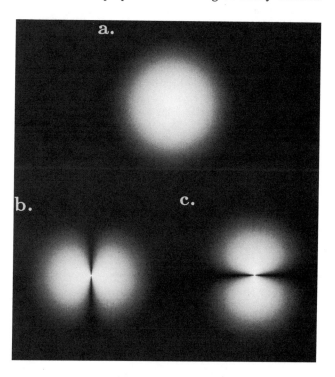

Fig. 3.12
Orientation tuning in Gaussian filters. (A) An isotropic Gaussian filter. (B) An anisotropic Gaussian filter, tuned to detect vertical energy (see equation 12). (C) The same filter, tuned to detect horizontal energy. The filters in (B) and (C) sum to produce the filter in (A).

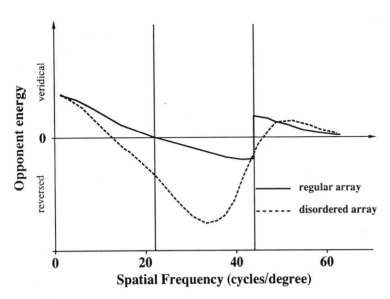

Fig. 3.13
The energy function obtained using the full-integration decision rule with cone aperture and bandwidth of the window of visibility set to the values known for 3.8° eccentricity. The dashed line corresponds to the disordered mosaic implemented in the model; the solid line corresponds to the crystalline triangular array with the same Nyquist frequency. The cone Nyquist frequency at this eccentricity in the human was taken to be 22 cycles/degree (with the cone sampling frequency at 44 cycles/degree), the standard deviation of the spatial bandwidth of a cone aperture was 32.5 cycles/degree, and the spatial bandwidth of the window of visibility was 10 cycles/degree.

energy. Note that the vertically oriented and horizontally oriented sub-windows obtained this way sum to the isotropic Gaussian filter.

In the next section we show the behavior of the model on the motion discrimination task and in the following section we show its behavior on the orientation discrimination task.

Results for Motion Direction Discrimination

In this section we determine whether the model can provide a reasonable quantitative description of the performance of human observers on the motion direction discrimination task when the model parameters are set to values taken from independent psychophysical and anatomical evidence. In particular, we are concerned with the question of whether the spacing of cones in the human mosaic at various retinal eccentricities is appropriate to produce the first and second motion nulls at the particular

spatial frequencies where they are observed in the psychophysical experiments. One prerequisite for linking cone spacing to these observed motion nulls would be that they remain stable despite large variations in the properties of the visual system prior to and following the sampling stage. We have examined this question by varying each of the parameters of the model in turn over a wide range, showing its effect on the model's performance. We will evaluate the influence of the following parameters: input spatial frequency, the spatial bandwidth of the cone aperture, cone Nyquist frequency, the spatial bandwidth of the window of visibility, and the amount of energy integration at the decision stage.

The output of the model is the opponent energy computed as a function of spatial frequency. Examples of two such opponent energy functions computed using parameters for an eccentricity of 3.8° are shown in figure 3.13. The decision rule used was the integration scheme in which the integrated leftward and rightward energies were subtracted to compute the opponent energy. The energy units in the vertical axis are arbitrary. For spatial frequencies that produce opponent energy greater than zero, the model decides the stimulus is moving in the true direction, but for negative opponent energies, the model produces a motion reversal. The dashed line corresponds to the disordered mosaic implemented in the model; the solid line corresponds to the crystalline triangular array with the same Nyquist frequency. Both curves bear a qualitative resemblance to the psychometric function obtained psychophysically (see figure 3.1). At low spatial

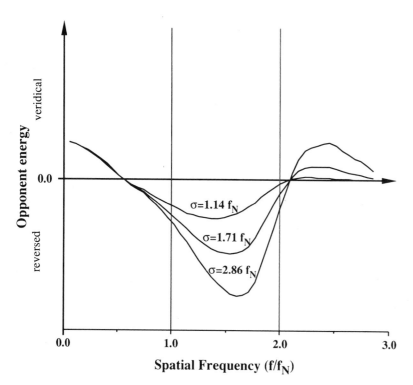

Fig. 3.14

The effect of cone aperture. The opponent energy functions were generated using the disordered mosaic and the full-integration scheme. The units on the vertical axis are arbitrary. Notice that the zero crossings remain constant for all cone apertures. Also, the energy functions are increasingly attenuated as spatial frequency increases. The aperture bandwidths used in these plots are as marked (in multiples of f_N). Actual cones at this eccentricity (3.8°) have an estimated aperture bandwidth of 1.48 f_N.

frequencies the model output is veridical, followed by a range in which motion is reversed. At still higher frequencies. the motion becomes veridical again, and finally, the opponent energy falls to zero and no motion is reported at the highest frequencies. A complete comparison of this function with the psychophysical motion data would require a method of expressing the two sets of data using a common ordinate. One could transform opponent energy into percent correct performance if the way in which noise limits the decision process were known. However, for the present purposes, we can treat the zero crossings of the opponent energy functions as directly comparable to the motion nulls of the psychophysical data, since the locations of the zero crossings are independent of assumptions about noise.

Note that for the crystalline array the first and second zero crossings agree precisely with the Nyquist frequency

and sampling frequency respectively. However, the effect of disorder in the array is to displace the zero crossings from these values. The second zero crossing remains reasonably near the mosaic sampling frequency but the first zero crossing has been displaced to much lower values than the Nyquist frequency.

Effect of Cone Aperture

In figure 3.14 we have plotted the opponent energy function for cone apertures of various diameters where all the remaining parameters in the model were fixed at the values for 3.8° eccentricity. The integration scheme was used to compute the energy function, and the disordered mosaic was used. The steeper curves in figure 3.14 apply to the smaller cone apertures and the shallower curves apply to the larger apertures. These plots show that the cone aperture (or any lowpass filtering of this kind, prior to the sampling stage) has *no effect* on the position of the zero crossings. This is because the cone aperture simply reduces the input stimulus contrast, increasingly so with increasing spatial frequency. To the extent that the model correctly simulates the situation in the human visual system, the cone aperture would not have an important impact on the locations of the motion nulls. This would not be true if the cone aperture were so large that the grating contrast were reduced below detection threshold, in which case the motion reversal would be obliterated. However, the actual estimate of the cone aperture yields a spatial bandwidth that is apparently high enough not to obscure either the first or second motion nulls.

Effect of Cone Spacing

To evaluate the effect of cone spacing we ran the simulations with all the parameters fixed except in absolute spatial frequency terms but the Nyquist frequency of the disordered mosaic was varied over a large range. As before, the decision rule used was the full integration scheme. Figure 3.15 shows the effects of varying the Nyquist frequency on the first and second zero crossings of the opponent energy function. Note that the second zero crossing remains relatively stable and equal to the sampling frequency, while the first zero crossing is unstable and never matches the Nyquist frequency. This behavior of the first zero crossing represents a departure of the model results from the observed psychophysical performance (see figure 3.2). The departure can be removed by adjusting the decision rule in the model, as shown below.

Effect of the Spatial Bandwidth of the Window of Visibility and Decision Rule

Despite the annulus of energy in the mosaic spectrum visible on a coarse scale, on a finer scale the amplitude of the mosaic transform is erratic. One consequence of this is that the opponent energy functions appear noisy when the bandwidth of the window of visibility becomes small compared with the Nyquist frequency. In the model, this made it more difficult to estimate the first and second zero crossings with smaller window bandwidths. This may account for the behavior of the psychometric functions obtained in the psychophysical experiments: We found that it was difficult to obtain reliable motion reversals at very large eccentricities, where the window bandwidth is small (Chen, Makous & Williams, 1989).

The bandwidth of the window of visibility is an important parameter in the model, and indeed, except for photoreceptor spacing, it has the greatest effect on the position of the zero crossings. Figure 3.16 shows the spatial frequencies at which zero crossings occur in the energy functions as a function of window bandwidth for three different decision rules. The curves show that the second motion null frequency stays relatively constant

under variation of window bandwidth and decision rule, while the behavior of the first motion null frequency is strongly affected by both these factors and in complex ways. Nonetheless, we have found a decision rule (namely patch integration) that will cause the first zero crossing to roughly equal the Nyquist frequency, in agreement with the psychophysical results. Recall that the patch integration scheme is an intermediate case between peak detection and full integration.

An important observation to make here is that as eccentricity is increased beyond $3.8°$, psychophysical data show that the contrast sensitivity function bandwidth decreases at a faster rate than the Nyquist frequency of the mosaic. This corresponds to increasing spatial summation as one moves into the periphery. For all amounts of integration we tried at the decision stage of the model, decreasing the window bandwidth below that used at $3.8°$ tends to shift the first zero crossing to lower spatial frequencies, below the cone Nyquist frequency. The first motion null observed psychophysically shows the same qualitative behavior. Thus the strong dependence of the first zero crossing on postreceptoral factors suggests that the first motion null measured psychophysically is a poor predictor of the spatial sampling rate of visual system. The second motion null, however, is stable and may serve as a good predictor. The psychophysical data on the second motion null also show a tendency to depart from the Nyquist frequency at the largest eccentricities (lowest Nyquist frequencies in figure 3.2), and our model predictions suggest that this cannot be accounted for by either pre- or postreceptoral spatial filtering. It could be evidence for subsampling at a subsequent stage of the visual system, but the psychophysical data are too sparse to make a firm case.

Results for Orientation Discrimination

The plausibility of the model to account for motion discrimination would be increased if, with minor modifications, the model could also predict the results of the orientation discrimination experiment. To tailor the model to the task of orientation discrimination, all stages were kept the same except that the window of visibility now consists of two filters, one oriented horizontally and one vertically (the sum of these two filters is the isotropic Gaussian filter we used previously). The decision rule is

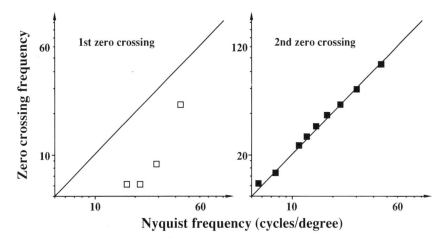

Fig. 3.15
The effects of varying the Nyquist frequency on the first and second
zero crossings of the opponent energy function.

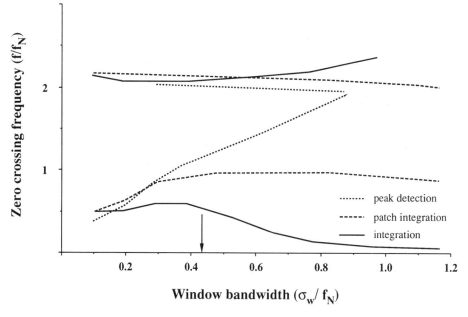

Fig. 3.16
The effect of bandwidth of the postreceptoral window of visibility.
The first and second motion null frequencies (normalized in units of
f_N) plotted against postreceptoral filter standard deviation (also in
units of f_N). The dotted curve is for the peak detection scheme, the
solid curve is for the full integration scheme and the dashed curve is
for the patch integration scheme, using a patch size equal to 4.8
cycles/degree. The postreceptoral filter shape was gaussian, applied
to the 3.8° retinal patch. The postreceptoral filter size matched to the
size of the neural c.s.f. is $\sigma = 0.43 f_N$. For the peak detection scheme
the effective bin width was 1.25 cycles/degree. The dotted curves
referring to the first and second zero crossing for the peak detection
scheme only extend to about 0.9 f_N, since the first zero crossing

frequency at window bandwidths greater than this value has reached
the value of the second zero crossing frequency. In addition, noise in
the energy functions prevented us from obtaining a reliable
estimation of the second zero-crossing frequency for the peak
detection rule at the narrowest window bandwidths.

again an opponent one, except that in this case, the opponency is between the horizontally and vertically oriented energies in the sampled stimulus' transform, rather than between the energy on either side of the f_y-axis of the spatial frequency plane. Coletta and Williams (1987) argued that cone sampling should produce an orientation reversal, which is most obvious at the cone sampling frequency, twice f_N. The present model provides a more precise test of this claim.

Figure 3.17 shows an opponent energy function for the orientation task, obtained with the disordered mosaic and the full integration scheme at 3.8 eccentricity, just as before. At low frequencies the model discriminates orientation veridically, but an orientation reversal occurs, producing an opponent energy minimum near the cone sampling frequency (44 cycles/degree). The behavior of the model closely follows the psychometric function for the orientation task shown in figure 3.1.

In figure 3.18 we have shown the frequencies at which orientation reversals occur for varying bandwidth of the window of visibility for the three decision rules. In this case the orientation reversal frequency computed from the model hovers closely around sampling frequency under all conditions.

Conclusions

We have explored whether a computational, opponent energy model of the visual system based on sampling by arrays of irregularly packed photoreceptors can predict the results of the psychophysical task of motion direction discrimination and orientation discrimination.

We have found that filtering prior to sampling as is the case for the photoreceptor aperture probably plays a small role in the performance of the task, except that its blurring effect decreases the signal to noise ratio at higher spatial frequencies. The photoreceptor aperture plays no part in the frequencies at which the perceived *direction of motion* of the stimulus reverses (nor on the frequencies at which the perceived orientation of the stimulus changes from horizontal to vertical, or vice versa). This agrees with the conclusion reached by Miller and Bernard (1983) and Williams (1988) that the *foveal* cone aperture has a minor effect on foveal aliasing.

Despite the disorder that is present in actual extrafoveal cone mosaics, there is sufficient regularity to produce a motion reversal phenomenon similar to what one would expect from a crystalline array. The main difference between these two cases is that for the extrafoveal (disordered) sampling arrays the aliasing energy in the spatial frequency domain is well dispersed over spatial frequency, rather than concentrated at and around particular spatial frequency values, which is the case for regular sampling arrays.

When the model is applied to the motion task, the second zero crossing is relatively stable at the cone sampling frequency, despite large changes in window bandwidth and decision rule. As can be seen in the fourth panel of figure 3.11, this immunity arises because the relevant energy lies at low spatial frequencies where the properties of the window are relatively constant. Furthermore, the leftward and rightward energy have similar spectra: Both are dispersed in the spatial frequency plane. These same considerations account for the stability of the minimum in the opponent energy function for the orientation task, which lies near the sampling frequency as does the second motion zero crossing. The immunity of these two aspects of the model output to postreceptoral effects strengthens the case that they provide an accurate measure of sample spacing. Thus the agreement between the second motion null, the orientation reversal frequency, and the cone sampling frequency at all the retinal eccentricities we examined psychophysically strongly implicates the cone mosaic as the source of these two perceptual phenomena.

There are two reasons why the first zero crossing in the motion opponent energy function is susceptible to post-receptoral effects. First, as can be seen by referring back to the second panel of figure 3.11, the model must compare the signal associated with the grating itself with an oppositely moving signal associated with the aliased energy. One pattern is periodic and confined in the frequency plane while the other is aperiodic and dispersed in the frequency plane. Changing the properties of the post-sampling stages can tend to favor one of these signals over the other. For example, the peak detection scheme tends to favor the grating so that the zero crossing shifts to higher frequencies. The integration scheme, on the other hand, favors the dispersed aliasing energy, shifting the first zero crossing to lower frequencies. Furthermore, the relevant energy for the discrimination lies near the edge of the window of visibility, so that small changes in the high frequency behavior of the window can have a large impact on the opponent energy balance.

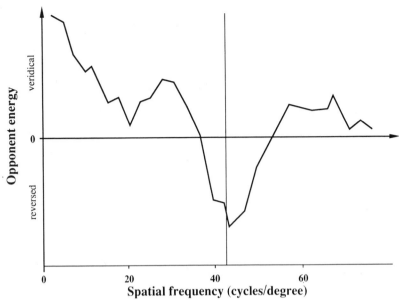

Fig. 3.17
An opponent energy function for the orientation task, obtained with
the disordered mosaic and the full integration scheme at 3.8°
eccentricity. The anatomical value for twice the Nyquist frequency
from the data of Curcio et al. (1987) is marked by the vertical line.

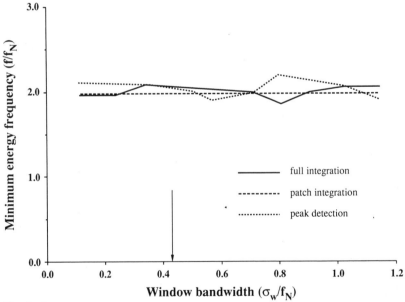

Fig. 3.18
The orientation reversal frequency (normalized in units of f_N) plotted
against standard deviation of the window of visibility (also in units of
f_N). The dashed curve is for the full integration scheme, the dotted
curve is for the patch integration scheme and the solid curve is for
the peak detection scheme. The arrow marks the spatial frequency
bandwidth of the window at 3.8° eccentricity (from c.s.f. data
collected by Williams & Coletta, 1987).

The model does not incorporate the effects of eye movements, which probably add noise to the actual psychophysical task. It seems highly unlikely that the visual system has accurate enough information about its small eye movements to compensate for them. Therefore, a grating drifting at a fixed velocity could produce a retinal slip of lesser or greater velocity, depending on the eye movement during the stimulus presentation. The retinal slip could even be in the wrong direction, particularly for very fine gratings. Indeed, the motion reversal was difficult to observe in the fovea, perhaps because the period of the interference fringe was very small with respect to the size of eye movements. Foveal aliases tended to dance and scintillate, rather than to drift systematically in one direction or the other.

The model described here only incorporates a single sampling stage, namely the cone mosaic. However, the early visual system is actually a cascade of spatial filtering and spatial sampling stages. For example, the photoreceptor output is resampled by the ganglion cell array for transmission to the lateral geniculate nucleus, and at large eccentricities the ganglion cell array is clearly sparser than the cone mosaic. Subsequent sampling arrays will only produce aliasing if they are unprotected by spatial filtering in the receptive fields that constitute these arrays. In such a situation, the observed aliasing effects would be a combination of aliasing by both the cone mosaic and these subsequent sampling stages. This could shift the motion nulls to lower frequencies. We found no convincing psychophysical evidence for it over the range of eccentricities we examined (out to 30°), although there may be a hint of this behavior at the largest eccentricities. The model presumably works over this range either because the spatial sampling rate set by cones is maintained at higher levels, or these levels are protected from aliasing by large receptive field centers compared with their sample spacing. This does not rule out the possibility of 'neural' aliasing at larger eccentricities, or even that there is a small contribution from later stages at smaller eccentricities. The good match between the second motion null, the orientation reversal, and the anatomical cone sampling frequency implicates the first sampling stage, the cone mosaic. The deviation between the first psychophysical motion null and the cone Nyquist frequency at large eccentricities cannot be attributed to neural aliasing with any certainty, because the model showed that this motion null could also be quite susceptible to other effects such as postreceptoral spatial filtering or the decision rule. For example, at 30°, the largest eccentricity we studied psychophysically, an increase in receptive field center size by a factor of only 2.5 would be sufficient to reduce the first motion null from the cone Nyquist frequency to the value observed in the psychophysical experiment.

The decision stage of the model is necessary to make it possible to compare the behavior of the model with the psychophysical data obtained from the two-alternative, forced choice experimental paradigm. A global judgment on the direction of motion or orientation of the stimulus has to be made on the basis of characteristics of the stimulus that are distributed throughout the visual field. As we have pointed out, the stimulus can contain aliasing noise locally moving in many different directions, or at many different orientations. For our psychophysical observers, perhaps the most compelling evidence in favor of the model comes from animated sequences we produced of the model output to drifting gratings of various spatial frequencies. The decision stage of the model was deleted, and the output of the window of visibility was observed in the space-time domain. Our observers reported that these animations provided an excellent rendition of the appearance of fine extrafoveal gratings, and both the motion and orientation reversals could be clearly seen.

Summary

This chapter provides a quantitative theory of the appearance of interference fringes imaged on the human perifoveal retina. A single computational model is constructed that accounts for two perceptual phenomena that occur when the spatial frequency of the fringes is high: the *motion reversal* phenomenon and the *orientation reversal* phenomenon. Over a certain range of spatial frequencies, interference fringes drifting in one direction can appear as spatial noise drifting in the opposite direction (Coletta, Williams & Tiana, 1990). In a slightly different but overlapping range of spatial frequencies, stationary interference fringes look like anisotropic spatial noise with a predominant orientation perpendicular to their actual orientation (Coletta & Williams, 1987). We have developed a computational model based on the photoreceptor sampling models proposed by Coletta and Williams (1987) and Williams (1988) that correctly predicts the ranges of spatial frequencies over which the orientation and motion reversals occur at various retinal eccentricities. The model consists of three stages: (1) a sampling stage (the primate cone mosaic, with cones of particular aperture, spacing, and packing arrangement); (2) a postreceptoral spatial filter of variable spatial frequency bandwidth and orientation; and (3) a decision stage. We have identified particular aspects of the motion and orientation reversal phenomena that provide measures of the spacing between sampling elements in the visual system. Furthermore, by systematically exploring the effects of the parameters of the model, these measures prove to be stable with large variation in the bandwidth of low-pass spatial filters either prior to or following the sampling operation. Over the range of eccentricities we have examined, the sampling elements responsible for these two aliasing phenomena are probably the cone photoreceptors.

Acknowledgments

We would like to thank Albert Ahumada, David Brainard, and Michael Landy for helpful comments on the manuscript.

The model presented in this chapter consists of the Master's Thesis work of the first author (University of Rochester, 1989).

This research was supported by US Air Force Office of Scientific Research Grant AFOSR-85-0019 and by National Institutes of Health grants EY04367 and RCDA EY00269 to David Williams, and by National Institutes of Health grant EY01319 to the Center for Visual Science.

References

Adelson, E. H. & Bergen, J. R. (1985). Spatio-temporal energy models for the perception of motion. *Journal of the Optical Society of America A, 2*, 284–299.

Byram, G. M. (1944). The physical and photochemical basis of resolving power. II: Visual acuity and the photochemistry of the retina. *Journal of the Optical Society of America, 34*, 718–737.

Campbell, F. W. & Green, D. G. (1965). Optical and retinal factors affecting visual resolution. *Journal of Physiology*, London, *181*, 576–593.

Chen, B., Makous, W. & Williams, D. R. (1989). A nonlinearity localized in the outer plexiform layer. *ARVO Annual Meeting Abstracts, 30*, 52.

Coletta, N. J. & Williams, D. R. (1987). Psychophysical estimate of extrafoveal cone spacing. *Journal of the Optical Society of America A, 4*, 1503–1513.

Coletta, N. J., Williams, D. R. & Tiana, C. L. M. (1990). Consequences of spatial sampling for human motion perception. *Vision Research, 30*, 1631–1648.

Curcio, C, A., Sloan, K. R., Packer, O., Hendrickson, A. E. & Kalina, R. E. (1987). Distribution of cones in human and monkey retina: Individual variability and radial asymmetry. *Science, 236*, 579–582.

Derrington, A. M. & Lennie, P. (1984). Spatial and temporal contrast sensitivities of neurones in lateral geniculate of macaque. *Journal of Physiology, 357*, 219–240.

Gavel, L. von (1939). Die kritische streifenbreite als mass der sehscharfe bei drosophila melanogaster. *Zeitschrift fur vergl. Physiologie, 27*, 80–135.

Geisler, W. S. (1989). Sequential ideal-observer analysis of visual discriminations. *Psychological Review, 96*, 267–314.

Goetz, K. G. (1965). Behavioral analysis of the visual system of the fruitfly drosophila. *Proceedings of the Symposium on Information Processing in Sight Sensory Systems*, pp. 85–100.

Helmholtz, H. (1962). *Helmholtz's treatise on physiological optics* (3rd ed.). New York: Dover, (Southall, J.P.C., ed.)

Hirsch, J. & Miller, W. H. (1987). Does cone positional disorder limit resolution? *Journal of the Optical Society of America A, 4*, 1481–1492.

MacLeod, D. I. A., Williams, D. R. & Makous, W. (in press). Visual nonlinearity fed by single cones. *Vision Research*.

Miller, W. H. & Bernard, G. D. (1983). Averaging over the foveal receptor aperture curtails aliasing. *Vision Research, 23*, 1365–1369.

Østerberg, G. (1935). Topography of the layer of rods and cones in the human retina. *Acta Opthalmologica (Suppl.), 6*, 11–103.

Pearson, D. E. (1975). *Transmission and display of pictorial information*. New York: Wiley.

Perry, V. H. & Cowey, A. (1985). The ganglion cell and cone distributions in the monkey's retina: Implications for central magnification factors. *Vision Research, 25*, 1795–1810.

Saleh, B. E. A. (1982). Optical information processing and the human visual system. In *Applications of optical Fourier transforms* (H. Stark, Ed.) (pp. 432–460). New York: Academic Press.

Smith, R. A. & Cass, P. F. (1987a). Aliasing in the parafovea with incoherent light. *Journal of the Optical Society of America A, 4*, 1530–1534.

Smith, R. A. & Cass, P. F. (1987b). Perceived motion reversal in parafoveal aliasing. *Journal of the Optical Society of America A, 4*, P80.

Thibos, L. N., Cheney, F. E. & Walsh, D. J. (1987). Retinal limits to the detection and resolution of gratings. *Journal of the Optical Society of America A, 4*, 1524–1529.

Thibos, L. N., Walsh, D. J. & Cheney, F. E. (1987). Vision beyond the resolution limit: Aliasing in the periphery. *Vision Research, 27,* 2193–2197.

Watson, A. B., Ahumada, A. J. & Farrell, J. E. (1986). Window of visibility: A psychophysical theory of fidelity in time-sampled visual motion displays. *Journal of the Optical Society of America A, 3,* 300–307.

Williams, D. R. (1985a). Aliasing in human foveal vision. *Vision Research, 25,* 195–205.

Williams, D. R. (1985b). Visibility of interference fringes near the resolution limit. *Journal of the Optical Society of America A, 2,* 1087–1093.

Williams, D. R. (1986). Seeing through the photoreceptor mosaic. *Trends in Neurosciences, 9,* 193–198.

Williams, D. R. (1988). Topography of the foveal cone mosaic in the living human eye. *Vision Research, 28,* 433–454.

Williams, D. R. & Coletta, N. J. (1987). Cone spacing and the visual resolution limit. *Journal of the Optical Society of America A, 4,* 1514–1523.

Williams, D. R., Collier, R. & Thompson, B. J. (1983). Spatial resolution of the short wavelength mechanism. In *Colour Vision: Physiology and Psychophysics.* (J. D. Mollon & L. T. Sharpe, Eds.). (pp. 487–503). London: Academic Press.

Yellott, J. I., Jr. (1982). Spectral analysis of spatial sampling by photoreceptors: Topological disorder prevents aliasing. *Vision Research, 22,* 1205–1210.

Yellott, J. I., Jr. (1983). Spectral consequences of photoreceptor sampling in the rhesus retina. *Science, 221,* 382–385.

4

Models of Human Rod Receptors and the ERG

Donald C. Hood and David G. Birch

Uncertainty remains about the role our receptors play both in the normal and in the diseased retina. For example, the receptors' involvement in such basic visual processing as our adjustment to different ambient light levels is still incompletely understood (for reviews see Adelson, 1982; Hood & Greenstein, 1990; Hood & Finkelstein, 1986; Shapley & Enroth-Cugell, 1984; Walraven, Enroth-Cugell, Hood, MacLeod & Schnapf, 1989). Further, for a variety of retinal diseases, both the extent of receptoral involvement and the nature of the disease action on the receptors are still debated. Many of the alternative hypotheses can be phrased in terms of the parameters of receptor functioning. For example, on a macro level a retinal disease can reduce the amount of photopigment, disorient the receptor, or cause a loss of receptors through cell death (e.g., Birch & Fish, 1987; Hood, 1988; Hood & Greenstein, 1990), and on a micro level the production or release of synaptic transmitter, the polarization of the cell, or one or more of the biochemical reactions between the absorption of light and the closure of light-sensitive conductance channels can be affected.

To answer these questions, we need a measure of human receptor activity that can be quantitatively related to underlying parameters of our receptors. To determine whether the initial portion of the electroretinogram (ERG) can provide this measure, we compared its behavior to a computational model of rod receptor activity.

The ERG

The electroretinogram (ERG) is a gross electrical potential easily recorded from the corneal surface of the human eye. In figure 4.1, the solid curve is a record of a human ERG elicited by a reasonably intense, 10-μsec flash. The vertebrate ERG shows two prominent peaks in potential, the a- and b-waves. These peaks result from the algebraic sum of a number of individual underlying components. For example, the a-wave is assumed to result from the

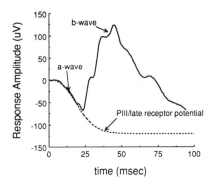

Fig. 4.1
The solid curve is a rod ERG response from a human eye. The stimulus was a short-wave, 10-μs flash of 2.0 log td-sec. The dashed curve is the presumed underlying receptor component. (From Hood & Birch, 1990a).

algebraic summation of the potential produced by the receptors with potentials produced by the cells of the inner nuclear layer (Brown, 1968; Granit, 1933, 1947; Heynen & van Norren, 1985). The potential generated by the receptors, shown in figure 4.1 as the dashed curve, was called PIII by Granit and the "rod late receptor potential" by Brown (1968). According to these analyses, the leading edge of the a-wave is the summed activity of the receptors.

The ERG records in figure 4.2 are from a normal adult. Each record is the computer average of 20 responses to a 10-μsec flash of a single intensity; the flash ranged in intensity over 4 log units. The figure caption contains some of the technical details. At low flash intensities only the b-wave is present while for higher flash intensities, both the a- and b-waves can be seen. The waveform and the amplitude of the leading edge of the a-wave change with flash intensity. Here we compare this portion of the ERG to receptor activity.

If the leading edge of the a-wave can be shown to be linearly related to receptor activity, then it will provide a quantitative measure of receptor activity necessary to test hypotheses about receptor functioning. We have tested whether this potential is linearly related to receptor activity by comparing its behavior to a computational model of the activity of the mammalian rod receptor.

A Computational Model of Rod Receptor Activity

Two studies of the mammalian rod include models of the time course of the response of the rod receptor as a

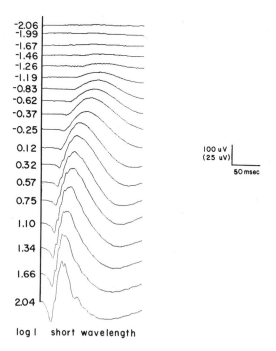

Fig. 4.2
Full-field ERGs from a normal observer. All stimuli were 10 μsec in duration and of braodband blue light (Wratten 47A). The methods used for obtaining full-field ERGs are relatively standard (see Birch, & Fish, 1987 for details). Responses were obtained from the anesthetized cornea with a Burian-Allen bipolar contact lens electrode. Responses were computer averaged ($n = 20$) and the rod component to flashes above 1.0 log scot td-sec was isolated by computer subtracting the response to a photometrically matched long-wave stimulus (50% cut-on at 605 nm). Thus, all responses were generated by the rod system. (Modified from Birch et al., 1987.)

function of flash intensity (Baylor, Nunn & Schnapf, 1984; Penn & Hagins, 1972). Although these studies employed different techniques and studied different species, they came to similar conclusions. Penn and Hagins recorded the voltage across the receptors of a rat retina. With their technique, the electrical activity of a large number of receptors was measured. Baylor, Nunn, and Schnapf recorded the current flow of single rod outer segments in a monkey retina. Both studies conclude that for a wide range of flash intensities, the rod response can be described by a two-component model. The first component is a linear process and the second component is a static (instantaneous) nonlinearity. These components are described below.

There is now a general agreement on the molecular events intervening between the isomerization of the pigment molecule by the absorption of a quantum of light and the change in membrane conductance producing the receptor potential (e.g., Lamb, 1986; Pugh & Cobbs, 1986; Stryer, 1986). According to what is being called "the cyclic GMP cascade theory," light-sensitive conductance channels are held open in the dark by an "internal transmitter," cyclic GMP. The absorption of a quantum of light by a pigment molecule initiates a cascade of biochemical steps resulting in an activation of phosphodiesterase. The activation of phosphodiesterase decreases the concentration of cyclic GMP, closing some of the channels and resulting in a hyperpolarization. The two-component model can be viewed in the context of this theory. The transduction process is no longer believed to be either a strictly linear process or a process in which the number of stages is simply related to the number of stages in the filter. But the initial molecular events up to the activation of phosphodiesterase can probably be described, over a wide range of light intensities, by a linear, low-pass filter with n stages (Baylor, Hodgkin & Lamb, 1974; Cobbs & Pugh, 1987; Penn & Hagins, 1972; Sneyd & Tranchina, 1989). In particular, to a first approximation, the initial chain of events can be considered linear for flash energies at least up to 4 log scot td-sec (Penn & Hagins, 1972) and the low-pass filter a convenient way to describe the time course of the output of this process.

If the output of the linear filter is $r(t)$, where t is the time in seconds, then

$$r(t) = I(t) * g(t), \qquad (1)$$

where $I(t)$ is the intensity expressed in trolands, $g(t)$ is the impulse response of the low-pass filter, and * indicates the convolution operation. For Baylor et al. (1984), the impulse response function for the low-pass filter, normalized such that the peak response equals 1.0, is given by

$$g(t) = [(t/t_p) \cdot e^{(1-(t/t_p))}]^{(n-1)} \qquad (2)$$

where t_p is the time to peak response and n is the number of stages, each with a time constant τ. (Note that t_p equals $(n-1)\tau$.) The impulse response function of Penn and Hagins' linear process can also be approximated by equation 2 (Hood & Birch, 1990b). In this form, the two models have similar values of t_p (Hood & Birch, 1990d). The primary difference between these two models is the number of stages in the filter, six (Baylor et al.) versus four (Penn & Hagins). As will be seen below, this produces a slightly different time course.

The second component of these models is a nonlinear response function that relates the output of the rod to the output of the linear filter at each point in time. In the context of the cyclic GMP cascade theory, the static nonlinear process probably captures the nonlinearities inherent in the limited number of light-sensitive conductance channels and, perhaps, nonlinearities in the changes in cyclic GMP with phosphodiesterase. For example, when the output of the linear component is small, doubling the intensity will double the number of channels closed. For more intense light, the number of channels closed approaches those available and doubling the light intensity will produce a smaller increase in the response. Presumably, this nonlinearity can be approximated by a static process because of the relatively rapid opening and closing of the light-sensitive conductance channel by the internal transmitter, cyclic GMP (see Cobbs & Pugh, 1987 for references).

The output R of the second component of the model is the receptor's response and is a nonlinear function of $r(t)$, the output of the low-pass filter. Baylor et al. assumed a nonlinear function of the form of equation 3 and Penn and Hagins a function of the form of equation 4 below. In particular,

$$R(t) = [1 - e^{-(\ln 2/K_a) \cdot r(t)}] \cdot R_m \qquad (3)$$

or

$$R(t) = \frac{r(t)}{r(t) + K_a} R_{m'} \qquad (4)$$

where K_a is the semisaturation constant and R_m the maximum receptor response. When $r(t)$ equals the semisaturation constant K_a, then $R(t)$ is one-half of R_m. Note that for an instantaneous flash, $r(t) = i \cdot g(t)$ where i is the energy of the brief flash. Thus, when the flash energy equals K_a, then $r(t_p) = K_a$ and the response R at time t_p is one-half of R_m. The nonlinear components in the two models are similar. Equations 3 and 4 produce functions similar in form and the semisaturation parameters given by the two studies are very close; about 30 isomerization/rod/flash. A semisaturation constant of 30 isomerization/rod/flash corresponds to about 0.85 log td-sec (Baylor et al., 1984).

Simulations

Figure 4.3A, B shows simulations of the two versions of the model. Each curve is for a different intensity of a brief

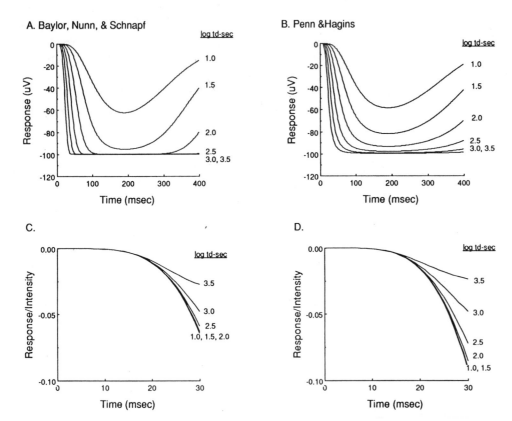

Fig. 4.3
Predicted receptor responses for the Baylor et al. (A and C) and Penn and Hagins models (C and D). In panels A and B the first 400 msec of the response for six flash energies are shown. In (C) and (D), the first 30 msec of these responses divided by the energy of the flash are shown. (From Hood & Birch, 1990b.)

flash. Since Baylor et al. and Penn and Hagins specify values for the parameters n, t_p, and K_a, to generate the theoretical responses in figure 4.3 only R_m, the maximum response amplitude, had to be specified. For the theoretical curves in figure 4.3A, B, the value of R_m was set to 100 for both models. Notice that only the first 400 msec of the response is shown in parts A and B.

A particularly useful way of comparing the predictions of these models to each other and to the ERG data is to divide the response at any point in time, $R(t)$, by the energy of the flash. Figure 4.3C, D shows the first 30 msec, the range over which the leading edge of the a-wave can be observed (see figure 4.1), of the predicted responses from parts A and B divided by flash energy. (See figure caption for details.) The curves for all flashes superimpose immediately following the onset of the flash because over this range of time, the output of the low-

pass filter is sufficiently small so as to be uninfluenced by the static nonlinearity. For weak flashes and/or at times immediately following the onset of the flash, the receptor's output is a linear function of flash energy. When the response amplitude is a linear function of energy, then the value of $R(t)/i$ is the same for all flash energies i. The curves deviate from the common curve at shorter times as the flash energy is increased. The primary difference between the predictions of the two models is the slope of the leading edge of the curves in figure 4.3

The Model and ERG Data

Application of the Model to Clinical Data

Intensity response series similar to the one in figure 4.2 exist for hundreds of patients. One of us (D.B.) has recorded such data from over 200 patients with retinitis pigmentosa. Similar data exist from other laboratories. We can apply the computational model to the specific questions: What can be learned about the parameters of the rod receptor from data such those in figure 4.2? Can

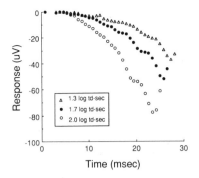

Fig. 4.4
The first 30 msec of the records in figure 4.2 for the three most intense flashes.

the leading edge of the a-wave be described by the model?

The data points in figure 4.4 are the first 30 msec of the response to the three most intense flashes in figure 4.2. These responses are truncated at the point that the b-wave intrudes. Because the cone contribution has been computer subtracted (see caption of figure 4.2), we can assume that these responses are rod driven. In figure 4.5A these are plotted as response amplitude divided by the energy of the flash, as in figure 4.3C, D. Figure 4.5 B–D shows the data for three additional normal observers.

These clinical Ganzfeld data are in qualitative agree-

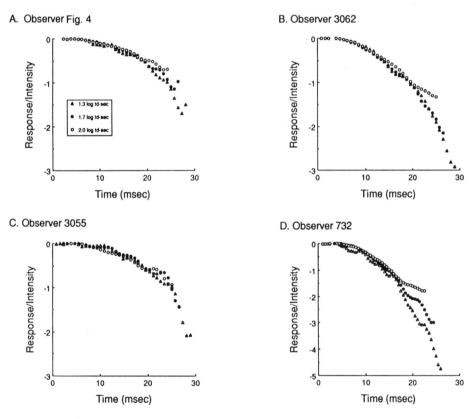

Fig. 4.5
(A) The ERG amplitudes from figure 4.4 were divided by flash energy. The different symbols are for different flash energies (see legend on figure). (B–D) As described in (A) for observers 3062, 3055, 732. (From Hood & Birch, 1990b.)

ment with the models of the rod receptor. The models predict that the curves for the three flash energies should fall together immediately after the onset of the flash. The data do fall along a common curve when plotted as response divided by energy. For this range of energies and times, there is clear evidence of a linear process. There is also a suggestion in parts B and D that the response to the 2.0 log td-sec flash is influenced by the nonlinear process beyond 20 msec.

Before considering how the data from the clinical Ganzfeld dome can be analyzed to assess receptor function, let us ask whether the nonlinear process can be observed with more intense stimulation. If it cannot, then the analysis of the a-wave in terms of these models must be questioned.

Testing the Model at Higher Intensities

An optical system was built to produce full-field (Ganzfeld) stimulation at intensities higher than those possible with the typical clinical Ganzfeld domes (Hood & Birch, 1990b). Computer-averaged ERGs are shown in figure 4.6 for the same observer whose records appear in figures 4.2 and 4.4. Each trace is the ERG response to a different intensity of a 10-msec flash. Notice that as the flash was increased in energy from 2.1 log scot td-sec, the lowest flash energy, to 4.2 log scot td-sec, the highest energy, there was a substantial change in the size of the a-wave. Over this range of flash intensities, the leading edge of the a-wave becomes larger and steeper. The first 25 msec of these responses are shown in figure 4.7A as the data points. The responses are truncated at the point that the b-wave intrudes.

To test for linearity, the amplitude of the response at each point in time was divided by the energy of the flash as in figure 4.5. The data points in figure 4.7B are the responses from figure 4.7A displayed in this way. As in figure 4.5, the data points for all flashes superimpose immediately following the onset of the flash. However, at longer times and for the more intense flashes, the data deviate from the common curve. According to the model (see figure 4.3C, D), for longer times following the onset of the relatively more intense flashes, the output of the linear component is large relative to the parameters of the nonlinear process and the size of the response per unit of energy is smaller. The model predicts that the responses will deviate from a common curve at shorter times as the

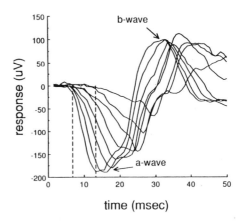

Fig. 4.6
Each record is the computer average of 20 ERG responses to 10 msec flashes of a single intensity. The energy of the flash ranged from 2.1 to 4.2 log td-sec. (From Hood & Birch, 1990d.)

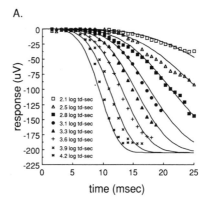

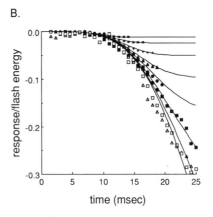

Fig. 4.7
(A) The first 25 msec of the records in figure 4.6 are shown with the responses truncated before the b-wave intrudes. The set of smooth curves is the fit of a model. (B) The ERG amplitudes from (A) were divided by flash energy. The different symbols are for different flash energies. The set of smooth curves is the fit of a model. (From Hood & Birch, 1990d.)

flash intensity is increased. The responses in figure 4.7B agree with this prediction.

To test for the presence of a static nonlinearity, the responses at fixed times after the onset of the flash are plotted against flash energy in figure 4.8A. The responses are plotted in the positive direction. The times, brief enough to exclude the influence of the b-wave, fall between the vertical dotted lines in figure 4.6. Because the nonlinear process is instantaneous (static), the response should become nonlinear at approximately the same voltage independent of time or intensity. For each time, a straight line (solid line in figure 4.8A) was fitted to the data points below 50 μV. At all five times, the response amplitude is described by this line for amplitudes less than 50 μV, while the larger responses fall below the extension of these lines (dashed lines) and reveal a compressive nonlinearity. In particular, the larger responses are smaller than predicted from a linear process. A further test of a static nonlinear process is provided by plotting the data on a log intensity axis as in figure 4.8B (Baylor et al., 1974). The model predicts that the data for different times are horizontally translated on a log axis. The smooth curve in figure 4.8B is the same nonlinear function (equation 3), translated horizontally to fit the data. The data are consistent with a static nonlinear process affecting the responses at longer times and higher intensities.

Fitting the High-intensity Data

The data exhibit the general characteristics of the two-component model of the receptor's response. To assess whether this model can be fitted to the data with plausible parameters, the general form of the functions used by Baylor et al. were assumed for the two components. In particular, we assumed that equation 2 described the linear transduction process and that equation 3 described the static nonlinearity. The value of K_a was set to 0.85 log td-sec, following both Baylor et al. and Penn and Hagins. Using these equations and parameters, values of R_m, n, and t_p were determined that would provide a best fit to the data. The smooth curves in figure 4.7 show the responses predicted by the model. The fit is quite good. The value of n of 4.4 falls within the range of values used by Baylor et al. and Penn and Hagins. The value of t_p of 149 msec is at the lower end of the range of values, 150 to 260 msec, measured for individual rods (Baylor et al., 1984). We set K_a equal to $10^{0.85}$ td-sec, as it was the

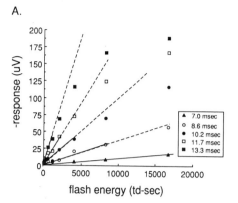

A.

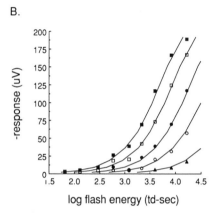

B.

Fig. 4.8
(A) The ERG amplitudes from figure 4.7 (A) plotted as a function of flash energy for fixed times after the onset of the flash. (From Hood & Birch, 1990d.) (B) The data points are the responses from panel A plotted on a log flash energy axis. The smooth curve is the function $R = (1 - e^{-ki})R_{max}$. The value of R_{max} was set to -205 μV, the value found for best fit of the data in figure 4.7. The value of k was arbitrarily set for a best fit. (From Hood & Birch, 1990c.)

parameter agreed upon by the physiologists; it also gives plausible values for the other parameters. Equally good fits can be obtained with values of K_a between 10^0 and $10^{2.5}$ td-sec. The best fitting values of n and t_p depend upon the value of K_a. For the values of K_a between $10^{0.5}$ and $10^{1.5}$, the estimate of n increases from 4.3 to 4.8, while the value of t_p decreases from 204 to 80 msec.

For the highest two flash intensities, 3.9 and 4.2 log td-sec, there is a consistent deviation from the model during the first 5 to 10 msec after the onset of the flash. The output of the model is larger than the observed amplitude of the a-wave. Penn and Hagins found that the leading edge of the rat's receptor potential deviated from the model in the same range of intensities. A similar discrepancy between theory and data was observed in the

Models of Human Rod Receptors and the ERG

turtle cones for the first 10 msec of the responses to intense flashes (Baylor et al., 1974). In both studies, a second nonlinearity was hypothesized to account for these findings; this nonlinearity was attributed to the electrical properties of the receptor's membrane (Baylor et al., 1974; Penn & Hagins, 1972), although voltage clamp experiments (Cobbs & Pugh, 1987) indicate that kinetic limitations in the biochemical steps preceding the conductance change can also produce a rate nonlinearity. In either case, there is a limit to how fast the receptor can respond and it appears that we are approaching this limit with our most intense flashes.

Does the a-wave have Properties Consistent with the Model of the Rod Receptor?

The amplitude of the leading edge of the a-wave varies with time and flash intensity in ways consistent with current models of the mammalian rod. This analysis suggests that the hypothesis that the leading edge of the a-wave is linearly related to the pooled response of the rod receptors cannot be rejected. We can return to the question of what can be said about abnormal receptor responses from clinically available data.

The Effects of Retinal Disease and the Computational Model

Can we test hypotheses about the site and mechanisms of disease action using the a-wave? In other words, can we estimate the parameters of human rod receptors from a-wave data and relate changes in these parameters to hypotheses about disease action? The model of the rod has four parameters: (1) the number n of stages in the low-pass filter, (2) the time to peak response t_p, which can be related to the time constant of the individual stages, (3) the semisaturation constant K_a of the nonlinear mechanism, and (4) the maximum amplitude of the response of the individual rods R_m. We will assume that the amplitude of the a-wave is linearly related to the underlying response of the individual receptors. In particular, assume that the amplitude of the a-wave $A(t)$ is given by

$$A(t) = \alpha c R(t) \tag{5}$$

and the maximum a-wave amplitude A_m by

$$A_m = \alpha c R_m$$

where $R(t)$ is the amplitude of the potential of a single rod, c is a constant that depends upon the number of rods recorded from, and α is a constant that depends upon the placement of the electrode, the size of the eye, and other factors in the recording situation that may produce variation among individuals with normal rods. We assume that for normal observers only α varies.

Different hypotheses about the cause of sensitivity loss with retinal disease make different predictions about changes in the model's parameters (e.g., Birch & Fish, 1987; Hood, 1988; Hood & Greenstein, 1990). For example, a simple loss of quantal absorbing ability secondary to pigment loss or preretinal filtering acts like an increase in K_a. On the other hand, a less responsive rod secondary to hypoxia may result in a decrease in R_m. To determine whether a change in K_a can be distinguished from a change in R_m, we assume that the model fitted to the 10 msec data describes the human rod response. Figure 4.9 shows the effects of increasing K_a or decreasing R_m by a factor of 4. The first 25 msec of the predicted a-wave responses to a flash of 2.0 log td-sec (parts A and C) and 3.5 log td-sec (parts B and D) are shown. The predicted responses are in linear coordinates in parts A and B and in log-log coordinates in parts C and D. For the 2.0 log td-sec flash, changes in K_a cannot be distinguished from changes in R_m. Thus, with the stimulus conditions commonly used in clinical research, we conclude that these receptor parameters cannot be reliably estimated.

For the 3.5 log td-sec flash, the changes in K_a and R_m produce different predictions. On the log-log plot (part D) the change in R_m appears as a vertical shift in the normal curve and the change in K_a by a horizontal shift. Although we can distinguish R_m from K_a changes, changes in the transduction process can mimic K_a changes. For example, increasing t_p from 123 msec to 185 msec produces a response indistinguishable, over the first 25 msec of the response, from the increase in K_a by a factor of 4. It is possible, however, to obtain estimates of three out of four of the parameters from these data.

The Effects of Steady Ambient Lights and the Computational Model

Steady lights markedly reduce the sensitivity of the human rod system. According to both Penn and Hagins and Baylor et al., rod receptor adaption is described, to a first

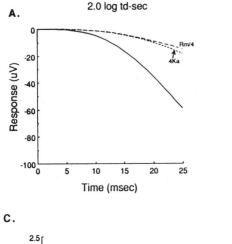

A. 2.0 log td-sec

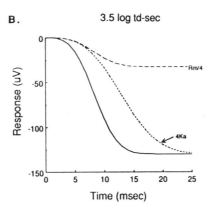

B. 3.5 log td-sec

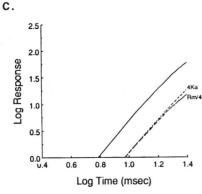

C.

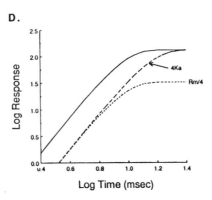

D.

Fig. 4.9
(A) The first 25 msec of the response predicted from the model in figure 4.8 to a 2.0 log td-sec flash. The solid curve is the normal response for the parameters used in the fit to the data in figure 4.8. The interrupted curves show the effects on this response of increasing K_a or decreasing R_m by a factor of 4. (B) As in (A) for a 3.5 log td-sec flash. (C) The responses in (A) on log-log axes. (D) The responses in panel B on log-log axes. (From Hood & Birch, 1990b.)

approximation, by the model described above with no need for a new parameter. In particular, the incremental response ΔR to a flash of intensity F presented upon a steady background of intensity A is given by

$$\Delta R(t) = R_{(A+F)}(t) - R_A(\infty)$$

where $R_{(A+F)}$ is the response to the combined flash and background light and $R_A(\infty)$ is the response to the steady field. Note that there is no time-dependent adaptation or desensitization in this model. Incremental responses are reduced in amplitude by steady adapting fields of sufficient intensity because of the static nonlinearity. The steady adapting field restricts or compresses the response range. This model of receptor adaptation was first de-

scribed by Boynton and Whitten (1970), who called it "response compression."

To test the model, a 100-msec, 4.6 log td-sec flash was presented on each of five adapting field intensities. Figure 4.10 presents the first 17 msec of the responses to the flash. The responses on the adapting fields of the three lowest intensities are approximately the same size. As the field approaches 1.5 log td, there is a discernible decrease in amplitude. For the 2.5 log td field, the response is markedly reduced in amplitude.

To fit the model to these data, the values of K_a, n, and t_p were set to $10^{0.85}$ scot td-sec, 4.4, and 149 msec, the same values found to fit the data in figure 4.7. The value of R_m, which depends on local recording conditions, was estimated for best fit to the dark-adapted response. The predicted responses for the other fields, shown by the solid lines, are determined by the model. For clarity, the predicted curve for the -0.5 log td field is omitted; it falls between the lowest two curves. Qualitatively, the model does well. The model predicts little change in the response for field up to 0.5 log td-sec and the data agree. The model, however, overestimates the decrease in ampli-

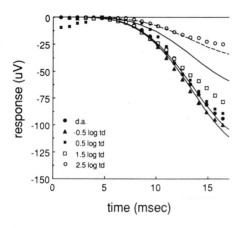

Fig. 4.10

The data points are the first 17 msec of the response to a 100 msec, 4.6 log td-sec flash presented upon a steady adapting field of the intensity shown in the legend. The smooth curves are the predictions of the computational model described in the text. For clarity, predictions are shown for only two of the three lowest adapting fields, d.a. and 0.5 log td. The dashed curve shows the predicted fit to response on the 2.5 log td field if K_a were increased to $10^{1.5}$ td-sec.

tude for the 1.5 and 2.5 log td fields. The open symbols fall well below the associated predictions, the upper two solid curves.

The computational model does not fit the a-wave data at high adapting field intensities. There is a similar discrepancy between the predictions of the model and human psychophysical data (Adelson, 1982). To compare the predictions of the model to psychophysical data, we define K(steady) as the value of a steady field that decreases the peak amplitude of the incremental response by one half. The value of K(steady) in trolands is equal to K_a(td-sec)/tsum, where tsum is the area under the impulse response function (equation 2). For the parameters of the model as fit to the data in figures 4.6 and 4.7, K(steady) equals $10^{1.5}$ td, approximately the same as the value estimated by Baylor et al.'s. To fit the psychophysical data at high adapting field intensities requires a minimum value of K(steady) for the human rods of between $10^{2.0}$ and $10^{3.0}$ td (see, Adelson, 1982; Aguilar & Stiles, 1954; Hayhoe, MacLeod & Bruch, 1976; Sakitt, 1976; Walraven & Valeton, 1984). Thus if human rods had a value of K(steady) of $10^{1.5}$ td, then our receptors would saturate at lower adapting field intensities than our rod system. This is clearly not possible. Our ERG data agree with the psychophysical data and argue for a larger K(steady) for higher adapting field intensities than predicted by the model. Increasing the value of K(steady) to about $10^{2.2}$ td

allows for a reasonable fit to the response on the 2.5 log td field, as shown by the dotted curve. Interestingly, as pointed out by Adelson (1982), the Penn and Hagins data also show a deviation from the model at high intensities. Thus, our analysis in figure 4.10, the Penn and Hagins data, and a recent study of individual cat rods (Tamura, Nakatani & Yau, 1989), all suggest that the computational model requires the addition of time-dependent changes at high adapting intensities.

Conclusions and Future Directions for the Computational Model

Collectively, the evidence suggests that the leading edge of the rod a-wave is linearly related to the underlying rod receptor response. The model found to describe the response of individual rod receptors describes the human a-wave elicited by flashes in the dark. Further, the deviations from the model at high flash energies and for incremental responses upon adapting fields of high intensity resemble the deviations observed by the physiologists.

Within the near future it should be possible to replace the two-component model with a computational model based on the biochemical events intervening between quantal absorption and the change in potential produced by the closure of light sensitive channels. A few laboratories (Cobbs & Pugh, 1987; Sneyd & Tranchina, 1989; Schnapf, Nunn, Meister & Baylor, 1990) have recently proposed models, in terms of biochemical events, of the first 50 msec or so of the receptor's response. Thus, the ERG elicited with flashes of relatively high intensity, as shown here, combined with current models of transduction, will provide an opportunity for testing quantitative hypotheses about the actions of normal and diseased rods. Such hypotheses might include changes in cyclic nucleotide or phosphodiesterase activity, metabolic pump activity, loss of receptor membrane and loss of receptors as well as the loss of quantal absorption secondary to a number of diseases processes.

References

Adelson, E. H. (1982). Saturation and adaptation in the rod system. *Vision Research, 22,* 1299–1312.

Aguilar, M. & Stiles, W. S. (1954). Saturation of the rod mechanism of the retina at high levels of illumination. *Optica Acta, 1,* 59–65.

Baylor, D. A., Hodgkin, A. L. & Lamb, T. D. (1974), The electrical response of turtle cones to flashes and steps of light. *Journal of Physiology, 242*, 685–727.

Baylor, D. A., Nunn, B. J. & Schnapf, J. L. (1984). The photocurrent, noise, and spectral sensitivity of rods of the monkey *Macaca fascicularis. Journal of Phyisology, 357*, 575–607.

Birch, D. G. & Fish, G. E. (1987). Rod ERGs in retinitis pigmentosa and cone-rod degeneration. *Investigative Ophthalmology and Visual Science, 28*, 140–150.

Birch, D. G., Herman, W. K., deFaller, J. M., Disbrow, D. T. & Birch, E. E. (1987). The relationship between rod perimetric thresholds and full-field rod ERGs in retinitis pigmentosa. *Investigative Ophthalmology and Visual Science, 28*, 954–965.

Boynton, R. M. & Whitten, D. N. (1970). Visual adaptation in monkey cones: Recordings of late receptor potentials. *Science,170*, 1423–1426.

Brown, K. T. (1968). The electroretinogram: Its components and their origin. *Vision Research, 8*, 633–678.

Cobbs, W. H. & Pugh, Jr., E. N. (1987). Kinetics and components of the flash photocurrent of isolated retinal rods of the larval salamander, *Ambystoma tigrinum. Journal of Physiology, 394*, 529–572.

Granit, R. (1933). The components of the retinal action potential in mammals and their relation to the discharge in the optic nerve. *Journal of Physiology, 77*, 207–239.

Granit, R. (1947). *Sensory Mechanism of the Retina*. London: Oxford University Press.

Hayhoe, M. M., MacLeod, D. I. A. & Bruch, T. A. (1976). Rod-cone independence in dark adaptation. *Vision Research, 16*, 591–600.

Heynen, H. G. M. & van Norren, D. (1985). Origin of the electroretinogram in the intact macaque eye-I. Principle component analysis. *Vision Research, 25*, 697–707.

Hood, D. C. (1988). Testing hypotheses about development with ERG and incremental threshold data. *Journal of the Optical Society of America, 5*, 2159–2165.

Hood, D. C. & Birch, D. G. (1990a). The relationship between models of receptor activity and the a-wave of the human ERG. *Clinical Vision Science, 5*, 293–297.

Hood, D. C. & Birch, D. G. (1990b). The a-wave of the human ERG and rod receptor function. *Investigative Ophthalmology and Visual Science, 31*, 2070–2081.

Hood, D. C. & Birch, D. G. (1990c). The a-wave of the ERG as a quantitative measure of human receptor activity. *OSA Technical Digest Series, 3*, 66–69.

Hood, D. C. & Birch, D. G. (1990d). A quantitative measure of the electrical activity of human rod photoreceptors using electroretinography. *Visual Neuroscience, 5*, 379–387.

Hood, D. C. & Finkelstein, M. A. (1986), Sensitivity to Light. In K. Boff, L. Kaufman & J. Thomas (Eds.), *Handbook of perception and human performance.* (pp. 5.1–5.66). New York: Wiley.

Hood, D. C. & Greenstein, V. (1990). Models of the normal and abnormal rod system. *Vision Research, 30*, 51–68.

Lamb, T. D. (1986). Transduction in vertebrate photoreceptors: The roles of cyclic GMP and calcium. *Trends in Neuroscience, 9*, 224–228.

Penn, R. D. & Hagins, W. A. (1972). Kinetics of the photocurrent of retinal rods. *Biophysical Journal, 12*, 1073–1094.

Pugh Jr., E. N. & Cobbs, W. H. (1986). Visual transduction in vertebrate rods and cones: A tale of two transmitters, calcium and cyclic GMP. *Vision Research, 26*, 1613–1643.

Sakitt, B. (1976). Psychophysical correlates of photoreceptor activity. *Vision Research, 16*, 129–140.

Schnapf, J. L., Nunn, B. J., Meister, M. & Baylor, D. A. (1990). Visual transduction in cones of the monkey *Macaca fascicularis. Journal of Physiology, 427*, 681–713.

Shapley, R. & Enroth-Cugell, C. (1984). Visual adaptation and retinal gain controls. *Progress in Retinal Research, 3*, 263–346.

Sneyd, J. & Tranchina, D. (1989). Phototransduction in cones: An inverse problem in enzyme kinetics. *Bulletin of Mathematical Biology, 51*, 749–784.

Stryer, L. (1986). The cyclic GMP cascade of vision. *Annual Review of Neuroscience, 9*, 87–119.

Tamura, T., Nakatani, K. & Yau, K.-W. (1989). Light adaptation in cat retinal rods. *Science, 245*, 755–758.

Walraven, J., Enroth-Cugell, C., Hood, D. C., MacLeod, D. I. A. & Schnapf, J. (1989) The control of visual sensitivity: Receptoral and postreceptoral processes. In L. Spillman & J. Werner (Ed.), *Visual Perception: The neurophysiological foundations* (pp. 53–101). New York: Springer-Verlag.

Walraven, J. & Valeton, J. M. (1984). Visual adaptation and response saturation. In A. J. Van Doorn, W. A. Van de Grind & J. J. Koenderink (Eds.), *Limits in perception.* Utrecht: VNU Science Press.

Part III

Models of Neural Function

One of the most gratifying aspects of modern visual science is the close and continued relationship between studies of computational and psychophysical mechanisms on the one hand, and studies of the underlying neurobiology on the other. Notable examples exist in the close relationship between psychophysical studies of visual spatial detection (part IV) and neurobiological analysis of the spatial filtering properties of single visual neurons. Neurophysiological studies inspired by the landmark work of Enroth-Cugell and Robson (1984) have applied the methods and concepts of spatial image analysis to the properties of neurons at many levels of the visual system and used the results to infer the nature of connections and functional interaction among many levels of "early" visual processing. The neurophysiological results in turn have inspired a good deal of work seeking to uncover perceptual signs of the mechanisms found in the "wetware." One example of this has been the extensive effort devoted to analyzing the perceptual correlates of the so-called M and P streams of early visual processing, which are thought to segregate and separately process color and luminance signals.

The P stream of visual information processing contains neurons having relatively small receptive fields that receive differential signals from cones of different color types, yielding a color-opponent code for the chromatic content of the retinal image. It has long been an intriguing problem to relate the apparent specificity of the connections from cones to central neurons with what is known about the circuitry of the retina. Here, Lennie and his colleagues explore the notion that the specificity is more apparent than real, and that the properties of chromatic receptive fields might be derived from a random, rather than orderly wiring of signals from cones.

All visual receptive fields can be formally described by the transformations undergone by the signals from each of the photoreceptors that comprise its receptive field, but students of central neural processing have tended to pay little attention to the consequences of the cone sampling mosaic for the structure of receptive fields. Hawken and Parker have undertaken a challenging series of experiments in which they relate receptive field structure to the underlying cone mosaic, thereby approaching the desirable situation in which central receptive fields might be described by writing down the most complete possible description—the wiring diagram between the cones and the central neuron. Watson's chapter gives a formal treatment of this same problem by providing an elegant set of formalisms for describing the construction of visual receptive fields by successive transformations of cone signals and using these in a model that accounts for variations in the measured sensitivity and resolution of neurons at different levels of the system.

A property of considerable interest and importance that emerges first in the visual cortex is directional movement selectivity. Shapley and Reid show that this property may emerge at least in part from the same kind of successive spatiotemporal filtering operations that are thought to lead to spatial receptive fields. They also present a new and exceptionally useful method for estimating spatiotemporal receptive fields. Heeger has also approached the problem of cortical neural organization, but from a somewhat different viewpoint. Lennie, Hawken and Parker, and Watson approach the visual signal transformations between photoreceptor and central neuron in a fundamentally linear manner; Shapley and Reid's analysis is also fundamentally linear, although they discern an important contribution from nonlinear mechanisms. Heeger considers data from a variety of sources that suggest the existence of a nonlinear central "gain control" that sets the contrast operating range of cortical neurons in the same way that light adaptation sets the gain of photoreceptors. His model is concise and startlingly accurate in its prediction of a variety of aspects of cortical neuronal behavior.

Reference

Enroth-Cugell, C. & Robson, J. G. (1984). Functional characteristics and diversity of cat retinal ganglion cells. *Investigative Ophthalmology and Visual Science*, 25, 250–267.

5

The Design of Chromatically Opponent Receptive Fields

Peter Lennie, P. William Haake, and David R. Williams

There are two major classes of primate ganglion cell, variously known as midget or parvocellular (P) cells and parasol or magnocellular (M) cells. P cells are thought to be important for color vision because they have chromatically opponent receptive fields: Illumination of certain spectral composition excites the cell, while illumination of a different composition inhibits it. Some M cells have chromatically opponent receptive fields, but that opponency is weak and inconsistent. There seem to be two principal types of P cell. One, loosely described as a red-green opponent cell, appears to receive inputs from long-wavelength–sensitive (R) cones opposed to inputs from middle-wavelength–sensitive (G) cones. The other type, loosely described as a blue-yellow opponent cell, appears to receive inputs from short-wavelength–sensitive (B) cones opposed to some mixture of signals from R and G cones (DeMonasterio & Gouras, 1975; Gouras, 1968). In red-green cells the opposed inputs seem to be segregated in center and surround of the receptive field. The defocus of short wavelengths that results from chromatic aberration makes it harder to establish the spatial organization of receptive fields of blue-yellow cells, but such measurements as there are suggest that spatial opponency is less pronounced, perhaps absent, in the blue-yellow cells. The problem to be explained is how chromatically opponent P cells make what appear to be rather specific connections with the different classes of cones. In this chapter we develop a model of the receptive field of a P cell, and show that the apparently precisely organized chromatic opponency found in the two classes of cells can result from their connections to cones depending principally on the positions of cones in the mosaic and not on the photopigments they contain.

Background

Several lines of evidence encourage the idea that the chromatic properties of P cells result from indiscriminate connections to cones. First, it seems likely from both psychophysical and anatomical analyses that for eccentricities of up to perhaps 8° to 10°, most P cells have receptive fields with centers driven by a single cone. Perceptual experiments (Coletta & Williams, 1987) show that from the fovea out to eccentricities beyond 10° the lowest-density sampling of the visual image is undertaken by a mosaic with the spacing of cones. Ganglion cells must therefore sample the image at least as densely as do cones. Anatomical observations bolster the case: After allowing for the displacement of ganglion cells near the fovea, for eccentricities up to perhaps as much as 8° to 10° there appear to be at least two ganglion cells per cone in the macaque's retina (Schein, 1988; Wässle, Grünert, Röhrenbeck & Boycott, 1989). Each cone probably drives two midget bipolar cells, one off-center, the other on-center (Kolb, 1970); each P cell is probably connected through a midget bipolar cell to a single cone that provides the drive to the center of the receptive field (Boycott & Dowling, 1969). That being the case, one can produce chromatically opponent neurons without any systematic selection of cones that drive the surround of the receptive field.

The surround is thought to be formed through the accumulation of signals in horizontal cells, fed to the ganglion cell through its bipolar cell. The primate's retina contains two morphological types of horizontal cell (H1 and H2). These are distinguished by the branching patterns of their dendrites and by the contacts made by their axon terminal systems: The terminals of an H1 cell contacts only cones, those of an H2 cell only rods. The dendrites of both types make contact only with cones (Kolb, Mariani & Gallego, 1980). Boycott, Hopkins, and Sperling (1987) and Wässle, Boycott, and Röhrenbeck (1989) found that both types of horizontal cell (H1 and H2) in the macaque's retina appear to make contact with all cones that lie under their dendritic trees. Indiscriminate connections of this sort would result in a P cell having a chromatically opponent receptive field.

Previous work (Lennie, 1980; Paulus & Kröger-Paulus, 1983; Shapley & Perry, 1986) has noted the possibility that indiscriminate wiring of the surround, coupled with center input from a single cone, could give rise to a chromatically opponent receptive field, but no one has pursued the idea quantitatively to see if it can account for the properties of cells observed in physiological experiments. Young and Marrocco (1989) have derived some

predictions of chromatic opponency from a model that assumes random connections to cones, but that model does not embody the physiological and anatomical constraints that we examine here.

Assumptions

We start with a real mosaic of foveal cones, from *Macaca fascicularis* (kindly provided by Hugh Perry), and tag cones as R or G or B. The proportion of B cones is relatively firmly established by anatomical and psychophysical work (DeMonasterio, Schein & McCrane, 1981; Williams, MacLeod & Hayhoe, 1981), and in the present analysis is fixed at 10 percent. (We assume a uniform distribution of B cones in the mosaic; we consider later the consequence of there being no B cones in the center of the fovea.) B cones are arranged in a quasicrystalline lattice, and in our simulations we mark as B cones those nearest the intersections of an imaginary triangular lattice laid on the mosaic. R and G cones cannot be distinguished anatomically, but psychophysical estimates (Cicerone & Nerger, 1989; Vimal, Pokorny, Smith & Shevell, 1989) suggest that in the human retina R cones outnumber G cones by about a factor of 2, on average. Observations by Lennie, Krauskopf, and Sclar (1990) on the weights assigned by cortical neurons to inputs from the three classes of cones are consistent with a factor of 2, but other evidence is more equivocal. Microspectrophotometric measurements of absorption spectra in cones from old-world monkeys yield a R : G ratio of 0.85 : 1 (J. Mollon & J. Bowmaker, personal communication). We have examined the consequences of the mosaic having several different proportions of R and G cones. Nothing is known about the arrangement of R and G cones in the mosaic, so we have examined the consequences of having both a random arrangement of cones and regular arrangement in a triangular lattice. The example in figure 5.1 shows a foveal mosaic in which R and G cones occur in equal numbers and are arranged randomly.

We use the Smith-Pokorny fundamentals (Smith & Pokorny, 1975) to characterize the spectral sensitivities of cones, since our simulation is to be compared with physiological measurements made with normal prereceptoral absorption. We represent the receptive field as the difference of two two-dimensional Gaussian weighting functions of different sizes, the smaller representing the center,

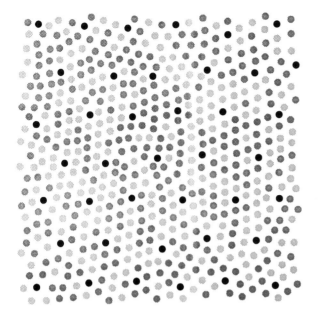

Fig. 5.1
Mosaic of cones (provided by V. H. Perry) from the center of the fovea of *Macaca fascicularis*. Cones are tagged as R (*lightest shading*) and G (*darker shading*) randomly and in equal proportions. Ten percent of cones, lying nearest the intersections of an imaginary triangular lattice, are tagged as B cones (*black*).

the larger the surround (Enroth-Cugell & Robson, 1966; Rodieck, 1965). Thus the point-weighting function of the receptive field is given by

$$W_x = k_c \exp[-(x/r_c)^2] - k_s \exp[-(x/r_s)^2], \qquad (1)$$

where r_c and r_s are the space-constants of center and surround and k_c and k_s are the peak values of the weighting functions. A center driven by a single cone is a special case, and is not represented by a Gaussian weighting function. To calculate the effect of stimulation by spatially uniform illumination of the receptive field, for both center and surround we sum (up to 3 SD from peak) the appropriately weighted signals from all cones. We assume that signals from cones vary linearly with the quantal catch (this is known to be the case for modest excursions about a steady adapting light) and we assume that, after allowing for preretinal absorption, all cones are equally sensitive to white light. We can vary the space constants of the center (r_c) and surround (r_s), and the relative strength of the surround ($k_s r_s^2 / k_c r_c^2$). (We define the strength of each mechanism as the sum of the weighted signals it receives from all the cones to which it is connected, given

that each cone is excited to the same degree. One can think of the relative strength of the surround as the ratio of surround to center signals when the receptive field is uniformly illuminated with light that equally excites all cones. In real neurons this ratio is almost always less than 1.) We can also vary the rule that each mechanism follows in sampling from the different classes of cones—for example, the center draws only from R cones, the surround only from G cones.

For the purposes of the present analysis we treat a P cell as though it were connected directly to cones, and in comparing the properties of synthetic cells with those measured in physiological experiments we do not distinguish P ganglion cells and P cells in lateral geniculate nucleus (LGN). We express the space constants of center and surround in cone separations rather than in degrees of visual angle. This compensates for enlargement of receptive fields with decreasing cone density, and allows us to ignore the effects of eccentricity in examining the implications of the model.

Figure 5.2 illustrates the general principles of the analysis. Part A is a schematic representation of a receptive field, superimposed on the mosaic of foveal cones. The (excitatory) center of standard deviation 1 cone separation draws from only G cones and the surround of standard deviation 4 cone separations draws from only R cones. The relative strength of the surround is set at 0.95. Part B shows the spectral sensitivity of the cell to a spatially uniform field that equally stimulates center and surround. This is the stimulus typically used in the analysis of chromatic opponency, because it optimally stimulates both center and surround. Part C shows the chromatic characteristics in a different form. The aggregate signal from G cones (w_g) is plotted against the aggregate signal from R cones (w_r), both normalized by the sum of the absolute values of the signals from R, G, and B cones. The quantities plotted are W_r and W_g where

$$W_r = w_r/(|w_r| + |w_g| + |w_b|) \qquad (2)$$

and likewise for W_g. Any cell that receives input from only R and G cones will be represented by a point lying on one of the unit diagonals. If the cell receives R and G inputs of the same sign it will be represented by a point in the first or third quadrants; if (as in the present example) the inputs are of opposite sign, the cell is represented by a point in the second or fourth quadrants. A canonical

The Design of Chromatically Opponent Receptive Fields

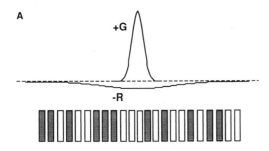

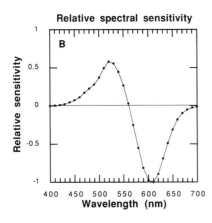

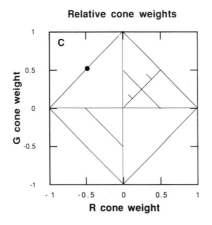

Relative spectral sensitivity

Relative cone weights

Fig. 5.2

(A) Gaussian weighting functions representing the center and surround of the ganglion cell's receptive field, superimposed upon the mosaic of foveal cones. In this example the center (standard deviation 1 cone separation) draws only from G cones (*unshaded*) and the surround (standard deviation 4 cone separations) only from R cones (*shaded*). The relative strength of the surround is 0.95. (B) Relative spectral sensitivity of an on-center cell constructed as in (A). (C) Relative weights assigned by the cell in A to inputs from the three classes of cones. These weights are calculated from equation 2 and assume that the receptive field is stimulated uniformly. Any cell that receives input only from R and/or G cones will be represented by a point lying on one of the diagonals defined by $R + G = 1$ or $R + G = -1$. Any neuron that receives input from B cones will be represented by a point lying inside these diagonals. In a diagram of this sort the weights assigned to inputs from R and G cones are represented explicitly; the absolute value (but not the sign) of the weight assigned to B cones can be deduced from the scale running from the origin to the diagonal in the first quadrant. B cone weight is constant along any line parallel to the bounding diagonals.

"red-green" opponent cell is represented by a point at 0.5, −0.5 (if R input is positive) or −0.5, 0.5 (if R input is negative). In a plot of this kind the relative magnitude of any input from B cones (though not its sign) is given by the distance along any perpendicular from a unit diagonal. A canonical "blue-yellow" cell that receives B cone input opposed to an equal mixture of inputs from R and G cones is represented by a point at −0.25, −0.25 (if B input is positive) or 0.25, 0.25 (if B input is negative). Results in either of the forms shown in part B and C can be compared with those found in physiological experiments. In what follows we have used the latter, since it provides sharper insights into the properties of the model.

Simulations

Figure 5.3 shows the properties of three synthetic cells that have receptive fields formed by drawing on a single cone (R, G, or B) for excitatory input to the center and on all cones indiscriminately for inhibitory input to the surround. In this and following simulations, R and G cones were distributed randomly with equal frequency. The standard deviation of the surround was 2.5 cone separations, a value consistent with estimates obtained

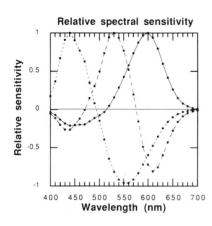

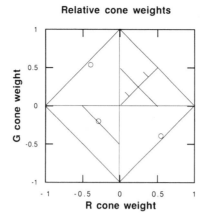

Fig. 5.3

(A) Relative spectral sensitivities of three on-center cells that received center input from a single R cone (*solid line*), a single G cone (*longer dashes*) or a single B cone (*shorter dashes*). The surround (of standard deviation 2.5 cone separations and relative strength 0.95) drew indiscriminately on all cones. (B) Graph of relative weights assigned to inputs from the three classes of cone. Conventions as in figure 5.2C. Note how the points that represent the cells that receive center input from R and G cones lie just inside the long diagonals.

physiologically and with estimates based on anatomical observations of the number of foveal cones contacted by an H1 or H2 horizontal cell. The relative strength of the surround was set to 0.91, the average value for P cells found by Derrington and Lennie (1984).

Two features of the figure are noteworthy. First, with center input constrained to a single cone, well-developed chromatic opponency can be produced even if the surround draws indiscriminately from all classes of cones. The spectral sensitivity curves in part A of figure 5.3 show this clearly for the cells that receive center input from G and B cones, though less clearly for the center driven by the R cone, and the analysis of cone weights in part B shows that all three types of cells have strong and well-balanced chromatic opponency.

Second, figure 5.3A shows that the spectral sensitivity curves of cells that receive R or G cone input to the center are not simply reflections of one another: The cell with a center driven by a G cone is overtly opponent, in the sense that it is inhibited by lights of long wavelength; the cell with the center driven by an R cone is not nearly so strongly inhibited at short wavelengths. There is no corresponding asymmetry in the relative weights of the signals from different classes of cones (figure 5.3B). The asymmetry in the spectral sensitivity curves has little to

do with the fact that the surround draws indiscriminately from all classes of cones. Rather, it results from the fact that R cones are relatively much more sensitive to short wavelengths than are G cones to long wavelengths. Thus only when G cones drive a cell through the center (which carries more weight than does the surround) does the cell have a clearly biphasic spectral sensitivity curve. This property may explain some puzzling discrepancies between experimental studies of the chromatic properties of P cells. Wiesel and Hubel (1966) in their early work on the LGN, and many investigators since, recognized a class of P cell that they called type III (spectrally nonopponent). These cells were identified through their responses to monochromatic or narrow-band lights. However, in later work that used nonspectral lights to analyze the weights with which the different classes of cone contribute to the receptive field, Derrington, Krauskopf, and Lennie (1984) found that essentially all P cells were chromatically opponent.

With a connection scheme of the kind examined in figure 5.3, the chromatic properties of a neuron are determined entirely by the class of cone that drives the center—the surround has a constant average spectral sensitivity. Because the surround signal is dominated by R and G cones, and these have similar spectral sensitivities, the chromatic properties of the average neuron with a center driven by an R (or G) cone will differ little from those of a cell whose surround drew on the other class exclusively. The principle illustrated in figure 5.3 also precludes certain types of receptive field organization: for example, it forbids a "blue-yellow" receptive field in which the "blue" input comes from the surround.

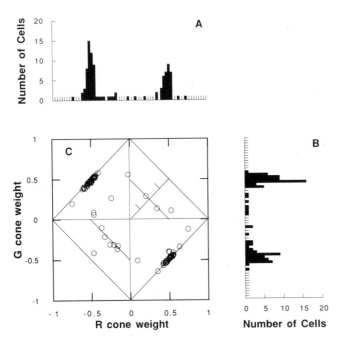

Fig. 5.4
Relative weights assigned by P cells in the LGN to inputs from the three classes of cones. Data replotted from Derrington, Krauskopf, and Lennie (1984). The histogram above the scatter plot shows the distribution of R cone weights; the histogram to the right of the scatter plot shows the distribution of G cone weights.

Comparison with Physiology

As long as the center of the receptive field receives input from a single cone, completely indiscriminate connections will give rise to qualitatively satisfactory chromatic opponency. However, it would be useful to show that the model is quantitatively satisfactory, and in particular that it can generate the variability of the physiological measurements shown in figure 5.4, which is redrawn from Derrington et al. (1984). We also need to see whether we obtain a quantitatively satisfactory account of the physiological results using physiologically reasonable values of parameters. Our approach to this has been to run large-scale simulations in which we create several hundred P cells, each with its receptive field centered on a different cone drawn from a pool in the middle of the mosaic shown in figure 5.1. We show the chromatic signature of each synthetic cell by a point on a plot of cone weights and compare the distributions of cone weights with those established physiologically.

The major simulations were run with R and G cones occurring equally frequently and arranged randomly in

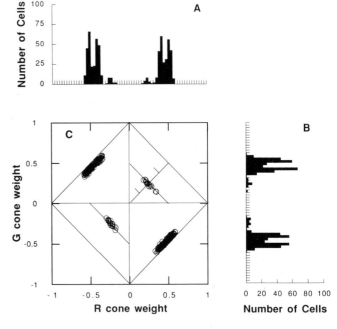

Fig. 5.5
Relative weights assigned by a population of synthetic cells to input from the three classes of cones. In this simulation the center of each receptive field drew on a single cone, and the surround (standard deviation 2.5 cones ± 0.4 cone separations, relative weight 0.95 ± 0.05) drew indiscriminately on all classes of cones. The population was randomly divided into equal-sized groups of on- and off-center cells.

the mosaic. This randomness gives rise to rather little variation in the chromatic signatures of the population of cells, because even a relatively small surround will accumulate signals from a large number of cones. To create a population with sufficient scatter of cone weights, we allowed variation from cell to cell in the space constant of the surround (r_s) and in its relative strength ($k_s r_s^2 / k_c r_c^2$). Figure 5.5 shows the results of a simulation that captures some major features of the physiological results. The caption to the figure provides values of parameters.

Although the simulation shown in Figure 5.5 is qualitatively satisfactory, it does not properly represent the physiological results. Part of the problem may be that some of the neurons represented in figure 5.4 had centers driven by more than one cone. In such cases, as we show later, cells can be represented by points anywhere within the bounds of the plot. There are also three more specific problems. First, the synthetic R-G cells (clustered near the diagonals in the second and fourth quadrants) attach too much weight to signals received from B cones. This can

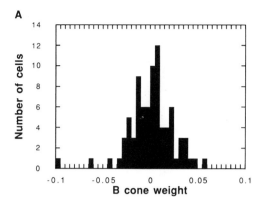

A

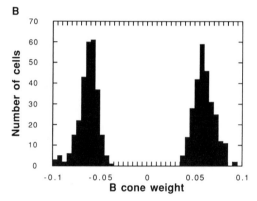

B

Fig. 5.6
Distributions of B cone weights for P-cells in LGN (A) and the synthetic population of cells represented in figure 5.5 (B). Correction of the synthetic distribution to account for the decreased density of B cones within the central 1° does not remove the discrepancy.

be seen by comparing figure 5.4 and 5.5, but is most clearly illustrated in figure 5.6, which shows the distributions of weights attached to signals from B cones, for real P cells (A) and simulated ones (B). The distributions differ greatly. The synthetic one can be made to resemble the real one by reducing the average weight of B cones to less than 1 percent. If we retain our assumption that individual cones all have the same quantal sensitivity, an aggregate B cone weight as low as 1 percent could arise naturally if the receptive fields of the real cells lay in the central 1° within which the density of B cones declines progressively. However, relatively few cells had receptive fields in this central region. The physiological results can be most easily explained by supposing that B cones carry little or no weight in the surround of the receptive field.

Second, for model R-G cells the distributions of R and G cone weights are clearly bimodal. This bimodality simply reflects the fact that whenever a particular class of cone

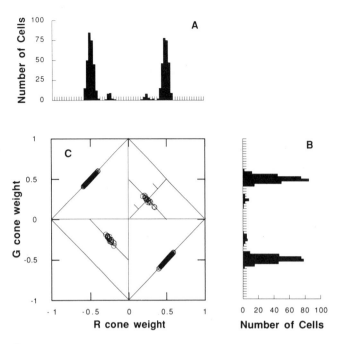

Fig. 5.7
Relative weights assigned by a population of synthetic cells to input from the three classes of cones, when the surround is constrained to draw only from R and G cones. Other details as for figure 5.5.

(R or G) drives the center of an R-G cell, it will always have more weight than when it drives the surround. The bimodality depends somewhat on the selection rule used in accumulating cone signals in the surround: If the surround does not draw on signals from B cones, more weight is attached to signals from R and G cones. For surrounds of the strengths simulated in figure 5.5, the bimodality disappears when we exclude B cones (figure 5.7).

The third weakness of the simulation represented in figure 5.5 is that it does not fully represent the variability in the subpopulation of cells that receive substantial input from B cones. Some physiological observations suggest that such cells have less pronounced center-surround organization than do R-G cells (Wiesel & Hubel, 1966). This might result from the center drawing selectively from more than one B cone, a possibility suggested by Mariani's (1984) analysis of the connections between B cones and bipolar cells. On the other hand, uncorrected chromatic aberration that defocusses short wavelengths may lead to erroneous estimates of the receptive field dimensions of cells with centers driven by B cones, and variations (both within and between animals) in macular pigment density over different receptive fields make our estimates of cone weights less certain. If we allowed the surround and center to be more nearly the same size (but still allowed only B cone input to the center and indiscriminate input to the surround), we could capture more of the variability in the physiological measurements.

Robustness

The synthetic distributions of cone weights are sensitive to variations in several parameters of our model. We explore these in the following paragraphs. We have already established that we cannot satisfactorily represent the properties of R-G cells if B cones contribute more than negligibly to the surround, so in all the following illustrations we have permitted the surround to draw only from R and G cones. All parameters except the one under consideration were fixed at the values used in generating figure 5.7.

Relative Strength of Center and Surround

As the average value of $k_s r_s^2 / k_c r_c^2$ falls below 1, the distributions of cone weights become progressively bimodal, because a particular class of cone will have considerable weight if it contributes to the center, and little if it does not. For the distribution of $k_s r_s^2 / k_c r_c^2$ permitted in the simulation of figure 5.7, the distributions of weights are unimodal, but they become bimodal (figure 5.8) if we adopt the lower values of $k_s r_s^2 / k_c r_c^2$ estimated from measurements made by Derrington and Lennie (1984) of spatial contrast sensitivity for achromatic gratings. This finding does not lessen the value of the simulation; rather, it suggests that estimates of $k_s r_s^2 / k_c r_c^2$ obtained from measurements of spatial contrast sensitivity for achromatic patterns do not adequately predict the behavior of a cell driven by chromatically modulated patterns. We do not yet know the source of the inconsistency. The conditions under which Derrington and Lennie characterized the spatial properties of neurons were not exactly like those used by Derrington et al. (1984) to characterize chromatic properties: The average chromaticity of the displays differed, and the measurements of spatial properties were made at higher mean luminance and slightly higher temporal frequency. We have no reason to suppose that these differences account for the inconsistency, which raises the possibility that the spatial organization of the recep-

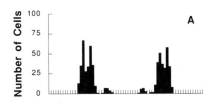
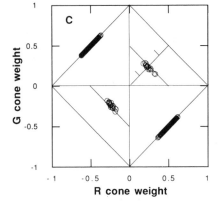

Fig. 5.8

Effect of surround strength on the distribution of cone weights for cells that receive center input from a single cone and surround input indiscriminately from R and G cones. Reducing the relative strength of the surround to 0.9 gives rise to bimodal distributions of weights assigned to R and G cones (*top* and *right*). In each case the mode with the larger absolute value represents cells that received center input from that class of cone. Other details as for figure 5.7.

tive field—and consequently the full weight of the surround—is not properly captured by the simple difference of Gaussians model. For example, the surround might be elongated in one dimension, an asymmetry that would not be discovered by measurements of spatial tuning made with gratings in a single orientation.

Space Constants

The space constant of the surround (r_s) used in our simulation was the average value estimated from physiological measurements of spatial contrast sensitivity, expressed as cone separations at the average eccentricity of the population of receptive fields studied (2.5 cones). Surrounds with space constants of 3 cone separations draw on so many cones that further enlargement has very little effect on the distributions. The distributions of R and G cone weights become progressively broader as r_s falls below 2 cone separations.

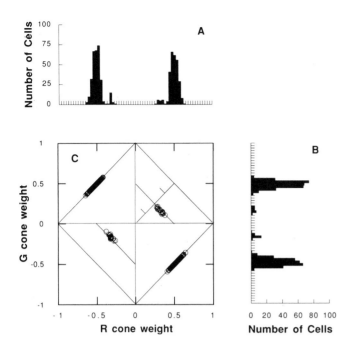

Fig. 5.9

Effect of varying the relative numbers of R and G cones on the distribution of cone weights for cells that receive center input from a single cone and surround input indiscriminately from R and G cones. In this example the ratio of R to G cones is 2:1. Other parameters as in figure 5.7. Changing the R:G ratio over a wide range has little effect upon the distributions of weights in cells that receive center input from R or G cones, but is directly reflected in the weights for cells that receive center input from B cones: a 2:1 ratio of R:G cones results in R cones in the surround having twice the weight of G cones.

Proportions of Cones of Different Classes

Plausible variations in the proportions of R and G cones in the mosaic bring about corresponding variations in the *numbers* of R-G cells whose centers are driven by each class of cone, but have modest effect on the corresponding distributions of normalized cone weights. Figure 5.9 shows the results of a simulation in which the ratio of R to G cones was 2:1. Other parameters were the same as those used in figure 5.7, for which the ratio of R to G cones was 1:1. In our model $k_s r_s^2 / k_c r_c^2$ is fixed at some value close to unity, so a change in the proportion of one class of cone in the surround is to a large degree automatically discounted. Consider a simple numerical example: A cell receives R cone input to the center and R and G cone input to the surround, which has a relative strength of 0.95. If the surround draws from a mosaic in which the R:G ratio is 1:1, the relative weights (center −

surround) are 1R − 0.95(.5R + .5G), which when normalized by equation 2 yield R and G weights of 0.525 and −0.475 respectively. If the ratio of R to G cones is 3:1, the relative weights are 1R − 0.95(.75R + .25G), giving normalized R and G weights of 0.548 and −0.452, respectively.

A change in the ratio of R to G cones markedly affects the chromatic properties of B − R and G cells. As the ratio departs from unity, the distributions of cone weights of B − R and G cells move towards the axis of the preponderant class of cone. This is clearly evident in figure 5.9. To the extent that our model adequately characterizes the receptive field, our simulations show that Derrington and colleagues' (1984) physiological measurements of cone weights are inconsistent with a 2:1 ratio of R to G cones.

Arrangement of Cones

Except when the surround is very small, the precise arrangement of the different classes of cones in the mosaic has no effect on the chromatic properties of cells stimulated by spatially uniform fields of light. If the surround draws on very few cones, the distributions of cone weights obtained with regularly arranged cones are less variable than those obtained with a random arrangement. The arrangement of cones could be more important when receptive fields are stimulated by heterochromatic gratings. A regular arrangement might lead to the distributions of cone weights depending on the orientation of the stimulus on the receptive field, though only at very high spatial frequencies.

More Than One Cone in the Center

The next issue to examine is the consequence of allowing the center to draw on more than one cone. There is no clear anatomical evidence on how cones are recruited, and we have assumed that if more than one is involved, a Gaussian weighting function is applied. Figure 5.10 shows the results of four simulations in which the standard deviation of the center, which drew indiscriminately on all cone types, varied from 0.5 cone separations to 2 cone separations. With even the smallest enlargement of the center beyond a single cone the opponency becomes very variable (figure 5.10A), and further enlargement progressively creates more units that have nonopponent receptive fields (represented by points in the first and third quadrants of the graphs). The distributions

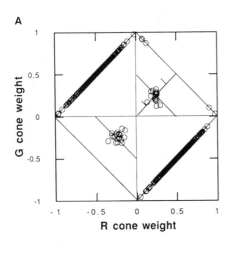

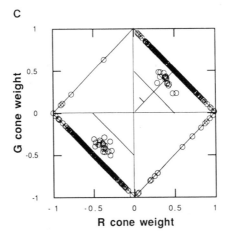

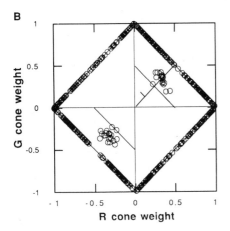

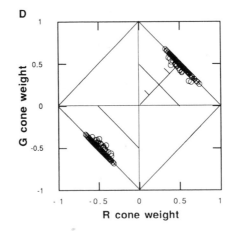

Fig. 5.10
Effect on the distribution of cone weights of varying the size of the center of the receptive field and allowing the center to draw indiscriminately on all cones. In all cases the standard deviation of the surround was 2.5 ± 0.4 cone separations. (A) Center standard deviation 0.5 cone separations. (B) Center standard deviation 0.75 cone separations. (C) Center standard deviation 1.0 cone separations. (D) Center standard deviation 2 cone separations.

of cone weights shown in figure 5.10A and B are not unlike those found for M cells (Derrington et al., 1984), but are quite unlike those found for P cells (figure 5.4), which show essentially no cells that receive R and G cone input of the same sign. To obtain distributions of cone weights like those observed in P cells, it seems a neuron must receive center input from a single class of cone. In the central visual field this is achieved by the ganglion cell drawing on only one cone. In more peripheral retina, where P cells receive center input from more than one cone, it remains to be seen whether this input is from a

single class. We have little physiological information on the chromatic properties of peripheral P cells, although psychophysical observations point clearly to peripheral color vision being poorer than that in the central visual field (Abramov & Gordon, 1977; Moreland, 1972).

Conclusions

Our simulation shows that the chromatic properties of most P cells in the central retina could arise through the application of two simple principles: Each cell receives center input from a single cone and surround input from R and G cones within its spatial domain. With physiologically plausible values of receptive field parameters, many of these cells will show little overt chromatic opponency, in the sense that they are excited by some wavelengths and inhibited by others, although the opponent inputs are clearly seen in the distributions of cone weights.

Our simulations do not adequately characterize all cells: The physiological results reveal a few P cells that receive mixtures of cone inputs unlike those produced by our simulation. Perhaps these cells receive center input from more than one cone.

The chromatic properties of cells are robust to large variations in the proportions of R and G cones in the mosaic and to variations in the arrangement of these cones. If the center is permitted to draw on more than one cone, then it must sample selectively from a single class; indiscriminate connections to cones in the center give rise to distributions of cone weights unlike those observed in populations of real P cells.

It has generally been thought that the formation of chromatically opponent receptive fields in the primate requires the selection of cones both by position and by class—a developmental problem of some complexity. Our analysis suggests that the problem is much simpler: A red-green opponent system and also a blue-yellow one can be formed without distinguishing R and G cones. The visual system apparently does need to identify B cones, which appear to be excluded from the surrounds of R-G neurons. Certain aspects of the organization of the blue-yellow system (the apparently close match of center and surround sizes, and the relative paucity of cells in which B cones provide an "off" input) also endorse the idea that B cones are identified.

Acknowledgments

David Brainard kindly commented on the manuscript. This work was supported by NIH grants EY 04440, EY01319, RR03825, and AFOSR-88-0292.

References

Abramov, I. & Gordon, J. (1977). Color vision in the peripheral retina. II. Hue and saturation. *Journal of the Optical Society of America, 67*, 202–207.

Boycott, B. B. & Dowling, J. E. (1969). Organization of the primate retina: Light microscopy. *Philosophical Transactions of the Royal Society B, 225*, 109–184.

Boycott, B. B., Hopkins, J. M. & Sperling, H. G. (1987). Cone connections of the horizontal cells of the rhesus monkey's retina. *Proceedings of the Royal Society of London B, 229*, 345–379.

Cicerone, C. M. & Nerger, J. L. (1989). The relative numbers of long-wavelength-sensitive to middle-wavelength-sensitive cones in the human fovea centralis. *Vision Research, 29*, 115–128.

Coletta, N. J. & Williams, D. R. (1987). Psychophysical estimate of extrafoveal cone spacing. *Journal of the Optical Society of America A, 4*, 1503–1513.

DeMonasterio, F. M. & Gouras, P. (1975). Functional properties of ganglion cells of the rhesus monkey retina. *Journal of Physiology, 257*, 155–170.

DeMonasterio, F. M., Schein, S. J. & McCrane, E. P. (1981). Staining of blue-sensitive cones of the macaque retina by fluorescent dye. *Science, 213*, 1278–1281.

Derrington, A. M., Krauskopf, J. & Lennie, P. (1984). Chromatic mechanisms in lateral geniculate nucleus of macaque. *Journal of Physiology, 357*, 241–265.

Derrington, A. M. & Lennie, P. (1984). Spatial and temporal contrast sensitivities of neurones in lateral geniculate nucleus of macaque. *Journal of Physiology, 357*, 219–240.

Enroth-Cugell, C. & Robson, J. G. (1966). Th contrast sensitivity of retinal ganglion cells of the cat. *Journal Physiology, 187*, 517–552.

Gouras, P. (1968). Identification of cone mechanisms in monkey ganglion cells. *Journal of Physiology, 199*, 533–547.

Kolb, H. (1970). Organization of the outer plexiform layer of the primate retina: Electron microscopy of Golgi-impregnated cells. *Philosophical Transactions of the Royal Society B, 258*, 261–283.

Kolb, H., Mariani, A. & Gallego, A. (1980). A second type of horizontal cell in the monkey retina. *Journal of Comparative Neurology, 189*, 31–44.

Lennie, P. (1980). Parallel visual pathways. *Vision Research, 20*, 561–594.

Lennie, P., Krauskopf, J. & Sclar, G. (1990). Chromatic mechanisms in striate cortex of macaque. *Journal of Neuroscience, 10*, 649–669.

Mariani, A. (1984). Bipolar cells in monkey retina selective for the cones likely to be blue-sensitive. *Nature, 308*, 184–186.

Moreland, J. D. (1972). Peripheral color vision. In Jameson, D. & Hurvich, L. M. (Eds.), *Handbook of Sensory Physiology, Vol VII/4. Visual Psychophysics*. Berlin: Springer-Verlag.

Paulus, W. & Kröger-Paulus, A. (1983). A new concept in the retinal color coding. *Vision Research, 23*, 529–540.

Rodieck, R. W. (1965). Quantitative analysis of cat retinal ganglion cell response to visual stimuli. *Vision Research, 5*, 583–601.

Schein, S. J. (1988). Anatomy of macaque fovea and spatial densities of neurons in foveal representation. *Journal of Comparative Neurology, 269*, 479–505.

Shapley, R. M. & Perry, V. H. (1986). Cat and monkey retinal ganglion cells and their visual functional roles. *Trends in Neuroscience, 9*, 229–235.

Smith, V. C. & Pokorny, J. (1975). Spectral sensitivity of the foveal cone photopigments between 400 and 500 nm. *Vision Research, 15,* 161–171.

Vimal, R. L. P., Pokorny, J., Smith, V. C. & Shevell, S. K. (1989). Foveal cone thresholds. *Vision Research, 29,* 61–78.

Wässle, H., Boycott, B. B. & Röhrenbeck, J. (1989). Horizontal cells in the monkey retina: cone connections and dendritic network. *European Journal of Neuroscience, 1,* 421–435.

Wässle, H., Grünert, U., Röhrenbeck, J. & Boycott, B. B. (1989). Cortical magnification factor and the ganglion cell density of the primate retina. *Nature, 341,* 643–646.

Wiesel, T. N. & Hubel, D. H. (1966). Spatial and chromatic interactions in the lateral geniculate body of the rhesus monkey. *Journal of Neurophysiology, 29,* 1115–1156.

Williams, D. R., MacLeod, D. I. A. & Hayhoe, M. M. (1981). Punctate sensitivity of the blue-sensitive mechanism. *Vision Research, 21,* 1357–1375.

Young, R. A. & Marrocco, R. T. (1989). Predictions about chromatic receptive fields assuming random cone connections. *Journal of Theoretical Biology, 141,* 23–40.

6

Spatial Receptive Field Organization in Monkey V1 and its Relationship to the Cone Mosaic

Michael J. Hawken and
Andrew J. Parker

Receptive fields at different levels of the visual pathway have vastly different shapes, sizes, and functional attributes. Exactly how each receptive field scales with respect to others at the same eccentricity and across different eccentricities is unknown. To investigate the spatial structure of receptive fields and their interrelationships, it may be more advantageous to consider spatial dimensions in terms of a retinal scale rather than the more familiar spatial coordinates of degrees of visual angle. This kind of scale would reflect the neural connections that have to be formed to support the receptive field structures found at higher levels in the visual pathway. Since the density of cone photoreceptors provides the initial spatial scale for retinal sampling of the visual image in photopic vision, then the spatial sensitivity of visual receptive fields could be expressed in terms of the spatial distribution of the underlying cones. In this chapter we discuss some of the factors that are important in connecting the substructure of lateral geniculate nucleus (LGN) and V1 neuron receptive fields to a spatial scale based on cone density. Then we extend this analysis to consider the projection of the cones onto the retinotopic map of V1 and explore the implications for the organization of receptive fields and the anatomical connections required to support them.

A number of areas need to be considered. One of these involves how to obtain quantitative measurements of receptive field dimensions and how these can be accurately projected onto the retinal surface. Therefore, in the first part of this chapter we introduce a number of models of the spatial structure of receptive fields, indicating how they can be used to derive quantitative estimates of the size and sensitivity of spatial subunits of receptive fields. This section also points out the advantages of using models of LGN and Vl receptive fields because it is relatively easy to compare subunit sizes and their sensitivities at different levels of the visual pathway. The results of applying these models to the spatial contrast sensitivity functions of neurons are then developed, along with consideration of the effects of optical attenuation, which must be factored out of the measurements to obtain an accurate estimate of the receptive field on the retina. This is particularly important for cells with small receptive fields that are close to the fovea.

An area of further importance in using cone density as a spatial scale is the measurement of cone density itself. Some of the main factors that influence the accuracy of the map of cone density are considered in the next section of the chapter, along with data that indicate considerable variability of cone density in the foveal region and, by contrast, homogeneity in the parafoveal and peripheral retina. These findings are then combined with the receptive field measures to give an account of the important factors in mapping the fields and their subunits onto the cones.

Background

In primates there are distinct functional differences between retinal ganglion cells projecting to the magnocellular and parvocellular divisions of the LGN, M and P cells respectively. Some of the key differences may be preserved in V1 (see Shapley, 1990 for a review). Receptive field structure of monkey M and P cells as well as V1 simple cells have been studied by measuring contrast sensitivity functions with sinewave grating stimuli (DeValois, Albrecht & Thorell, 1982; Derrington & Lennie, 1984; Hawken & Parker, 1987; Kaplan & Shapley, 1982; Parker & Hawken, 1988). One advantage of measuring spatial contrast sensitivity is that quantitative comparisons over retinal, geniculate, and V1 receptive fields becomes relatively straightforward. For example, in both the retina and LGN, M or P cell receptive fields can be described by a difference of Gaussians (DOG) center/surround mechanism, so the space constants and sensitivities of different cell classes in the retina and LGN can be compared quantitatively. Expressing spatial measures, such as the width of a subregion of a receptive field, in terms of the numbers of cones underlying that region means that comparison between receptive fields can be made across eccentricities and even between species while using the same metric. In this way, common organizational features in the neural elements of primate visual pathways can be sought independently of the factors that

do not reflect neural connectivity such as eye size, optics and variations in cone density.

Anatomical studies indicate that the ratio of retinal P cells to cones is at least 2:1 for central vision (Perry & Cowey, 1988; Schein, 1988; Wässle, Grünert, Röhrenbeck & Boycott, 1989), which provides the foundation for a 1:1 relationship between individual cones and both "on" and "off" retinal ganglion cells. Therefore, there is a solid anatomical basis for a single cone to provide the input to the center mechanism of at least two midget ganglion cells. There is also evidence that the numbers of retinal ganglion cells and LGN relay cells are similar, indicating that there is not a major convergence or divergence at the level of the LGN (Connolly & van Essen, 1984). Therefore, it may be reasonable to assume that there are LGN neurons that have single cone inputs to their receptive field centers, and this would be one of the sets of inputs into V1. We take this as support for the notion of scaling receptive field size in terms of the number of cones.

Models

One of the measures that is often used to characterize the spatial organization of receptive fields is the sensitivity or responsiveness to a point of light at each position in the receptive field, often called the point weighting or spatial weighting function. This measure not only gives the area of visual space over which a cell is responsive, but the magnitude and sign of the response as well. Although it is possible to make these measurements directly with small spots of light, there are a number of advantages in analyzing the spatial organization of receptive fields in the frequency domain (Enroth-Cugell & Robson, 1984). The spatial weighting of receptive fields can be recovered as the inverse transform of the spatial frequency tuning function, or obtained by the application of model functions to the tuning curves. The use of models has the advantage that simple combinations of spatial subunits can be incorporated into them.

For example, most primate retinal ganglion cells exhibit a center/surround organization of their receptive fields, where the center and surround responses are antagonistic. In the monkey retinal ganglion cell layer and LGN, the relative spatial dimensions of the center and surround depend on the cell type (Wiesel & Hubel, 1966). Most commonly, the central region is flanked by an antagonistic surrounding region that is spatially more extensive than the central region. As discussed below, the center and surround regions can be described by a Gaussian function and combined to form a model of the receptive field based on the difference of these two Gaussians. Using a model function and applying it to the sensitivity data allows the extraction of the parameters of the center and surround mechanisms that define the spatial organization of receptive fields at different levels of the visual pathway.

Lateral Geniculate

The best known physiologically based receptive field model is the DOG, which was introduced by Rodieck (1965) to describe the spatial tuning of retinal ganglion cells, then extended from the spatial to the spatial frequency domain by Enroth-Cugell and Robson (1966). The DOG model has also been modified to account for the changes in receptive field organization of cat retinal ganglion cells when different rates of temporal modulation of the stimulus are used (Dawis, Shapley, Kaplan & Tranchina, 1984; Enroth-Cugell, Robson, Schweitzer-Tong & Watson, 1983) and to account for the elliptical shape of some receptive fields (Soodak, Shapley & Kaplan, 1987). Additionally, the DOG function has been successfully used to model receptive fields of both cat and monkey LGN X-cells (Derrington & Lennie, 1982, 1984) and the linear components of Y cell receptive fields.

Figure 6.1A shows the best-fitting DOG function to the measurements of contrast sensitivity (CS) as a function of spatial frequency (f) for an LGN neuron. The smooth curve is given by:

$$CS(f) = k_c \pi r_c^2 \exp(-(r_c f \pi)^2) - k_s \pi r_s^2 \exp(-(r_s f \pi)^2). \quad (1)$$

In this equation the space constants of the center and surround Gaussians are denoted by r_c and r_s, and the sensitivities are k_c and k_s, respectively. In the cat, some retinal and geniculate X cells have elliptical receptive field centers, requiring separate space constants for the major and minor axes of the ellipse (Soodak et al., 1987). At present it is not known if retinal or LGN P and M cells in the primate show significant deviation from radial symmetry, so we assume for the present that they are radial. However, it should be noted that if there is a single cone to midget ganglion cell connection for the center mechanism of neurons in the parvocellular pathway, for foveal and parafoveal vision, then radial symmetry is likely to be a good approximation.

Cortex

One of the first applications of modeling V1 receptive field shape came from the work of Campbell, Cooper, and Enroth-Cugell (1969). They applied an exponential function to the spatial frequency tuning curves of cat cortical cells. This function fit the high frequency limb of the spatial frequency tuning curve quite well but did not account for the sharpness of the low frequency cut-off. More recently, the Gabor function has been successfully applied to modeling cat V1 simple cells (Field & Tolhurst, 1986; Jones & Palmer, 1987; Marcelja, 1980). In the monkey the Gabor model fails to fit the contrast sensitivity curves of a significant number of V1 neurons (Hawken & Parker, 1987). Moreover, it does not reduce to a set of subunits that are easily related to the form of the geniculate input to V1. Since it has been shown, to a first approximation, that LGN receptive fields can be modeled by DOG functions, then it is straightforward to formalize the suggestion, originally made by Hubel and Wiesel (1962, 1968), that V1 simple cell receptive fields can be specified by an assembly of neighboring LGN neuron receptive fields.

Hawken and Parker (1987) constructed receptive fields from combinations of spatially offset DOG functions in the direction orthogonal to the preferred orientation and to model the sensitivity along the preferred orientation by a Gaussian sensitivity profile. Each subunit of the simple cell receptive field can be thought of as a row of DOG functions, and for each subunit, the size of the center and surround of each of the DOG's is constant. For neighboring subunits, the size of the center and surround may be different. This is a basic departure from the Gabor model in which the size of each subunit is explicitly the same, as defined by the frequency of the sinusoidal component.

For the difference of Gaussians with separation (d-DOG-s), as applied to the contrast sensitivity (CS) of V1 neurons as a function of the spatial frequency (f) of gratings of the preferred orientation, we have:

$$CS(f) = \{[A_{c_1} \exp(-(x_{c_1} \pi f)^2) - A_{s_1} \exp(-(x_{s_1} \pi f)^2)$$
$$- [A_{c_2} \exp(-(x_{c_2} \pi f)^2)$$
$$- A_{s_2} \exp(-(x_{s_2} \pi f)^2)] \cos(2\pi fS)]^2$$
$$+ ((1 - 2g)[A_{c_2} \exp(-(x_{c_2} \pi f)^2)$$
$$- A_{s_2} \exp(-(x_{s_2} \pi f)^2)] \sin(2\pi fS))^2\}^{1/2}, \quad (2)$$

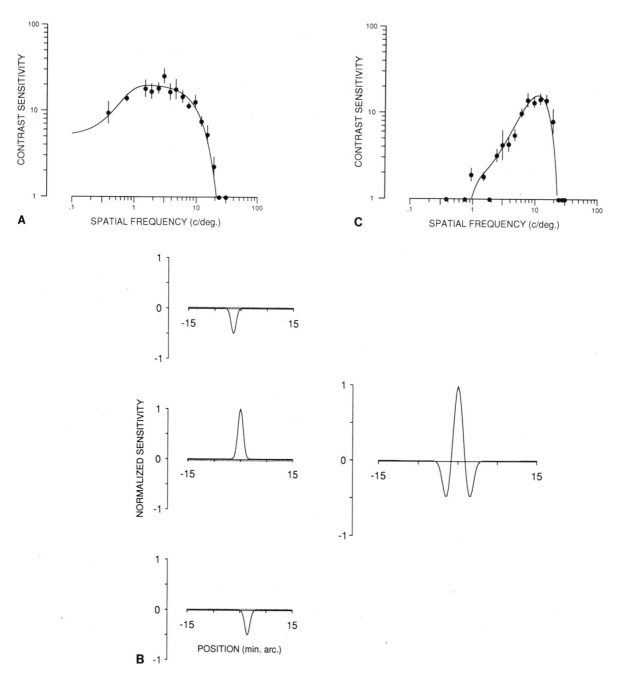

Fig. 6.1

(A) Spatial contrast sensitivity measurements of an M cell from the LGN of a juvenile cynomolgus monkey. The circles show the mean contrast sensitivity of the neuron derived from a staircase procedure based on 24 reversals. The error bars are ± 1 SD. The solid curve shows the best-fitting DOG function. Parameter values: $r_c = 1.57'$, $r_s = 26.8'$, $k_c = 9311$, $k_s = 23.7$ (Data from Hawken, Morley & Blakemore, unpublished). (B) Spatial components of the d-DOG-s model. The parameters are derived from the fit to the contrast sensitivity data shown in (C). The left-hand column shows the

individual Gaussian mechanisms; the top and bottom graphs show the flanking subunits, while the middle graph shows the central subunit. The right-hand graph shows the linear combination of the three subunits, to give the spatial profile of the receptive field. (C) Contrast sensitivity as a function of spatial frequency for a layer $4c\beta$ simple cell. The measures of contrast sensitivity and details are as for (A). The solid curves are the best-fitting version of the d-DOG-s model (equation 2) of receptive field organization whose parameters are: $x_{c_1} = 1.10'$, $x_{s_1} = 30.3'$, $x_{c_2} = 1.03'$, $x_{s_2} = 32.7'$, $A_{c_1} = 13.3$, $A_{s_1} = 15.9$, $A_{c_2} = 12.0$, $A_{s_2} = 14.6$, $g = 0.5$, and $S = 2.21'$.

where x_{c_1}, x_{c_2}, x_{s_1}, and x_{s_2} are the space constants of the Gaussians and A_{c_1}, A_{c_2}, A_{s_1}, and A_{s_2} control the sensitivity of the Gaussians. This equation is for a receptive field consisting of a central DOG mechanism (with parameters A_{c_1}, A_{s_1}, x_{c_1}, and x_{s_1}), and DOG mechanisms on either side (with parameters A_{c_2}, A_{s_2}, x_{c_2}, and x_{s_2}) separated from the center subunit by a distance S. The parameter g determines the surround symmetry. A value of $g = 0$ specifies an even symmetric receptive field, and a value of 1 specifies odd symmetry (Hawken & Parker, 1987).

Figure 6.1B shows the spatial arrangement of the individual Gaussian components of the d-DOG-s model, described by equation 2. Each individual subunit in the model is a DOG function, with the overall arrangement as described above. The values of the space constants of the Gaussians, the symmetry and separation parameters are derived from the best fit of equation 2 to the simple cell's contrast sensitivity data shown in figure 6.1C. The amplitude has been normalized. The top and bottom graphs of the left-hand column show the flanking subunits. Each has the same center space constant (x_{c_2}) of 1.0 min arc which is offset from the central subunit by the separation parameter ($S = 2.2$ min arc). For this fit the symmetry parameter (g) is $\frac{1}{2}$, so that the flanking subunits are equal in amplitude. The central subunit shown in the middle left graph is centered at the origin, its center Gaussian has a space constant (x_{c_1}) of 1.1 min arc. The surround space constant of the center subunit (x_{s_1}) is 30 min arc, which is almost the same value as that returned for the surround space constant of the flanking subunits (x_{s_2}). The surrounds are shown by the low-amplitude dotted Gaussians in each of the left-hand graphs. For this cell the surrounds effectively cancel each other, consequently neither makes a substantial contribution to the overall fit. However, for contrast sensitivity functions from other cells, especially where the low-frequency attenuation is relatively steep, the surround of each subunit is essential in producing a good fit. The linear combination of the three subunits gives the overall spatial weighting of the receptive field orthogonal to the preferred orientation, which is shown in the right-hand graph.

Figure 6.1C shows an example of the d-DOG-s function fitted to the spatial contrast sensitivity data of a layer 4 simple cell. Note that in this particular case, the dimensions of either of the DOGs that make up the V1 receptive field could almost be taken directly from the spatial

weighting of the LGN neuron's receptive field that is shown in figure 6.1A. Both cells were recorded within $0.5°$ from the fovea. The sensitivity of the subunits of the DOG and d-DOG-s models can be related by their point weighting sensitivities. For the d-DOG-s the integrated sensitivity of the center Gaussian mechanism A_{c_1} (i.e., the total volume under that Gaussian) is given by:

$$A_{c_1} = k_{c_1} \pi x_{c_1} y_h \tag{3}$$

where k_{c_1} is the point weighting and y_h is the space constant of the height Gaussian (Parker & Hawken, 1988). The sensitivities of the individual mechanisms for LGN and V1 receptive fields can be compared by their point weighting amplitudes.

Receptive Fields and the Cone Mosaic

It has been argued earlier that the cone mosaic could provide a standard spatial scale against which the size and spatial distribution of receptive fields at different levels of the visual pathway can be evaluated. The number and size of foveal and parafoveal cone photoreceptors are similar in different species of macaque monkeys and in man. The main difference between macaques and man is in eye size and consequently the number of microns on the retina per degree of visual angle. For the standard human eye, the retinal distance for $1°$ is 291 μm, while for the cynomolgus monkey it is only 201 μm. Photoreceptors 3 μm in diameter in the foveolar region would subtend 37 sec arc in man and 53 sec arc in the cynomolgus monkey. Assuming a regular packing of cones, with 3 μm center-to-center spacing in a hexagonal array for both species, the Nyquist sampling frequency for humans would be 83 cycles/degree and for cynomolgus monkey 58 cycles/degree. Under normal viewing conditions, however, the Nyquist frequencies are seldom reached because the optics of the eye low-pass filter the image. The cut-off frequency of the optics in the human eye is around 60 cycles/degree (Campbell & Green, 1965; Campbell & Gubisch, 1966).

A major consequence of the external image passing through the optics is a substantial reduction in the image contrast on the retina, especially for high spatial frequency components of the image. The contrast attenuation can be expressed in terms of the spatial frequency modulation transfer function (MTF) of the optics. The MTF of the human eye depends on a variety of factors (Campbell & Gubisch, 1966). Since we are attempting to establish a relationship between receptive field dimensions and the cone mosaic, we need to determine the receptive field dimensions when projected onto the retina. Experimentally, measurements were made through the optics and, therefore, any estimates of contrast sensitivity include a component that is due to the optical MTF. In the following section, we describe the measurements of receptive field dimensions by fitting the DOG and d-DOG-s models to contrast sensitivity data expressed in terms of retinal contrast. After that the cone mosaic is discussed and then the relationship between the cone spacing and the receptive fields is considered.

Receptive Field Structure

To estimate the substructure of the receptive fields in monkey geniculate or V1, the DOG or d-DOG-s model is applied to the spatial contrast sensitivity function (see under Models). Contrast sensitivity, rather than response at a fixed contrast, is measured across different spatial frequencies so that the cell's output is maintained around a constant mean level of response, in the linear region of the contrast response function. This reduces the likelihood of changes in gain or saturation contributing to the measurements, therefore eliminating a potential output nonlinearity that might distort an otherwise linear response. Another advantage of contrast threshold as an indicator of response is that it becomes relatively simple to account for the purely optical contribution to a neuron's spatial frequency tuning. During an experiment, the actual retinal contrast required to bring the cell to a criterion response, for each spatial frequency, is the external stimulus contrast attenuated by the optical MTF. For low spatial frequencies there is little optical attenuation, and the stimulus and retinal contrasts are almost identical. However, at higher frequencies there is a significant reduction in the image contrast at the retina.

Effective retinal contrast can be determined by correcting for the optical attenuation. The best estimates of the MTF available are for the human eye (Campbell & Green, 1965; Campbell & Gubisch, 1966), so we assume that this provides an adequate model for the Old World monkey eye. To calculate the retinal contrast as a function of

spatial frequency, for a 3-mm pupil and 570-nm light, data from the normalized MTF of the human eye from Campbell and Gubisch (1966) was used. The retinal contrast sensitivity is then the measured contrast sensitivity divided by the optical MTF. Figure 6.2A shows retinal contrast sensitivity (filled squares) for the same neuron whose stimulus contrast sensitivity values were shown in figure 6.1A. The spatial contrast sensitivity measures were obtained by using a threshold tracking procedure (Derrington & Lennie, 1982; Hawken & Parker, 1987). The best-fitting DOG function was obtained by minimizing the squared logarithmic error using a nonlinear minimization routine (E04VDF) from the Numerical Algorithms Group library. The lower curve in figure 6.2A is the DOG function from figure 6.1A, while the upper curve is that estimated by fitting the retinal contrast sensitivity data. The major difference between external stimulus sensitivity and retinal sensitivity is seen at the higher spatial frequencies where the two curves diverge. This is reflected by the parameters of the DOG's center Gaussian, which dominates the high frequency limb of the spatial contrast sensitivity function. The value of r_c for external stimulus contrast sensitivity data is 1.57 min arc while r_c for the retinal contrast sensitivity data is 0.95 min arc, corresponding to 5.2 μm and 3.1 μm on the retina, respectively. The point sensitivity (k_c) from the retinal data is more than three times that for the external sensitivity data.

This difference is significant because the retinal measure reflects the performance of the neural elements supporting sensitivity to contrast. As noted psychophysically by Campbell and Green (1965), this becomes especially important when attempting to make comparisons between the sensitivities of the center and surround components of the DOG function, because these components have different spatial frequency performance. As a consequence, for a standard receptive field with center and surround mechanisms, the only region of spatial frequency in which the performance of the center mechanism can be determined is exactly that region which is most affected by the optical factors. At low frequencies, where the optics affect contrast sensitivity rather less, the cell's response is a mixture of factors from the center and the surround.

Figure 6.2B illustrates the retinal contrast sensitivity for the simple cell whose external sensitivity data are shown

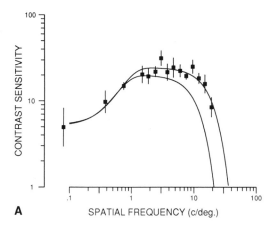

A

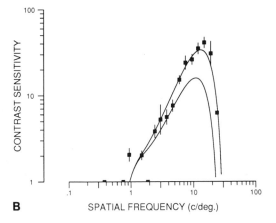

B

Fig. 6.2

(A, B) Contrast sensitivity as a function of spatial frequency for the same data as shown in figure 6.1; here the sensitivity is shown in terms of retinal contrast. At high spatial frequencies there are substantial effects of optical attenuation on the contrast sensitivity estimates. The upper curves in both graphs are the best fitting versions of the DOG and d-DOG-s models fitted to the data points, while the lower curves are those shown in figure 6.1 and shown here for comparison. The parameters for (A) are: $r_c = 0.95'$, $r_s = 22.2'$, $k_c = 30980$, $k_s = 44.6$; and for (B): $x_{c_1} = 1.0'$, $x_{s_1} = 30.9'$, $x_{c_2} = 0.91'$, $x_{s_2} = 34.6'$, $A_{c_1} = 29.4$, $A_{s_1} = 10.7$, $A_{c_2} = 28.4$, $A_{s_2} = 9.1$, $g = 0.5$, and $S = 1.80'$.

in Figure 6.1C. The fitted function is the best-fitting version of the d-DOG-s model to the retinal sensitivity data. As expected, the major difference is seen at the higher spatial frequencies. But for this example a comparison of the parameters for each of the component mechanisms shows that there is a modest reduction in the center space constants of the opposing mechanisms, with most of the difference accounted for by a substantial increase in the

sensitivity of each of the mechanisms. See the figure legends for the values of each of the parameters. To check the uniqueness of the amplitude parameters in the d-DOG-s fit to the retinal contrast sensitivity data, we evaluated the error for a range of values of A_{c_1}, A_{s_1}, A_{c_2}, A_{s_2}, from 10 to 45. The error only reached the global minimum at amplitude values of around 30, indicating that the increased contrast sensitivity of the Gaussian mechanisms is required to produce a good fit to the data.

Cone Density

There are a number of recent reports of the variation in cone density within and between species of primates, including man (Curcio, Sloan, Kalina & Hendrickson, 1990; Curcio, Sloan, Packer, Hendrickson & Kalina, 1987; Hawken, Perry & Parker, 1988; Perry & Cowey, 1985). This variability, which can be substantial, must be taken into account when relating receptive field substructure to the spatial grain defined by the underlying cone mosaic. Within the macaques, commonly used for physiological studies, there are reports of differences in cone density between different species (Perry & Cowey, 1985), although it is not yet clear whether these differences are significant for foveal and parafoveal regions alone or over the whole retina. Some of the more recent investigations report the peak foveal cone density of *Macaca mulatta* (rhesus monkey) to be in the range of 150,000 to 220,000 mm^{-2} (Perry & Cowey, 1985) and of *Macaca nemestrina* (pigtail macaque) to be 170,000 to 250,000 mm^{-2} (Packer, Hendrickson & Curcio, 1989). For *Macaca fascicularis* (cynomolgus macaque) reports give peak density ranges of 110,000 to 145,000 mm^{-2} (Perry & Cowey, 1985), 200,000 mm^{-2} (Schein, 1988), and 150,000 to 250,000 mm^{-2} (Wässle et al., 1989). However, the exact values of peak density depend, to some extent, on the size of the sampling window. This can be especially significant at the foveal pit, where the density is changing fastest. For example, Perry and Cowey (1985) used a 90 μm by 90 μm grid for their samples; 90 μm corresponds to just less than 30 min arc on the retina in *Macaca fascicularis*. In the foveal region there are significant changes in photoreceptor density at a smaller scale than 30 min arc (see Curcio et al., 1990). Therefore, foveal estimates will be blurred by using a relatively large sampling window.

There is also growing evidence of substantial variability in the peak density and distribution of foveal cones within a single species. When comparing the cone density of eight human eyes, Curcio and coworkers (1990) found significant variability between individuals, a factor of 3.3 in density. Although there is individual variation at the fovea, the cone density in the parafovea and near periphery is uniform across individuals. Since most of our physiological studies were in the cynomolgus macaque, we initially set out to produce a standard cone density distribution.

The cone density was measured from the foveal pit along the horizontal meridian in temporal retina from eight eyes from seven *Macaca fascicularis*. In one animal the cone density was measured in both eyes, and is shown in Figure 6.3A. There is very little difference between the two eyes from the fovea out to 64° in the temporal retina. However, when the cone densities of different individuals are compared (Figure 6.3B), there can be significant variation in the foveal counts. In both parafoveal and peripheral retina there is relatively little individual variation when comparison is made along the temporal region of the horizontal meridian. It is well established that there are differences in density between nasal and temporal retina, although it is not clear that these are seen in the foveal region (Perry & Cowey, 1985; Curcio et al., 1987, 1990).

To obtain an accurate estimate of the number of cones underlying each receptive field subunit in the foveal region it is necessary to measure the cone density and the receptive field dimensions in the same animal. This is the case because the variation in cone spacing found in the foveal region is as large as 2.45, even when considered in linear terms as opposed to areal measures. This is certainly important when considering the relationship between receptive field center size and cone spacing for the smallest receptive fields. However, the range of densities of the six retinae for which we had counts at 2° was only a factor of 1.4, a linear variation of 1.2. Similar values for five retinae at 4° were found; the linear difference in the range was again 1.2. Densities in parafoveal retina seem much less prone to individual variation and even in the perifovea there is a reasonably small variation.

Mapping Receptive Fields onto Cones

The consequence of foveal variability in cone density is that the exact distribution of cones underlying each re-

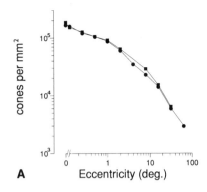

A

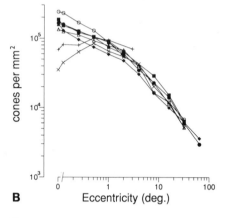

B

Fig. 6.3

(A) The density of cones in the temporal retina from the left and right eyes of an adult cynomolgus monkey. The densities across all eccentricities are closely matched between the two eyes. The counts were obtained from photomicrographs of flat-mounted retinae, cleared with DMSO, and viewed through Nomarski optics. (B) The cone density plotted against eccentricity for eight eyes from *M. fascicularis*. Counts were made from photographs of the retinal mosaic like the one shown in figure 6.4. It can be seen that there is considerable variation between animals over the central retina but quite similar densities in the parafovea and periphery. The highest foveal cone density predicts a Nyquist limit of 62 cycles/degree, while the lowest predicts 20 cycles/degree. For some of the flatmounts we only had the central area available for counting while in others there were certain positions where the quality of the preparation was not sufficiently well visualized to be able to make clear photographs.

ceptive field needs to be evaluated on an individual basis for neurons with central receptive fields. For example, after correcting for some of the optical attenuation, the space constants of the center mechanisms (r_c for LGN cells; x_{c_1} and x_{c_2} for cortical cells) of the two neurons illustrated in figure 6.2, when projected onto the retina are 3.2, 3.4, and 3.1 μm respectively. The full width (2 standard deviations of the center Gaussian) of these

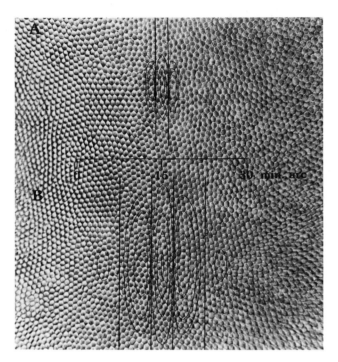

Fig. 6.4

(A, B) Contour plots of the two-dimensional sensitivity profiles of two simple cells from layer 4c of V1. To gain an impression of the relationship between the receptive field and the underlying cone distribution the contours have been reproduced on acetate sheet and overlaid onto a photomicrograph of cone inner segments at 0.5° from the fovea (from a different animal). The cone density in the photograph matches the average cone density determined at 0.5° from the eight eyes in figure 6.2. Both the receptive field plots and the photograph are at the same scale.

mechanisms would be 6 to 7 μm on the retina. This can be compared with the cone spacing at the same eccentricity. From figure 6.3 the range of center-to-center spacings is 3.0 to 5.0 μm, so each of the mechanisms could be 1 to 2 cone diameters.

This point is further illustrated in figure 6.4A, where the two-dimensional spatial profiles of two layer 4 cells are overlaid onto a cone mosaic. Each of the flanking subfield centers also covers 1 to 2 cones across their width. However, without knowledge of the chromatic properties of this receptive field's subregions it is not possible to decide if the input comes from a single cone type or if there is a dual input (red and green). Thus, the variation in cone spacing means that for a more exact match the measures need to be made in the same animal.

Mapping Cones onto V1

The relationship between cone density and the visuotopic map of V1 also allows us to consider the dimensions of receptive fields in terms of possible geniculocortical and intracortical connections. Anatomical studies show that the afferent arborization of single LGN P cells, in layer 4cβ of V1, is restricted to a single eye dominance column, while some LGN M cell afferents branch to give terminal arbors, in layer 4cα, which span two or three neighboring ocular dominance columns from the same eye (Blasdel & Lund, 1983). The orderliness and degree of overlap of the visuotopic representation for neighboring regions of V1 presumably depend, to some extent, on which cortical layer is being considered. On both physiological and anatomical grounds, it would be expected that the P cell to layer 4cβ pathway would show a finer spatial grain than the M cell to layer 4cα pathway. However, it should be noted that even at this early stage in cortical processing, there is some overlap of afferent arbors from the P cell and M cell pathways around the 4cα/4cβ border, giving rise to the possibility of mixed input to some cells in this region.

For the simple cell shown in figure 6.4A, the number of cones along the length of the receptive field is between 10 and 12, if the border is set by the outer contour, or between 6 and 8 cones, if the border is the middle contour. The cell was recorded in layer 4cβ and its field was located at 0.5° from the fovea. Figure 6.5 shows that the number of cones across a single eye dominance column at 0.5° eccentricity is between 6 and 9. If this simple cell's receptive field is constructed by summation of P cell inputs along its length, each of which has a single cone center mechanism, then the anatomical wiring required to achieve this organization could be derived from within a single eye dominance column (LeVay, Connolly, Houde & van Essen, 1985). Similarly, by taking a horizontal section through the center of the receptive field shown in figure 6.4A, it can be seen that the outer borders of the flanking subregions of this cell are 5 to 7 cones apart. So, the intracortical connections that would be necessary to account for the full two-dimensional spatial extent of this receptive field fall within the limits of a single eye dominance column.

In contrast, both the length and the width of the simple cell's receptive field, which is illustrated in figure 6.4B,

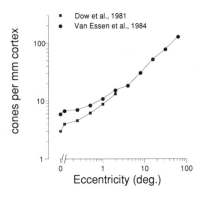

Fig. 6.5

The number of cones mapped onto each millimeter of cortex in monkey V1 is shown for eccentricities out to 64°. The estimates, which were made using the cortical magnification factor determined by Dow, Snyder, Vautin and Bauer (1981), are shown by the filled squares, while the data derived using the magnification factor of van Essen, Newsome and Maunsell (1984) are shown by the filled circles. It should be noted that the magnification factor regression equation of van Essen *et al.* was obtained from measurements made outside the central 2.5°, so that values for central retina are extrapolated.

exceed the estimated number of cones across a single eye dominance column by a factor of 3 or more. This simple cell was recorded in layer 4cα, again at an eccentricity of 0.5°. The limits of the visuotopic representation within layer 4cα are complicated by two main factors. Firstly, the receptive field centers of LGN M cells, the predominant input to 4cα, are larger than those of the P cells projecting to 4cβ (Derrington & Lennie, 1984) and their coverage factor is unknown. Secondly, each M cell can branch to give an input to neighboring eye dominance columns. Since the magnitude of the effect of these factors on the precision of the visuotopic map in layer 4cα is unknown, then the limits of the anatomical connections required to account for the receptive field in figure 6.4B can not be specified.

There is substantial evidence for lateral intra-cortical connections between neighboring hypercolumns in V1 (Lund, 1989), providing an anatomical basis for the generation of receptive fields where the spatial extent is greater than the visuotopic representation in a single eye dominance column. However, as discussed above, both the scatter of anatomical connections and the range of receptive field sizes of the input neurons are critical factors in linking cortical anatomy to functional receptive field organization. So, to extend the links between recep-

tive field structure and anatomical circuits within V1, we require a visuotopic map of each major layer and sublayer in conjunction with the cone density and receptive field structure.

Acknowledgments

The research was supported by grant 7900491 to C. Blakemore from the MRC, NATO grant 85/0167, Wellcome Trust major equipment grant and USAF grant AFOSR-85-0296.

References

Blasdel, G. G. & Lund, J. S. (1983). Termination of afferent axons in macaque striate cortex. *Journal of Neuroscience, 3*, 1389–1413.

Campbell, F. W. & Green, D. G. (1965). Optical and retinal factors affecting resolution. *Journal of Physiology, 181*, 576–593.

Campbell, F. W. & Gubisch, R. W. (1966). Optical quality of the human eye. *Journal of Physiology, 186*, 558–578.

Campbell, F. W., Cooper, G. F. & Enroth-Cugell, C. (1969). The spatial selectivity of visual cells in the cat. *Journal of Physiology, 203*, 223–235.

Connolly, M. & van Essen, D. C. (1984). The representation of the visual field in parvocellular and magnocellular laminae of the lateral geniculate nucleus of the macaque monkey. *Journal of Comparative Neurology, 171*, 544–564.

Curcio, C. A., Sloan, K. R., Kalina, R. E. & Hendrickson, A. E. (1990). Human photoreceptor topography. *Journal of Comparative Neurology, 292*, 497–523.

Curcio, C. A., Sloan, K. R., Packer, O., Hendrickson, A. E. & Kalina, R. E. (1987). Distribution of cones in human and monkey retina: Individual variability and radial asymmetry. *Science, 236*, 579–582.

Dawis, S., Shapley, R. M., Kaplan, E. & Tranchina, D. (1984). The receptive field organization of X-cells in the cat: Spatiotemporal coupling and asymmetry. *Vision Research, 24*, 549–564.

Derrington, A. M. & Lennie, P. (1982). The influence of temporal frequency and adaptation level on receptive field organization of retinal ganglion cells in the cat. *Journal of Physiology, 333*, 343–366.

Derrington, A. M. & Lennie, P. (1984). Spatial and temporal contrast sensitivities of neurones in the lateral geniculate nucleus of the macaque. *Journal of Physiology, 357*, 219–240.

DeValois, R. L., Albrecht, D. G. & Thorell, L. G. (1982). Spatial frequency selectivity of cells in the macaque visual cortex. *Vision Research, 22*, 545–559.

Dow, B. M., Snyder, A. W., Vautin, R. G. & Bauer, R. (1981). Magnification factor and receptive field size in foveal striate cortex of the monkey. *Experimental Brain Research, 44*, 213−228.

Enroth-Cugell, C. & Robson, J. G. (1966). The contrast sensitivity of the retinal ganglion cells of the cat. *Journal of Physiology, 187*, 517−552.

Enroth-Cugell, C. & Robson, J. G. (1984). Functional characteristics and diversity of cat retinal ganglion cells. *Investigative Ophthalmology and Visual Science, 25*, 250−267.

Enroth-Cugell, C., Robson, J. G., Schweitzer-Tong, D. E. & Watson, A. B. (1983). Spatiotemporal interactions in cat retinal ganglion cells showing linear spatial summation. *Journal of Physiology, 341*, 279−307.

Field, D. J. & Tolhurst, D. J. (1986). The structure and symmetry of simple-cell receptive-field profiles in the cat's visual cortex. *Proceedings of the Royal Society B, 228*, 379−400.

Hawken, M. J. & Parker, A. J. (1987). Spatial properties of neurons in monkey striate cortex. *Proceedings of the Royal Society B, 231*, 251−288.

Hawken, M. J., Perry, V. H. & Parker, A. J. (1988). Structural relationship of photoreceptors to V1 receptive fields in the primate. *Investigative Ophthalmology and Visual Science, 29* (Suppl.), 297.

Hubel, D. H. & Wiesel, T. N. (1962). Receptive fields, binocular interaction and functional architecture in cat's visual cortex. *Journal of Physiology, 160*, 106−154.

Hubel, D. H. & Wiesel, T. N. (1968). Receptive fields and functional architecture of monkey striate cortex. *Journal of Physiology, 195*, 215−243.

Jones, J. P. & Palmer, L. A. (1987). An evaluation of the two dimensional Gabor filter model of simple receptive fields in cat striate cortex. *Journal of Neurophysiology, 57*, 1233−1258.

Kaplan, E. & Shapley, R. M. (1982). X & Y cells in the lateral geniculate nucleus of macaque monkeys. *Journal of Physiology, 330*, 125−143.

LeVay, S., Connolly, M., Houde, J. & van Essen, D. C. (1985). The complete patterns of ocular dominance stripes in the striate cortex and visual field of the macaque monkey. *Journal of Neuroscience, 5*, 486−501.

Lund, J. S. (1989). Excitatory and inhibitory circuitry and laminar mapping strategies in primary visual cortex of the monkey. In Edelman, G. M., Gall, W. E. & Cowan, M. W. (Eds.), *Signal and Sense: Local and Global Order in Perceptual Maps.* New York: John Wiley & Sons.

Marcelja, S. (1980). Mathematical description of the responses of simple cortical cells. *Journal of the Optical Society of America A, 2*, 1297−1300.

Packer, O., Hendrickson, A. E. & Curcio, C. A. (1989). Photoreceptor topography of the adult pigtail macaque (Macaca nemestrina) retina. *Journal of Comparative Neurology, 288*, 165−183.

Parker, A. J. & Hawken, M. J. (1988). Two-dimensional spatial structure of receptive fields in the monkey striate cortex. *Journal of the Optical Society of America A, 5*, 598−605.

Perry, V. H. & Cowey, A. (1985). The ganglion cell and cone distributions in the monkey's retina: Implications for central magnification factors. *Vision Research, 25*, 1795−1810.

Perry, V. H. & Cowey, A. (1988). The lengths of the fibres of Henle in the retina of macaque monkeys: Implications for vision. *Neuroscience, 25*, 225−236.

Rodieck, R. W. (1965). Quantitative analysis of cat retinal ganglion cell response to visual stimulation. *Vision Research, 5*, 583−601.

Schein, S. J. (1988). Anatomy of macaque fovea and spatial densities of neurons in foveal representation. *Journal of Comparative Neurology, 269*, 479−505.

Shapley, R. M. (1990). Visual sensitivity and parallel retinocortical channels. *Annual Review of Psychology, 41*, 635−658.

Soodak, R. E., Shapley, R. M. & Kaplan, E. (1987). Linear mechanisms of orientation tuning in the retina and lateral geniculate nucleus of the cat. *Journal of Neurophysiology, 58*, 267−275.

van Essen, D. C., Newsome, W. T. & Maunsell, J. H. R. (1984). The visual field representation in striate cortex of macaque monkey: Asymmetries, anisotropies, and individual variability. *Vision Research, 24*, 429−448.

Wässle, H., Grünert, U., Röhrenbeck, J. and Boycott, B. B. (1989). Cortical magnification factor and the ganglion cell density of primate retina. *Nature, 341*, 643−646.

Wiesel, T. N. & Hubel, D. H. (1966). Spatial and chromatic interactions in the lateral geniculate body of the rhesus monkey. *Journal of Neurophysiology, 29*, 1115−1156.

7

Neural Contrast Sensitivity

Andrew B. Watson

As we worry away at the puzzle of vision, we collect clues from many sources, such as psychophysics, anatomy, electrophysiology, and mathematical theory. In the area of electrophysiology, recordings are made from individual neurons as the retina is exposed to light. A fundamental way of characterizing a particular neuron, or class of neurons, is in terms of its sensitivity to some aspect of the distribution of light. For example, a neuron may respond preferentially to a particular band of wavelengths or to a particular area of the visual field. A systematic study of the responsiveness of a neuron to the full range of light distributions would appear to be the way to fully understand the cell. The problem is that this range is infinite, while our experimental time is very finite. A solution to this quandary is available if the neuron is linear. A linear neuron obeys the laws of superposition and homogeneity, which state respectively that the response to a sum of stimuli is the sum of the responses to the individual stimuli, and that the response to an amplified stimulus is an equally amplified response. When a neuron is linear, it suffices to measure sensitivity to a finite number of stimuli and, from those measurements, to deduce all others. The sort of measurements that are typically taken are sensitivities to sinusoids of various frequencies, and the collection of such measures has become known as a *contrast sensitivity function*. To characterize sensitivity to spatial patterns, these should be sinusoids over space; to temporal patterns, sinusoids over time; to both space and time, sinusoidal modulation in both space and time.

The measurement of contrast sensitivity functions is most common in psychophysics but has more recently been applied to individual visual neurons. When applied to a neuron, it may give some insight into the role of that neuron in the visual process. For example, a neuron that responds selectively to motion in one direction might be thought to play a role in the sensing of motion. A second reason for interest in neural contrast sensitivity is that it may give some insight into which neurons are connected to which others. In this way, contrast sensitivity can assist anatomical observations. A third reason for interest is that estimates of neural contrast sensitivity may help us to understand the sensitivity of the human observer.

The goal of this chapter is to set forth some elementary theoretical principles that govern the contrast sensitivity of individual neurons. This will be done in the context of a simple model of the linear visual neuron and of networks of such neurons. I hope that the reader will come away with a basic understanding of the problem and with a few useful tools. The chapter is organized in three parts. The first sketches a picture of the neuron as a linear system and introduces the quantities contrast gain, noise, and contrast sensitivity. It further describes how these quantities are revealed in a typical electrophysiological experiment. The second part considers a visual pathway consisting of layers of linear neurons feeding signal and noise from one layer to the next. Formulas are derived that show how sensitivity is altered as one passes through the various levels of the network. The third part applies these principles to the prediction of cortical contrast sensitivity from the sensitivity of parvocellular lateral geniculate nucleus (LGN) neurons. The presentation here is intended to be brief and general; additional details are available elsewhere (Watson, 1990, 1991). I assume that the reader is familiar with elementary linear systems theory and Fourier transforms (Bracewell, 1978) and with the basics of probability and random processes (Papoulis, 1965).

The Neuron as a Linear System

Receptive Fields, Impulse Responses, and Transfer Functions

A visual neuron collects light over some region of space and time, subjects the collected signal to some spatial and temporal processing, and generates an electrical response. For a linear neuron it is possible to completely characterize this input-output relation by means of the spatiotemporal *receptive field*. This is ordinarily written as a function $f(\mathbf{x}, t)$ of two spatial and one time dimensions, which expresses the contribution of contrast at each point in space and time to the response of a neuron at location [0, 0] at time 0. An equivalent characterization is provided by the *spectral receptive field* $F(\mathbf{u}, w)$, where $\mathbf{u}$ is a spatial frequency vector in cycles/degree and w is temporal frequency in Hertz. The spectral receptive field is the Fourier transform of the receptive field, and it specifies the amplitude and phase of the response evoked by sinusoidal modulations of particular spatial and temporal frequency.

Mathematically, it is often more convenient to work with the *impulse response* of the neuron, which is simply the reflection of the receptive field, $h(\mathbf{x}, t) = f(-\mathbf{x}, -t)$. This has a Fourier transform $H(\mathbf{u}, w)$ that is called the *transfer function* of the neuron. The *contrast gain* of the neuron is the modulus of the transfer function

$$G(\mathbf{u}, w) = |H(\mathbf{u}, w)|. \qquad (1)$$

It specifies the magnitude of the response to a sinusoid of unit contrast when drifted across the receptive field (Enroth-Cugell, Robson, Schweitzer-Tong & Watson, 1983). It also specifies the slope of the contrast-response function (Kaplan & Shapley, 1986). It is measured in units of impulse $\sec^{-1}$ (we omit the dimensionless unit of contrast).

Contrast gain would appear to be a good measure of the sensitivity of a neuron to spatial and temporal contrast, and indeed it has been the most widely used measure. But it fails to represent the noisiness of the response, and therefore cannot tell us whether the neuron can detect a particular signal. Contrast sensitivity, on the other hand, is a measure of the ability of the neuron (or an observer) to detect contrast. To relate the sensitivity of neurons and observers, it is clear that we need a neural measure of contrast sensitivity, since there is no way to measure contrast gain from the performance of an observer.

Neural Contrast Sensitivity

How might we measure the ability of a neuron to detect contrast? Fortunately, this question has been answered for us by several authors (Derrington & Lennie, 1982, 1984; Hawken & Parker, 1984; Troy, 1983a). The basic idea is to find, for a particular spatial and temporal frequency, the contrast that produces a response that just exceeds the noise. In what follows, we will formalize this idea and show how it leads to a specific expression for neural contrast sensitivity.

What measure shall we take of the response of the neuron? If the signal is at temporal frequency w Hz, then the linear response must also be at w Hz. It is therefore sensible to measure the amplitude of the response at w Hz. To do this, we first collect a record of duration T sec.

While not essential, we assume that the record is sampled into bins of some brief duration. Each bin count is divided by the bin duration to give a measure of instantaneous rate in imp sec^{-1}. Each record is then multiplied, sample by sample, by a cosine function of temporal frequency w Hz. The resulting sequence is added up, and divided by $\sqrt{T}$ to produce a cosine term c. The process is repeated with a sinusoid to produce a sine term s. The two terms are squared and added, and the square root is taken, to yield a single amplitude measure.

Note that this same quantity can be used to measure noise-alone responses, obtained when the stimulus contrast is zero, and signal + noise responses to non-zero stimulus contrast. At what contrast will the signal + noise response exceed the noise-alone response? Because of variability, this question can only be answered probabilistically, in the context of the distributions of signal + noise and noise-alone responses. To derive these distributions, we must adopt a model for the variability or noise in the neuron.

We model the noise in the response of each neuron as a stationary random process: roughly speaking, a random variable that is a function of time. By "stationary" we mean that its statistical properties do not vary over time. The reader is referred to Papoulis (1965) for a complete introduction to random processes. This random process is characterized by a power spectral density $N(w)$. The power spectral density is a measure of the amount of noise at each temporal frequency w, in units of imp^2 sec^{-2} Hz^{-1}.

In the context of this noise model, what are the distributions of noise-alone and signal + noise responses? First, consider distributions of sine and cosine coefficients, c and s. We assume that each coefficient has a normal distribution. This is plausible, given that each is a linear combination of identically distributed random variables. Because the phase of the noise component is random, the two coefficients are independent. Time stationarity implies that the two coefficients have equal variance σ^2. For mathematical convenience, we normalize the individual sine and cosine terms by their common standard deviation, σ. These normalized sine and cosine coefficients are

then independent, normally distributed random variables with unit variance. To obtain the normalized amplitude, we take the square root of the sum of their squares

$$y = \frac{1}{\sigma}\sqrt{c^2 + s^2}. \tag{2}$$

This normalized amplitude has a probability density function,

$$f_y(y) = y \exp\left(\frac{-y^2 - \eta^2}{2}\right) I_0(y\eta) U(y), \tag{3}$$

where $I_0(\ )$ is the modified Bessel function of order 0, and $U(\ )$ is the unit step function[1] (Papoulis, 1965, p. 196). The parameter η is the square root of the sum of the squared normalized means of the distributions of s and c.

What are these means? Suppose that the signal has contrast r. Then the deterministic response will be

$$a \cos[2\pi wt] + b \sin[2\pi wt], \tag{4}$$

where

$$a^2 + b^2 = r^2 G^2(\mathbf{u}, w), \tag{5}$$

where $G(\mathbf{u}, w)$ is the contrast gain defined in equation 1. Multiplying this response by sine and cosine functions, integrating, and dividing by $\sqrt{T}$, we get sine and cosine terms of $a\sqrt{T}/2$ and $b\sqrt{T}/2$. Since the noise is additive, these coefficients will be the mean coefficients when noise is present. Thus the parameter η of the normalized amplitude density is equal to

$$\eta = \frac{\sqrt{T}}{2\sigma}\sqrt{a^2 + b^2} = r\frac{\sqrt{T}}{2\sigma}G(\mathbf{u}, w). \tag{6}$$

This expression tells us what distribution of amplitudes will result from any particular contrast r. When $r = 0$, it yields the density for noise-alone. We can now answer the question posed earlier: What contrast will produce a response just greater than noise. But we must be a little more precise about what we mean by "just greater." Here we make use of signal detection theory. We wish to establish a criterion amplitude λ that will distinguish signal from noise. To do this we establish a false alarm rate, p_f,

---

1. When $\eta = 0$, this is a Rayleigh density, or a Chi density with 2 degrees of freedom. When $\eta \neq 0$, it is the square root of a noncentral Chi square with 2 degrees of freedom.

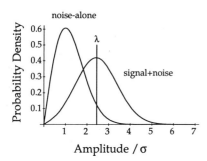

Fig. 7.1
Distributions of amplitude for noise-alone and signal + noise when the signal is at threshold. The false alarm rate is $p_f = 0.05$, and the hit rate is $p_h = 0.5$.

specifying the probability that noise-alone responses will exceed the criterion. A typical example is $p_f = 0.05$. Then the criterion can be easily obtained by evaluating at p_f the inverse cumulative distribution for noise-alone responses.

Then we choose a hit rate p_h, specifying with what probability we wish the signal responses to exceed the criterion λ. A typical example is $p_h = 0.5$. Then we must find the value of the parameter η that will push a fraction p_h of the signal + noise density over the criterion λ. This may be accomplished through iterative techniques. The resulting situation is pictured in Figure 7.1.

This situation is one example of what we mean by the signal "just exceeding" the noise. There are other situations, however, characterized by different values of p_f and p_h, that we might equally well take as specifying "threshold." What is important in each situation is the value of the parameter η, which we may therefore think of as a performance parameter. For a particular value, we can derive an expression for the contrast required to achieve this threshold. The inverse of this contrast is our definition of contrast sensitivity. Rearranging equation 6 we find

$$\frac{1}{r} = \frac{\sqrt{T}G(\mathbf{u}, w)}{2\eta\sigma}. \tag{7}$$

Finally, we introduce a relationship between the variance of the sine and cosine coefficients, and the power spectral density. When the measurement interval T is reasonably long, it can be shown that

$$\sigma^2 = \frac{1}{2}N(w), \tag{8}$$

where w is the signal frequency (Papoulis, 1965; Watson,

Table 7.1
Values of the performance parameter η for the yes/no procedure for various hit and false alarm rates

		False alarm	
		0.05	0.10
Hit	0.5	2.226	1.886
	0.75	2.931	2.602

1990). Combining equations 7 and 8, we arrive at a final expression for contrast sensitivity which we now write explicitly as a function of spatial and temporal frequency,

$$C(\mathbf{u}, w) = \frac{\sqrt{T}G(\mathbf{u}, w)}{\sqrt{2\eta}\sqrt{N(w)}}. \tag{9}$$

We see that contrast sensitivity is essentially a signal to noise ratio. For future reference, table 7.1 provides values of η for several hit and false alarm rates.

The method of estimating neural contrast sensitivity that I have described may be likened to a "yes/no" method in psychophysics. Another method, analogous to forced choice, can also be derived, along with appropriate values of η (Watson, 1990).

To summarize this section, I have derived the distribution of amplitude estimates for an arbitrary contrast, including zero contrast. I then made use of elementary concepts from signal detection theory to define a detection threshold for the neuron. This allowed me to derive an expression for contrast sensitivity (the inverse of threshold contrast) in terms of contrast gain, noise power spectrum, duration of measurement, and a parameter reflecting the level of performance.

Contrast Sensitivity in Linear Networks

The previous section illustrated how the contrast gain and the noise power spectrum of a neuron affect its contrast sensitivity. In this section we will use these principles to examine how contrast sensitivity flows through the various levels of a linear visual network.

Linear Visual Networks and Level Transfer Functions

We model a visual pathway as a series of neural levels, each with its own source of noise, and with signals and noise flowing in one direction from level to level (figure 7.2).

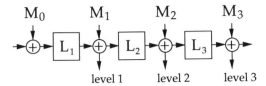

Fig. 7.2
The early visual pathway depicted as a cascade of linear filters (L) with additive noise (M) at each level.

In this model, each level k is characterized by a noise power spectrum $M_k(\mathbf{u}, w)$, and by a *level transfer function* (LTF), $L_k(\mathbf{u}, w)$. The connections, weights, and dynamics that exist between each pair of levels are encapsulated in the LTF. The LTF is in fact the Fourier transform of the spatiotemporal weighting function between each pair of levels.

This model of visual processing assumes that all neurons at one level are alike except for the spatial positions of their receptive fields. This appears to be approximately true for certain common types of neuron in the retina, LGN and cortex, at least when the population is drawn from a local region of the visual field. Over larger areas, receptive field sizes grow with eccentricity. This model is thus an approximation that may be valid for one type of neuron in a local area.

Transfer of Contrast Sensitivity

We have seen that neural contrast sensitivity depends upon contrast gain and noise power spectrum, so we consider in turn how each of these is manifest in the network. The transfer function of a neuron at level k is equal to the product of all the level transfer functions up to that level,

$$H_k(\mathbf{u}, w) = \prod_{j=1}^{k} L_j(\mathbf{u}, w). \tag{10}$$

Consequently, the ratio of contrast gains between two adjacent levels is equal to the modulus of the LTF

$$\frac{G_k(\mathbf{u}, w)}{G_{k-1}(\mathbf{u}, w)} = |L_{k-1}(\mathbf{u}, w)|. \tag{11}$$

Thus contrast gain flows through the network by incrementally multiplying by the contrast gain of each stage (the modulus of the LTF).

The transfer of noise is equally simple. A filtered random process has a power spectrum equal to the product of the original power spectrum and the squared modulus

of the filter (Papoulis, 1965). And if the noise sources are independent, then the power spectra will add. Thus the noise at each level is shaped by all the filters it passes through and added to the noise from all other sources. For example, the total noise at level k will be

$$N_k(\mathbf{u}, w) = M_k(\mathbf{u}, w) + |L_k(\mathbf{u}, w)|^2 N_{k-1}(\mathbf{u}, w). \tag{12}$$

Note that I use the symbol M for the noise added at each level, and the symbol N for the total noise at each level.

I have modeled the output of each layer as a function of both space and time in order to represent a continuous "sheet" of neurons. Consequently, I have also modeled the noise at each level as a random process over both space and time. However, when we record from a single neuron, the output is only a function of time. This measurement is a spatial sampling process, and the temporal power spectrum of its noise given by

$$N_k(w) = \int_{-\infty}^{\infty} N_k(\mathbf{u}, w) \, d\mathbf{u}. \tag{13}$$

Taking the ratio of contrast sensitivities at levels k and $k - 1$, as given by equation 9, we see that contrast sensitivities at two levels are related by the level contrast gain and the square root of the ratio of power spectra,

$$C_k(\mathbf{u}, w) = C_{k-1}(\mathbf{u}, w)|L_k(\mathbf{u}, w)| \sqrt{\frac{N_{k-1}(w)}{N_k(w)}}. \tag{14}$$

The noise at level k can be expanded by way of equations 12 and 13,

$$N_k(w) = M_k(w) + \int_{-\infty}^{\infty} |L_k(\mathbf{u}, w)|^2 N_{k-1}(\mathbf{u}, w) \, d\mathbf{u} \tag{15}$$

and the result substituted into equation 14

$$C_k(\mathbf{u}, w) = C_{k-1}(\mathbf{u}, w)|L_k(\mathbf{u}, w)| \tag{16}$$

$$\sqrt{\frac{N_{k-1}(w)}{M_k(w) + \int_{-\infty}^{\infty} |L_k(\mathbf{u}, w)|^2 N_{k-1}(\mathbf{u}, w) \, d\mathbf{u}}}.$$

This formula predicts sensitivity at one level from sensitivity at the previous level. In the following section, we will apply it to the specific problem of predicting cortical cell sensitivity from the sensitivity of cells of the LGN.

Predicting Cortical Sensitivity

Neurons in the parvocellular portion of the LGN typically have rather low peak contrast sensitivities of around 10 or below (Derrington & Lennie, 1984; Hicks, Lee & Vidyasagar, 1983; Kaplan & Shapley, 1982). In contrast, many simple cells in primary visual cortex (V1) have sensitivities of 100 or better (Hawken & Parker, 1984, 1987). Likewise, peak psychophysical contrast sensitivities (for gratings with few cycles) are around 100 (Banks, Geisler & Bennett, 1987; Pointer & Hess, 1990; Watson, 1987). This has led some authors to conclude that parvocellular LGN neurons cannot be the precursors of sensitive simple cells and psychophysical thresholds. Here we will use the model developed above to determine what sensitivities can be expected of cortical cells driven exclusively by parvocellular neurons.

In what follows, levels $k - 1$ and k are now associated with LGN and cortex, respectively, The subscripts (lgn, cor) will be used to make this explicit.

Model of LGN Neuron

For computational convenience, we assume space-time separability of the LGN contrast sensitivity function. Following Derrington and Lennie (1984), we model the LGN spatial contrast sensitivity as a difference of Gaussians,

$$C_{lgn}(\mathbf{u}) = a[\exp(-\pi s|\mathbf{u}|^2) - r_a \exp(-\pi s r_s|\mathbf{u}|^2)]. \qquad (17)$$

This is the Fourier transform of a spatial difference of Gaussians in which the center Gaussian has a spatial scale of s degrees, and a volume of a, and the surround Gaussian has a spatial scale of $s\, r_s$ degrees and a volume of $a\, r_a$. Parameters r_a and r_s are thus the ratios of volumes and spatial scales for surround and center. The parameter r_a may also be regarded as the ratio of peak amplitudes of the two Gaussians in the frequency domain, as is evident in equation 17. Parameters describing an average foveal cell have been derived from data of Derrington and Lennie (Derrington & Lennie, 1984; Watson, 1991). Parameters a, r_a, and r_s have been averaged from six individual estimates, while the value of s was obtained by extrapolating their figure 6 to the fovea. The resulting values are $a = 13.66$, $s = 0.025°$, $r_s = 4.98$, $r_a = 0.65$, and the corresponding contrast sensitivity function is pictured in figure 7.3.

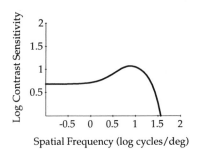

Fig. 7.3
Spatial contrast sensitivity function for an average foveal primate parvocellular LGN neuron.

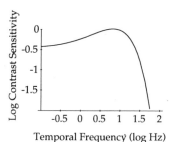

Fig. 7.4
Temporal contrast sensitivity function of a primate parvocellular LGN neuron.

An estimate of the parvocellular temporal contrast sensitivity function has also been taken from (Derrington & Lennie, 1984). Of their two cells, we have taken the more sustained. The transfer function is given by

$$C_{lgn}(w) = (517 \exp[-0.128w]$$
$$- 513 \exp[-0.135w])/11.5. \qquad (18)$$

The normalizing constant 11.5 is the contrast sensitivity at the temporal frequency (5.2 Hz) at which the spatial contrast sensitivity measurements were made, so that spatiotemporal contrast sensitivity is now the product $C_{lgn}(w)$ $C_{lgn}(\mathbf{u})$. The model LGN temporal contrast sensitivity is pictured in figure 7.4

Temporal noise power spectra for primate LGN neurons are not available, but Troy has published data from a cat LGN cell (Troy, 1983b) from which a power spectrum can be estimated (Watson, 1990) as shown in figure 7.5. The smooth curve is a third order polynomial (in log-log coordinates), fit by least squares, that we will use for interpolation,

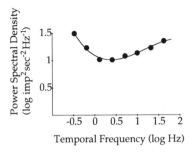

Fig. 7.5
Noise power spectral density for a cat LGN cell. Points are estimates, curve is a polynomial fit. Values are estimated from data of Troy (1983b).

$$N_{lgn}(w) = 10^{[1.097 - 0.460 \log(w) + 0.696 \log(w)^2 - 0.196 \log(w)^3]}.$$
(19)

While direct comparisons have not been made, the use of similar criteria (λ, see page 97) in the two species suggests that their power spectra are similar, and justifies our adoption of equation 19 as the model primate LGN temporal noise power spectrum.

For our predictions we need to know the complete spatiotemporal LGN noise power spectrum (see equation 16). What we have in figure 7.5 is the temporal noise power spectrum, which is the integral over spatial frequency of this full spectrum. To estimate the full spectrum, one would need to simultaneously measure from multiple neurons at various distances from one another. Few data of this sort are available. We therefore assume that the autocorrelation (and power spectrum) is separable in space and time, and that the spatial component $n_{lgn}(\mathbf{x})$ is a two-dimensional Gaussian with spatial scale ρ deg. Then $N_{lgn}(\mathbf{u})$ is constrained by equation (13) to have unit volume, and consequently a height of ρ^2,

$$N_{lgn}(\mathbf{u}) = \rho^2 \exp[-\pi \rho^2 |\mathbf{u}|^2].$$
(20)

Since $N_{lgn}(\mathbf{u})$ has unit volume, $n_{lgn}(\mathbf{x})$ has a peak value of 1 at $\mathbf{x} = [0, 0]$ and can therefore be regarded as the correlation between two LGNs separated by a distance vector $\mathbf{x}$. For this reason, we will call the parameter ρ the *correlation distance*.

Cortical Level Transfer Function

Note that the cortical LTF is the ratio of cortical and LGN transfer functions (equation 10). Thus in designing the model cortical LTF we consider how the cortical transfer function differs from that of the LGN. Notably, cortical cells are more sluggish in time, oriented, and more narrowly tuned in spatial frequency than cells in the LGN. Thus we desire an LTF that is lowpass in time, oriented, and bandpass in spatial frequency.

We assume that the LTF is separable in space and time,

$$L_{cor}(\mathbf{u}, w) = \gamma L_{cor}(\mathbf{u}) L_{cor}(w).$$
(21)

This is roughly so for many cortical cells (Tolhurst & Movshon, 1975) and fails primarily in cases of direction selective cells, which may be modeled as the sum of two separable functions (Hamilton, Albrecht & Geisler, 1989; Watson & Ahumada, 1983). For mathematical convenience, we normalize spatial and temporal LTFs and include a *level gain factor* γ. This γ is thus the peak gain of the spatiotemporal LTF.

We assume the spatial LTF is a pair of two-dimensional Gaussians, centered at $\mathbf{u}_0$ and $-\mathbf{u}_0$, which corresponds to a spatial weighting function that is a Gabor function. The Gabor function is widely used as a model of the cortical receptive field (Daugman, 1980; Hawken & Parker, 1987; Jones & Palmer, 1987; Kulikowski, Marcelja & Bishop, 1982; Marcelja, 1980). We adopt it as a convenient and plausible way of creating a cell tuned for spatial frequency and orientation; details of its shape are not important here. As noted above, we normalize the spatial transfer function, which is then

$$L_{cor}(\mathbf{u}) = \exp\left[-\pi\left(\frac{p}{u_0}\right)^2 |\mathbf{u} + \mathbf{u}_0|^2\right] + \exp\left[-\pi\left(\frac{p}{u_0}\right)^2 |\mathbf{u} - \mathbf{u}_0|^2\right].$$
(22)

The parameter p is the spatial scale (halfwidth at 0.043%) of the LTF in cycles of u_0. If we suppose that each neuron has a constant logarithmic bandwidth of b octaves, then p is constant and equal to

$$p = \frac{2^b + 1}{2^b - 1} \sqrt{\frac{\ln 2}{\pi}}.$$
(23)

In what follows, we will fix this bandwidth at 1.4 octaves, which is the mean estimate for primate V1 simple cells (De Valois, Albrecht & Thorell, 1982), and which corresponds to $p = 1.043$ cycles.

Since V1 cortical cells typically are temporally much more lowpass than LGN cells, we assume that the temporal level transfer function is an exponential lowpass

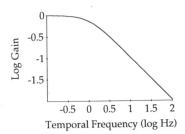

Fig. 7.6
Model cortical temporal level transfer function magnitude. The exponential time constant is 0.15 sec.

filter with time constant τ sec. An example is pictured in figure 7.6.

Predicting Cortical Contrast Sensitivity

Before embarking on any calculations, we show a slightly expanded version of equation 16, to show the effect of the various preceding assumptions,

$$C_{cor}(\mathbf{u}, w) = C_{lgn}(\mathbf{u}, w)|L_{cor}(\mathbf{u})|$$
$$\times \left[\frac{M_{cor}(w)}{\gamma^2 N_{lgn}(w)|L_{cor}(w)|^2} + \sigma_{s,lgn}^2 \right]^{-1/2} \quad (24)$$

where

$$\sigma_{s,lgn}^2 = \int_{-\infty}^{\infty} |L_{cor}(\mathbf{u})|^2 N_{lgn}(\mathbf{u}) \, d\mathbf{u}. \quad (25)$$

The variance term $\sigma_{s,lgn}^2$ is the portion of the LGN spatial power spectrum that is "seen" by the cortical cell through its spatial LTF.

We begin our exploration of this function by considering the case in which there is no cortical noise ($M_{cor}(w) = 0$). In this case, the first bracketed term, which includes the only appearance of the temporal transfer function, disappears, and we are left with

$$C_{cor}(\mathbf{u}, w) = C_{lgn}(\mathbf{u}, w)|L_{cor}(\mathbf{u})|/\sigma_{s,lgn}. \quad (26)$$

In the model we have constructed, the variance term $\sigma_{s,lgn}^2$ is the integral of the product of two Gaussians and therefore has a closed-form solution

$$\sigma_{s,lgn}^2(u_0) = \alpha \exp(-\pi \alpha p^2), \quad (27)$$

where

$$\alpha = \left[\frac{1}{2} + \left(\frac{p}{\rho u_0} \right)^2 \right]^{-1} \quad (28)$$

When the correlation distance ρ is small relative to the dimensions of the cortical receptive field ($\rho \ll p/u_0$), this variance is approximately equal to $\left(\frac{\rho u_0}{p} \right)^2$.

While the contrast sensitivity of individual neurons is of interest, we would also like to know the *peak contrast sensitivity function* describing the peak sensitivity of a neuron tuned to u_0, as a function of u_0. This is the upper envelope of a collection of neurons of various spatial frequencies. Under the approximation considered in the previous paragraph, this peak function will be

$$\hat{C}_{cor}(\mathbf{u}, w) = C_{lgn}(\mathbf{u}, w)/\sigma_{s,lgn} \approx C_{lgn}(\mathbf{u}, w) \frac{p}{\rho|\mathbf{u}|}. \quad (29)$$

This very simple prediction illustrates a number of important facts about the transfer of sensitivity from LGN to cortex. First, for a bandwidth of $b = 1.47$ octaves (close to the median reported for primate cortical simple cells (De Valois et al., 1982)), $p = 1$. If the spacing of LGN centers is equivalent to that of receptors (Packer, Hendrickson & Curcio, 1989; Samy & Hirsch, 1989), and if they are essentially uncorrelated (as would be true if all noise were added at the LGN output), then $\rho \approx 0.01$ degree. Peak cortical sensitivity at frequency u_0 cycles/degree would then be $100/u_0$ times LGN sensitivity at that frequency. For example, at 1 cycle/degree it would be two log units above LGN sensitivity! Thus a fundamental observation is that *cortical sensitivity can in principle be vastly higher than that of the cells that provide its input.*

These large gains in sensitivity are the result of spatial pooling of LGN cells. To continue the example, at 1 cycle/degree, $p = 1$ implies a circular pooling area of $1°$ radius, which when LGNs are spaced at $0.01°$ implies roughly $\pi \, 100^2 = 31,415$ LGN inputs! This number is undoubtedly an overestimate, since it does not take into account the decline in LGN cell density with eccentricity, but it nonetheless gives a sense of the massive amount of spatial pooling that must be involved.

To get a more detailed look at the constraints on cortical sensitivity, we compute contrast sensitivity functions for individual cortical neurons, as well as the peak function, under various conditions. These calculations are based on equations 27 and 28, and do not use the approximation in equation 29. In what follows, we fix the cortical bandwidth at 1.4 octaves, which is the mean estimate for primate V1 simple cells (De Valois et al., 1982). Figure 7.7

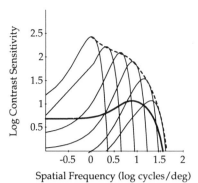

Fig. 7.7
Predicted cortical sensitivity when there is no cortical noise. Other parameters: $\rho = 0.02°$, $b = 1.4$ octaves, $w_0 = 5.2$ Hz. Thin solid lines show sensitivities of individual cells at frequencies of 1, 2, 4, 8, 16, and 32 cycles/degree. Dashed curve is the peak function (the envelope of peak sensitivities). Heavy solid curve is sensitivity of the underlying parvocellular LGN neuron.

shows predicted cortical sensitivity in the case of no cortical noise, and an LGN correlation distance of $\rho = 0.02°$. The figure shows the sensitivities of individual neurons at octave intervals from 1 to 32 cycles/degree, as well as the peak function and the contrast sensitivity of the LGN input. The approximation given in equation 29 differs by at most 0.15 log unit from the peak function shown (the dashed curve).

As noted above, predicted cortical sensitivity is well above LGN sensitivity. At the lowest frequencies, the peak function ascends with decreasing frequency at a slope of -1. This ascent will of course be limited by the size of the lowest frequency neuron, which in the fovea might be at about 1 cycle/degree (Hawken, Parker & Lund, 1988). The true peak function would then follow down the left shoulder of this neuron's sensitivity curve. In the following figures we do not correct for this effect, but consider sensitivities only above 1 cycle/degree.

Figure 7.8 shows the effect of varying the correlation distance ρ. At low to medium spatial frequencies, and small, plausible values of ρ, sensitivity is proportional to ρ^{-1}, as we expect from equation 29. At high frequencies, sensitivity is actually enhanced by increasing ρ. This is because increasing ρ lowers the cut-off frequency of the spatial noise power spectrum, so that sensors at high spatial frequencies see less and less noise.

Pelli (1990) has argued that, except at low spatiotemporal frequenices (below 4 Hz and 4 cycles/degree), psy-

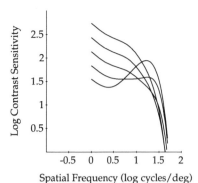

Fig. 7.8
Peak cortical sensitivity for no cortical noise and varying LGN correlation distances: $\rho = 0.01°$, $0.02°$, $0.04°$, $0.08°$, and $0.16°$. Other parameters: $b = 1.4$ octaves, $w_0 = 5.2$ Hz.

chophysical sensitivity is limited by quantum fluctuations. This would imply that at threshold contrasts, cortical cells add little noise of their own over most of the frequency range. At low frequencies, he found an added neural noise component, which would tend to lower the peak function in this region. But though cortical noise may not be limiting over much of the spatiotemporal spectrum, we should nevertheless like to understand what effects it will have when it does intrude. We therefore consider predictions of cortical sensitivity in the presence of added cortical noise.

We have little information on the power spectrum of the noise added at the cortical level, $M_k(w)$. We therefore assume it is constant over the frequency range of interest.

The absence of cortical noise completely removes any effect of the level gain factor γ, because both signal and noise are amplified equally by the LTF (equation 24). If cortical noise is present, some assumption must be made regarding γ. Note that this gain could be quite different for neurons of different spatial frequencies, following some *level gain function* $\gamma(u_0)$, allowing an almost arbitrary shape for the resulting peak function (though it must always lie below the no-cortical-noise curve). Empirically, some insight into this function might be offered by comparison of the LGN contrast gain at some visual field location and the contrast gain of cortical cells of various frequencies drawn from the same location. However, such data appear not to be available.

Here we will consider only one of the multiplicity of possible assumptions regarding the level gain function $\gamma(u_0)$. We assume that level gain is set in such a way that each cortical neuron has the same peak contrast gain, regardless of its peak spatial frequency. This rule will optimize the use of the available response range of each neuron. Neurons have a rather limited dynamic range, those in the LGN and cortex typically responding at less than 100 impulses/sec (Sclar, Maunsell & Lennie, 1990). The maximum response produced by our linear model neuron is equal to the peak contrast gain times the maximum contrast. The little available evidence (Field, 1987) suggests that the spatial contrast amplitude spectrum of natural imagery is proportional to $1/u$. This corresponds to equal energy within spectral regions of constant log bandwidth. Since our model cortical neurons are designed to have a constant log bandwidth, they will, if given equal peak gain, have equal expected energy in their outputs. This in turn means that each neuron, exposed to an ensemble of natural images, will produce a distribution of responses with equal standard deviation. The gain of the neuron should be set in such a way that the maximum response is proportional to this standard deviation. Therefore, to match the dynamic range of each neuron to the expected natural contrast distribution, the peak gains of neurons at different frequencies should be equated. We lack specific values for the absolute magnitude of the natural contrast power spectrum, so we will be content to adopt a constant cortical peak gain of γ_{cor}. Then the gain factor of a neuron at spatial frequency u_0 will be

$$\gamma(u_0) = \frac{\gamma_{cor}}{|L_{cor}(w_1)||G_{lgn}(u_0, w_1)|}. \tag{30}$$

This gain function yields a constant peak contrast gain for each cortical neuron (at some temporal frequency w_1) by compensating for the variations in gain introduced by the LGN neuron. It may be thought of as a "deblurring" operation applied to the ensemble of cortical neurons.

Figure 7.9 shows peak sensitivity for various amounts of cortical noise under the above assumption regarding level gain. Increasing cortical noise has two effects: Sensitivity is reduced at middle and low frequencies, and the curve becomes flatter in this frequency range. The flattening of the curve is explained as follows. Under the adaptive gain assumption, all neurons have the same peak gain regardless of their spatial frequency. Furthermore, we have assumed a flat cortical spatial noise spectrum. Thus as cortical noise comes to dominate the total noise, contrast sensitivity becomes independent of spatial frequency.

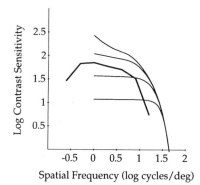

Fig. 7.9
Peak contrast sensitivity for model cortical neurons at four levels of cortical noise, $M_{cor} = 0$, 0.1, 1, and 10 impulses^2 sec^{-2} Hz^{-1}. Other parameters, $\rho = 0.02$, $b = 1.4$, $w_0 = 5.2$ Hz, $w_1 = 6.5$ Hz, $\gamma_{cor} = 100$. The solid curve is psychophysical data for a human observer.

I have justified this assumption about cortical gain on functional grounds, but it is consistent with the finding that average semisaturation constants of primate contrast response functions are roughly constant as a function of the spatial frequency of the neuron (Albrecht & Hamilton, 1982).

Relation to Psychophysics

Figure 7.9 also shows contrast sensitivity for a human observer detecting Gabor functions of various frequencies (Watson, 1987). For an observer relying on the output of a single neuron and making no use of the phase of the response, we expect agreement between neural and psychophysical contrast sensitivity. A detailed comparison of cortical and psychophysical sensitivity is beyond the scope of this chapter, but several comments are in order. First, the highest sensitivities attained by the observer, in the middle frequency range, are consistent with predictions that include a modest amount of cortical noise. This illustrates that parvocellular neurons are in principle capable of providing the basis for psychophysical contrast thresholds. Second, under these particular assumptions, predicted sensitivity at the highest spatial frequencies is greater than that measured. Differences in species and measurement conditions prevent us from making too much of this discrepancy, but it does suggest the need for data that more directly address the issue, and for further exploration of the model.

Discussion

In this chapter we have (1) derived a mathematical expression for contrast sensitivity in a linear visual neuron, (2) shown how this contrast sensitivity is dependent upon contrast gain, noise, and conditions of measurement, and (3) shown how contrast sensitivity behaves in feedforward networks of homogeneous linear neurons. These theoretical concepts have been illustrated in the specific case of predicting contrast sensitivity of V1 simple cells (and perhaps psychophysical contrast sensitivity) from the sensitivity of parvocellular LGN neurons.

It is appropriate to discuss some limitations of our analysis. First, it is restricted to linear neurons. In primate, at least, this appears to include a majority of visual neurons up to the level of visual cortex. Cortical simple cells are typically nonlinear, primarily because they have low or nonexistent maintained discharges, and hence cannot signal negative values. However, for small responses they behave like a linear neuron subject to an output half-wave rectification. The cortical predictions above are of this linear internal response.

Another complication is the possible nonlinear adaptation of the cortical gain to the ambient contrast (see chapter 9; Albrecht, Farrar & Hamilton, 1984; Maddess, McCourt, Blakeslee & Cunningham, 1988; Ohzawa & Freeman, 1985). However, this process, while quite powerful in the cat, may be much less evident in primates. It would not, at any rate, have much effect for the near-threshold stimuli employed in measurements of contrast sensitivity.

A third limitation is the assumption of spatial homogeneity. This has two aspects: local disorder in spacing and size of receptive fields, and systematic increase in size and spacing with eccentricity. The former is unlikely to have large effects in foveal vision. As to the latter, human and monkey cone diameter and spacing increase by about 70 to 90 percent over an eccentricity of $1°$ (Packer et al., 1989; Samy & Hirsch, 1989). This inhomogeneity will have its greatest effect at the lower frequencies. Lower frequency cells require larger receptive fields (assuming constant log bandwidth), and thus must pool over a larger, more inhomogeneous region, in which the mean spacing is below that at the fovea. Relative to the homogeneous prediction, then, inhomogeneous predictions would be somewhat lower at the low frequency end. It should also

be noted that the more fundamental relationships between gain, noise, and contrast sensitivity introduced here are not dependent upon homogeneity, and inhomogeneous predictions could be derived from them.

A fourth limitation concerns the relation between neural and psychophysical contrast sensitivity. Under certain assumptions (one cell, phase-uncertain ideal observer), neural contrast sensitivity is a direct predictor of psychophysical sensitivity. Experiments can be designed that increase the reasonableness of these assumptions, for example, by matching the size of the stimulus and the target cell. Various departures from these assumptions can be imagined, however, such as use of information from many cells, phase knowledge, or less than ideal detection. Nevertheless, the direct prediction is an important benchmark, from which these departures are relatively minor amendments.

Another apparent complication is that in this analysis we have treated the LTF as a continuous function of space. While this is mathematically convenient, it is at odds with our conventional picture of the connections from one cell to the next, namely, that these connections take the form of discrete synapses. Each synapse would be made with a particular prior neuron whose receptive field has a particular location. This situation may be represented by sampling the continuous LTF at these locations. These samples represent the discrete weights associated with each synapse. This sampling will replicate the LTF, but this replicated LTF is multiplied by functions such as the contrast sensitivity and noise power spectral density of the previous level, both of which are likely to be lowpass functions. Provided that the replicas are outside the passband of these functions, sampling will have no effect on the shape of the predicted contrast sensitivity function, but will introduce a scalar factor equal to the sample density D (cells/degree) multiplying each instance of the spatial LTF (Watson, 1991). This factor cancels out entirely when there is no cortical noise or when the peak cortical gain is assumed to be constant over cell spatial frequency, as in figure 7.9. Consequently, the issue of sampling may be safely ignored in these calculations, provided that the sample density is sufficiently high.

A final caveat is that in looking at the relation between LGN and cortical sensitivity we have considered only one class of LGN cell, the parvocellular neurons, and have ignored the magnocellular neurons. A similar analysis could of course be applied to the latter class to provide a more complete picture of what to expect in the sensitivity of cortical cells.

Despite the cautions mentioned above, several rather strong conclusions emerge. The first is that the rather insensitive parvocellular neurons can feed very sensitive cortical cells and can be the basis for very high psychophysical sensitivities. This explains the once rather puzzling result that loss of P ganglion cells (the precursors of parvocellular LGN cells) reduces psychophysical sensitivity everywhere except at the lowest spatial and highest temporal frequencies (Merigan & Eskin, 1986).

A more general conclusion is that relationships between sensitivities at various levels in the visual pathway depend strongly upon the level transfer function, the noise at each level, and correlations among nearby cells. The formulae discussed here allow these factors to be combined to generate meaningful predictions.

A final observation is that the measurement of contrast gain, noise, and sensitivity of neurons at various levels may provide a new and powerful way of dissecting the functional anatomy of visual pathways, and of understanding of the relationship between neural and psychophysical contrast sensitivity.

References

Albrecht, D. G., Farrar, S. & Hamilton, D. B. (1984). Spatial contrast adaptation characteristics of neurons recorded in the cat's visual cortex. *Journal of Physiology, 347,* 713–739.

Albrecht, D. G. & Hamilton, D. B. (1982). Striate cortex of monkey and cat: Contrast response function. *Journal of Neurophysiology, 48,* 217–237.

Banks, M. S., Geisler, W. S. & Bennett, P. J. (1987). The physical limits of grating visibility. *Vision Research, 27,* 1915–1924.

Bracewell, R. N. (1978). *The Fourier transform and its applications.* New York: McGraw-Hill.

Daugman, J. G. (1980). Two-dimensional spectral analysis of cortical receptive field profiles. *Vision Research, 20,* 847–856.

De Valois, R. L., Albrecht, D. G. & Thorell, L. G. (1982). Spatial frequency selectivity of cells in macaque visual cortex. *Vision Research, 22,* 545–559.

Derrington, A. M. & Lennie, P. (1982). The influence of temporal frequency and adaptation level on receptive field organization of retinal ganglion cells in cat. *Journal of Physiology, 333,* 343–366.

Derrington, A. M. & Lennie, P. (1984). Spatial and temporal contrast sensitivities of neurones in lateral geniculate nucleus of macaque. *Journal of Physiology, 357,* 219–240.

Enroth-Cugell, C., Robson, J. G., Schweitzer-Tong, D. & Watson, A. B. (1983). Spatio-temporal interactions in cat retinal ganglion cells showing linear spatial summation. *Journal of Physiology, 341,* 279–307.

Field, D. J. (1987). Relations between the statistics of natural images and the responses properties of cortical cells. *Journal of the Optical Society of America A, 4,* 2379–2394.

Hamilton, D. B., Albrecht, D. G. & Geisler, W. S. (1989). Visual cortical receptive fields in monkey and cat: Spatial and temporal phase transfer function. *Vision Research, 29,* 1285–1308.

Hawken, M. J. & Parker, A. J. (1984). Contrast sensitivity and orientation selectivity in lamina IV of the striate cortex of old world monkeys. *Experimental Brain Research, 54,* 367–372.

Hawken, M. J. & Parker, A. J. (1987). Spatial properties of neurons in the monkey striate cortex. *Proceedings of the Royal Society London B, 231,* 251–288.

Hawken, M. J., Parker, A. J. & Lund, J. S. (1988). Laminar organization and contrast sensitivity of direction-selective cells in the striate cortex of the old world monkey. *Journal of Neuroscience, 8,* 3541–3548.

Hicks, T. P., Lee, B. B. & Vidyasagar, T. R. (1983). The responses of cells in the macaque lateral geniculate nucleus to sinusoidal gratings. *Journal of Physiology (London), 337,* 183–200.

Jones, J. P. & Palmer, L. A. (1987). An evaluation of the two-dimensional gabor filter model of simple receptive fields in cat striate cortex. *Journal of Neurophysiology, 58,* 1233–1258.

Kaplan, E. & Shapley, R. M. (1982). X- and Y cells in the lateral geniculate nucleus of macaque monkeys. *Journal of Physiology (London), 330,* 125–143.

Kaplan, E. & Shapley, R. M. (1986). The primate retina contains two types of ganglion cells, with high and low contrast sensitivity. *Proceeding of the National Academy of Science USA, 83,* 2755–2757.

Kulikowski, J. J., Marcelja, S. & Bishop, P. O. (1982). Theory of spatial position and spatial frequency relations in the receptive fields of simple cells in the visual cortex. *Biological Cybernetics, 43,* 187–198.

Maddess, T., McCourt, M. E., Blakeslee, B. & Cunningham, R. B. (1988). Factors governing the adaptation of cells in area-17 of the cat visual cortex. *Biological Cybernetics, 59,* 229–236.

Marcelja, S. (1980). Mathematical description of the responses of simple cortical cells. *Journal of the Optical Society of America, 70,* 1297–1300.

Merigan, W. H. & Eskin, T. A. (1986). Spatio-temporal vision of macaques with severe loss of P-beta retinal ganglion cells. *Vision Research, 26,* 1751–1761.

Ohzawa, I. & Freeman, R. D. (1985). Contrast gain control in the cat visual system. *Journal of Neurophysiology, 54,* 651–665.

Packer, O., Hendrickson, A. & Curcio, C. A. (1989). Photoreceptor topography of the retina in the adult pigtail macaque (Macaca nemestrina). *Journal of Comparative Neurology, 288,* 165–183.

Papoulis, A. (1965). *Probability, random variables, and stochastic processes*. New York: McGraw-Hill.

Pelli, D. G. (1990). The quantum efficiency of vision. In C. B. Blakemore (Ed.), *Vision: Coding and efficiency*. Cambridge, UK: Cambridge University Press.

Pointer, J. S. & Hess, R. F. (1990). The contrast sensitivity gradient across the major oblique meridians of the human visual field. *Vision Research, 30,* 497–501.

Samy, C. N. & Hirsch, J. (1989). Comparison of human and monkey retinal photoreceptor sampling mosaics. *Visual Neuroscience, 3,* 281–285.

Sclar, G., Maunsell, J. H. R. & Lennie, P. (1990). Coding of image contrast in central visual pathways of the macaque monkey. *Vision Research, 30,* 1–10.

Tolhurst, D. J. & Movshon, J. A. (1975). Spatial and temporal contrast sensitivity of striate cortical neurons. *Nature, 257,* 674–675.

Troy, J. B. (1983a). Spatial contrast sensitivities of X and Y type neurones in the cat's dorsal lateral geniculate nucleus. *Journal of Physiology, 344,* 399–417.

Troy, J. B. (1983b). Spatio-temporal interaction in neurones of the cat's dorsal lateral geniculate nucleus. *Journal of Physiology, 344,* 419–432.

Watson, A. B. (1987). Estimation of local spatial scale. *Journal of the Optical Society of America A, 4,* 1579–1582.

Watson, A. B. (1990). Gain, noise, and contrast sensitivity of linear visual neurons. *Visual Neuroscience, 4,* 147–157.

Watson, A. B. (1991). Transfer of contrast sensitivity in linear visual networks. *Visual Neuroscience,* in press.

Watson, A. B. & Ahumada, A. J., Jr. (1983). A look at motion in the frequency domain. In J. K. Tsotsos (Ed.), *Motion: Perception and representation* (pp. 1–10). New York: Association for Computing Machinery.

8

Spatiotemporal Receptive Fields and Direction Selectivity

Robert Shapley,
R. Clay Reid,
and Robert Soodak

Visual neurons from the retina to primary visual cortex act like transducers of spatial and temporal visual stimuli. They transform patterns of modulation of light, in space and time, into trains of nerve impulses. To understand the function of visual neurons, we must investigate how this transformation is achieved with neural mechanisms and also in what way a particular transformation accomplishes the goals of visual perception. In this chapter, we will consider the neural mechanisms of direction selectivity in the primary visual cortex of the cat and will review recent research we have done on this subject (Reid, Soodak & Shapley, 1987, 1991).

Visual perception of motion depends on a computation of spatiotemporal change and computation of direction. Models of the perception of motion always include a stage at which direction is calculated (for example, Adelson & Bergen, 1985; Reichardt, 1961; van Santen & Sperling, 1985; Watson & Ahumada, 1985; see also Nakayama, 1985 for a comprehensive review). Some recent psychophysical models include a stage at which direction is computed by linear systems with specific spatiotemporal properties (Adelson & Bergen, 1985; Burr, Morrone & Ross, 1986; Watson & Ahumada, 1985). However, nonlinear combination of signals has also been proposed in other models (Barlow & Levick, 1965). Therefore, one theoretical issue that has concerned us is whether nonlinear interaction must be invoked in order to explain directional computations in visual cortical neurons, or whether linear spatiotemporal mechanisms may do the job (cf. Soodak, 1986). Since not all direction selectivity in simple cells can be explained by linear mechanisms alone, we have begun to investigate the nature of nonlinear cortical interactions in simple cortical cells. We will describe a new experimental procedure we are beginning to use to solve this second problem.

The experimental data on computation of direction we are considering come from simple cells in the primary visual cortex, area 17, of the cat. These neurons are defined as "simple" by tests of receptive field properties that are, at least qualitatively, diagnostic for linearity of spatial summation (Hubel & Wiesel, 1962; Movshon, Thompson & Tolhurst, 1978; Spitzer & Hochstein, 1985). For instance, simple cells give only a single sign of response to localized increments or decrements of light and never the frequency-doubled "on-off" response that characterizes complex cells. Furthermore, linear predictions of responses to complicated spatial stimuli are possible in simple cells from their responses to localized stimuli, and these linear predictions are sometimes accurate. However, there is evidence from many laboratories that simple cells may not be so simple and linear. For example, Bishop, Coombs, and Henry (1973) found evidence for nonlinear, suppressive regions in simple cell receptive fields. Morrone, Burr, and Maffei (1982) have found a nonlinear cross-orientation inhibition mainly in simple cells of cat primary visual cortex. Moreover, Ohzawa, Sclar, and Freeman (1985) have demonstrated the existence of a highly nonlinear gain-control mechanism that normalizes the response to contrast in cat simple cells. With the knowledge that simple cells may be qualitatively linear spatiotemporal transducers but that nonlinear spatial interactions may also play a role, we have designed experiments to test the hypothesis that directional selectivity may be generated in simple cells by linear spatiotemporal interactions.

Direction Selectivity

At this point we need to define the concept of *direction selectivity*. Direction selectivity means a sensory preference for stimuli moving in one direction, independent of the sign of contrast. Directionally selective neurons must be distinguished from directionally asymmetric neurons, the directional preference of which switches with sign of contrast (Emerson & Gerstein, 1977). A directionally asymmetric cell will respond preferentially to one direction of motion of a bright bar, and to the opposite direction of motion of a dark bar. While a minority of feline simple cells are directionally asymmetric, the majority are directionally selective (Bishop et al., 1973). Directionally asymmetric cells will not respond preferentially to drifting sinusoidal grating patterns in any direction, because such patterns have no net sign of contrast but are modulated equally above and below their mean level. However, directionally selective neurons do respond preferentially

to sine gratings drifted in their preferred directions. If an ensemble of such directionally selective neurons constituted the front end of spatiotemporal filters for a spatiotemporal energy model like that of Adelson and Bergen (1985), they would enable the model to compute correctly the direction of motion of arbitrary grating patterns.

Spatiotemporal Separability and Spatiotemporal Coupling

Direction selectivity emerges as a property of linear, spatiotemporal filters when the spatial and temporal filtering characteristics are coupled rather than independent of one another. If the spatiotemporal impulse response of a filter, denoted $W(x, t)$, can be written as the product of spatial and temporal impulse responses, $g(x)$ and $h(t)$, respectively, then the filter is said to have a *spatiotemporally separable* spatiotemporal impulse response, and

$$W(x, t) = g(x)h(t). \qquad (1)$$

However, if the temporal properties at different positions of the spatial impulse response are different, then the filter's spatiotemporal impulse response cannot be written as in equation 1, and the spatiotemporal impulse response is *inseparable*, also termed *spatiotemporally coupled*. In simple cells of the visual cortex, spatiotemporal coupling might arise from convergence of excitation from afferents with different dynamics of response, as suggested recently by Saul and Humphrey (1989), or by different intracortical temporal filtering of signals that originate from different spatial loci in the neuron's receptive field.

The relation of spatiotemporal separability and inseparability (or coupling) to direction selectivity is illustrated by graphs of neural response versus position and time, so-called x-t plots. One such graph is shown in figure 8.1 (cf. Adelson & Bergen, 1985; Burr, 1981; among others). In an x-t plot, a spatiotemporally separable field has axes of symmetry that are parallel to the x- and t-axes, because of equation 1. For example, consider the two positions A and B in figure 8.1, column I. The spatiotemporal impulse responses for these two times will be, respectively, $g(A)$ $h(t)$ and $g(B)$ $h(t)$, and so the temporal impulse response will be the same $h(t)$ for these two times. This is indicated in figure 8.1A, B.

However, a spatiotemporally coupled field may be tilted in the x-t plot, with its axes of symmetry parallel to

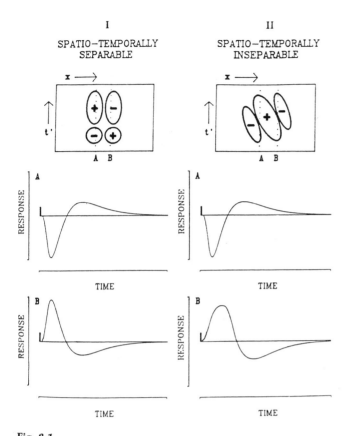

I

SPATIO—TEMPORALLY
SEPARABLE

II

SPATIO—TEMPORALLY
INSEPARABLE

Fig. 8.1
Space-time (x-t) plots of hypothetical spatiotemporally separable and inseparable neurons. In these graphs one dimension of space is plotted to the right, and time is increasing from below. Regions are labeled with sign of response. The dotted lines in each graph are slices through the response surface at particular positions labeled A and B. (I) Separable. This is the graph for a spatiotemporally separable receptive field. Time functions (impulse responses) at A and B are identical except for sign inversion. (II) Inseparable. A spatiotemporally inseparable field is graphed here and again slices at two positions are compared. It is evident that the impulse response at A is different from that at B, as indicated by inspection of the x-t plot. (From Reid et al., 1991.)

lines that follow the equation: $x = vt$ where v is the preferred velocity. This is shown in figure 8.1, column II. Patterns that move with velocity v will produce a large response from such a spatiotemporally coupled field, while patterns that move with a velocity $-v$, in the nonpreferred or "null" direction, will produce a smaller response from a spatiotemporally coupled field.

In previous work on simple cells located in area 17 of the cat's visual cortex, Tolhurst and Movshon (1975) found support for spatiotemporal separability in experiments in which they used as stimuli sine grating patterns drifting in a single (usually the optimal) direction. They used the Fourier transformed version of equation 1, as follows:

$$W(k,f) = g(k)\, h(f), \qquad (2)$$

where k is spatial frequency in cycles/degree, and f is temporal frequency in cycles per second, or Hertz. Tolhurst and Movshon observed that for different values of temporal frequency f, the amplitude of the spatiotemporal frequency response $W(k,f)$ appeared to have the same dependence on spatial frequency k, thus seeming to follow the amplitude of a separable spatial frequency response $g(k)$. This experiment was not designed to account for directional selectivity but mainly to compare with earlier psychophysical tests of separability. However, measurement of the amplitude of the spatiotemporal frequency response to gratings drifting in one direction is not a sufficient test for spatiotemporal separability, as was pointed out by Dawis, Shapley, Kaplan, and Tranchina (1984) in their study of spatiotemporal separability and coupling in lateral geniculate nucleus (LGN) neurons. The reason it is not sufficient can be seen clearly from an example. Consider a neuron which sums from an even-odd quadrature pair of neurons, like those in the Adelson-Bergen model. Then,

$$W_{\text{sum}}(k,f) = g_e(k)\, h_e(f) + g_o(k)\, h_o(f), \qquad (3)$$

where $g_e(k)$ is the spatial frequency response of the even spatial profile and $g_o(k)$ is the odd profile's spatial frequency response.

Let each element of the pair have the same amplitude of spatial frequency response as a function of spatial frequency k, $g(k)$, but of course with different values for the phase of $g(k)$ corresponding to the different symmetries: The phase of the even spatial frequency response g_e will be zero because the Fourier transform of an even function is real valued, while the phase of the spatial frequency response of the odd profile will be 90°. Similarly, suppose the temporal responses h_e and h_o have the same amplitude as a function of temporal frequency f, but are also in quadrature. Then, in an experiment with drifting sine gratings moving in the preferred direction, the spatial frequency response will always be the same at all temporal frequencies. Yet, the spatiotemporal transfer function in equation 3 is *not* spatiotemporally separable; it cannot be written as a simple product of one spatial frequency response and one temporal frequency response. In fact, a neurons with the spatiotemporal transfer function in equation 3 would be completely directionally selective, responding maximally in one direction and with zero amplitude of response in the other direction. The question is, what sort of experiment would reveal such spatiotemporal coupling and allow its contribution to direction selectivity to be calculated?

Sinusoidal Gratings: Contrast Reversal and Drift

We have used a combination of two experiments to measure linear spatiotemporal coupling and its contribution to direction selectivity, quantitatively. The first experiment is measurement of the response amplitude and phase of a simple cell when the stimulus is a sine grating undergoing sinusoidal contrast reversal. The stimulus in such an experiment is,

$$S_{CR}(x,t) = L_0[1 + C\sin(2\pi kx + \phi)\sin(2\pi ft)], \qquad (4)$$

where L_0 is the mean luminance, C is the contrast, k the spatial frequency, and f the temporal frequency. In this experiment, the most important stimulus variable is ϕ, the spatial phase or position of the grating. The stimulus contrast C was chosen to be in the range 0.1 to 0.4 and was determined to lie within the linear range of the response vs. contrast function for each cell.

In the second kind of experiment we have measured the response amplitude to sine gratings drifting in two directions: preferred and "null." The stimulus in this case for the preferred direction is,

$$S_{D-P}(x, t) = L_0[1 + C\sin(2\pi kx - 2\pi ft)], \qquad (5a)$$

and for the "null," or antipreferred, direction it is,

$$S_{D-N}(x, t) = L_0[1 + C\sin(2\pi kx + 2\pi ft)]. \qquad (5b)$$

The amount of directional selectivity in the drifting grating experiment is quantified in terms of a *directional index*, which is defined as:

$$DI = (R_P - R_N)/(R_P + R_N) \qquad (6)$$

where R_P is the amplitude of response in the preferred direction of motion, and R_N is the amplitude of response in the "null" direction. A nondirectional neuron has a directional index of 0, while a completely directionally

selective neuron, one which only responds to one direction of drift, has a directional index of 1.

Linearity and Elliptical Polar Plots

Evidence for linear spatial summation in simple cells can be found in the pattern of these cells' responses to contrast reversal of gratings. Suppose such a simple neuron sums its inputs linearly, and the time courses of all its spatial inputs are identical (the condition of spatiotemporal separability). However, further suppose that simple cells have a threshold for spike firing that is so high that there is either no mean rate in the absence of stimulation, or a very low mean rate. The spike firing threshold acts like a static rectifier, to a first approximation. Then the neuron's response amplitude to contrast reversal of a sine grating will be a rectified sinusoidal function of spatial phase and the temporal phase of the response will be constant except for a jump of half a cycle near the zeroes of response (the so-called null positions; Enroth-Cugell & Robson, 1966; Hochstein & Shapley, 1976). A fraction of the simple cells in cat primary cortex behave in this manner (Movshon et al., 1978; Reid et al., 1987), resembling retinal ganglion cells and LGN neurons of the X type (Hochstein & Shapley, 1976; Shapley & Hochstein, 1975). However, the amplitudes of response of most cat simple cells do not follow a sinusoidal function of spatial phase at all spatial and temporal frequencies in their response range, and their temporal phases can vary continuously with the spatial phase of the stimulus grating in the contrast reversal experiment (Reid et al., 1987). Movshon and colleagues (1978) found that many cat simple cells' responses in the contrast reversal experiment traced out an *ellipse* when plotted as vectors in the complex plane and showed that this was theoretically predicted for a spatiotemporally coupled simple cell. We confirmed this result and have presented an additional algebraic proof (Reid et al., 1987) and a geometrical proof (Reid, 1988; Reid, Soodak & Shapley, 1991) for the proposition that this behavior was to be expected from a linear neuron that did not have a spatiotemporally separable receptive field. The responses as a function of spatial phase of a cat simple cell with a spatiotemporally inseparable field are shown in figure 8.2, and it can be seen that they form an ellipse. We have used these response ellipses as a criterion for linearity of simple cell responses. Furthermore, one can use the ellipses to

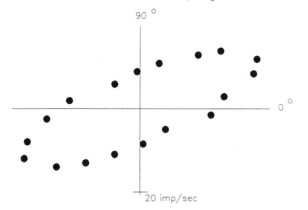

Contrast Reversal 0.8 c/deg, 1 Hz

Fig. 8.2
Polar plot of response amplitude and temporal phase, parametric in spatial phase. The response of a simple cell to contrast reversal is plotted as a complex number from the response amplitude and temporal phase lead with respect to the stimulus. The points trace out an ellipse, as described in the text. This was from a simple cell stimulated by a 0.8 cycles/degree sine grating, contrast reversed sinusoidally at 1 Hz. The amplitude calibration is indicated on the bottom of the vertical axis.

make quantitative predictions of the directional index, and also the response magnitudes in the preferred and anti-preferred, or "null," directions of motion (Reid et al., 1987). Similar ideas have been put forward by Movshon and Tolhurst (Movshon & Tolhurst, personal communications).

Linear Predictions of Direction Selectivity

One can compute a linear prediction for the amount of directional selectivity in the drifting grating experiment from the dependence of response amplitude and phase on the stimulus spatial phase in the contrast reversal experiment. The advantage of comparing responses to drifting and contrast reversal grating stimuli is that any nonlinearities of the visual cortex are elicited equally by the two stimuli except for those having to do specifically with image motion. Thus the equal contrast and spatial extent of the drifting and contrast reversing stimuli should be equally effective at evoking signals in the cortical contrast gain control (Ohzawa et al., 1985) or from other suppressive nondirectional interactions.

It can be shown (Reid et al., 1987) that the magnitude of the major axis of the contrast reversal-ellipse, denoted r_1, equals the sum of the amplitudes of response in the preferred and "null" (antipreferred) directions:

$$r_1 = r_p + r_n, \tag{7}$$

while the minor axis, r_2, is equal to the difference of the amplitudes of the two directional responses to drift; thus:

$$r_2 = r_p - r_n. \tag{8}$$

It follows that a linear prediction of the directional index is the ratio of the minor to major axes of the ellipse:

$$DI^{lp} = r_2/r_1. \tag{9}$$

A direct test of this linear prediction is offered in figure 8.3, which shows the predicted directional index for a population of cat simple cells and also the directly measured directional index. A scatter plot of these data was given in an earlier paper (Reid et al., 1987). The average directional indices indicate that the measured directionality of simple cells is partially accounted for by linearity of spatial summation and spatiotemporal inseparability, but that some nonlinearities of spatial summation must augment the magnitude of directional selectivity. The analysis of the scatter plot in our earlier paper led to the same conclusion because the directional indices of the neurons, measured and predicted, were qualitatively, but not quantitatively, similar.

The nature of the nonlinear enhancement of directional selectivity can be deduced from the linear predictions of drifting grating responses from the contrast reversal-ellipse. From equations 7 and 8 above, one can derive linear predictions for the response amplitudes in the preferred and "null" directions:

$$r_p^{lp} = (r_1 + r_2)/2, \tag{10a}$$

$$r_n^{lp} = (r_1 - r_2)/2, \tag{10b}$$

where the superscripts indicate that equations 10a and b are linear predictions of the preferred and "null" response amplitudes from the magnitudes of the major and minor axes of the contrast reversal ellipse, r_1 and r_2. A comparison of this linear prediction with measured directional responses of a simple cell is offered in figure 8.4. Here, as in most directional simple cells, the linear prediction is very accurate for the response in the preferred direction but is too large for the response in the "null" direction. This indicates that the major nonlinearity that enhances directional selectivity in simple cells is suppressive, reducing the response amplitude in the "null" direction. We reached this conclusion earlier from an analysis of a popu-

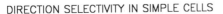

DIRECTION SELECTIVITY IN SIMPLE CELLS

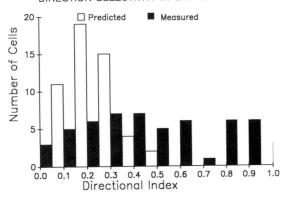

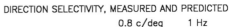

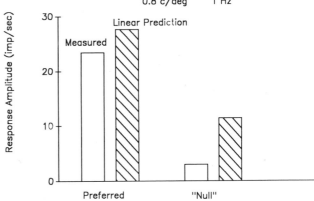

Fig. 8.3

Linear predictions and measurements of directional index. The predicted directional indices were based on the ellipse axis ratio, as described in the text, equation 9. The measured directional indices were from drifting grating experiments on 19 simple cells and the linear predictions were derived from the same neurons, from measurements of their response ellipses when the stimulus was grating contrast reversal. The measurements of directional index were done at several spatiotemporal pairs in most cells, so that 55 different conditions are included in the histogram. The predicted indices are graphed with empty bars while the measured indices are indicated by the filled bars in the histogram. The horizontal locations of the keyed squares labeled "Predicted" and "Measured" in the graph are at the values of the mean directional index for the predicted (0.18) and measured (0.48) population, respectively. In all of the experiments described in this chapter, the mean luminance of the display was 50 to 100 cd/m^2, and this was seen through an artifical pupil of 7 mm^2. Thus the retinal illumination was photopic for the cat. Contrast was chosen to be in a linear response vs. contrast range of operation of the cell; usually contrast of 0.2 was used.

lation of directional simple cells (Reid et al., 1987). We believe that many properties of cat simple cells are affected by suppressive nonlinearities of the kind needed to explain the discrepancy of the prediction from measurement in figure 8.4. This belief is discussed somewhat more in what follows.

M-sequences and the Measurement of Spatiotemporal Receptive Fields

In order to understand the nature of direction selectivity comprehensively, we have embarked on a program of measurement of the two-dimensional spatiotemporal weighting functions of directional neurons. The aim is to characterize the neuron's linear space-time properties and from these to make a linear prediction of the response

Fig. 8.4

Linear prediction of preferred and null responses. The preferred and "null" direction responses were measured on a simple cell at 0.8 cycles/degree and 1 Hz. This was the optimal stimulus for this neuron. The linear prediction is based on responses to contrast reversal of the same sine grating using equations 10a, b in the text. As is evident, the linear prediction of the preferred response is more accurate than the prediction of the "null" response.

to moving stimuli. In this paper we report some preliminary observations and predictions that support the earlier research reviewed above. These observations, however, lead to new ideas about the significance of nonlinear spatial interactions in simple cells.

Although the defining characteristics of simple cells concern linearity of spatial summation, significant nonlinearities in cortical circuitry require the use of techniques from nonlinear systems analysis for the measurement of spatiotemporal weighting functions. This working hypothesis, justified by our subsequent measurements, motivated the development of equipment and software for the computation of spatiotemporal weighting functions, or kernels, by means of orthogonal functional analysis (Emerson, Citron, Vaughn & Klein, 1987; Marmarelis & Marmarelis, 1978; Victor and Knight, 1979; Victor and Shapley, 1980).

We have adapted an approach to spatiotemporal functional analysis pioneered by Erich Sutter (1987), called maximal length shift register sequences, or m-sequences. An m-sequence of *order n* is a sequence of -1's and 1's of length $2^n - 1$ within which no strings of length n or longer are duplicated. Thus, an m-sequence is the binary sequence of maximal diversity for its length. In our experiments, each picture element or pixel in a 16 by 16 array is modulated in time by a sixteenth order m-sequence. The sequences are derived by a computation to be described elsewhere with a technique similar to that described by Sutter (1987). One important property of the m-sequence is that its power spectrum is white, and therefore the value of the m-sequence at any moment is uncorrelated with any time shift of itself. Such a signal can be used to recover the temporal weighting function of a linear system by cross-correlation (Marmarelis & Marmarelis, 1978). Following Sutter (1987), we have exploited the whiteness of the m-sequences by making each of the 256 pixels in the 16 by 16 array a time-shifted version of the same basic m-sequence. Therefore, the temporal stimulus at each spatial position is uncorrelated with all the others for all times less than the time-shift between pixels (usually 4 sec). Then the temporal weighting function at each of the positions in the array can be recovered by computation of a single cross-correlation between neuron output and m-sequence input. The first order response from each pixel occurs at a separate, predetermined time in the cross-correlation function. Another advantage of m-sequences is that the correlation functions of all orders may be recovered with a single rapid computation referred to as the fast m-transform (Sutter, 1990). Thus, first and second order spatiotemporal kernels may be computed very rapidly. There are practical limits to this approach. Overlap of low order with high order kernels could be a problem, as could overlap of second order with first order responses if there were widespread strong second order interactions across long distances. Prolonged temporal impulse responses could also be a problem. However, these practical difficulties are infrequent and occur in deterministic ways which can be dealt with effectively. We have reported on some of the results of our experiments with m-sequences at the 1989 Neuroscience meeting (Reid, Victor & Shapley, 1989).

To illustrate the usefulness of spatial m-sequence analysis, we offer results from a well-studied and highly tuned simple cell from cat primary visual cortex. A time slice from the first order m-kernel is drawn in figure 8.5 as a contour plot representing the two-dimensional spatial surface of responsiveness of the neuron. This is equivalent to the pointspread function of the best-fitting linear system (cf. Marmarelis & Marmarelis, 1978, and Victor & Shapley, 1980 for a discussion of the interpretation of first order kernels). The first order kernel of the cortical simple cell has many of the properties that have been obtained with other two-dimensional mapping techniques, such as narrow, long receptive field regions that respond to sti-

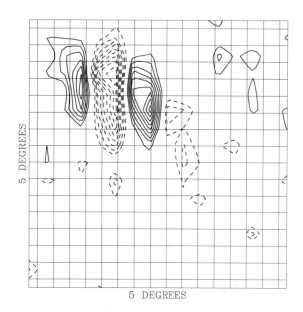

5 DEGREES

Fig. 8.5

M-sequence two-dimensional spatial first order kernel for a directional simple cell. This is the first order kernel in two spatial dimensions at one instant in time, 73 msec after stimulus occurrence. The contour plots represent the kernel's surface; each contour is a response increment of 0.02 impulse/sec. The solid contours represent excitation by incremental stimuli; the dashed contours excitation by decrements. The m-sequence was binary valued with the magnitude of the contrast of the incremental and decremental pixels set to 1.0. The duration of each pixel was 16 msec, and this was clearly smaller than the neuron's integration time (see figure 8.6). Thus, the effective contrast for the cortical neuron was considerably less than 1.0 because of temporal summation of positive and negative contrasts within the integration time (Reid & Shapley, unpublished).

muli of a single sign (ON or OFF), and an organization of responsive regions of opposite sign that will lead to orientation tuning and spatial frequency tuning (Hubel & Wiesel, 1962; Jones & Palmer, 1987; McLean & Palmer, 1989). The kernel is shown for a particular moment in time, 73 msec from stimulus onset. Since this is a spatiotemporal first order kernel, there is a distinct spatial kernel surface for each moment in time.

The time evolution of the first order kernel is illustrated in the x-t plot of the kernel surface in figure 8.6. First order kernels in cortical simple cells typically show little response in the first 40 msec, then a growth of response then gradual decay of response until the kernel is virtually zero after about 250 msec. Noticeable in figure 8.6 is the tilt in the first order kernel at longer times and longer distances from the spatial origin. This is an indication of spatiotemporal inseparability and indicates that the first

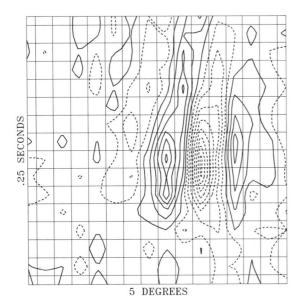

.25 SECONDS

5 DEGREES

Fig. 8.6
Space-time or x-t plot of the first order kernel. In this graph from the same simple cell as in figure 8.5, first order kernel values along one spatial dimension, the long axis of the neuron, have been added together and plotted along the single spatial dimension of this graph, and the time evolution of the kernel values plotted along the other dimension. The time and space origins are located at the lower left corner of the graph. Each contour stands for an increment in the magnitude of response by 0.06 impulse/sec. As in figure 8.5, the dashed contours are excitatory responses to decrements, while the solid contours are excitatory responses to increments. The tilt in the x-t plot, especially at long times, is an indication of space-time inseparability, as in the schematic plot of figure 8.1, column II.

order spatiotemporal m-kernel would predict directional selectivity in this simple cell (cf. McLean & Palmer, 1989). This prediction is made quantitative in figure 8.7. The prediction was accomplished by a three-dimensional (two space, one time) Fourier transform of the spatiotemporal kernel into a spatiotemporal frequency response. At the temporal frequency and spatial frequency used in the experiments, the orientation tuning was predicted all around the clock.

The predicted and measured orientational tuning of this simple cell are very high, as indicated in figure 8.7. Qualitatively, the linear prediction is correct with respect to orientational preference and directional preference. But it is very clear that the magnitude of predicted response is much smaller than measured. We believe this is because the total contrast was much higher in the m-sequence measurement, on which the prediction is based, than in the experiment with drifting sine gratings with which

ORIENTATION TUNING AT 1 C/DEG

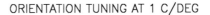

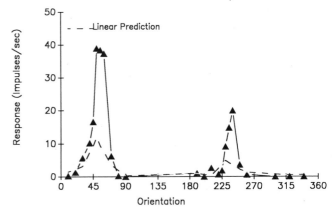

Fig. 8.7
Predicted and measured orientation tuning. The orientation tuning of the simple cell, the first order kernel of which is depicted in figure 8.5 and 8.6, was predicted by Fourier transforming the kernel and collecting the terms at the spatial frequency, temporal frequency and orientations of the measurements. In this case the orientation tuning curve was measured with drifting gratings of 0.2 contrast, 1 cycle/degree spatial frequency, and 4 Hz temporal frequency. The responses were taken as the fundamental Fourier coefficient in the response of the neuron at the temporal drift rate, 4 Hz. The dashed curve is the linear prediction from the first order kernel. The measured orientation tuning data are plotted as filled triangles and connected with the solid line.

orientation tuning was measured. The total spatial contrast may be integrated by the cortical contrast gain control (Ohzawa et al., 1985) and thus used to suppress the amplitude of response.

The spatial frequency responses at the optimal orientation and in the preferred and "null" directions were also predicted from m-sequence kernels. These are given in figure 8.8 along with direct measurements of the spatial frequency responses with drifting gratings. As with the orientation tuning curves, the predicted response amplitudes are lower and the predicted tuning curves here are considerably broader than the measured functions. Direction selectivity is approximately accounted for by the linear prediction in this case. However, the sharpening of spatial frequency tuning requires an explanation in terms of spatial nonlinearities within the cortical circuitry. A possible explanation is that there are nonlinear suppressive effects generated mainly by stimuli of low spatial frequency, and that this spatial-frequency–specific suppression controls the sharper tuning in the spatial frequency response measured with gratings.

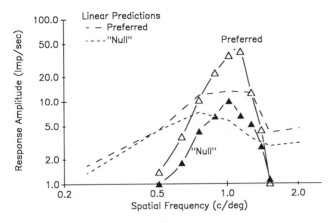

SPATIAL FREQUENCY TUNING AT BEST ORIENTATION

Fig. 8.8
Predicted and measured spatial frequency tuning. As in figure 8.7, the spatial frequency response of the simple cell was calculated from the first order kernel and compared with the measured spatial frequency tuning at the optimal orientation, in the two directions of drift: preferred (empty triangles) and "null" (filled triangles). The temporal frequency was 4 Hz. The spatial frequency tuning was measured at a contrast of 0.2. The linear predictions from the first order kernel are indicated in the graph as the dashed and dotted curves. The predictions were corrected for the finite sampling by the 16 by 16 lattice of pixels in the m-sequence. Note that this is a standard log-log plot, whereas figure 8.7 is plotted on linear coordinates.

A complete account of all the spatial and temporal nonlinear mechanisms in cerebral cortex is beyond the scope of this paper. However, our initial measurements and computations with the m-sequence kernels indicate that nonlinear gain control mechanisms are very powerful determinants of cortical responses and therefore of spatio-temporal tuning functions. It is interesting that the dominant nonlinearity revealed with the comparison of m-kernel predictions and direct measurements is that of a non-directional gain control. The kernel prediction of directional selectivity is like the measured value, even though the shapes of the tuning functions of orientation and spatial frequency deviate greatly from the linear predictions. In order to get at the question of linearity or nonlinearity of the directionally selective process, one has to use stimuli that are nearly equivalent for the dominant gain-control nonlinearity. This was accomplished in the previous experiments from our lab with drifting and contrast reversal gratings (Reid et al., 1987). It is the reason that we were able to reveal the less strong but nevertheless significant suppressive directional nonlinearity discussed above.

In conclusion, linear spatiotemporally inseparable interactions contribute to the directional selectivity seen in cortical simple cells. However, there is a directionally sensitive suppressive nonlinearity that heightens the amount of directional selectivity as quantified by the directional index. Preliminary measurements of first order spatiotemporal kernels with m-sequences allow another kind of linear prediction of directional selectivity, as well as linear predictions of orientation and spatial frequency tuning. Direction selectivity is qualitatively well predicted from the m-sequence kernels, but magnitudes of peak response are predicted to be too small. The sharpness of the spatial tuning functions is greater than predicted from the kernels. This indicates the possibility for nonlinear suppressive sharpening mechanisms for all spatial tuning functions of cortical simple cells.

Acknowledgments

For electronic hardware and computer software development needed for this project we thank Norman Milkman and Michelangelo Rossetto at Rockefeller University. Dr. Jonathan Victor of Cornell University Medical College gave theoretical and technical support and help, for both of which we are grateful. Dr. Michael Hawken worked together with us on experiments. This work was supported by grants from the National Eye Institute, EY 01472, the National Science Foundation BNS 8708606, and a grant from the Sloan Foundation.

References

Adelson, E. H. & Bergen, J. R. (1985). Spatiotemporal energy models for the perception of motion. *Journal of the Optical Society of America A, 2*, 285–299.

Barlow, H. B. & Levick, W. R. (1965). The mechanism of directionally selective units in the rabbit's retina. *Journal of Physiology, 178*, 477–504.

Bishop, PO, Coombs, G. H. & Henry, G. H. (1973). Receptive fields of simple cells in cat striate cortex. *Journal of Physiology, 231*, 31–60.

Burr, D. C. (1981). Temporal summation of moving images by the human visual system. *Proceeding of the Royal Society B, 211*, 321–339.

Burr, D. C., Morrone, M. C. & Ross, J. (1986). Seeing objects in motion. *Proceeding of the Royal Society B, 227*, 249–265.

Dawis, S., Shapley, R., Kaplan, E. & Tranchina, D. (1984). The receptive field organization of X-cells in the cat: spatiotemporal coupling and asymmetry. *Vision Research, 24*, 549–561.

Emerson R. C. & Gerstein, G. L. (1977). Simple striate neurons in the cat. II. Mechanisms underlying directional asymmetry and directional selectivity. *Journal of Neurophysiology, 40*, 136–155.

Emerson, R. C., Citron, M. C., Vaughn, W. J. & Klein, S. A. (1987). Nonlinear directionally selective subunits in complex cells of cat striate cortex. *Journal of Neurophysiology, 58*, 33–65.

Enroth-Cugell, C. & Robson, J. G. (1966). The contrast sensitivity of retinal ganglion cells of the cat. *Journal of Physiology, 187*, 517–552.

Hochstein, S. & Shapley, R. (1976). Linear and nonlinear spatial subunits in Y cat retinal ganglion cells. *Journal of Physiology, 262*, 265–284.

Hubel, D. H. & Wiesel, T. N. (1962). Receptive fields, binocular interaction and functional architecture in cat's visual cortex. *Journal of Physiology, 160*, 106–154.

Jones, J. P. & Palmer, L. A. (1987). The two-dimensional spatial structure of simple receptive fields in cat striate cortex. *Journal of Neurophysiology, 58*, 1187–1211.

McLean, J. & Palmer, L. A. (1989). Contribution of linear spatiotemporal receptive field structure to velocity selectivity of simple cells in area 17 of cat. *Vision Research, 29*, 675–679.

Marmarelis, P. & Marmarelis, V. (1978). *Analysis of physiological systems*. New York: Plenum Press.

Morrone, M. C., Burr, D. C. & Maffei, L. (1982). Functional implications of cross-orientation inhibition of cortical visual cells. I. Neurophysiological evidence. *Proceedings of the Royal Society B, 215*, 335–354.

Movshon, J. A., Thompson, I. D. & Tolhurst, D. J. (1978). Spatial summation in the receptive fields of simple cells in the cat's striate cortex. *Journal of Physiology, 283*, 53–77.

Nakayama, K. (1985). Biological image motion processing: A review. *Vision Research, 25*, 625–660.

Ohzawa, I., Sclar, G. & Freeman, R. D. (1985). Contrast gain-control in the cat's visual system. *Journal of Neurophysiology, 54*, 651–667.

Reichardt, W. (1961). Autocorrelation, a principle for the evaluation of sensory information by the central nervous system. In W. A. Rosenblith (Ed.), *Sensory communication*. New York: Wiley.

Reid, R. C. (1988). Directional selectivity and the spatiotemporal structure of the receptive fields of simple cells in cat striate cortex. Ph.D. Thesis, Rockefeller University.

Reid, R., Soodak, R. & Shapley, R. (1987). Linear mechanisms of directional selectivity in simple cell of cat striate cortex. *Proceedings of the National Academy of Science, 84*, 8740–8744.

Reid, R. C., Soodak, R. & Shapley, R. (1991). Directional selectivity and the spatiotemporal structure of the receptive field of simple cells in cat striate cortex. *Journal of Neurophysiology*, in press.

Reid, R. C., Victor, J. D. & Shapley, R. (1989). A new two-dimensional pseudorandam stimulus for the study of receptive fields in the LGN and striate cortex. *Society of Neuroscience Abstracts 15*, 323.

Saul, A. B. & Humphrey, A. L. (1989). Phase differences in the cat LGN and cortical direction selectivity. *Society of Neuroscience Abstracts, 15*, 1394.

Shapley, R. & Hochstein, S. (1975). Visual spatial summation in two classes of geniculate cells. *Nature, 256*, 411–413.

Soodak, R. E. (1986). Two dimensional modeling of visual receptive fields using Gaussian subunits. *Proceedings of the National Academy of Sciences USA, 83*, 9259–9263.

Spitzer, H. & Hochstein, S. (1985). Simple and complex-cell response dependences on stimulation parameters. *Journal of Neurophysiology, 53*, 1244–1265.

Sutter, E. (1987). A practical non-stochastic approach to nonlinear time-domain analysis. *Advances in Methods of Physiological Systems Modelling*, vol 1. University of Southern California.

Sutter, E. (1990). The fast m-transform: A fast computation of cross-correlations with binary m-sequences. SIAM *Journal on Computing*, in press.

Tolhurst, D. J. & Movshon, J. A. (1975) Spatial and temporal contrast sensitivity of striate cortical neurons. *Nature, 257*, 674–675.

van Santen, J. P. H. & Sperling, G. (1985). Elaborated Reichardt detectors. *Journal of the Optical Society of America A, 2*, 300–321.

Victor, J. D. & Knight, B. W. (1979). Nonlinear analysis with an arbitrary stimulus ensemble. *Quarterly Journal of Applied Mathematics, 37*, 113–136.

Victor, J. D. & Shapley, R. (1980). A method of nonlinear analysis in the frequency domain. *Biophysical Journal, 29*, 459–484.

Watson, A. B. & Ahumada, A. J. (1985). Models of human visual-motion sensing. *Journal of the Optical Society of America A, 2*, 322–342.

9

Nonlinear Model of Neural Responses in Cat Visual Cortex

David J. Heeger

The first description of the physiological responses of neurons in the cat's primary (striate) visual cortex was provided by Hubel and Wiesel in 1962. They were able to divide striate cells into two groups, simple and complex. Simple cells have receptive fields that are, like those of the retina and lateral geniculate nucleus (LGN), divided into distinct excitatory and inhibitory regions. Hubel and Wiesel found that "summation occurred within either type of region," and that "when the two opposite regions were illuminated together their effects tended to cancel." This suggests that simple cells sum linearly over their receptive fields. Complex cells, on the other hand, do not have excitatory and inhibitory subregions and do not sum linearly over their receptive fields. Rather, complex cells generally respond to either an increase or a decrease in the intensity of a properly oriented stimulus placed anywhere within the receptive field. Hubel and Wiesel suggested that complex cell receptive fields might result from combinations of simple cell inputs.

Since the pioneering work of Hubel and Wiesel, vision scientists have used the tools of linear systems analysis to investigate the properties of visual neurons. In 1968, Campbell and Robson reported psychophysical evidence for linear mechanisms selectively sensitive to a limited range of spatial frequencies. At about the same time, physiological experiments (Campbell, Cooper & Enroth-Cugell, 1968, 1969) demonstrated that cells (both simple and complex) in cat striate cortex are selective for spatial frequency and for orientation.

The linear systems approach to cortical function is attractive because if correct, the response of a linear cell can be completely characterized with a relatively small number of measurements. A linear cell's response to any stimulus can be predicted from its responses to impulses (spots of light) flashed throughout its receptive field. Sine grating stimuli also play an important role in the linear systems approach because a linear cell transforms an input sinusoid into an output sinusoid of the same frequency; only the amplitude and phase may change.

A popular view is that simple cells act like halfwave-rectified linear operators, at least over a limited range of stimulus contrasts. The rectification is due to the fact that neurons can give only positive responses. A popular model for complex cells is that they act like energy mechanisms that compute the sum of the squared outputs of a quadrature pair of linear subunits (Adelson & Bergen, 1985).

The linear systems approach has found success in psychophysical modeling as well. It is now generally believed that the detection and identification of simple spatial patterns is mediated by linear mechanisms tuned for spatial frequency. More recently, energy mechanisms have been used to model psychophysical data on human texture discrimination (see chapters 17 and 18) and on the perception of Mach bands (Ross, Morrone & Burr, 1989).

Linear filters and energy mechanisms have also been useful in machine vision research. Quadrature pair linear filters have been used for optical flow measurement (e.g., Heeger, 1987; Watson & Ahumada, 1985; see chapter 16), texture discrimination (Bergen & Adelson, 1988; Malik & Perona, 1990; Turner, 1986), shape from shading (Pentland, 1989), and stereo disparity estimation (Sanger, 1988).

The linear systems approach has gone a long way toward explaining visual physiology, psychophysics, and machine vision. It is clear, however, that the linear/energy model falls short of a complete account of early vision. Even so, there is good reason to pursue the linear/energy paradigm. Rather than throw away the model, researchers have proposed modifying it in various ways.

One of several major objections to the linear/energy model comes from experiments that test for linearity in simple cells. Although some of the experimental data (discussed below) is consistent with linearity, some of it is not. This has led physiologists (for example, Tadmor & Tolhurst, 1989; Movshon, Thompson & Tolhurst, 1978a) to suggest replacing halfwave-rectification with over-rectification at the output of the model simple cells (half-wave-rectification clips responses less than zero whereas over-rectification clips responses less than some fixed positive threshold). In this chapter, I propose using half-squaring instead (half-squaring is halfwave-rectification followed by squaring).

A second objection to the linear/energy model comes from experiments that reveal nonspecific suppression in cortical cells. Excitation of cortical cells is highly stimulus specific, that is, cells are selective for stimulus orientation, spatial frequency, and direction of motion. The excitatory response to a preferred stimulus can be suppressed by superimposing an additional stimulus (e.g., Bonds. 1989). This suppression has been found to be largely nonspecific; it is independent of direction of motion, it is largely independent of orientation, it is broadly tuned for spatial frequency, and it is broadly tuned for spatial position.

A third objection to the linear/energy model is the fact that cell responses saturate at high contrasts. The responses of ideal linear operators and energy mechanisms, on the other hand, increase with increased stimulus contrast over the entire range of contrasts.

To explain nonspecific suppression and response saturation, several physiologists (for example, Bonds, 1989; Robson, 1988) have suggested that striate cells mutually inhibit one another, effectively normalizing their responses with respect to stimulus contrast.

In this chapter, I show that the linear/energy model taken together with half-squaring and contrast normalization yields a simple and mathematically elegant model that explains a large body of physiological data. In the next section, I explain the model: linear operators, energy mechanisms, half-squaring, and contrast normalization. In the following section, I compare model cell responses with responses of real cells for a variety of physiological measurements. Some of the experimental results can be explained simply with the linear/energy model. For these cases, I show that including half-squaring and contrast normalization does just as well. Some of the experimental results are inconsistent with the linear/energy model. I show that these results can be explained by including half-squaring and contrast normalization.

This chapter treats the visual system as a black box up to the level of striate cortex. I pay no attention to the responses of retinal or geniculate cells, but rather relate cortical cell responses directly to the time-varying stimulus intensities. In doing so I implicitly assume that the retina is at a fixed state of light adaptation.

The Model

Linear Operators and Energy Mechanisms

An operator is linear, by definition, if it obeys the property of superposition. That is, the response of the operator to a linear combination of two stimuli is equal to the linear combination of the responses to each of the component stimuli. If the response of the operator is given by $R(I)$ for stimulus I, then this property is expressed mathematically as:

$$R(aI_1 + bI_2) = aR(I_1) + bR(I_2),$$

for any constants a and b, and for any stimuli I_1 and I_2.

It is straightforward to show that a visual neuron is a linear operator (obeying the superposition property) if and only if its response is a weighted sum of the stimulus intensities. Let (x, y) denote position in the visual field, $f(x, y)$ be the receptive field of a linear operator, and $I(x, y)$ be a stimulus. The response, $R(I)$, of the cell is expressed as the inner product of the receptive field and the stimulus,

$$R(I) = f(x, y) \cdot I(x, y) = \int\int_{-\infty}^{\infty} f(x, y)I(x, y)\,dx\,dy.$$

The impulse response, $h(x, y)$, of the operator is simply related to its receptive field:

$$h(x, y) = f(-x, -y).$$

The response of the operator can be expressed as convolution with the impulse response:

$$R(I) = h(x, y) * I(x, y)|_{(x,y)=(x_0,y_0)}$$

$$= \int\int_{-\infty}^{\infty} h(\xi, \eta)I(x - \xi, y - \eta)\,d\xi\,d\eta \Big|_{(x,y)=(x_0,y_0)}$$

where $*$ denotes convolution, and where $f(x)|_{x_0} = f(x_0)$. If there were copies of the operator centered at each location in the visual field then convolving, $h(x, y) * I(x, y)$, would give their collective outputs. We consider the response of one operator by sampling the convolved output at (x_0, y_0), the center of the receptive field.

An example of a linear operator is the two-dimensional Gabor operator (see Daugman, 1980; Gabor, 1946). The receptive field of a Gabor operator is a sine grating multiplied by a two-dimensional Gaussian window, and as such it is made up of alternating excitatory and inhibitory subregions. A Gabor operator responds well to stimuli in the excitatory subregions that are brighter than the mean luminance and to stimuli in the inhibitory subregions that are darker than the mean luminance. The number of alternating subregions, the width and orientation of the subregions, and the symmetry (phase) of the operator can all be varied by changing the parameters of the sine grating and the Gaussian window that make up the Gabor operator.

The transfer function of a linear operator is defined as the Fourier transform of its impulse response, and it is made up of two parts, the amplitude response and the phase response. A linear operator is completely characterized by either its impulse response or its transfer function. For a Gabor operator, there is a peak in the amplitude response corresponding to the operator's preferred spatial frequency and orientation. The spatial frequency and orientation of a Gabor operator's underlying sine grating determine the peak in the amplitude response, and the width of the operator's Gaussian window is inversely proportional to the width (bandwidth) of the amplitude response. The phase response depends on the symmetry of the operator. For example, an operator with a central excitatory subregion flanked on either side by equal inhibitory subregions has even phase, and an operator with excitatory and inhibitory subregions to either side of center has odd phase.

Two linear operators with the same amplitude response but with phase responses that are shifted $90°$ in phase relative to one another are called a quadrature pair (or Hilbert transform pair). Intuitively, one often thinks of even- and odd-phase operators, like cosine- and sine-phase Gabor operators, as standard examples of quadrature pairs. Strictly speaking however, sine- and cosine-phase Gabor operators are not quadrature pairs because cosine phase Gabor operators always have some dc response (i.e., they will respond to a constant, zero contrast input), whereas sine phase Gabor operators do not. Even so, there are examples of quadrature pair operators that look very much like sine- and cosine-phase Gabor operators.

A mechanism that sums the squared outputs of a quadrature pair is called an energy mechanism (Adelson & Bergen, 1985). Its response depends only on the Fourier energy (squared magnitude of the Fourier transform) of the stimulus, not on the stimulus phase. The amplitude response of an energy mechanism is equal to the squared amplitude response of the component linear operators.

Spatiotemporal Mechanisms

The responses of striate cells depend not only on the spatial distribution of light in a stimulus, but also on its temporal presentation. Striate cells are best thought of as spatiotemporal mechanisms.

A 3D (space-time) Gabor operator is a three-dimensional sine grating multiplied by a three-dimensional Gaussian window. The spatiotemporal frequency tuning of the operator is specified by the spatial and temporal frequencies of the underlying sine grating, and its spatial and temporal bandwidths are specified by the spread of the operator's Gaussian window. The operator looks something like a stack of plates with small plates at the top and bottom of the stack and larger plates in the middle of the stack. The plates correspond to excitatory subregions of the receptive field, and the spaces between the plates correspond to inhibitory subregions. The stack can be tilted in any orientation in space-time, each different orientation corresponding to an operator with a different spatiotemporal frequency tuning.

A spatiotemporal linear operator that is tilted along an oblique axis in space-time is direction selective. It is now well recognized that stimulus motion is like orientation in space-time, and that spatiotemporally oriented filters can be used to detect and measure it. A number of authors have proposed spatiotemporal linear operators and spatiotemporal energy mechanisms as models of the early stages of motion perception (for examples, see Adelson & Bergen, 1985; Heeger, 1987; van Santen & Sperling, 1985; Watson & Ahumada, 1983, 1985; see also chapter 16).

Mathematically, the response, $R(t)$, of a spatiotemporal linear operator is the inner product in space and the reverse correlation in time of a stimulus, $I(x, y, t)$, with the receptive field of the operator, $f(x, y, t)$,

$$R(t) = \int \int \int_{-\infty}^{\infty} f(x, y, \tau) I(x, y, \tau - t) \, dx \, dy \, d\tau. \tag{1}$$

The response can also be expressed using convolution with the impulse response:

$$R(t) = h(x, y, t) * I(x, y, t)|_{(x,y)=(x_0, y_0)}$$

$$= \int \int \int_{-\infty}^{\infty} h(\xi, \eta, \tau) I(x - \xi, y - \eta, t - \tau)$$

$$\times \, d\xi \, d\eta \, d\tau \bigg|_{(x,y)=(x_0, y_0)}$$

where $h(x, y, t) = f(-x, -y, -t)$ is the impulse response, and where (x_0, y_0) is the center of the receptive field. The

response waveform, $R(t)$, is the model equivalent of a post-stimulus time histogram (PSTH). The PSTH is a measure of a cell's average response per unit time.

The receptive field of a spatiotemporal linear cell is measured as the time-varying response to impulses flashed at each point in the visual field. The transfer function of a spatiotemporal linear cell is measured using drifting sine gratings. For each stimulus spatial and temporal frequency, the response $R(t)$ is sinusoidal with frequency equal to the temporal frequency of the stimulus. The amplitudes (peak height) of the output sinusoids give the amplitude response, and the phases (relative peak latency) of the output sinusoids give the phase response.

Halfwave-Rectification and Half-Squaring

Cell firing rates are always positive, whereas linear operators can have positive or negative outputs. For a linear cell with a high maintained firing rate the positive and negative values correspond to responses above and below the maintained response. Cortical cells have very little maintained discharge so they can not truly act as linear operators.

The positive and negative outputs of a linear operator can be encoded by two halfwave-rectified linear operators. One mechanism encodes the positive outputs of the underlying linear operator, and the other one encodes the negative outputs. The two mechanisms are complements of one another, that is, the excitatory subregions of one receptive field are replaced by inhibitory subregions in the other. In other words, the two mechanisms are shifted $180°$ in phase relative to one another. Due to the rectification, only one of the two has a non-zero response at any given time.

For a halfwave-rectified linear cell, the receptive field of the underlying linear operator is measured using impulses of opposite polarity. Positive impulses (brighter than the mean luminance) are used to map the excitatory subregions of the receptive field, and negative impulses (darker than the mean luminance) are used to map the inhibitory subregions. The responses to dark impulses are interpreted with negative sign. The transfer function of the underlying linear operator is measured using sine grating stimuli. The response of the halfwave-rectified operator is a truncated sinusoid. The amplitude (peak height) and phase (relative peak latency) of the response are unaffected by halfwave-rectification.

A popular model of simple cells is that they are half-wave-rectified linear operators. It is suggested in this chapter that half-squaring (halfwave-rectification followed by squaring) is a more accurate model of the output nonlinearity. The output of a half-squared linear operator is given by:

$$A(t) = \left\lfloor \int\int\int_{-\infty}^{\infty} f(x, y, \tau) I(x, y, \tau - t) \, dx \, dy \, d\tau \right\rfloor^2, \quad (2)$$

where $\lfloor x \rfloor = \max(x, 0)$ is taken to mean halfwave-rectification, $I(x, y)$ is the stimulus, $f(x, y, t)$ is the receptive field of the linear operator, and where the integral expression is copied from equation 1.

Care must be taken when interpreting measurements of the receptive field and transfer function of a half-squared linear cell. Responses to impulses and gratings do not give the receptive field and transfer function of the underlying linear operator. The amplitude (peak height) of the response waveform for a drifting grating stimulus is the square of the amplitude of the underlying linear operator. The phase (relative peak latency) of the response waveform is unaffected by the squaring. The response to positive impulses minus the response to negative impulses gives the signed-square of the receptive field of the underlying linear operator. That is,

$$R'(t) = \begin{cases} R^2(t) & \text{if } R(t) > 0 \\ -R^2(t) & \text{if } R(t) < 0, \end{cases}$$

where $R'(t)$ is the signed-square of $R(t)$, and $R(t)$ is the response of the underlying linear operator.

Although the term "amplitude response" should be reserved for linear operators, I use it in this chapter when writing about half-squared operators and energy mechanisms as well. In both cases, the "amplitude response" is measured using sine grating stimuli. For half-squared linear operators we measure the Fourier amplitude of the fundamental component of the response waveform (this is proportional to the peak height of the response waveform). Energy mechanisms give an unmodulated response to sine gratings so we measure the dc response.

An energy mechanism can be constructed as the average of the outputs of four half-squared linear operators, all four with the same "amplitude response," but with phases in steps of $90°$. The energy output, $E(t)$, is expressed as:

$$E(t) = (1/4)[A^0(t) + A^{90}(t) + A^{180}(t) + A^{270}(t)], \quad (3)$$

where $A^\phi(t)$ is the response of a half-squared linear operator, and where the superscript, ϕ, specifies the operator's phase in degrees. The "amplitude response" of the energy mechanism is the same as the "amplitude response" of each of the input half-squared linear operators.

Contrast Normalization

The responses of linear and energy mechanisms increase with stimulus contrast over the entire range of contrasts. Information about a visual stimulus, other than its contrast, is represented as the relative response of a collection of mechanisms. For example, the orientation of a grating is represented as the relative response of a collection of energy mechanisms, each with a different orientation tuning. The ratio of the responses of two of the mechanisms is fixed, independent of stimulus contrast. Likewise, consider the response of one mechanism when presented with two differently oriented gratings. If the contrast of both gratings is changed by the same factor then the ratio of the responses to the orientations remains unchanged.

It is possible that the visual system also represents visual information as the relative response of collections of cells. For this to be the case, it is crucial that the ratio of a cell's responses to two stimuli be independent of contrast. But cortical cells, unlike linear or energy mechanisms, have a limited dynamic range, so their responses saturate for high contrasts. How is it possible for response ratios to be independent of stimulus contrast, in the face of response saturation? I propose in this chapter that cell responses are normalized for stimulus contrast.

The contrast-normalization mechanism discussed here is analogous to models of retinal light adaptation and gain-control (see Sperling & Sondhi, 1968 for an example, and Shapley & Enroth-Cugell, 1984 for a review), the purpose of which is to keep the retinal response approximately the same when the level of illumination changes. That way, the brain can proceed to process visual information without having to attend to the light level. The consequence of retinal light adaptation is that much of our perception is invariant with respect to intensity, over a wide range of light levels. For example, the perceived contrast of a grating stimulus is largely invariant with respect to intensity.

Likewise, contrast-normalization allows the brain to process visual information without having to attend further to the contrast. For example, the perceived orienta-

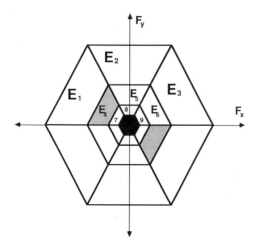

Fig. 9.1
Diagram of the frequency domain, partitioned by nine oriented energy mechanisms. Each subregion, labeled E_1 through E_9, represents the "amplitude response" of one energy mechanism. For example, the E_2 mechanism responds to high frequency horizontal gratings. The "amplitude responses" are drawn schematically here; for actual energy mechanisms the regions are more rounded and they overlap somewhat.

tion of a grating stimulus is largely invariant with respect to contrast.

Figure 9.1 illustrates the partition of the frequency domain by a collection of energy mechansims. Each region in the diagram corresponds to the "amplitude response" of one energy mechanism. Contrast normalization of each mechanism is realized by dividing its output by the total energy at all orientations and nearby spatial frequencies. The normalized energy, $\bar{E}_i(t)$, is given by:

$$\bar{E}_i(t) = \frac{E_i(t)}{\sigma^2 + \sum_{j=1}^{9} E_j(t)}, \qquad (4)$$

where σ is a constant in the denominator, known as the semisaturation constant. As long as σ is nonzero, the normalized output will always be finite, even for a zero contrast stimulus. In fact, the normalized output will always have a value between 0 and 1, saturating for high contrasts.

The underlying linear operators can be chosen so that the sum of their squared amplitude responses is the unit constant function (everywhere equal to one). Then the summation in the denominator gives the total Fourier energy in an annulus of spatial frequencies.

Operators tuned to different orientations (e.g., corresponding to each of the regions labeled E_4, E_5, and E_6 in

figure 9.1) are all normalized together. That is, each is divided by the sum of all nine energy outputs at all orientations and nearby spatial frequencies, plus σ^2. Within each spatial frequency band, the ratio of the outputs of two normalized operators is invariant with respect to stimulus contrast. The ratio is maintained even though the normalized outputs saturate at high contrasts. E_1, E_2, and E_3 are normalized by a different set including higher frequencies and excluding E_7, E_8, and E_9. Likewise for the lower frequency operators.

Feedback Normalization

Contrast normalization given by equations 2, 3, and 4 is expressed in feedforward manner. First, the A_i^ϕ's are computed, then they are combined to give the E_i's, and then the E_i's are combined to give the $\bar{E}_i$'s. However, the unnormalized A_i^ϕ's and E_i's cannot be represented by mechanisms (e.g., neurons or 8-bit computers) with limited dynamic range.

The solution is to use a feedback network to do the normalization. Then, the A_i^ϕ's and E_i's need not be explicitly represented as cell output firing rates. The details of the feedback normalization network are beyond the scope of this chapter, but will be discussed in a forthcoming paper.

One consequence of using a feedback network to achieve the normalization is that the feedback signal must be averaged over space and/or time to avoid unstable oscillations in the output. For spatially extended periodic stimuli, the feedback reaches a steady state after a brief period of time. The spatial and temporal pooling of the contrast normalization signal is left unspecified in this chapter, since it only deals with steady state responses.

Model Simple and Complex Cells

The model in its entirety is depicted in figure 9.2. Simple cells are modeled as contrast normalized and half-squared linear operators. Model complex cells are built on outputs of model simple cells. The contrast normalization feedback signal is combined from all orientations and nearby spatial frequencies.

The various stages of the model are as follows. Linear operators of four different phases are applied to the stimulus. The outputs of these operators are then half-squared and normalized to give the model simple cell responses:

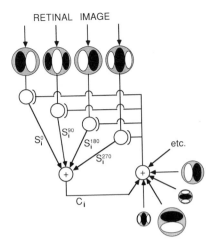

RETINAL IMAGE

S_i^0 S_i^{90} S_i^{180} S_i^{270} etc.

C_i

Fig. 9.2
Illustration of the various stages of the model. Linear receptive fields are depicted as circles, subdivided into bright and dark subregions. The S_i^ϕ labels represent simple cell outputs, and the C_i label represents a complex cell output. The feedback signal is the combined energy at all orientations and nearby spatial frequencies, averaged over space and time. The feedback signal suppresses the simple cell responses by way of divisive inhibition.

$$S_i^\phi(t) = k \frac{A_i^\phi(t)}{\sigma^2 + \frac{1}{4}\sum_j \sum_\phi A_j^\phi(t)}$$

$$= k \frac{A_i^\phi(t)}{\sigma^2 + \sum_j E_j(t)}, \qquad (5)$$

where S_i^ϕ is the response of a model simple cell with phase, ϕ, σ is the semisaturation constant, k is a constant scale factor that determines the maximum attainable firing rate, and $A_i^\phi(t)$ is defined in equation 2. The subscript i is an index used to specify the "amplitude response" of each operator. The model complex cell responses are computed by averaging the simple cell responses:

$$C_i(t) = (1/4)\sum_\phi S_i^\phi(t)$$

$$= (k/4)\sum_\phi \frac{A_i^\phi(t)}{\sigma^2 + \frac{1}{4}\sum_j \sum_\phi A_j^\phi(t)}$$

$$= k \frac{E_i(t)}{\sigma^2 + \sum_j E_j(t)}. \qquad (6)$$

Note again that if the underlying linear operators are chosen correctly then the denominator of equations 5 and 6 gives the Fourier energy of the stimulus within an annulus of spatial frequencies. As mentioned above, space-time averaging of the contrast-normalization is not

included in the above equations because this chapter deals only with steady state responses.

Striate Cell Responses

The previous section describes a nonlinear model of striate cell responses. This section reviews some of the electrophysiological data on the responses of simple and complex cells in cat striate cortex and compares model cell responses, given by equations 5 and 6, with electrophysiological data.

The results in this section demonstrate that simple cells behave more like half-squared linear operators than like halfwave-rectified linear operators. The results in this section also demonstrate that response saturation can be attributed to contrast normalization.

Simple Cells

Receptive Field

Simple cells have clearly defined excitatory and inhibitory subregions. Bright (brighter than the mean luminance) light in an excitatory region or dim light in an inhibitory region enhances a simple cell's response, whereas bright light in an inhibitory region or dim light in excitatory region inhibits its response. The excitatory and inhibitory subregions are also called "on" and "off" regions; the cell responds to light increment (the onset of a bright stimulus) in an "on" region, and to light decrement (the offset of a bright stimulus) in an "off" region. Superimposed on each "on" subregion is "off" inhibition and vice versa.

Although many physiologists have used oriented bars, edges, and gratings to generate one-dimensional maps of receptive fields, relatively few (e.g., Jones & Palmer, 1987) have measured the two-dimensional spatial structure of receptive fields. Some researchers have mapped the three-dimensional spatiotemporal structure of simple cell receptive fields (Hamilton, Albrecht & Geisler, 1989; McLean & Palmer, 1989; see chapter 8).

Frequency Domain vs. Space Domain

Many experimenters (Andrews & Pollen, 1979; Kulikowski & Bishop, 1981; Maffei, Morrone, Pirchio & Sandini, 1979; Movshon et al., 1978a; Tadmor & Tolhurst, 1989) have tested for linearity of simple cells by comparing cells' transfer functions with their impulse responses. The

Nonlinear Model of Neural Responses in Cat Visual Cortex

logic of these experiments is straightforward. The response of a linear cell to the sum of two stimuli is equal to the sum of the responses to each of the component stimuli. Since a grating is composed of the sum of a number of impulses, the response of a linear cell to a grating is predictable from its response to impulses. Likewise, since an impulse can be thought of as the sum of a number of gratings, the response to an impulse is predictable from the response to gratings.

The results of these experiments show that simple cell response to gratings and their response to impulses look very nearly like Fourier transforms of one another, up to an arbitrary scale factor. These results have been taken as evidence for linearity.

Most of these researchers found, however, that the response to gratings and the response to impulses are not precise transforms of one another. In many cases, the inverse transform of the response to gratings gives a receptive field profile with additional side bands beyond those measured directly. In addition, the measured response to gratings is often more narrowly tuned than predicted from the Fourier transform of the response to impulses.

Several experimenters (e.g., Tadmor & Tolhurst, 1989) suggest that the discrepancy between the frequency and space domain measurements can be explained by over-rectification. If the neuron has to reach a certain level of excitation before any activity is seen, there will be a disproportionate decrease in small responses.

The results are also predicted by half-squaring. With half-squaring instead of halfwave-rectification, the response to impulses and the response to gratings are not transforms of one another. But in spite of the nonlinearity, the inverse transform of the response to gratings still looks very similar to the response to impulses, when they are rescaled relative to one another by an appropriate scale factor. As shown in figure 9.3A, the inverse transform of the response to gratings has some extra (low amplitude) side bands, in agreement with much of the physiological data. As shown in figure 9.3B, the response to gratings is more narrowly tuned than predicted from the response to impulses, also in agreement with physiological data.

The point of this demonstration is that the experiments do not distinguish well between halfwave-rectification, over-rectification, and half-squaring. The experimental re-

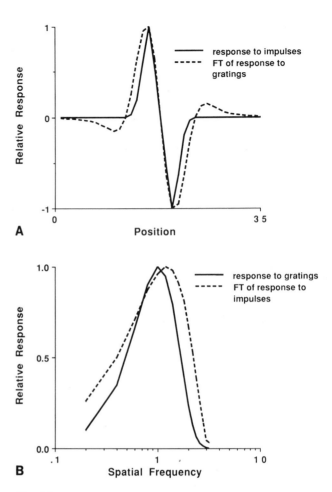

Fig. 9.3
A comparison between the response to impulses and the response to gratings of a half-squared Gabor operator. Response to gratings measured as the Fourier amplitude of the response, for each stimulus spatial frequency. Response to impulses measured as the signed-square of the underlying linear operator. Since the operator is nonlinear, the response to impulses and response to gratings are not transforms of one another. (A) Response to impulses superimposed with the inverse Fourier transform of response to gratings.
(B) Response to gratings superimposed with the magnitude of the Fourier transform of response to impulses. The response to gratings is more narrowly tuned than predicted from the response to impulses, and the response to impulses is more narrowly tuned than predicted from the response to gratings. This is in agreement with much of the physiological data.

sults can not be taken as evidence to favor one model over the other.

Responses to Counterphase Gratings

Simple cells exhibit characteristic responses to temporally modulated (e.g., counterphase) sine gratings. The response varies over time with the temporal modulation of the stimulus, and the amplitude and phase of modulation both depend on the spatial phase of the grating (Kulikowski & Bishop, 1981; Maffei & Fiorentini, 1973; Movshon et al., 1978a; Reid et al, 1987; see chapter 8). Reid et al. (1987) and Movshon et al. (1978a) have measured response amplitude and response phase of simple cells while varying the spatial phase of counterphase gratings. They have both shown (mathematically) that for a halfwave-rectified spatiotemporal linear operator, a polar plot of the response amplitude as a function of the response phase is elliptical in shape. Their experimental results, however, are typically not quite elliptical. Rather the results have been described as "wasp-waisted ellipses" since the amplitudes near the minor axes are smaller than they should be to fit an ellipse. Movshon et al. proposed that this deviation could be explained by over-rectification.

The wasp-waisted elliptical shape is also predicted by half-squaring. In figure 9.4, the output of a spatiotemporal Gabor operator was computed for counterphase gratings of various spatial and temporal frequencies, and various spatial phases. The response waveforms were then half-squared, and the amplitude and phase of the fundamental Fourier component (equal to the temporal frequency of the stimulus) were measured. Figure 9.4 plots relative response amplitude as a function of response phase for two different spatial and temporal frequencies. The plots are similar in shape to physiological data. Like the results discussed above, this experiment does not distinguish well between over-rectification and half-squaring.

Counterphase vs. Drifting Gratings

By comparing the responses to counterphase stimuli with responses to drifting grating stimuli, Reid et al. (1987) have demonstrated that there is a nonlinear contribution to the direction selectivity of simple cells. They computed a directional index given by $(R_p - R_a)/(R_p + R_a)$, where R_p and R_a are, respectively, the responses for gratings drifting in the preferred and antipreferred directions. Reid et al. showed that for a halfwave-rectified spatiotemporal

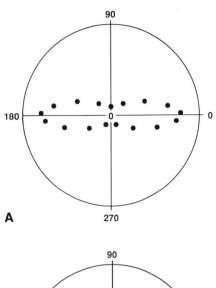

A

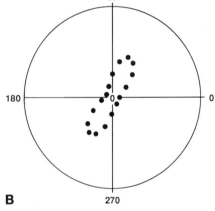

B

Fig. 9.4
Responses of a half-squared linear operator for counterphase grating stimuli of varying spatial phase. The amplitude of the fundamental component of the response is represented radially, while the angular coordinate indicates the temporal phase of the response. The stimulus spatial and temporal frequencies are different for the two plots. These polar plots of response amplitude versus response phase are shaped like wasp-waisted ellipses, in agreement with physiological data.

linear operator this directional index is predictable from the responses to counterphase gratings. Specifically, the directional index is equal to the ratio of the axes of the ellipse obtained, as described above, from counterphase grating stimuli. However, Reid et al. found that these two measures of the directional index do not agree; the prediction from counterphase stimuli underestimates the index by about half.

Half-squaring explains this result reasonably well. Figure 9.5 plots the ratio of the axes of the best fitting ellipse derived from counterphase stimuli against the directional

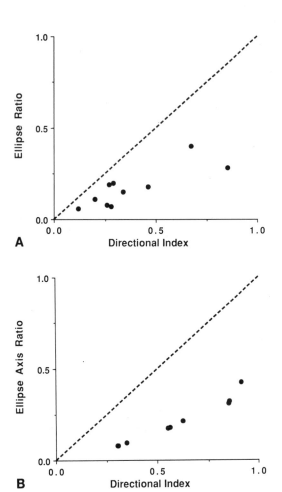

Fig. 9.5

Directional index predicted from counterphase grating stimuli versus that measured directly from drifting gratings for: (A) a direction selective simple cell (replotted from Reid et al., 1987), and (B) a half-squared spatiotemporal Gabor operator. Each point is for a different stimulus spatial and temporal frequency. The dotted line is the prediction of a halfwave-rectified linear operator. For both model cells and real cells, the directional index predicted from counterphase stimuli underestimates that measured directly with drifting gratings.

index measured with drifting grating stimuli. The figure shows that for a half-squared Gabor operator, the directional index predicted from counterphase stimuli underestimates that measured directly with drifting gratings, in a manner very similar to the experimental results.

Complex Cells

Complex cells are clearly nonlinear as they respond to either a bright or a dim stimulus placed anywhere within their receptive fields. In experiments performed by Movshon et al. (1978b) a bar fixed in one position was flashed

simultaneously with a second bar, of the same or opposite polarity, that could appear in one of several positions around the location of the fixed bar. By measuring the influence of the second bar upon the response to the first, Movshon et al. were able to demonstrate that complex cell receptive fields are composed of subunits. The subunits have clearly defined spatial profiles with excitatory and inhibitory subregions. The subunit outputs are rectified before being combined into the complex cell response. In addition, Movshon et al. measured complex cell responses to grating stimuli. They determined that the inverse Fourier transform of the response to gratings matches the spatial profile of the underlying subunits, up to an arbitrary scale factor. The present model is in general agreement with these results. The subunits of model complex cells are model simple cells with identical "amplitude response."

Emerson and coworkers (1987, 1991) analyzed responses of complex cells to stimuli made up of pairs of bars flashed in sequence. The response to a pair of bars is different from the sum of the responses to each individual bar. For some spatial and temporal separations between the bars the cell response is greater than the linear prediction, and for other separations it is less than the linear prediction. Emerson et al. (1991) have shown that the nonlinear interaction between pairs of bars is consistent with that predicted by energy mechanisms.

A variety of other experiments also indicate that energy mechanisms are reasonable models of complex cells. An energy mechanism has an unmodulated response to drifting sine grating stimuli, as do the majority of complex cells (Maffei & Fiorentini, 1973; Movshon 1978b). For counterphase grating stimuli, both complex cells and energy mechanisms have responses that vary over time at twice the temporal frequency of the stimulus (Movshon et al., 1978b). In addition, responses to counterphase gratings do not depend on the spatial phase of the stimulus (Maffei & Fiorentini, 1973; Movshon et al., 1978b).

Contrast-Response

The inclusion of contrast normalization in the model results in response saturation. The contrast-response function (that is, response as a function of log contrast for sine grating stimuli of optimal spatial frequency and orientation) for model cells is qualitatively similar to typical experimentally measured contrast-response relationships in both cat and primate (Albrecht & Hamilton, 1982; Dean, 1981; Maffei & Fiorentini, 1973; Ohzawa, Sclar & Freeman, 1985; Sclar, Maunsell & Lennie, 1990).

The constrast-response functions for striate cells in both cat and primate have been fitted by the hyperbolic ratio function (Albrecht & Hamilton, 1982; Li & Creutzfeldt, 1984; Sclar et al., 1990):

$$R = R_{max} \frac{c^n}{\sigma^n + c^n} + M, \tag{7}$$

where R is the evoked response, c is the contrast of the test grating, M is maintained discharge, n is a constant, σ is the semisaturation constant, and R_{max} is the maximum attainable response.

With parameters $n = 2$ and $M = 0$, the contrast-response function given by equation 7 is equivalent to that of model cells given by equations 5 and 6. The equivalence is easily demonstrated by recalling that the summation in the denominator of equations 5 and 6 is proportional to c^2.

Physiological data from both cat and primate show that the exponent in the contrast-response function does not differ significantly between populations of simple and complex cells (Albrecht & Hamilton, 1982; Dean, 1981). The exponent is 2 on average, but there is variability from cell to cell (Albrecht & Hamilton, 1982; Sclar et al., 1990).

In the present model, the contrast-response functions of both simple and complex cells have exponents of 2, because of half-squaring. If the model simple cells were halfwave-rectified rather than half-squared, then their exponent would instead be 1.

Contrast Dependence of Tuning

The contrast-response curve of a model cells shifts downward (on log-log axes) if the orientation of the test grating is non-optimal. This property of model cells is easily explained by equations 5 and 6. In each of these equations the value of the numerator depends on stimulus orientation because the underlying linear operator is orientation tuned. The value of the denominator does not depend on stimulus orientation because the suppression is pooled equally over all orientations. If the suppression was broadly tuned for orientation then the contrast-response curves would shift downward and rightward. The relative

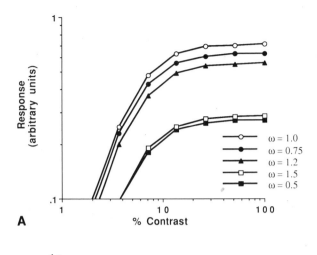

A

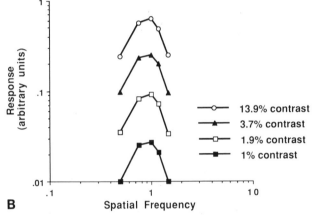

B

Fig. 9.6

Model complex cell response for grating stimuli of various contrasts and spatial frequencies. (A) and (B) show the same data plotted in different ways. (A) Response versus contrast as the spatial frequency, ω, of the stimulus is varied. The contrast-response curve shifts downward and very slightly rightward (not visible in the graph) in the log-log plot if the spatial frequency of the test grating is nonoptimal. (B) Spatial frequency tuning curves as the contrast of the stimulus is varied. Tuning width is largely invariant with respect to contrast. Width broadens very slightly (not visible in the graph) with increased contrast. Both of these results are in agreement with physiological data.

amount of rightward shift depends on the breadth of the tuning.

Figure 9.6A shows the contrast-response curves of a model cell for various stimulus spatial frequencies. The curves shift downward and slightly rightward for non-optimal spatial frequencies. The small rightward shift occurs because the suppression from contrast normalization is broadly tuned for spatial frequency. If the suppression were equal for all spatial frequencies then there would be no rightward shift.

Downward shifts of contrast-response have been measured physiologically by Li and Creutzfeldt (1984) for stimuli of nonoptimal orientation, for stimuli of nonpreferred direction of motion, and for stimuli in the nondominant eye. Li and Creutzfeldt, and other authors, interpreted these results as demonstrating that saturation of the contrast-response curve is already present at the precortical level and therefore not due to intracortical mechanisms. On the contrary, the model predicts the downward shift precisely because of the mutual suppression between cortical cells. Albrecht and Hamilton (1982) recorded similar downward shifts of contrast-response curves for stimuli of nonoptimal spatial frequency, but they also found a slight rightward shift of the curves, in agreement with the present model.

The orientation tuning width of model cells is invariant with respect to contrast. Changing the stimulus contrast scales the response by a constant factor over all orientations. In other words, the ratio of the responses produced by different orientations remains fixed, independent of contrast. Contrast has no impact on tuning width because the suppression from contrast normalization is equal for all stimulus orientations. If the suppression was broadly tuned for orientation then the model cell's tuning width would depend on contrast.

Figure 9.6B shows the spatial frequency tuning curves of a model cell for various contrasts. The spatial frequency bandwidth broadens very slightly with increased contrast, because the suppression from contrast normalization is broadly tuned for spatial frequency. Experimental results demonstrate that real cells behave similarly. In spite of response saturation, orientation and spatial frequency tuning widths vary little with contrast (Albrecht & Hamiltom, 1982; Li & Creutzfeldt, 1984; Sclar & Freeman, 1982).

Discussion

For some years, simple cells have been modeled as halfwave-rectified linear operators. It has also become popular to model complex cells as energy mechanisms. A variety of experimental results provide evidence in support of the linear/energy model, but a variety of other experimental results can not be explained by the linear/energy model.

In this chapter I have suggested two modifications to the linear/energy model in order to explain a larger body of physiological data. One modification is the use of half-squaring instead of halfwave-rectification (or over-rectification) at the output of the model simple cells. The other modification is to include a contrast normalization nonlinearity.

With contrast normalization and squaring, the contrast-response curves of model cells are very similar to physiological measurements. Contrast-response curves of model cells shift mostly downward for nonoptimal stimuli, and the tuning widths of model cells are largely independent of contrast (figure 9.6). In other words, the ratio of the responses produced by two different stimuli is largely invariant with respect to stimulus contrast. In this way, information about a visual stimulus, other than its contrast, can be represented as the relative responses of a collection of cells.

Contrast normalization explains some additional properties typical of striate cells including nonspecific suppression (e.g., Bonds. 1989) mentioned in the introduction to this chapter, and contrast adaptation (e.g., Ohzawa et al., 1985). These issues will be addressed in a forthcoming paper.

In addition, the results of a variety of psychophysical experiments have been modeled using contrast normalization. For example, both Bergen and Landy (see chapter 17), and Graham (see chapter 18) include contrast normalization steps in their models of texture discrimination.

In this chapter, I discuss three models of simple cell rectification: halfwave-rectification, over-rectification, and half-squaring. While there is ample evidence to reject halfwave-rectification, the experiments to date are generally consistent with both over-rectification and half-squaring. This is not surprising since these two nonlinearities are approximately the same over a restricted operating range. Mathematically, the two nonlinearities are expressed as:

$$N_1(x) = a_1 \lfloor x \rfloor^2$$

$$N_2(x) = a_2 \lfloor x - T \rfloor,$$

where $N_1(x)$ and $N_2(x)$ are half-squaring and over-rectification, respectively, a_1 and a_2 are scale factors, T is a threshold, and $\lfloor x \rfloor = \max(x, 0)$ is taken to mean halfwave rectification. By choosing a_2 and T appropriately, $N_2(x)$ can be made to approximate $N_1(x)$ for a certain range of x values.

These two functions approximate one another only for a certain range of values, so it may be possible to discriminate between them experimentally. For example, the results of the Reid et al. experiment (figure 9.5) can be reanalyzed to test the different hypotheses. One can compensate for the effect of half-squaring by taking the square root of the responses. After taking square roots, the directional indices measured from drifting gratings should be equal to the ellipse ratios measured from counterphase gratings. Likewise, one can compensate for the effect of over-rectification by adding a fixed constant value to the responses. More generally, one could try fitting the experimental data using the following nonlinearity:

$$N(x) = a\lfloor x - T \rfloor^n. \tag{8}$$

The choice of exponent, n, and threshold, T, that yield the best fit would be measured from the data. Half-squaring corresponds to the case in which $n = 2$ and $T = 0$. Over-rectification corresponds to the case in which $n = 1$ and $T \neq 0$.

Although the present model explains a large body of physiological data, there is variability in the behavior from one cell to the next. Some, but not all, of the variability between cells can be accounted for by the present model's parameters. For example, there are some complex cells that, unlike energy mechanisms, have modulated responses to gratings of certain spatial frequencies.

As another example, half-squaring predicts that polar plots of response to counterphase gratings are shaped like wasp-waisted ellipses (figure 9.4). Half-squaring also predicts that the ellipse axis ratio underestimate the directional index (figure 9.5). For some cells, however, the ellipse axis ratio underestimates the directional index even though polar plots of response to counterphase gratings are well fit by ellipses (not wasp-waisted).

Future research will aim to enhance the model so that it might account for some of the variability between cells. For example, it is possible to account for some of the variability in contrast-response measurements by adding a threshold parameter to the model. Contrast-response of model cells would then be given by:

$$R = R_{\max} \frac{\lfloor c - T \rfloor^n}{\sigma^n + c^n} + M. \tag{9}$$

If T is negative and M is positive then the cell would have a nonzero maintained discharge. If T is positive and M is negative then the cell would be over-rectified.

Varying T in equation 9 not only changes the level of maintained discharge, but also changes the shape of the contrast-response curve. Varying T and σ simultaneously can look very much like a change in the exponent, n. This suggests the possibililty of fitting contrast-response data with a fixed exponent of 2, accounting for the variability from cell to cell by changing the value of T.

For a particular cell, the parameters of the model can be measured and compared using different experiments. For example, the exponent, n, and threshold, T, can be measured by fitting contrast-response data to equation 9. These parameters can also be measured, as discussed above, by using equation 8 to fit the data of Reid et al.

As another example, recall that the contrast-response curve of model cells shifts downward and slightly rightward if the spatial-frequency of the test grating is non-optimal. The amount of rightward shift depends on the breadth of tuning of the contrast-normalization suppression. For a particular cell, one could measure both the breadth of tuning and the shift in contrast-response, and then compare the two.

The ultimate goal of modeling visual neurons is to be able to predict the response of a cell to any stimulus, based on a limited number of measurements. The success of this endeavor hinges on pinpointing the regularities in the behavior of visual neurons. A good model will have a small number of easily measured parameters and will be able to predict the responses of a large number of cells.

Acknowledgments

This chapter benefitted greatly from discussions with Ted Adelson, Beau Watson, Jim Bergen, John Robson, A. B. Bonds, and Tony Movshon.

References

Adelson, E. H. & Bergen, J. R. (1985). Spatiotemporal energy models for the perception of motion. *Journal of the Optical Society of America A*, 2, 284–299.

Albrecht, D. G. & Hamilton, D. B. (1982). Striate cortex of monkey and cat: Contrast response function. *Journal of Neurophysiology*, 48, 217–237.

Andrews, B. W. & Pollen, D. A. (1979). Relationship between spatial frequency selectivity and receptive field profile of simple cells. *Journal of Physiology (London), 287*, 163–176.

Bergen, J. R. & Adelson, E. H. (1988). Early vision and texture perception. *Nature, 333*, 363–367.

Bonds, A. B. (1989). Role of inhibition in the specification of orientation selectivity of cells in the cat striate cortex. *Visual Neuroscience, 2*, 41–55.

Campbell, F. W., Cooper, G. F. & Enroth-Cugell, C. (1968). The angular selectivity of visual cortical cells to moving gratings. *Journal of Physiology (London), 198*, 237–250.

Campbell, F. W., Cooper, G. F. & Enroth-Cugell, C. (1969). The spatial selectivity of visual cells of the cat. *Journal of Physiology (London), 203*, 223–235.

Campbell, F. W. & Robson, J. G. (1968). Application of Fourier analysis to the visibility of gratings. *Journal of Physiology (London), 197*, 551–556.

Daugman, J. G. (1980). Two-dimensional spectral analysis of cortical receptive field profiles. *Vision Research, 20*, 846–856.

Dean, A. F. (1981). The relationship between response amplitude and contrast for cat striate cortical neurons. *Journal of Physiology (London), 318*, 413–427.

Emerson, R. C., Bergen, J. R. & Adelson, E. H. (1991). Directionally selective complex cells and the computation of motion energy in cat visual cortex. *Vision Research*, in press.

Emerson, R. C., Citron, M. C., Vaughn, W. J. & Klein, S. A. (1987). Nonlinear directionally selective subunits in complex cells of cat striate cortex. *Journal of Neurophysiology, 58*, 33–65.

Gabor, D. (1946). Theory of communication. *JIEE (London), 93*, 429–457.

Hamilton, D. B., Albrecht, D. G. & Geisler, W. S. (1989). Visual cortical receptive fields in monkey and cat: Spatial and temporal phase transfer function. *Vision Research, 29*, 1285–1308.

Heeger, D. J. (1987). Model for the extraction of image flow. *Journal of the Optical Society of America A, 4*, 1455–1471.

Hubel, D. & Wiesel, T. (1962). Receptive fields, binocular interaction, and functional architecture in the cat's visual cortex. *Journal of Physiology (London), 160*, 106–154.

Jones, J. P. & Palmer, L. A. (1987). The two-dimensional spatial structure of simple receptive fields in cat striate cortex. *Journal of Neurophysiology, 58*, 1187–1211.

Kulikowski, J. J. & Bishop, P. O. (1981). Linear analysis of the response of simple cells in the cat visual cortex. *Experimental Brain Research, 44*, 386–400.

Li, C. & Creutzfeldt, O. (1984). The representation of contrast and other stimulus parameters by single neurons in area 17 of the cat. *Pflugers Archives, 401*, 304–314.

Maffei, L. & Fiorentini, A. (1973). The visual cortex as a spatial frequency analyzer. *Vision Research, 13*, 1255–1267.

Maffei, L., Morrone, C., Pirchio, M. & Sandini, G. (1979). Responses of visual cortical cells to periodic and nonperiodic stimuli. *Journal of Physiology (London), 296*, 27–47.

Malik, J. & Perona, P. (1990). Preattentive texture discrimination with early vision mechanisms. *Journal of the Optical Society of America A, 7*, 923–931.

McLean, J. & Palmer, L. A. (1989). Contribution of linear spatiotemporal receptive field structure to velocity selectivity of simple cells in area 17 of cat. *Vision Research, 29*, 675–679.

Movshon, J. A., Thompson, I. D. & Tolhurst, D. J. (1978a). Spatial summation in the receptive fields of simple cells in the cat's striate cortex. *Journal of Physiology (London), 283*, 53–77.

Movshon, J. A., Thompson, I. D. & Tolhurst, D. J. (1978b). Receptive field organization of complex cells in the cat's striate cortex. *Journal of Physiology (London), 283*, 79–99.

Ohzawa, I., Sclar, G. & Freeman, R. D. (1985). Contrast gain control in the cat's visual system. *Journal of Neurophysiology, 54*, 651–667.

Pentland, A. P. (1989). A possible neural mechanism for computing shape from shading. *Neural Computation, 1*, 208–217.

Reid, R. C., Soodak, R. E. & Shapley, R. M. (1987). Linear mechanisms of directional selectivity in simple cells of cat striate cortex. *Proceedings of the National Academy of Science, 84*, 8740–8744.

Robson, J. G. (1988). Linear and nonlinear operations in the visual system. *Investigative Ophthalmology and Visual Science Supplement, 29*, 117.

Ross, J., Morrone, M. C. & Burr, D. C. (1989). The conditions under which Mach bands are visible. *Vision Research, 29*, 699–715.

Sanger, T. (1988). Stereo disparity computation using Gabor filters. *Biological Cybernetics, 59*, 405–418.

Sclar, G. & Freeman, R. D. (1982). Orientation selectivity of the cat's striate cortex is invariant with stimulus contrast. *Experimental Brain Research, 46*, 457–461.

Sclar, G., Maunsell, J. H. R. & Lennie, P. (1990). Coding of image contrast in central visual pathways of the macaque monkey. *Vision Research, 30*, 1–10.

Shapley, R. & Enroth-Cugell, C. (1984). Visual adaptation and retinal gain control. *Progress in Retinal Research, 3*, 263–346.

Sperling, G. & Sondhi, M. M. (1968). Model for visual luminance discrimination and flicker detection. *Journal of the Optical Society of America, 58*, 1133–1145.

Tadmor, Y. & Tolhurst, D. J. (1989). The effect of threshold on the relationship between the receptive-field profile and the spatial-frequency tuning curve in simple cells of the cat's striate cortex. *Visual Neuroscience, 3*, 445–454.

Turner, M. R. (1986). Texture discrimination by Gabor functions. *Biological Cybernetics, 55*, 71–82.

van Santen, J. P. H. & Sperling, G. (1985). Elaborated Reichardt detectors. *Journal of the Optical Society of America A, 2*, 300–321.

Watson, A. B. & Ahumada, A. J. (1983). *A look at motion in the frequency domain*. Technical Report 84352, NASA-Ames Research Center.

Watson, A. B. & Ahumada, A. J. (1985). Model of human visual-motion sensing. *Journal of the Optical Society of America A, 2*, 322–342.

Part IV

Detection and
Discrimination

To understand how the visual system does the work of analyzing images, it is essential to know the fundamental limits that determine how much information, and of what kind, can be made available for central processing. In this section, we concentrate on models of spatial vision and, in particular, how one might model two psychophysical tasks: detecting a simple pattern, and discriminating simple patterns from one another. In a pattern discrimination task, an observer must choose among two or more patterns that differ slightly along one dimension, such as contrast, orientation, spatial frequency, or spatial location. In a detection task an observer must detect a stimulus whose intensity is made so low that it inhabits the hazy border zone between the seen and the unseen. The two tasks are formally similar—a detection task is essentially a discrimination between an absent stimulus and a present one. Between them, the two tasks capture many of the fundamental limitations on visual performance that must be known before more complex tasks can be understood; for a comprehensive recent review of the state of knowledge in this field, see Graham (1989).

A rich base of detection and discrimination data is available from many sources. Two recurring and important features of these data that require theoretical treatment are the themes that dominate the chapters in this section. First, experiments in which observers discriminate two patterns that differ from one another only in contrast generally produce an apparently paradoxical result: When both targets are clearly visible, discrimination thresholds grow roughly in proportion to the overall contrast, but when the targets are near contrast threshold, thresholds *fall* with increasing contrast. The function relating contrast discrimination thresholds to base contrast thus has a characteristic "dipper" shape, first falling and then growing again. Second, both for detection and discrimination, when pairs of simple patterns are used, similar patterns interact strongly, while dissimilar ones seem to be processed more-or-less independently. For example, detection of a vertically oriented grating pattern in the fovea is impeded by the addition of a vertical masking pattern of similar spatial structure, but is largely unaffected by added gratings of different orientation, spatial structure, retinal location, and so forth. Similar results are obtained from experiments using a variety of other experimental methods.

These results have suggested that the visual system contains multiple spatial frequency "channels" having different specificities for spatial pattern, and that these channels have particular contrast transduction properties that give rise to the apparently anomalous performance seen near the threshold of visibility. Although both of these phenomena have been modeled in the past, the treatments that work for one have not been consistent with data obtained for the other. It is only recently that satisfying theoretical frameworks have been presented for accounting for both, and for the other aspects of spatial detection and discrimination performance.

All of the chapters in this section speak to these issues. Nachmias describes a model designed to account for the effects of summing similar and dissimilar patterns that uses a model of multiple spatial channels formulated in a manner designed to be consistent with contrast discrimination data. Pelli examines the statistical characteristics of observer performance and suggests that with multiple channels examining the stimulus, it is possible to model detection and discrimination performance based on a type of model first devised to account for performance on multiple-pattern tasks. Finally, Wilson reviews some of his work modeling spatial pattern discriminations using a small set of spatial channels and concludes that an additional noise source is needed to model spatial position judgments: the disorder of the sampling lattice (cf. section II).

Reference

Graham, N. (1989). *Visual Pattern Analyzers*. New York: Oxford University Press.

10

A Template Matching Model of Subthreshold Summation

Jacob Nachmias

The last two decades have seen the development of ever more sophisticated and more successful models of detection of visual contrast patterns (Graham, 1989). Analyses of subthreshold summation experiments have played a major role in this endeavor. In subthreshold summation experiments one compares the detectability of two or more patterns when presented one at a time, to the detectability of those same patterns presented together. For k component patterns matched in detectability, the ratio of threshold contrasts under these two conditions of presentation is found empirically to vary from k to k raised to the power of $1/b$, where b is a number between 3 and 4. I will refer to such a ratio as a *summation ratio*. The actual value of the summation ratio depends on how much the component patterns differ in spatial or temporal location, or in other attributes such as spatial frequency or orientation. The ratio equals k only when the component patterns are identical; it starts dropping rapidly as they begin to separate in stimulus parameter space, and gradually approaches its lower asymptotic value as their separation increases further.

The form of the initial decline of the summation ratio was originally misinterpreted as being governed by the properties of the underlying sensors (Kulikowski & King-Smith, 1973; Quick & Reichart, 1975; Sachs, Nachmias & Robson, 1971) but is now understood to result from other causes having little or nothing to do with sensor properties (Graham & Robson, 1987; Hall & Sondhi, 1977; Quick, Mullins & Reichart, 1978)

On the other hand, the critical stimulus separation at which the summation ratio essentially reaches its asymptotic value, and that value itself, are commonly still attributed to sensor properties. In brief, the currently most widely accepted account goes as follows: (1) The summation ratio reaches its asymptotic value when the stimulus components are sufficiently different so that they stimulate entirely different sets of sensors; thus the critical stimulus-component separation serves as a rough measure of sensor bandwidth. (2) The value of the asymptotic summation ratio, which measures the increase in sensitivity due to subthreshold summation of highly disparate patterns, is due to probability summation alone. On this account, b—which controls the value of the asymptotic summation ratio itself—is equal to β, the Weibull parameter governing the slope of the "psychometric function" of the individual sensors (Nachmias, 1981). Because of the properties of Weibull functions, the value of β can be independently estimated from the observer's psychometric function for detection. It turns out that these two independent estimates of β agree quite well, which gives strong support to the probability summation account of subthreshold summation—despite the fact that the "high threshold theory" of detection on which this account is rooted has been repeatedly discredited in many other contexts (Green & Swets, 1966)

Pelli's Uncertainty Model

Recently, Pelli (1985) showed there was a different way to account for both the observed value of the asymptotic summation ratio and the value of β estimated from detection psychometric functions. He proposed an uncertainty model of detection similar to the one originally developed by Tanner (1961) in the context of psychoacoustics. The model assumes that the observer's task—whether the components are presented separately or together—is to detect one of M orthogonal signals. In other words, the observer is said to behave as if on every trial, any one of M uncorrelated stimuli has an equal likelihood of being presented. Corresponding to each possible stimulus, there is a matched sensor or channel, whose output is perturbed by independent Gaussian noise. The decision variable used by the observer is the largest sensor output. For present purposes, Pelli's major conclusions are the following:

1. *Uncertainty steepens psychometric functions.* For M sufficiently large—300 or so—the predicted value of β for two-alternative forced choice (2AFC) detection is a good approximation to that estimated from empirical results.

2. *Uncertainty reduces the amount of subthreshold summation.* When the ratio of the number of stimulus components presented to the total number of orthogonal stimulus components, k/M, is sufficiently small—around 1 percent—the asymptotic summation ratio should be approxima-

tely equal to k raised to the power $1/\beta$, in accord with many empirical findings.

The original motivation for the work to be reported here was dissatisfaction with the status of the probability summation concept. True, Pelli had shown that the concept was not inevitably tied to the oft-discredited high threshold theory of detection; signal detection theory, at least under certain conditions, can be made to yield predictions indistinguishable from those of probability summation. However, it is not clear what would result from extending Pelli's approach to more general conditions such as nonorthogonal sensors and stimuli. Furthermore, the "largest sensor output" approach is not easy to generalize to tasks other than contrast detection—to pattern discrimination or masking, for example.

Template Matching Model

The present computer simulations of subthreshold summation use a variant of a template matching model developed by Nielsen, Watson, and Ahumada (1985). This model seems at least in principle to avoid the limitations of Pelli's model. Unlike the sensors in Pelli's model, which have orthogonal receptive fields, those in the present model have receptive fields that overlap both in the two-dimensional space and the 2D Fourier domains. In fact, they are borrowed from Watson's 1983 model, which was inspired by the results of cortical electrophysiology (for details see Watson, 1983).

Another difference between the models is the hypothesized decision rule. In Pelli's model, decisions are based on the largest sensor output, hence only the magnitudes of the individual sensor outputs matter. By contrast, the statistical observer of the present model uses the pattern of outputs across all sensors to decide on each 2AFC trial whether any one of M possible (but not necessarily orthogonal) stimuli has in fact been presented in either the first or the second interval. In essence, the observer is assumed to compare the observation made on each trial to the templates for the stimuli that could have been presented in each interval of the 2AFC trial, and to select that interval in which the best match occurs.

The separate effects of each of these two departures from Pelli's model were briefly examined. However, this chapter will summarize only the more extensive simulations in which both differences were incorporated. It will be shown that a version of the template matching model accounts surprisingly well for most aspects of the reported results of psychophysical subthreshold summation experiments with widely separated components. It will then be argued that in light of this model, these psychophysical results might say very little about sensor properties, just as has turned out to be the case for the rate of decline of the summation ratio with component separation.

Method

The 2AFC detection psychometric functions were generated by Monte Carlo simulation in the following manner.[1]

The Basic Algorithm

1. Sensor responses were computed for each of the M possible stimuli which define this ideal observer's uncertainty. The response of each sensor was taken to be the crosscorrelation between the sensor's weighting function and the stimulus (where the stimulus is defined as the spatial distribution of local luminance minus overall mean luminance). The set of responses to any particular stimulus will be referred to as a *sensor response vector*. To each of these M vectors were appended null vectors of the same length, to represent the hypothesis that the given stimulus appears in the first interval of the 2AFC trial; similarly, null vectors were prepended to represent hypothetical stimuli appearing in the second interval. The resulting vectors were stored as the *template* vectors. Since each possible stimulus could appear in either interval of the 2AFC trial, M possible stimuli generated $2M$ template vectors, or M template vector pairs. (The terms *templates* and *template vectors* will be used interchangeably throughout this chapter.)

2. A sensor response vector was also computed for the stimulus actually presented, and a null vector was pre-pended (or appended) as above. This time, however, a different sample of zero mean, unit variance, Gaussian noise was added to each element of the entire vector on each trial. The resulting *trial vector* consequently differed slightly from trial to trial.[2] It should be noted that throughout this chapter, all vectors are defined in sensor response space. To put it more precisely, if there are N sensors in the model, then each sensor response vector has length (number of elements) equal to N, while template vectors and trial vectors have lengths of $2N$, because they take into account the two intervals of the temporal forced-choice trial.

3. On every trial, the Euclidean distance was computed between the trial vector and each of the $2M$ template vectors. The observer was assumed to decide in which interval the stimulus occurred by choosing the interval-hypothesis embodied in the template vector closest to the trial vector.

4. The process was repeated for 256 trials at each of 10 contrast levels of the test stimulus to generate a psychometric function (proportion of responses correct as a function of stimulus contrast). A maximum likelihood procedure originally developed by Watson (1979) was applied to the data to estimate the α and β parameters of the best fitting Weibull function.[3]

The stimuli used in these simulations were two small Gabor patches centered $1°$ on either side of the fixation point. The spread at half amplitude of each patch was $0.25°$, and the underlying sinusoidal luminance modulation was horizontal, at 2 cycles/degree. To increase the speed of the simulations, only a subset of Watson's sensors were used: the 292 sensors whose receptive fields fell within a $3°$ radius of the fixation point and that were tuned to 2 cycles/degree vertical gratings at the fovea. (In Watson's model, sensor properties are scaled with eccentricity.) Inclusion of the entire sensor set of Watson's model would have vastly increased the required CPU time for the simulations without affecting the results.

---

1. The source code for the programs can be obtained by anonymous ftp from cattell.psych.upenn.edu (internet number 128.91.2.173). Interested readers should log in as "anonymous" and use the password "guest." They will find the files in directory /pub/jn4.

2. Those familiar with Watson's original terminology should note that the terms *template vector* and *trial vector* used here correspond to his *mean vector* and *feature vector*, respectively.

3. The Weibull function used to fit data from two-alternative, forced-choice experiments has the form

$$P = 1 - .5 \exp(-[c/\alpha]^\beta)$$

where P stands for proportion correct, c for contrast; the parameters α and β represent contrast sensitivity and steepness of the psychometric function.

However, probably the only essential aspect of the chosen stimulus and sensor parameters is that the resulting sensor response vectors to each of the two stimulus patches are orthogonal. Under these circumstances, the magnitude[4] of the sensor response vectors to both patches together is root-2 times that to either patch alone. Thus if the magnitude of the sensor response vector were the sole determiner of detectability, then, as Nielsen and Wandell (1988) have recently shown, the expected summation ratio for two components would be 1.41, rather than the value of around 1.2 usually estimated from the results of subthreshold summation experiments with human observers. (According to the standard probability summation account elaborated at the start of this chapter, the summation ratio should be approximately 2 raised to the power of 1/3.5, or 1.22—which is indistinguishable from empirically obtained values.) To be sure, the difference between 1.2 and 1.41, though very reliable, is quite small. However, the size of the discrepancy increases with the number of components. For example, with eight components, the vector magnitude model predicts an asymptotic summation ratio of 2.83 (the square root of 8), whereas empirical results (Robson & Graham, 1981), suggest a value close to 1.8 (8 raised to the power of 1/3.5, as predicted by the standard probability summation account).

Types of Templates

Templates are internal representations of possible stimuli. Monte Carlo psychometric functions were obtained with two types of stimulus templates (that is, templates for possible stimuli like the presented stimuli): *matched* (optimal) templates, and *component* (suboptimal) templates.

1. *Matched templates.* Such a template is the internal representation of a hypothetical stimulus identical to the stimulus actually presented on that trial; hence by definition there is but a single matched template pair per trial. For example, if the stimulus was one patch to the left of fixation, then a matched template pair represents precisely the same type of patch located exactly in the same place as the presented stimulus in either interval of the 2AFC

trial; if the stimulus was a two-patch stimulus, the matched template pair represents a correctly positioned two-patch stimulus. It might be expected that with matched templates, at least in the absence of additional templates, detection performance will be determined solely by the magnitude of the sensor response vectors to the stimuli.

2. *Component templates.* Here the same templates were used whether a one- or a two-patch stimulus was presented. In both types of trials, there were two template pairs, each pair corresponding to one of the component patches presented alone. In other words, the observer *always* considered two hypotheses—one patch to the left or one patch to the right—whether the presented stimulus was actually one patch to the right (or to the left), or both patches together.

In most simulations, additional templates were also included to represent the observer's uncertainty about the stimulus.

3. *Spatial uncertainty templates.* In one set of simulations the observer was assumed to always expect the presentation of a one-patch stimulus, but to be very uncertain about its exact location. There were altogether 289 component (one-patch) template pairs to represent stimuli at different possible locations, the locations forming a 17 by 17 grid centered at the fixation point, with adjacent location midpoints separated by $0.25°$. Because of the overlap among the possible stimuli and among the sensors, the corresponding 289 pairs of template vectors were certainly not orthogonal.

4. *Noise templates.* To assure more nearly orthogonal template vectors, simulations were also run where the extraneous templates each represented a different sample of two-dimensional noise. More precisely, in addition to the stimulus template vectors, a certain number of random noise template vectors were included. Every element of these latter vectors was filled by drawing an independent sample from a zero mean, unit variance Gaussian noise distribution. Random noise templates were coupled with both matched and component templates.

Vector Magnitude Scaling

The magnitudes of the sensor response vectors for the hypothetical stimuli (templates) were scaled in the fol-

---

4. The magnitude of a vector is defined as the square root of the sum of the squared values of all of its elements.

lowing manner. For templates of hypothetical stimuli like the presented stimuli, that is, matched templates or component templates in the correct or incorrect location, the sensor response vectors were those that would have resulted from the actual presentation of the hypothesized stimulus at its current contrast level. In the case of the random noise templates, the magnitudes of their sensor response vectors were set equal to those for the component or matched templates which they accompanied.

Results

Eight independent psychometric functions were generated for each set of stimulus and uncertainty conditions. The means of all the corresponding α and β estimates are summarized in table 10.1. The α's are expressed as dB attenuation relative to some arbitrary reference contrast. The total number of template pairs, M, consists of one matched template pair and M-1 random noise template pairs, or two component template pairs and M-2 random noise template pairs (except in the last row of the table, where M comprises the 289 spatial uncertainty component template pairs).

Table 10.1
Effect of uncertainty on α and β

M	One-patch stimuli		Two-patch stimuli	
	α	β	α	β
Matched templates				
1	25.16	1.35	28.07	1.37
2	23.19	1.47	26.10	1.49
9	20.14	2.03	23.03	1.94
25	18.67	2.45	21.60	2.51
289	16.43	3.15	19.43	3.19
Component templates				
2	23.29	1.49	26.89	1.31
9	20.07	2.08	22.66	1.75
25	18.72	2.33	20.96	2.15
289	16.41	3.18	18.08	3.09
289*	18.05	2.29	20.35	2.27

*Spatial uncertainty

Effect of Uncertainty on α and β

The first thing to notice is the overall effect of uncertainty on α and β. It is clear that as the number of templates increases, contrast sensitivity (α) declines, and psychometric functions get steeper (β increases). In this regard, the present model behaves like Pelli's, even though the sensors and decision rules are apparently quite different in the two models. The effects are also quantitatively very similar. Comparison of results of simulations with matched templates reveals that as the total number of essentially orthogonal template pairs increases from 1 to 289, sensitivity for 1 patch stimuli is reduced by 8.73 dB and β is up from 1.35 to 3.15. By comparison, in Pelli's model, increasing the number of orthogonal sensors monitored from 1 to 300 brings about an α reduction of 8.72 dB, and β increases from 1.41 to 3.28. The β values predicted by both models for large uncertainty are close to those obtained from real observers in detection experiments.

It should be noted (last row of the table) that when component templates are coupled with spatial uncertainty, the effect of the set of 289 nonorthogonal template pairs is only equivalent to that of 25 orthogonal template pairs.[5] Since it takes something in the neighborhood of 300 orthogonal template pairs to generate β's comparable to those from human observers, it is apparent that even the large amount of spatial uncertainty incorporated in this condition is not nearly sufficient by itself to match performance of real observers.

As can also be seen from table 10.1, uncertainty seems to have roughly the same effect on β's estimated from one- and two-patch stimulus presentations. Standard probability summation theory predicts that one- and two-patch β's should be exactly the same, if both one-patch psychometric functions are Weibull with the same β. Actually, as can be seen in table 10.1, β's from two-patch simulations are consistently smaller than from one-patch simulation, but only when component templates are used. The effect is small and is unlikely to be reliably detected in psychometric functions based on the small number of trials dictated by the practical constraints of experiments with human observers.

---

5. The relative inefficacy of the 289 "spatial uncertainty" template pairs, compared to the like number of random noise templates, may also be due in part to the fact that magnitudes of the sensor response vectors for the former is not always equal to that for the stimulus presented in the correct location. See the discussion of "contrast uncertainty" in the discussion section for further consideration of the effects of relative sensor response vector magnitudes.

Table 10.2
Effect of uncertainty on the summation ratio

M	Template matching		Probability summation	
	dB	linear	dB	linear
Matched templates				
1	2.90	1.40	4.43	1.67
2	2.91	1.40	4.09	1.60
9	2.89	1.39	2.95	1.40
25	2.93	1.40	2.45	1.33
289	3.00	1.41	1.91	1.25
Component templates				
2	3.59	1.51	4.02	1.59
9	2.59	1.35	2.89	1.39
25	2.23	1.29	2.58	1.35
289	1.67	1.21	1.89	1.24
289*	2.30	1.30	2.62	1.35

*Spatial uncertainty

Effect of Uncertainty on Summation Ratio

The first two columns of table 10.2 summarize the amount of subthreshold summation found by Monte Carlo simulation of the template matching model. The difference between one- and two-patch α's from table 10.1 are listed in the first column. They are, in effect, summation ratios in "dB units," and their standard errors are about 0.13 dB. Summation ratios are expressed in linear units in the next column. The last two columns contain the corresponding quantities predicted from standard probability summation theory, using the one-patch β values in table 10.1.

Recall that the empirically obtained value of the summation ratio for two well-separated stimuli is in the neighborhood of 1.2, or about 1.7 dB. The baseline condition, with only matched templates, clearly exhibits too much summation—about 3 dB. However, uncertainty alone has no effect on the amount of summation. Increasing uncertainty by the addition of as many as 288 random noise template pairs does steepen the psychometric function and reduce contrast sensitivity (as shown in table 10.1) but leaves the summation ratio at its initial value of approximately 3 dB.

Replacing optimal (matched) with suboptimal (component) templates does not by itself reduce the summation ratio either; in fact it increases it, as can be seen in table 10.2. However, this effect seems to disappear as the total amount of uncertainty increases. In fact, for large uncertainty, the summation ratio with component templates

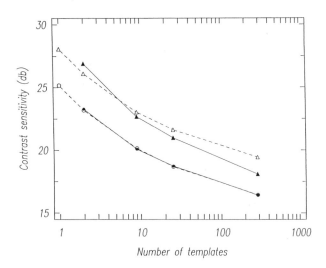

Fig. 10.1
Contrast sensitivity (dB re arbitrary reference level) plotted against number of orthogonal template pairs. Circles represent results for one-patch stimuli, triangles for two-patch stimuli, empty symbols and broken lines for template sets containing an exact match to the presented stimulus, filled symbols and dashed lines for sets containing instead templates for each component patch.

drops appreciably below 1.41 (3 dB). With a great deal of spatial uncertainty (single Gabor patches at 289 different possible locations) the summation ratio goes down to 1.30 (2.30 dB). When the orthogonality of the extraneous templates is increased by making them samples of random noise, the summation ratio drops further to 1.21 (1.67 dB).

Figure 10.1 may help clarify how this reduction in amount of subthreshold summation comes about. In this figure, contrast sensitivity (α) is plotted against number of orthogonal template pairs containing either templates matched to the presented stimulus, or to the component patches alone. Note that with one-patch stimuli, the variation of α with total number of templates is the same regardless of whether matched or component templates are included in the set. This is not surprising, because for one-patch stimuli, the two types of templates are really equivalent: one random noise template in the matched set is replaced, in the component set, by a template for a possible test patch 2° away from the presented stimulus. On the other hand, the two sets of templates are clearly not equivalent when two-patch stimuli are presented. In this case, to go from the matched to the component template sets, one has to trade in one matched and one random noise template for two component templates. The trade seems to improve performance when the total number of templates is small, but to harm it when the total number increases.

The value of the summation ratio obtained with 289 orthogonal template pairs which do not include a template matched to the two-patch stimulus compares very favorably with estimates from the data of human observers in similar experiments. It is also very similar to what would be expected from probability summation, given the β obtained from simulation of single-patch detection performance with these same templates.

Discussion

Relation to Pelli's Model

Pelli's uncertainty model and the template matching model considered in this paper seem to differ greatly with respect to both the assumed sensors and the observer's decision rule. Yet, as was shown above, they lead to identical predictions about the dependence of α and β on amount of orthogonal uncertainty. The reason is that in certain respects, the models are effectively identical. This becomes apparent if one considers the templates of the present model as coordinate with the sensors of Pelli's model. Then it can be shown that if the template vectors are orthogonal and of equal magnitude, the "maximum sensor output rule" of Pelli and the "smallest vector difference rule" of the present model lead to equivalent results.[6] In other words, Pelli's model is a special case of the template matching model.

A "Single Channel" Model with General Applicability

Although the simulations reported here were of spatial summation—detection of one vs. two spatially well-separated grating patches—the conclusions drawn from their results almost certainly apply to other cases of subthreshold summation as well. As was pointed out in the methods section, probably the only essential property of the sensors and stimuli used in these simulations was that they resulted in orthogonal sensor response vectors to the component stimuli. One way to attain vector orthogonality is indeed to choose stimulus components each of which activates completely nonoverlapping sets of sensors. A specific example of this case is the one examined here: stimulus patches whose spatial separation is large relative to receptive field extents of the underlying sensors sensitive to the stimuli. Another possible example, drawn from the majority of subthreshold summation experiments performed in the past, is two spatially superimposed component stimuli (e.g., gratings of different spatial frequency or orientation) chosen so as to stimulate different families of sensors narrowly "tuned" to each of the components.

However, it is not necessary to have different families of tuned sensors in order to generate orthogonal sensor response vectors, even with component stimuli that are spatially completely superimposed. Suppose the underlying sensors all had identical weighting functions, and the visual field were indefinitely large. Then any set of component gratings of nonidentical spatial frequencies would produce orthogonal sensor response vectors. For gratings and visual fields of finite size, and sensors whose sensitivities vary with position, the requisite component frequency separation would have to be greater than zero, by an amount that depends on the details of the stimuli and sensitivity variations. Note that if the assumptions of this template matching model are correct, the empirical fact that gratings differing greatly in spatial frequency and orientation are "detected independently" does not require the assumption of sensors tuned to these stimuli. Put another way, subthreshold summation performance of human observers does not reject this particular "single channel" model of contrast detection.[7]

The point is that even with one class of sensors and completely overlapping stimuli, it is possible to have (nearly) orthogonal sensor response vectors to those sti-

---

6. Pelli (personal communication) puts it this way: "Suppose we have a noisy stimulus and a set of expected stimuli. Let us represent them as vectors. Assume the expected signals all have equal energy. There are two calculations that we can imagine making to compare the noisy stimulus with each expected signal. (1) Evaluate the dot product (i.e., integrated product) of the stimulus with each expected signal. (This corresponds to using the expected signal as a receptive field and evaluating its response to the noisy stimulus.) (2) Evaluate the root-mean-square (RMS) difference between the stimulus and each expected signal.

If the expected signals all have equal energy then choosing the expected signal which maximizes the dot product ("maximum sensor response") is equivalent to choosing the expected signal that minimizes the RMS difference."

7. The terms *single channel* model and *multiple channel* model are used here in the same way as in the extensive subthreshold summation literature of the preceding two decades (see Graham, 1989).

muli. Given sufficient uncertainty and only component templates, the present model predicts very little subthreshold summation, in fact about as little as is found empirically, and as little as is predicted by "multiple channel" models[7] with probability summation.

Verisimilitude

Whether the assumptions of this model adequately capture the processes actually underlying contrast detection in human observers is another matter. One assumption is certainly false for most psychophysical experiments, namely, that there is no "contrast uncertainty." In the present implementation of the model, the magnitude of the sensor response vector to each hypothetical stimulus was matched either to that produced by the presented stimulus or by one of the components of the presented stimulus—in the correct location, or in the case of spatial uncertainty, in both the correct and incorrect locations. When the contrast of the presented stimulus was changed, the magnitudes of all the template vectors were scaled by the same factor. Actually, it turns out that the magnitude of template vectors otherwise "matched" to the stimulus do not affect detection performance. However, the magnitude of extraneous template vectors does affect β, and to a lesser extent, α. Future work will have to examine the effects, if any, of plausible ranges of uncertainty regarding the contrast of the extraneous templates.

Undoubtedly the most problematic assumptions of the model are those pertaining to the number and type of hypothesized templates. The number of templates required is large—even if they are orthogonal, about 300 template pairs are needed. If the templates are not orthogonal, then many more than 300 are needed. It is actually difficult to conjure up sufficient realistic sources of uncertainty to meet this requirement. That is why we resorted to the artifice of using samples of two-dimensional Gaussian noise as templates.

An even more curious requirement for the observer's template set is that it contain templates matched to the components but not to the composite stimulus itself. But the classification of stimuli as "components" and "composites" is somewhat arbitrary. Start with two stimuli, a and b. If they produce orthogonal sensor response vectors, so will $a + b$ and $a - b$. In the set $\langle a, b, a + b \rangle$, a would be designated a "component" stimulus. However, in the set $< (a + b)/2, (a - b)/2, a \rangle$, a would be designated a "com-

posite" stimulus. So the assumption required to make the template matching model work is not that the observer is only capable of using component templates, but rather that the observer is capable of using only *certain* templates. For those who wish to develop this model further, the challenge will be to discover the identity of these privileged templates, and understand why they alone are used.

Summary

1. Monte Carlo simulations were used to assess the ability of a template matching model to account for the properties of subthreshold summation displayed by human observers in contrast-pattern detection tasks with widely separated stimuli.

2. Although apparently differing greatly from Pelli's uncertainty model with regard to both sensor properties and observer's decision rule, the present model nevertheless predicts a very similar dependence of α and β on amount of orthogonal uncertainty. The reason for the similarity in predictions is that Pelli's model turns out to be a special case of the template matching model.

3. In the presence of matched (optimal) templates, uncertainty does not affect the summation ratio, which remains in the neighborhood of 1.41 (3 dB) for two-component stimuli.

4. In the absence of additional uncertainty, component (suboptimal) templates do not decrease the summation ratio, but actually increase it above 1.41.

5. With increasing uncertainty, component templates do yield summation ratios significantly below 1.41. With component templates and a large number of additional orthogonal templates, the behavior of the template matching model is very similar to that of human observers.

6. The success of this version of the template matching model does not require the assumption of several different families of sensors. This model thus constitutes a "single channel" model of subthreshold summation. It can be applied to any stimuli that produce orthogonal sensor response vectors. However, it does seem to require the assumption that observers are only capable of using certain types of templates.

Acknowledgment

This chapter is based on work started in 1986 at NASA/Ames, in collaboration with K. R. K. Nielsen and A. B. Watson. They also wrote the original software for the simulations, which was subsequently modified by Brian Madden at the University of Pennsylvania. Preparation of this chapter was partially supported by grant 2-307 from NASA/Ames to Stanford University.

References

Graham, N. (1989). *Visual pattern analyzers*. New York: Oxford.

Graham, N. & Robson, J. G. (1987). Summation of very close spatial frequencies: The importance of spatial probability summation. *Vision Research, 27*, 1997–2007.

Green, D. M. & Swets, J. A. (1966). *Signal detection theory and psychophysics*. New York: Wiley.

Hall, J. L. & Sondhi, M. M. (1977). Detection threshold for a two tone complex. *Journal of the Acoustical Society of America, 62*, 636–640.

Kulikowski, J. J. & King-Smith, P. E. (1973). Spatial arrangement of line, edge, and grating detectors revealed by subthreshold summation. *Vision Research, 13*, 1455–1478.

Nachmias, J. (1981). On the psychometric function for contrast detection. *Vision Research, 21*, 215–233.

Nielsen, K. R. K. & Wandell, B. (1988). Discrete analysis of spatial sensitivity models. *Journal of the Optical Society of America A, 5*, 743–755.

Nielsen, K. R. K., Watson, A. B. & Ahumada, Jr., A. J. (1985). Application of a computable model of spatial vision to phase discrimination. *Journal of the Optical Society of America A, 2*, 1600–1607.

Pelli, D. G. (1985). Uncertainty explains many aspects of visual contrast detection and discrimination. *Journal of the Optical Society of America A, 2*, 1508–1532.

Quick, R. F. & Reichart, T. A. (1975). Spatial-frequency selectivity in contrast detection. *Vision Research, 15*, 647–653.

Quick, R. F., Mullins, W. W. & Reichart, T. A. (1978). Spatial summation effects in two component grating thresholds. *Journal of the Optical Society of America, 68*, 116–121.

Robson, J. G. & Graham, N. (1981). Probability summation and regional variation in contrast sensitivity across the visual field. *Vision Research, 21*, 409–418.

Sachs, M. B., Nachmias, J. & Robson, J. G. (1971). Spatial frequency channels in human vision. *Journal of the Optical Society of America, 61*, 1176–1186.

Tanner, Jr., W. P. (1961). Physiological implications of psychophysical data. *Annals of the New York Academy of Sciences, 89*, 752–765.

Watson, A. B. (1979). Probability summation over time. *Vision Research, 19*, 515–522.

Watson, A. B. (1983). Detection and recognition of simple spatial forms. In O. J. Braddick & A. C. Sleigh (Eds.), *Physical and biological processing of images*. Berlin: Springer Verlag.

11

Noise in the Visual System May Be Early

Denis G. Pelli

Most models of visual performance incorporate random variations: noise. Sometimes the model maker injects this randomness as an afterthought, to account for trial-to-trial variations in subjects' responses. Sometimes the noise is an essential part of the model, as in probability summation, where the key idea is the random detection that can occur in any of many independent channels (e.g., Graham, 1977). Recent psychophysical evidence indicates that the main source of noise limiting visual detection is in the proximal stimulus: the photon noise arising from the random nature of light absorption (Banks, Geisler & Bennett, 1987; Cohn, 1976; Krauskopf & Reeves, 1980; Pelli, 1981, 1983, 1990). While noise undoubtedly arises at every stage of visual processing, it is a hallmark of well-engineered systems, and apparently of human vision (at near-threshold contrasts), that the gains of each stage are sufficient to amplify the unavoidable noise of the first stage (i.e., photon noise) so that it dwarfs the additional noises that arise at later stages.[1]

This chapter argues that psychophysical models of the visual system should incorporate noise at the first stage, an equivalent input noise added to the stimulus, rather than injecting an arbitrary noise later. The observer's equivalent input noise is susceptible to direct measurement psychophysically (Pelli, 1981, 1983, 1990), thus removing many degrees of freedom from the specification of the model (Ahumada, 1987; Ahumada & Watson, 1985). Physiological models may usefully represent noise arising at each stage, but with appropriate simplifying assumptions (e.g., linearity) these models will be equivalent to a black-

---

1. Previous claims that visual detection is photon noise limited (e.g., Rose, 1942, 1948) have been criticized on the grounds that the observer's overall efficiency, from stimulus to decision, is strongly dependent on the experimental conditions (Barlow, 1962). However, the observer's overall efficiency depends not only on the amount of noise in the system. It also depends on the efficiency of the observer's algorithm for reducing the multidimensional noisy data to a single number upon which a detection decision may be made. Our visual system's algorithms are not particularly well matched to the stimuli and tasks that we usually use to study vision, resulting in low efficiency strongly dependent on the stimulus conditions. For example, the observer's overall efficiency is very strongly dependent on disk size (Barlow, 1958; Jones, 1959) but the observer's equivalent input noise is independent of disk size (Pelli, 1981). (See Pelli, 1990.)

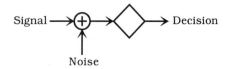

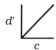

Fig. 11.1
The simplest case: ideal detection of a one-number signal in noise. The psychometric function, in the lower left hand corner, is linear.

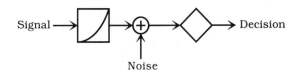

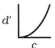

Fig. 11.2
Inserting a nonlinear tranformation before adding the noise results in a nonlinear psychometric function, which is needed to match the human observer. However, this assumes a late noise, which is inconsistent with evidence that visual detection is limited by photon noise.

box model with only an equivalent input noise (Pelli, 1990; see chapter 7).

The *theory of signal detectability* is a collection of theorems about the detectability of signals in noise (Peterson, Birdsall & Fox, 1954). This naturally formed the starting point for the first attempts to model sensory processes as noise-limited detectors. When considering the task faced by our visual system, it is instructive to begin by asking what would be the ideal way to detect a signal in noise. These sensory models, and many ad hoc modifications of them, have come to be called *signal detection theory*, after Green and Swet's (1974) textbook of that name. Unfortunately, many students of signal detection theory have mistakenly come to think that known human behavior is inconsistent with an early noise. This is because theorems proved for zero-dimensional models—whose stimulus is a single number—have been mistakenly assumed to generalize to the multidimensional case of real vision—whose stimulus is a dynamic image (i.e., many numbers).

Figure 11.1 illustrates the simplest possible detector. A signal, represented by a single number, is added to noise, a single random number, and the resulting sum is compared to a criterion (in the diamond box) to yield a detection decision, such as "Yes, it's there" or "No, it's not." Absence of the signal would correspond to a value of zero added to the noise. This decision rule, with the appropriate criterion, is the ideal way to decide whether or not the signal is present. Alternatively, in a two-alternative, forced-choice paradigm, the signal and zero would each be presented once, in random order, and the decision stage would choose the interval that produced the larger number. Again, the decision is ideal.

The graph in the lower left hand corner describes the performance of the detector. The horizontal scale is contrast c, in this case equal to the signal. The vertical scale is

detectability d', which describes the level of performance. d' is a simple transformation of one of the conventional measures of detection performance, such as proportion correct. d' is defined as the signal-to-noise ratio required by an ideal observer to equal the observed performance of the observer under study (Tanner & Birdsall, 1958). For this simple case the graph is linear, indicating that d' is proportional to the input contrast.

A linear relationship between d' and contrast is inconsistent with the nearly universal finding that for visual detection of simple patterns d' is a nonlinear accelerating function of contrast, that is, $d' \propto c^2$ (e.g., Nachmias, 1981; Nachmias & Sansbury, 1974). Modelers have ususally resolved this inconsistency by introducing a comparable nonlinearity into the model, as illustrated in figure 11.2. By applying a nonlinear transformation to the signal *before* the noise is added, the signal-to-noise ratio d' becomes a nonlinear function of contrast, as shown in the lower left hand corner of the figure.

The nonlinear transformation introduced in figure 11.2 bent the psychometric function (d' vs. c) appropriately, but it also nullified any claim that the model is ideal. An ideal detector would yield the best possible performance, limited solely by the statistics of the stimulus. In figure 11.2 the noise is assumed to arise inside the model, not to be part of the proximal stimulus, like photon noise.

Figure 11.3 shows what would happen if we were to introduce the nonlinearity *after* the signal and noise are summed. Nothing. It is traditional to call the number that is fed into the decision box the decision variable. The introduction of the monotonic nonlinearity will change the values of the decision variable, but it will preserve

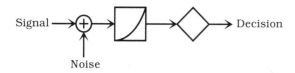

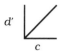

Fig. 11.3
Birdsall's theorem: Inserting the nonlinearity after the noise has no effect.

their ranking (which is greater than which). Since the model observer's decisions all depend solely on comparisons of values of the decision variable, the monotonic transformation will not affect any of the model observer's decisions. (For yes-no or rating-scale tasks, where the observer is comparing the decision variable with a remembered criterion, we are free to think of the criterion as a remembered value of the decision variable.) This immunity to monotonic transformation of the decision variable is sometimes called Birdsall's Theorem (Lasley & Cohn, 1981; Tanner, 1961).

Figures 11.1 to 11.3 might seem to imply that human observers must have a late noise. However, these figures apply only to the zero-dimensional case where the signal and noise are each simple numbers. Real vision is a three-dimensional problem: The stimulus is a pattern varying over two spatial dimensions and time. Such a stimulus may be thought of as a continuous function of three dimensions or may be represented by a large three-dimensional array of numbers; it cannot be represented reasonably by a single number. An early visual noise, such as photon noise, has the same high dimensionality.

Figure 11.4 illustrates the multidimensional version of figure 11.3. The large open arrows now represent the transmission of a multidimensional quantity—a movie—and the thin arrows continue to represent the transmission of single numbers. The multidimensional signal and noise are added together, and the multidimensional sum goes to an unspecified nonlinear transformation that some-

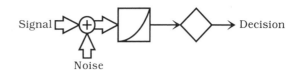

Fig. 11.4
When the signal and noise are multidimensional, as in real vision, then Birdsall's theorem no longer applies, and any psychometric function is possible.

how reduces it all to a single number, which is the basis for the decision. As indicated by the question mark in the lower left hand corner, such a model could have any psychometric function.

As an example, figure 11.5 illustrates a detector with early noise that nonetheless has a nonlinear psychometric function. This is the uncertainty model, so called because it arose in the context of theory of signal detectability as a nearly optimal way to detect one of M orthogonal signals in white noise (Nolte & Jaarsma, 1967; Pelli, 1985; Peterson, Birdsall & Fox, 1954; also see chapter 10).[2] We assume that there are M possible signals, that the signals are all orthogonal (i.e., have equal energy and zero correlation with each other). There are M filters (i.e., receptive fields), each matched to one of the possible signals. Each filter yields a single number, a measure of the likelihood that a particular signal was present. The decision is based on the largest of these numbers. If M is about 50 then d' will be proportional to squared contrast. Alternatively, if M is 1—no uncertainty—then d' will be proportional to contrast, that is, the psychometric function will be linear. In general, the exponent k in the power law $d' \propto c^k$, increases linearly with $\log M$ (Pelli, 1985).

Figure 11.6 shows a more physiologically plausible way to build the uncertainty model of figure 11.5. Each filter is implemented by a cell (e.g., a cortical cell) with the appropriate receptive field and temporal impulse response. Rather than having an explicit maximum oper-

---

2. Choosing the largest cross-correlation is optimal for identification, and nearly optimal for detection. The ideal detector is considerably more difficult to analyze. The simplifying assumptions of orthogonality of the signals could probably be dropped, provided that M were reduced appropriately, possibly to the number of orthogonal basis functions required to span the stimuli. Of

course, in real life one would not expect the signals to match the receptive fields. Pelli (1985) showed that allowing a signal to stimulate multiple filters in the uncertainty model provides a good account for the results of "probability" summation experiments. Also see chapter 10.

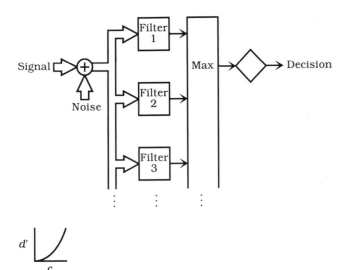

Fig. 11.5
An example: The uncertainty model has an early noise and yet results in a linear psychometric function if $M = 1$ and a nonlinear psychometric function if $M > 1$.

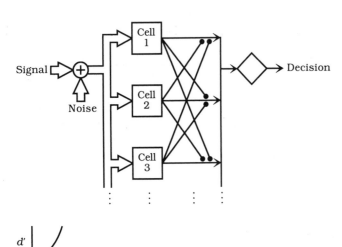

Fig. 11.6
A more physiologically plausible implemention uses mutually inhibitory interconnections to suppress all but the maximum response.

ator, we suppose that each cell sends an output to the final decision stage and that each output receives inhibition from all the other cells. We suppose that the inhibition is such that the output is suppressed unless the signal it is carrying exceeds that in each inhibitory connection. The decision stage will then receive only one signal, the maximum. There is substantial evidence that cortical cells receive input from far beyond their conventional receptive field (Gilbert & Wiesel, 1983, 1989), and are inhibited by a wider range of orientations than will excite them (Burr & Morrone, 1987; Morrone, Burr & Maffei, 1982; Ramoa, Shadlen, Skottun & Freeman, 1986). In the context of this model, that might implement a (nearly) ideal detector of a signal of unknown orientation.[3]

So don't be too quick to inject a late noise in your model. An early noise may be more consistent with what we know.

References

Ahumada, A. J., Jr. (1987). Putting the visual system noise back in the picture. *Journal of the Optical Society of America A, 4,* 2372–2378.

Ahumada, A. J., Jr. & Watson, A. B. (1985). Equivalent-noise model for contrast detection and discrimination. *Journal of the Optical Society of America A, 2,* 1133–1139.

Banks, M. S., Geisler, W. S. & Bennett, P. J. (1987). The physical limits of grating visibility. *Vision Research, 27,* 1915–1924.

Barlow, H. B. (1958). Temporal and spatial summation in human vision at different background intensities. *Journal of Physiology, 141,* 337–350.

Barlow, H. B. (1962). Measurements of the quantum efficiency of discrimination in human scotopic vision. *Journal of Physiology, 160,* 169–188.

Burr, D. C. & Morrone, M. C. (1987). Inhibitory interactions in the human vision system revealed in pattern-evoked potentials. *Journal of Physiology, 389,* 1–21.

Cohn, T. E. (1976). Quantum fluctuations limit foveal vision. *Vision Research, 16,* 573–579.

Gilbert, C. D. & Wiesel, T. N. (1983). Clustered intrinsic connections in cat visual cortex. *Journal of Neuroscience, 3,* 1116–1133.

3. This physiological model is only meant to illustrate the availability of the kind of hardware needed to implement this kind of decision rule, not to advocate this particular realization. In fact, uncertainty in orientation would generate only a modest M, perhaps 8, not enough to account for the steepness of human psychometric functions. Furthermore, neurometric functions have been measured for cortical cells in the cat and monkey, and they too are much shallower than human psychometric functions (Tolhurst, Movshon & Dean, 1983). Relkin and Pelli (1987) found a similar discrepancy in psychometric/neurometric slopes for auditory thresholds.

Gilbert, C. D. & Wiesel, T. N. (1989). Columnar specificity of intrinsic horizontal and corticocortical connections in cat visual cortex. *Journal of Neuroscience, 9,* 2432–2442.

Graham, N. (1977). Visual detection of aperiodic spatial stimuli by probability summation among narrow band channels. *Vision Research, 17,* 637–652.

Green, D. M. & Swets, J. A. (1974). *Signal detection theory and psychophysics.* Huntington, NY: Krieger.

Jones, R. C. (1959). Quantum efficiency of human vision. *Journal of the Optical Society of America, 49,* 645–653.

Krauskopf, J. & Reeves, A. (1980). Measurement of the effect of photon noise on detection. *Vision Research, 20,* 193–196.

Lasley, D. J. & Cohn, T. E. (1981). Why luminance discrimination may be better than detection. *Vision Research, 21,* 273–278.

Morrone, M. C., Burr, D. C. & Maffei, L. (1982). Functional implications of cross-orientation inhibition of cortical visual cells. I. Neurophysiological evidence. *Proceedings of the Royal Society of London [Biology], 216,* 335–354.

Nachmias, J. (1981). On the psychometric function for contrast detection. *Vision Research, 21,* 215–223.

Nachmias, J. & Sansbury, R. V. (1974). Grating contrast: Discrimination may be better than detection. *Vision Research, 14,* 1039–1042.

Nolte, L. W. & Jaarsma, D. (1967). More on the detection of one of M orthogonal signals. *Journal of the Acoustical Society of America, 41,* 497–505.

Pelli, D. G. (1981). *Effects of visual noise.* Ph. D. thesis. Cambridge University, Cambridge, England.

Pelli, D. G. (1983). The spatiotemporal spectrum of the equivalent noise of human vision. *Investigative Ophthalmology and Visual Science (Supplement), 4,* 46.

Pelli, D. G. (1985). Uncertainty explains many aspects of visual contrast detection and discrimination. *Journal of the Optical Society of America A, 2,* 1508–1532.

Pelli, D. G. (1990). The quantum efficiency of human vision. In C. Blakemore (Ed.), *Vision: Coding and efficiency.* Cambridge, England: Cambridge University Press.

Peterson, W. W., Birdsall, T. G. & Fox, W. C. (1954). Theory of signal detectability. *Transactions of the IRE PGIT, 4,* 171–212.

Ramoa, A. S., Shadlen, M., Skottun, B. C. & Freeman, R. D. (1986). A comparison of inhibition in orientation and spatial frequency selectivity of cat visual cortex. *Nature, 321,* 237–239.

Relkin, E. M. & Pelli, D. G. (1987). Probe tone thresholds in the auditory nerve measured by two-interval forced-choice procedures. *Journal of the Acoustical Society of America, 82,* 1679–1691.

Rose, A. (1942). The relative sensitivities of television pickup tubes, photographic film, and the human eye. *Proceedings of the IRE, 30,* 293–300.

Rose, A. (1948). The sensitivity performance of the human eye on an absolute scale. *Journal of the Optical Society of America, 38,* 196–208.

Tanner, W. P., Jr. (1961). Physiological implications of psychophysical data. *Annals of the New York Academy of Sciences, 89,* 752–765.

Tanner, W. P., Jr. & Birdsall, T. G. (1958). Definitions of d' and η as psychophysical measures. *Journal of the Acoustical Society of America, 30,* 922–928.

Tolhurst, D. J., Movshon, J. A. & Dean, A. F. (1983). The statistical reliability of signals in single neurons in cat and monkey visual cortex. *Vision Research, 23,* 775–785.

12

Pattern Discrimination, Visual Filters, and Spatial Sampling Irregularity

Hugh R. Wilson

Psychophysical research has demonstrated that images on the human retina are processed in parallel by a number of spatial filters or mechanisms each tuned for both orientation and size or spatial frequency.[1] Furthermore, the strong correlation between human spatial mechanisms and the receptive field properties of single cells in primate visual cortex leads to the hypothesis that the psychophysical mechanisms reflect the properties of orientation selective cells in human visual cortex (Wilson, 1991a; Wilson, Levi, Maffei, Rovamo & DeValois, 1990). This has made it possible to theoretically calculate the presumed cortical representation of any visual image by computing the responses of all mechanisms stimulated by the image. It might then be expected that the ability to discriminate among similar patterns would be dependent on the degree to which these patterns generate different levels of mechanism response, that is, on the difference between their cortical representations. A number of recent models for spatial pattern discrimination have successfully pursued this analysis (Klein & Levi, 1985; Nielsen, Watson & Ahumada, 1985; Watt & Morgan, 1985; Wilson, 1986; Wilson & Gelb, 1984).

Despite their success, pattern discrimination models based on visual filter responses have encountered difficulties in at least three areas. First, when discrimination requires comparison of features that are widely separated (e.g., two lines spaced 10° apart), the filtering approach requires modification, as there is no single spatial filter large enough to encompass all pattern elements (Burbeck, 1987). Thus there appear to be two strategies employed by the visual system: a filtering approach for local feature discrimination and a cortical measurement procedure for discrimination over long distances. Second, spatial discrimination tasks have been found to fall into two groups with respect to their dependence on stimulus contrast. In

---

1. The term "visual filter" refers to a two-dimensional spatial function that describes the weighting for a spatial convolution integral (see below). A "spatial mechanism" is composed of a visual filter plus an associated contrast nonlinearity.

the first group are tasks like vernier acuity, which improve with increasing contrast, while tasks like spatial frequency discrimination are largely independent of contrast. Finally, all of the current models tacitly assume that visual filters are regularly positioned at precisely known locations. While this idealization works reasonably well for foveal pattern discrimination, it fails for peripheral vision. Thus, it becomes important to assess the role of spatial sampling irregularity in peripheral pattern discrimination.

These three issues in spatial pattern discrimination are not independent, and they will be tightly interwoven throughout this chapter. For example, long distance cortical measurement processes may be limited by the spatial irregularity of peripheral sampling. Similarly, it will be argued that contrast-independent tasks involve cortical distance measurement limited by spatial irregularity, while tasks that improve with contrast are primarily dependent on local filter responses. These themes will be elucidated through the application of pattern discrimination models to hyperacuity, curvature, and spatial frequency discrimination tasks.

Local and Global Processing in Hyperacuity

Hyperacuity is the name coined by Westheimer (1979) for those pattern discrimination tasks yielding thresholds substantially smaller than the 30 to 35 sec arc spacing of the smallest foveal cones. The two hyperacuity tasks to be considered here are vernier acuity and two line separation discrimination, each of which yields thresholds of about 5 sec arc under optimal conditions. It will be shown that vernier acuity can be explained by local mechanism responses, and that spatial irregularity plays an important role in determining peripheral vernier thresholds. Separation discrimination, on the other hand, is limited by global distance measurement processes and spatial irregularity at large but not at small separations.

As a prelude to consideration of vernier acuity, let us briefly review the properties of psychophysically measured spatial filters. As discussed elsewhere, there is general agreement among results obtained with the three major methods of measurement: subthreshold summation, spatial frequency adaptation, and masking (Wilson, 1991a). These techniques all indicate that human visual filters are orientation selective with bandwidths averaging $\pm 20°$ at half amplitude, and they exhibit bandpass spatial fre-

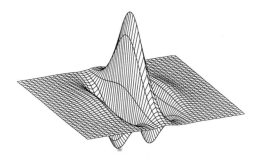

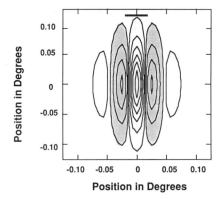

Fig. 12.1

Spatial sensitivity of the smallest visual filter revealed in psychophysical masking studies (Wilson, McFarlane & Phillips, 1983). At the top the sensitivity is shown as a three-dimensional surface plot, while at the bottom the same data are represented as a contour plot. The negative or inhibitory zones are shaded in the contour plot. As this filter is most sensitive to 16 cycles/degree, the central excitatory zone is about 1.9 min arc wide. For reference, the short horizontal bar at the top of the contour plot is 2 min arc in length. Despite these dimensions, calculations show that these filters can detect vernier offsets of about 5 sec arc. This is due to the rapid change in filter sensitivity with spatial position in the region near the transition from excitation to inhibition.

quency tuning with half amplitude bandwidths of 1 to 2 octaves. Wilson, McFarlane, and Phillips (1983) and Phillips and Wilson (1984) developed a masking technique to obtain detailed measurements of the orientation and spatial frequency tuning curves of six filters tuned to peak frequencies ranging from 0.8 to 16.0 cycles/degree in foveal vision. Figure 12.1 depicts the spatial sensitivity profile of a foveal filter tuned to 16 cycles/degree, which was the smallest filter found in these studies. Note that it is composed of an elongated excitatory region flanked on either side by parallel inhibitory zones. In addition, there are weak secondary excitatory zones beyond the inhibitory zones, as has also been reported for cortical cells in cats (Movshon, Thompson & Tolhurst, 1978) and monkeys (DeValois, Albrecht & Thorell, 1982). In fact, quantitative correlations between the properties of human visual filters from these studies and properties of simple cells in monkey striate cortex suggest that these filters reflect the properties of simple cells in the human visual system. Spatial filters tuned to lower spatial frequencies were found to be spaced about one octave apart in their tuning and were similar in shape to the filter in figure 12.1.

In order to calculate filter responses, it is necessary to have a mathematical description of the filter shape, and Wilson and Gelb (1984) found that the following expression provided an accurate fit to the data:

$$F(x, y) = A[e^{-x^2/\sigma_1^2} - Be^{-x^2/\sigma_2^2} + Ce^{-x^2/\sigma_3^2}]e^{-y^2/\sigma_y^2}. \quad (1)$$

This function, which represents a vertically oriented filter, is just the difference of three Gaussian functions in the x direction multiplied by a single Gaussian in the y direction. Filters at other orientations are obtained by simple rotation of coordinates. It is interesting to note that Phillips and Wilson (1984) found that $\sigma_y = 3.2\sigma_1$ for all filters measured, and this same ratio has been found for the majority of simple cells in monkey cortex (Parker & Hawken, 1988). Values of the parameters for all filters may be found elsewhere (Wilson, 1991a; Wilson & Gelb, 1984).

Masking studies have also revealed that there is a nonlinearity associated with the contrast response of visual mechanisms (Legge & Foley, 1980; Nachmias & Sansbury, 1974; Wilson, McFarlane & Phillips, 1983). This takes the form of an accelerating or threshold type nonlinearity at low contrasts followed by a compressive nonlinearity at higher contrasts. A mathematical description of this nonlinearity is provided by the function:

$$R(S) = \frac{S^2 + kS^{3-\varepsilon}}{k + S^2}, \quad (2)$$

where

$$S = \int_{-\infty}^{\infty} \int_{-\infty}^{\infty} F(x, y) I(x, y) \, dx \, dy. \quad (3)$$

In this expression, $I(x, y)$ is the intensity distribution in a spatial pattern. The parameter ε has been found empirically to be about 0.55 for low and intermediate spatial frequencies and about 0.25 at frequencies of 8 cycles/degree and above. Thus, the response of a visual mecha-

nism tuned to any orientation and spatial frequency, and centered at any point (x, y) in space can be calculated by a linear filtering operation followed by a contrast nonlinearity. As discussed elsewhere (Wilson et al., 1990), this human mechanism model is basically identical to quantitative models of cortical simple cell responses.

Given the presence of mechanisms tuned to a range of sizes or spatial frequencies and orientations, it follows that any local feature of a spatial pattern can be represented as a point in a multidimensional mechanism response space. One might expect, therefore, that the threshold for pattern discrimination would be dependent on the distance between the representations of patterns in this space. If the difference in response of mechanism i to a pair of patterns is ΔR_i, then the distance between representations of these patterns will be given by:

$$\Delta R = \sqrt{\sum_{\omega} \sum_{\theta} \sum_{\Delta x} |\Delta R_i^2|}. \quad (4)$$

Here the summation is over orientation (θ), size or spatial frequency (ω), and spatial nearest neighbors separated by a distance of $\pm\Delta x$. Note that this expression sums over all orientations and filter sizes at a point, while it only sums over spatial nearest neighbors rather than across all space. Thus, ΔR is a measure of the difference in representation of spatially localized pattern features. The model has been normalized so that $\Delta R = 1$ corresponds to 75 percent correct discrimination, with other points on the psychometric function depending monotonically on ΔR. As this model is formally similar to line element models for color discrimination, it has been termed a line element model for spatial pattern discrimination. Further details and lists of all parameter values have been published elsewhere (Wilson, 1986, 1991a; Wilson & Gelb, 1984).

A key concept in this model is that pattern discrimination is based on the change in response of visual mechanisms as a parameter of the pattern is varied. This is illustrated for the case of vernier acuity in figure 12.2. In a vernier task, the subject is required to discriminate the direction of offset of the top bar relative to the bottom. In parts A and B of figure 12.2, a vertically oriented visual filter is represented with the central excitatory region indicated by +'s and the inhibitory zones shown in gray. Note that this filter is displaced slightly to the left of the center of the vernier bars. In part A the vernier bars are aligned and fall entirely within the excitatory zone of the filter. As shown in part B, however, a small displacement of one bar causes it to overlap the inhibitory zone substantially, which will greatly reduce the visual response of this filter. Similar changes in response to a vernier offset are depicted in parts C and D, where the preferred orientation of the filter is at 15° relative to the vertical.

Calculations employing the equations above bear out this picture quantitatively, as is shown by the comparison between theory and data from a study by Westheimer and McKee (1977) in figure 12.3. Here vernier thresholds are plotted as a function of the length of the individual bars. When the bars are longer than the underlying visual filter (about 10 min arc for the smallest filter), thresholds are not affected by bar length, but as the bars become shorter than this filter, they provide a weaker stimulus, and thresholds are progressively elevated. Although the smallest filters are separated by the width of a single foveal cone (38 sec arc in the model) and have excitatory zones 1.9 min arc wide (see figure 12.1), they nevertheless predict vernier thresholds of about 5 sec arc.

In addition to the data shown in figure 12.3, Wilson (1986) has shown that the line element model for pattern discrimination correctly predicts the dependence of vernier acuity on the separation of the vernier bars as well as thresholds for variants of vernier acuity such as periodic vernier acuity (Tyler, 1973), chevron acuity (Westheimer & McKee, 1977), and conditions producing spatial interference with vernier acuity (Levi, Klein & Aitsebaomo, 1985; Westheimer & Hauske, 1975). The most important point for the current argument, however, is that the line element model predicts that vernier acuity will improve as a power law function of contrast with an exponent of about −0.5, and this prediction has been corroborated experimentally (Watt & Morgan, 1983; Wilson, 1986). The model makes this prediction as a result of the compressive power law dependence of mechanism responses at high contrasts (Legge and Foley, 1980; Nachmias & Sansbury, 1974; Wilson et al., 1983), which is embodied in equation 2 above. In fact, the contrast dependence of mechanism responses predicts that all pattern discrimination tasks that are limited by filter responses will improve with increasing contrast. As will be seen, the conditions under which this prediction fails will provide insight into a second visual pattern discrimination strategy: cortical distance measurement.

Vernier Acuity

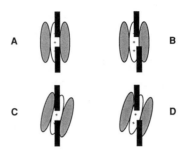

Fig. 12.2
Prediction of vernier thresholds based on local mechanism responses. In (A) and (B) vertically oriented filters are depicted with a central excitatory zone (+ + +) flanked by inhibitory zones (*shaded*; see figure 12.1 for a detailed contour plot of the smallest visual filter). The filters in (A) and (B) are offset slightly to one side of the vernier stimulus. For filters in this position a small shift of one vernier bar will move it from the excitatory zone (A) partially into the inhibitory zone (B), thus causing a significant change in mechanism response. (C) and (D) show that a filter oriented at 15° relative to the axis of the vernier target will also produce a significant change in response to a small offset of one bar. Calculations pooling the responses of filters in these locations predict vernier thresholds of 5.1 sec arc (see figure 12.3).

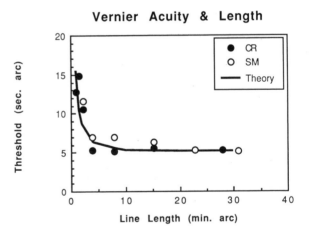

Fig. 12.3
Comparison of experimental and theoretical vernier thresholds as a function of bar length. Data are from Westheimer and McKee (1977). In agreement with the data, vernier thresholds are predicted to be independent of bar length for bars greater than about 10 min arc long. For shorter bars, thresholds increase for both data and theory. In the theoretical calculations this threshold increase begins at the point where the bars become shorter than the effective length of the smallest filters (figure 12.1), thereby progressively decreasing the level of stimulation of the smallest mechanisms.

A second hyperacuity task that has received considerable attention is discrimination of the separation between two parallel lines. Data from several studies (Watt & Morgan, 1983; Westheimer, 1984; Westheimer & McKee, 1977) are plotted as a function of base separation in figure 12.4. Note that minimum thresholds of about 5 sec arc are obtained for separations of 1 to 4 min arc, while thresholds increase roughly linearly with separation for greater separations and thus exhibit Weber's law behavior. The heavy solid line shows the prediction of the line element model based on localized mechanism responses. Clearly, this theoretical curve provides a reasonable fit over this range of separations given the variability of the data across subjects and studies. The explanation for the accuracy of the model predictions is qualitatively the same as that depicted in figure 12.2A, B for vernier acuity: For a given bar separation there will generally be some filter that is optimally positioned so that a small change in separation will occasion a large change in mechanism response.

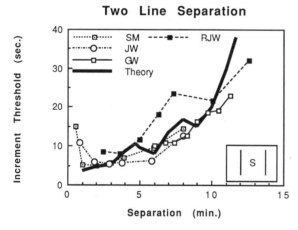

Fig. 12.4

Two line separation discrimination. As shown in the inset at the lower right, this hyperacuity task requires discrimination of the separation S between a pair of parallel bars. Data are plotted from several studies to illustrate intersubject variability: GW (Westheimer, 1984), RJW (Watt & Morgan, 1983), SM and JW (Westheimer & McKee, 1977). The theoretical curve (*heavy solid line*) was calculated from local mechanism responses using the line element model of Wilson (1986). The theory correctly predicts minimum thresholds of about 5 sec arc for separations near 2 min arc, followed by a progressive increase at greater separations. The notches in the theoretical curve are produced by transitions from one filter size to the next in the model.

Although the agreement between two line separation discrimination and theory is good over the range shown in figure 12.4, the theory fails in two major ways. First, it has been shown that Weber's law for two line separation thresholds is valid for separations up to at least 10° (Burbeck, 1987; Levi, Klein & Yap, 1988). Due to the existence of a limited range of filter sizes at each eccentricity, however, calculations based on local mechanism responses predict thresholds that are far too high at separations greater than about 10 min arc. This is because ΔR in equation 4 only pools responses of mechanisms centered at a point plus their spatially adjacent neighbors. Local mechanism predictions are illustrated in figure 12.5 (dashed line) for comparison with the large separation data of Levi, Klein, and Yap (1988). The failure of the local predictions beyond about 10 min arc (arrow) suggests that a second visual strategy is employed at larger separations. Although it might seem that simply extending the pooling in equation 4 to cover all of space would lead to accurate predictions at large separations, Klein and Levi (1987) have demonstrated that this produces thresholds that are far too low and that fail to exhibit the observed Weber's law behavior at large separations.

The second failure of the local line element prediction for two line separation involves contrast dependence. Due to the existence of the compressive nonlinearity at high contrasts (equation 2), separation discrimination based on local mechanism responses is predicted to improve as a power function of contrast, just as vernier acuity does. This prediction was tested by Morgan and Regan (1987), who found that discrimination improved with contrast at separations below about 5 min arc. However, at a separation of 10 min arc they discovered that two bar separation acuity was independent of contrast once the contrast was about three times the threshold for detecting the bars. Thus two different regimes for separation discrimination are also suggested based on the degree of improvement with contrast.

To summarize, spatially localized mechanism responses accurately predict two line separation thresholds and an improvement with contrast for separations below 10 min arc. At larger separations, however, they predict thresholds that are too high and fail to predict contrast independence above threshold. In addition to a local discrimination strategy mediated by contrast dependent mechanism responses, therefore, there is apparently a second strategy that is contrast independent and operates more globally.

Separation Discrimination

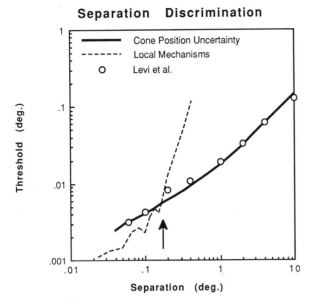

Fig. 12.5

Two line separation discrimination at large separations. Data are averages from Levi, Klein, and Yap (1988). In this task the subject fixated a central line and discriminated the separation between it and two flanking peripheral lines. Note that the data fall on a straight line with a slope of unity in this log-log plot, thus indicating Weber's law behavior for separations up to 10°. The dashed line shows the theoretical predictions based on local mechanism responses. While these predictions are very accurate at separations below 10 min arc (see figure 12.4), they become much too high for separations above 10 min arc (*arrow*), as a result of the limited range of filter sizes present in the fovea. The heavy solid line is the discrimination prediction for a distance measurement process that is limited by the cumulative spatial irregularity inherent in the cone mosaic (see text for details).

Klein and Levi (1987) have suggested that the second visual strategy is a cortical measurement process limited by the positional uncertainty of the retinocortical mapping. Qualitatively, the measurement hypothesis seems very plausible, as two widely separated bars will generate activity at two discrete cortical loci (in different cortical modules), and subsequent cortical processing must then be able to make some estimate of the distance between these loci. Accordingly, I shall adopt this hypothesis, but I shall provide evidence that the spatial irregularity limiting this process may arise in the photoreceptor mosaic.

Quantitative estimates of cone spacing and mosaic regularity have recently been published for one human and one primate retina (Hirsch & Curcio, 1989; Hirsch & Miller, 1987). Mean cone spacing for these two retinas is plotted as a function of eccentricity in figure 12.6 (solid

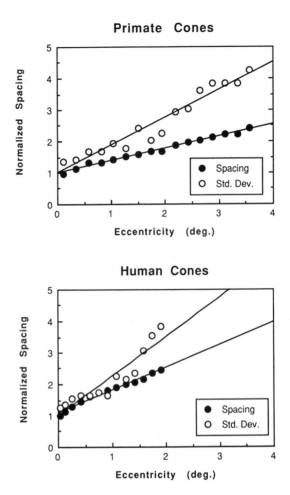

Fig. 12.6

Separation of cones in one primate (Hirsch & Miller, 1987) and one human retina (Hirsch & Curcio, 1989) for eccentricities near the fovea. The data on mean spacing (*solid circles*) and the standard deviation of spacing (*open circles*) have been plotted relative to the foveal values to emphasize the relative changes of these two measures with eccentricity. All data sets are very well fit by the linear regression lines shown (correlations all greater than 0.93). Although both mean spacing and the standard deviation of spacing increase with eccentricity, the latter increases about twice as rapidly: For the primate retina the slope ratio is 2.27; for the one human retina it is 1.74. Thus cone position irregularity is a larger fraction of spacing in the periphery than in the fovea.

circles). Also plotted are the standard deviations of spacing at each eccentricity (open circles). Both data sets have been normalized to unity at the foveal center in order to emphasize the difference in slope. The linear regression lines through the data indicate that the standard deviation of cone spacing increases about twice as fast as does the mean spacing with increasing eccentricity for both primate and human. Accordingly, the following equations will be used to describe the mean cone spacing, $S(E)$, and standard deviation, $\sigma(E)$, as functions of eccentricity E:

$$S(E) = 34.47\left(1 + \frac{E}{1.53°}\right), \tag{5}$$

$$\sigma(E) = 3.79\left(1 + \frac{E}{0.765°}\right). \tag{6}$$

Here S and σ are expressed in arc sec, and E is given in degrees. Given these relationships, it is possible to calculate the mean number of cones in a line from the center of the fovea to any eccentricity by choosing each successive value for E in equation 5 to be the sum of the preceding values of $S(E)$ until the sum equals the desired eccentricity. On the assumption that the uncertainty in successive cone spacings is uncorrelated, the cumulative standard deviation associated with this distance can then be calculated using the formula:

$$\sigma_{\text{total}} = \sqrt{\sum_i \sigma_i^2}, \tag{7}$$

where σ_i is the standard deviation associated with the ith cone interval. Representative values are listed in table 12.1. These values may be used to predict the effects of cone position uncertainty on two line separation thresholds, as separations differing by $0.95\sigma_{\text{total}}$ would produce 75 percent correct discrimination in a two-altenative, forced-choice paradigm. This prediction is shown by the solid line in figure 12.5, which provides a very good fit to the empirical data.

The use of cone position irregularity to predict two line separation discrimination in this manner is only valid if the retina of each individual subject effectively provides a statistical distribution of irregularities during the course

Table 12.1

Cones	Length	Standard deviation
10	0.10°	0.0035° (12.6″)
24	0.25°	0.0060° (21.6″)
45	0.50°	0.0093° (33.5″)
81	1.00°	0.0155° (55.8″)
134	2.00°	0.0274° (99″)
233	5.00°	0.0636° (229″)
324	10.0°	0.1244° (448″)

of each experiment. How could a single retina with fixed, albeit irregular, cone locations provide such an ensemble? A plausible answer is provided by the observation that eye movements will cause each experimental trial to stimulate a different retinal locus. Measurements of eye movements during fixation indicate that fixations on average cover an area of 64.0 (min arc)^2, which corresponds to a circle of 4.51 min arc radius (Steinman, Cunitz, Timberlake & Herman, 1967). In the foveal center, given hexagonal packing and a mean cone spacing of 0.6 min arc, this area would contain about 205 cones. Furthermore, the mean length of saccades during fixation was 8.18 min arc. Thus, eye movements should provide adequate retinal sampling to support the statistical treatment above.

These considerations support the hypothesis that two line separation acuity at large separations requires a distance measurement process that is limited by the spatial irregularity of the cone mosaic. This hypothesis gains added credence from the recent observation that the cortical magnification factor is directly related to both ganglion cell density and foveal cone density (Wässle, Grünert, Röhrenbeck & Boycott, 1989).

Vernier Acuity and Spatial Uncertainty

Sampling irregularity in the cone mosaic not only limits two line separation acuity but also serves to degrade peripheral vernier acuity. Westheimer (1982) measured both grating acuity and hyperacuity as a function of eccentricity and observed that although both were degraded in the periphery relative to the fovea, hyperacuity was much more strongly affected. In particular, at a horizontal eccentricity of 10° grating acuity was reduced by a factor of 4.5 relative to its foveal value, while hyperacuity was 10 times worse than foveal hyperacuity.

It has long been known that grating acuity decreases with eccentricity, and it has also been shown that this is associated with a shift of spatial filter tuning towards lower spatial frequencies (Swanson & Wilson, 1985). Can this increase in filter size alone explain the rapid degradation of peripheral vernier acuity? The answer is no, as the following simple considerations show. Suppose that at a particular eccentricity spatial processing was identical to that in the fovea, except that the size and spacing of all visual filters had been increased by a linear factor of **k** reflecting a **k**-fold reduction in grating acuity. The gain (*A* in equation 1) must also be multiplied by $(1/k)^2$ to reflect the reduced cone density and to keep the peak grating sensitivity of each mechanism constant with eccentricity, as has been observed experimentally (Rovamo, Virsu & Näsänen, 1978). If the linear dimensions of hyperacuity stimuli are each scaled up **k** times, then these stimuli will overlap visual filters by an amount identical to that in the fovea and thus will generate an identical mechanism response. Accordingly, hyperacuity thresholds should be scaled up by the same factor **k**. In other words, if both the stimulus and the responding visual mechanisms were simply enlarged by the same factor **k**, computation shows that hyperacuity thresholds would also be scaled by this same factor; yet hyperacuity degrades 2 to 3 time faster than this in the periphery.

As the dramatic increase in peripheral hyperacuity thresholds cannot be explained simply by an increase in visual filter size, additional factors must be involved. As the cone mosaic data in figure 12.6 indicate that the standard deviation of cone separation increases more rapidly than the separation itself in the periphery, it is natural to ask whether sampling irregularity can account for the degradation of hyperacuity in the periphery. French, Snyder, and Stavenga (1977) were the first to calculate the effects of spatial noise in the photoreceptor mosaic in degrading the retinal image, and the present calculations are in the same spirit as their analysis. However, the present analysis goes beyond theirs in two respects: It determines the effects of position uncertainty on the responses of orientation selective cortical mechanisms, and it predicts the reduction in hyperacuity produced by position uncertainty.

Suppose that only the mean position of orientation selective cortical filters is known and that there is an uncertainty in their location given by the two-dimensional normal distribution:

$$U(x, y) = \frac{1}{2\pi\sigma_u^2} e^{-(x^2+y^2)/2\sigma_u^2}, \quad (8)$$

where σ_u is the standard deviation of the position uncertainty. The effect of this spatial irregularity on the mean response of a visual filter (equation 1) may now be easily calculated by convolution:

$$F_u(x, y) = \int_{-\infty}^{\infty} \int_{-\infty}^{\infty} U(x - x', y - y')F(x', y') \, dx' \, dy'. \quad (9)$$

When $F_u(x, y)$ is convolved with any stimulus it will produce a response averaged over the distribution of position uncertainties. The effect of spatial irregularity on the variance $V(x, y)$ of the response to a stimulus at (x, y) must also be calculated, as pattern discrimination depends on the signal-to-noise ratio. From the definition of variance it follow that:

$$V(x, y) = \int_{-\infty}^{\infty} \int_{-\infty}^{\infty} U(x - x', y - y')F^2(x', y') \, dx' \, dy'$$
$$- F_u^2(x, y). \quad (10)$$

Equations 9 and 10 can be solved analytically, and those results have been reported elsewhere (Wilson, 1991b). The standard deviation of the filter response is then given by $\sqrt{1 + V}$, as thresholds in the absence of spatial irregularity have been normalized to unity variance.

The theoretical effects of spatial uncertainty in elevating hyperacuity thresholds are indicated by the solid line in figure 12.7. This theoretical calculation determined the accuracy with which a single thin line could be localized by the smallest visual filter measured by masking (see

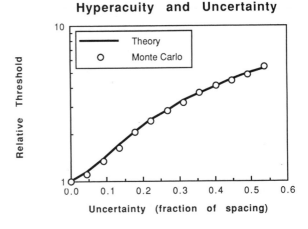

Fig. 12.7
Effects of position irregularity on hyperacuity. Thresholds are plotted relative to the case where there is no position irregularity. The abscissa indicates the standard deviation of the position distribution as a fraction of the normal spacing between neighboring units, which is given by equation 5 as a function of eccentricity. The solid line shows the results of the theoretical calculation in equations 9 and 10, while the open circles show the results of a Monte Carlo simulation with the same parameters. The agreement between theory and simulation supports the accuracy of equations 9 and 10. Both the theory and simulation were obtained for the smallest visual filter (see figure 12.1) with a mean location that was optimal for vernier position discrimination (figure 12.2A, B).

figure 12.1). For this calculation the mean location of the filter relative to the line was at the point of maximum change of sensitivity with position, that is, at the point for optimal position discrimination (see figure 12.2B). The open circles in the figure show the results of a Monte Carlo calculation in which the location of the visual filter was varied about its optimum from trial to trial based on the distribution in equation 8. The good agreement with the simulation supports the theoretical calculation. As discussed previously, the application of statistical averaging to a single retina rests upon the assumption that eye movements during fixation cause the hyperacuity target to fall on different groups of peripheral cones from trial to trial.

The abscissa in figure 12.7 indicates the uncertainty standard deviation σ_u as a fraction of the spacing between neighboring filters. When σ_u is about 20 percent of the spacing, position uncertainty raises hyperacuity thresholds by a factor of 2 relative to those in the absence of uncertainty, which is about the factor by which hyperacuity is degraded relative to grating acuity in the periphery. Reference to equations 5 and 6 indicates that a 20 percent uncertainty in neighboring cone spacing occurs by about 6° eccentricity, which is in reasonable agreement with the experimental data. Although these calculations have utilized only one filter and have ignored complications due to the contrast nonlinearity in equation 2, simulations with a multimechanism nonlinear model show virtually the same rise of vernier acuity thresholds as a function of increasing sampling irregularity.

These calculations show that the increased spatial irregularity in the peripheral retina can provide an explanation for the rapid degradation of peripheral hyperacuity beyond what would be expected based solely on increased filter size and spacing. Thus the same spatial uncertainty that limits two line separation discrimination at large separations (figure 12.5) also degrades peripheral hyperacuity. Levi, Klein, and Aitsebaomo (1985) first suggested that the degradation of peripheral hyperacuity might result from the increased mean spacing of visual filters and resultant spatial undersampling of the retinal image.

Curvature Discrimination

A careful analysis of two line separation acuity has suggested that the visual system employs both a local and a

Curvature Discrimination

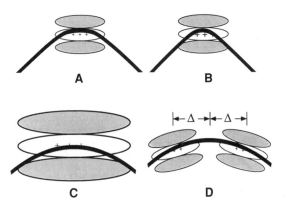

Fig. 12.8
Local mechanism responses in curvature discrimination. Contours of moderate and sharper curvature respectively are illustrated in (A) and (B) along with a high frequency visual filter optimally placed for discrimination. Note that for the sharper curvature (B) the contour encroaches on the shaded inhibitory zone, which causes a significant change in mechanism response relative to the moderate curvature in (A). (C) illustrates that the same strategy might be used for contours of low curvature if large, low spatial frequency filters were used for discrimination. Alternatively, the visual system might analyze low curvatures by calculating the orientation at two locations separated by $\pm \Delta$ along the tangent to the curve (D). Experiments with bandpass filtered contours have shown that the visual system processes low curvature contours using the nonlocal strategy in (D) (Wilson & Richards, 1989). The value of Δ is estimated to be about 8.2 min arc, which is similar to the value of 10 min arc at which the transition in figure 12.5 occurs.

global strategy in this task. Curvature discrimination is a second area in which clear evidence for two different visual strategies has recently emerged (Watt & Andrews, 1982; Wilson & Richards, 1989). Consider the illustrations in figure 12.8, which suggest different ways in which contour curvature might be encoded. As the contour in part B has a sharper curvature (i.e., a smaller radius of curvature), it encroaches on the inhibitory zones of the illustrated visual filter and thus will produce a significantly smaller mechanism response than the broader curve in part A. For curves that are broad relative to the dimensions of the smallest visual filters (see figure 12.1), two alternative approaches are possible. As illustrated in part C, larger filters might be used for discrimination in a manner identical to that in parts 8A and B. Alternatively, small filters might be used to estimate contour orientation at a pair of locations displaced by a small distance $\pm\Delta$ (part D).

Wilson (1985) first reported that curvature discrimination thresholds could be predicted by local mechanism responses as suggested in figure 12.8A, B. However, that study did not critically test the two different strategies in figure 12.8C, D for contours with low curvature. Accordingly, Wilson and Richards (1989) designed an experiment to discriminate between the two. As most contours bounding natural objects have isolated points of maximum curvature, the stimuli employed were sections of parabolas, which are the simplest curves having a single curvature maximum. These were joined smoothly to straight lines so that each stimulus had the same total range of orientations independent of curvature. The curved contours in figure 12.8 are examples of such stimuli. Data averaged over subjects are plotted as solid symbols in figure 12.9 for a wide range of curvatures. The dashed line shows that calculations based on local mechanism responses have the same general shape as the data and accurately predict thresholds for curvatures above 2/deg. However, the local mechanism predictions are too high by a factor of about 2.5 at low curvatures.

If low curvatures are analyzed locally, as illustrated in figure 12.8C, then large filters tuned to low spatial frequencies must be doing the processing. To test this, curvature discrimination thresholds were measured using curves that had been bandpass filtered with a peak frequency of 25 cycles/degree to remove all low spatial frequency information (Wilson & Richards, 1989). This filtering had no effect on curvature discrimination in the low curvature range, thus demonstrating that these curvatures clearly are not processed by large, low frequency mechanisms.

As high frequency mechanisms displaced along the contour would not be significantly affected by high pass filtering, these data lend support to the low curvature computation strategy shown in figure 12.8D. Accordingly, the highest frequency mechanisms (see figure 12.1) were used to calculate a quantitative fit to the low curvature data by choosing a single value of Δ. Computed thresholds obtained for $\Delta = 8.2$ min arc are plotted as a solid curve in figure 12.9 and provide a much better fit to the low curvature data.

Several points concerning this nonlocal curvature discrimination process are of interest. First, note that this

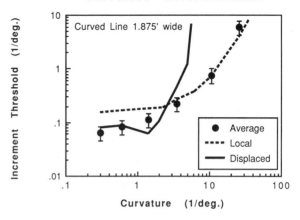

Curvature Discrimination

Fig. 12.9

Comparison of curvature discrimination data with theory. Thresholds for detecting the contour of sharper curvature (e.g., figure 12.8B vs A) in a two-alternative, forced-choice paradigm are plotted as a function of the mean curvature (Wilson & Richards, 1989). Curvature is the reciprocal of radius of curvature. The dashed line shows the curvature discrimination prediction based on local mechanism responses, as schematized in figure 12.8A and B, while the solid line shows the prediction based on small filters displaced by $\pm\Delta$ along the tangent to the contour (figure 12.8D). Note that local mechanism responses accurately predict curvature thresholds above about 2/degree, while responses of displaced filters predict thresholds below this point. Thus curvature discrimination involves both local and nonlocal strategies just as does separation discrimination (figure 12.5).

nonlocal process cannot analyze contours of high curvature, as such contours perforce change direction too rapidly to stimulate filters displaced by $\pm\Delta$ from the curvature extremum. Thus, the two different curvature strategies dovetail nicely to extend the range of accurate curvature discrimination. Second, the nonlocal process utilizes filters displaced by $\pm\Delta$ *along the tangent to the contour* rather than along the contour itself. Were the filters displaced *along* the contour, curvature estimates would first be needed to estimate arc length, thus leading to an infinite regress. On the other hand, local contour tangents are readily computed from the responses of orientation selective mechanisms. Finally, $\Delta = 8.2$ min arc is close to the 10 min arc at which two line separation thresholds begin to be determined by a non-local mechanism (see above). This suggests that the transition from a local to a global pattern discrimination strategy may be determined by a common spatial scale factor, a notion to be amplified subsequently.

Spatial Wavelength Discrimination

Spatial frequency discrimination provides a particularly interesting example in which the major themes of this chapter are merged. As a cosine grating is extended in space, two different discrimination strategies are possible in principle. Responses of spatial frequency tuned mechanisms might be used locally to provide a direct estimate of grating frequency. Alternatively, discrimination might be based on cortical measurement of the distance between peaks a fixed number of cycles apart. To put it otherwise, this task might be performed either as spatial frequency discrimination or as spatial wavelength discrimination. Hirsch and Hylton (1982) first suggested that performance was based on a measurement of the distance between adjacent peaks of the waveform, although they did not specify how the peaks were localized or the nature of the measurement process. Wilson and Gelb (1984), on the other hand, suggested a discrimination strategy based upon responses of localized, spatial frequency tuned mechanisms.

Predictions of spatial frequency discrimination thresholds calculated from local mechanism responses (Wilson and Gelb, 1984) are compared with data in figure 12.10A. Note that the data of Hirsch and Hylton (1982, open squares), obtained at 30 percent contrast, exhibit a scalloped appearance with alternating peaks and troughs. This same scalloping occurs in color discrimination, where it reflects the existence of just three cone photopigments (Bouman & Walraven, 1972). The scalloping present in the theoretical results is similarly a reflection of the existence of just six spatial frequency tuned mechanisms in the model. However, more recent evidence has failed to replicate the peaks and troughs in these data, as shown by the open circles (Mayer & Kim, 1986). These new data challenge models based on the localized responses of a small number of spatial frequency tuned mechanisms. However, a model with a small number of mechanisms whose spatial frequency tuning varied somewhat from fixation to fixation would produce a smooth theoretical curve. Nevertheless, the local mechanism theory does correctly predict thresholds of 2 to 4 percent over this spatial frequency range.

A second aspect of spatial frequency discrimination that has recently been examined is its dependence on grating contrast. Watson and Robson (1981) reported

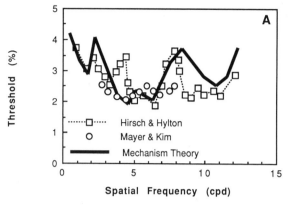

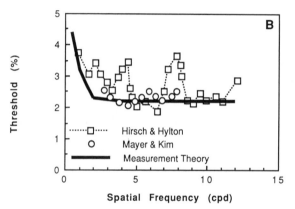

Fig. 12.10
Spatial frequency discrimination thresholds (percent) as a function of spatial frequency in cycles/degree. Data are from Hirsch and Hylton (1982, *open squares*) and Mayer and Kim (1986, *open circles*). Although both data sets show that thresholds fall in the 2 to 4 percent range, the open squares show alternate peaks and troughs of discriminability analogous to those in color discrimination, while the open circles fail to show this structure. The heavy solid line in (A) shows predictions based on local mechanism responses (Wilson & Gelb, 1984). Due to the presence of just six different foveal filter sizes, the local mechanism predictions exhibit a pattern of peaks and troughs similar to those in the Hirsch and Hylton (1982) data. The data are replotted in (B) together with predictions based on a cortical measurement process limited by the cumulative spatial irregularity inherent in the cone mosaic (see text for details). This prediction provides a better fit to the Mayer and Kim (1986) data.

that for threshold contrasts, spatial frequency discrimination thresholds were approximately one octave or 100 percent. As the data in figure 12.10A show thresholds in the 2 to 4 percent range for contrasts of 30 percent, it is apparent that there is improvement in discrimination performance with contrast. Campbell, Nachmias, and Jukes (1970) initially reported contrast independence above 3 times threshold. Bowne (1990) critically examined the contrast dependence of spatial frequency discrimination and compared it with the localized mechanism predictions of Wilson and Gelb (1984). His data, plotted in figure 12.11, show that spatial frequency discrimination is almost independent of contrast over the range from 2 to 50 percent.[2] The dashed line in the figure shows the contrast dependence predicted from responses of localized, spatial frequency tuned mechanisms. Although these predictions are reasonably close to the data above 10 percent contrast, they clearly fail at low contrasts and incorrectly predict a continuous improvement with contrast over the entire range. Also plotted on the same graph is the discrimination threshold measured by Watson and Robson (1981, solid square) at threshold contrast, and it is notable that the local mechanism responses predict this point quite well (Wilson & Gelb, 1984).

These observations make it clear that spatial frequency discrimination falls into the class of pattern discrimination tasks that are largely independent of contrast for contrasts 2 to 3 times threshold. From the previous consideration of two line separation acuity at large separations, therefore, it may be conjectured that spatial frequency discrimination entails a nonlocal distance measurement process. Suppose Δ represents the accuracy with which local mechanism responses can be used to localize the center of a grating bar. The uncertainty associated with measurement of the distance between this bar and a second bar N cycles away will then be given by σ_{total} from equation 7, if it is assumed that the measurement process is limited by cumulative cone position uncertainty. Values of σ_{total} for various distances are listed in table 12.1. If the spatial frequency of the standard grating is ω, then use of the usual formula for combination of standard deviations permits us to calculate that spatial wavelength $1/\omega$ can be

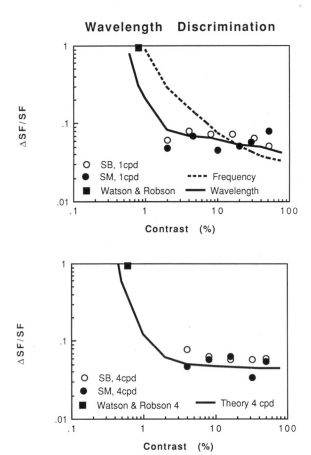

Fig. 12.11
Dependence of spatial frequency discrimination on contrast. Open and solid circles plot Weber fractions ($\Delta S/S$) for two subjects from a study by Bowne (1990) at a spatial frequency of 1 cycles/degree (*upper panel*) or 4 cycles/degree (*lower panel*). The solid square in each panel shows discrimination at threshold contrast (Watson & Robson, 1981). The dashed line in the top panel is the predicted contrast dependence based on local mechanism responses, while the solid lines in both panels are predictions based on a cortical measurement process limited by position irregularity in the cone mosaic. The cortical measurement process clearly provides a more accurate fit to the data, which suggests that spatial frequency discrimination might be better viewed as spatial wavelength discrimination.

---

2. The generally higher discrimination thresholds (5 to 8 percent) obtained by Bowne (1990) are due to the fact that his measurements are for 92 percent correct discrimination rather than 75 percent, which is more common.

discriminated from:

$$\frac{1}{N}\left(\frac{N}{\omega} - k\sqrt{2\Delta^2 + \sigma_{total}^2}\right) = \frac{N - k\omega\sqrt{2\Delta^2 + \sigma_{total}^2}}{N\omega}. \quad (11)$$

In this equation $2\Delta^2$ appears due to the fact that it is necessary to localize two bars of the grating if a measurement process is to operate. The expression on the left is multiplied by $1/N$ to give the correct wavelength change per cycle. Finally, the constant k indicates the number of standard deviations necessary for any given percent correct performance (e.g., 0.95 for 75 percent; 1.98 for 92 percent). As the Weber fraction is generally reported for spatial frequency discrimination, this equation may be easily manipulated to yield:

$$\begin{aligned}\frac{\Delta\omega}{\omega} &= \frac{1}{\omega}\left[\frac{N\omega}{N - k\omega\sqrt{2\Delta^2 + \sigma_{total}^2}} - \omega\right] \\ &= \frac{k\omega\sqrt{2\Delta^2 + \sigma_{total}^2}}{N - k\omega\sqrt{2\Delta^2 + \sigma_{total}^2}}. \end{aligned} \quad (12)$$

In applying this formula to spatial frequency discrimination data it must be emphasized that it is only the local mechanism responses that are contrast dependent, and thus Δ is the only quantity in the equation that decreases with contrast. The cumulative standard deviation σ_{total} depends only on the spatial uncertainty inherent in the cone mosaic and thus will be independent of contrast. The solid lines in figure 12.11 plot values of $\Delta\omega/\omega$ as a function of contrast for spatial frequencies of 1 and 4 cycles/degree. The contrast dependence of Δ was calculated using the Wilson and Gelb (1984) model to determine the threshold for localizing a bar of a cosine grating. In agreement with the data, the predictions for spatial frequency discrimination show a rapid improvement with contrast up to about three times threshold followed by a region of almost complete contrast independence. From equation 12 it is evident that the reason for this behavior is that the contrast dependence of Δ limits discrimination performance at low contrasts, but this term rapidly becomes smaller than σ_{total}, which provides a contrast independent limit at high contrasts.

Equation 12 may also be used to predict spatial frequency discrimination thresholds as a function of frequency. To do this, it is first necessary to choose a value of N, the number of cycles upon which discrimination is based. Hirsch and Hylton (1982) provided data suggesting that spatial frequency discrimination was independent of the number of cycles once about 2.5 cycles of the grating were present. As pointed out by Wilson and Gelb (1984), this is about the number of cycles necessary to provide optimal stimulation for spatial filters, and spatial frequency discrimination thresholds calculated from local mechanism responses are in fact independent of grating width beyond 2.5 cycles. However, recent studies have found that spatial frequency discrimination thresholds continue to improve over several cycles (Heeley, 1987; Heeley & Thompson, 1989). This is further evidence against a local mechanism computation of spatial frequency discrimination, and it indicates that values of N greater than unity should be used in equation 12.

The dependence of equation 12 on N requires brief comment. Although it may appear that $\Delta\omega/\omega$ would be proportional to N^{-1} for large N, this fails to take into account the dependence of σ_{total} on N. If cone spacing were uniform across the central retina, then σ_{total} would be proportional to $N^{.5}$, and thus $\Delta\omega/\omega$ would vary with $N^{-.5}$ for large N. Due to the increased spacing and position uncertainty at increasing eccentricities (equations 5 and 6), however, $\Delta\omega/\omega$ actually decreases less rapidly than $N^{-.5}$ and eventually reaches an asymptotic level. Calculations show that this asymptotic level is 1.45 percent and is independent of spatial frequency from 0.5 to 12.0 cycles/degree. Reference to figure 12.10 shows that this asymptotic value falls somewhat below the actual data. It may be noted, however, that Heeley and Thompson (1989) found that discrimination improved as the number of cycles was increased up to a limit of about 8, and calculated thresholds are just about at the asymptotic limit for $N = 8$.

A better fit to the data is obtained on the assumption that discrimination is based on the number of cycles spanning a fixed spatial extent. If frequencies below 2 cycles/degree are discriminated based on the width of one cycle, while thresholds above 2 cycles/degree are based on the number of cycles spanning $0.5°$, equation 12 predicts the thresholds shown by the solid line in figure 12.10B. In agreement with the data of Mayer and Kim (1986), $\Delta\omega/\omega$ is predicted to be constant at 2.2 percent over most of the spatial frequency range. This constancy of $\Delta\omega/\omega$ is achieved even though spatial filters of only six different sizes are included in the computations.

It may be concluded that both the contrast independence of spatial frequency discrimination and spatial frequency Weber fractions as a function of wavelength can be predicted by a model consisting of a local mechanism computation to localize grating bars plus a cortical measurement process limited by the cumulative position uncertainty in the cone mosaic. This model is in the spirit of models suggested by Hirsch and Hylton (1982) and Heeley (1987) for spatial frequency discrimination. However, it goes beyond them by including the contrast dependent responses of localized spatial mechanisms plus the spatial irregularity and inhomogeneity of cone spacing.

Discussion

Examination of vernier acuity, two line separation discrimination, curvature discrimination, and spatial frequency discrimination indicates that the visual system utilizes two different pattern discrimination strategies. The essence of these strategies may be captured in three propositions:

1. The analysis of local stimulus features is based on the contrast dependent responses of spatial mechanisms.

2. Discrimination of distances between local stimulus features entails a cortical measurement process.

3. Both discrimination processes are limited by the spatial irregularity inherent in the cone mosaic.

Due to the contrast nonlinearity in spatial mechanism responses, it immediately follows that pattern discrimination will improve as a power function of contrast for strictly local discrimination processes, such as vernier acuity and two bar separation discrimination for separations less than about 10 min arc. As the cortical measurement process is independent of contrast, however, global discrimination tasks, such as spatial frequency discrimination and discrimination of the spacing of widely separated bars, will be independent of contrast once the contrast is 2 to 3 times threshold. For large separations at high contrast, two line separation discrimination is limited by the cumulative spatial irregularity in the cone mosaic. In addition, the relatively rapid degradation of vernier acuity in the periphery is due to the fact that the uncertainty in cone spacing increases more rapidly than mean cone spacing with increasing eccentricity. These conclusions rest on the assumption that eye movements during fixation (Steinman et al., 1967) serve to statistically sample the retina during the course of an experiment.

Both two line separation acuity (Morgan & Regan, 1987) and curvature discrimination (Wilson & Richards, 1989) indicate that the visual system employs a global measurement strategy when the relevant stimulus information is separated by 8 to 10 min arc in the fovea. This is strikingly similar to estimates that an individual cortical module or "hypercolumn" in the central fovea processes a 6 to 10 min arc patch of the retinal image (Daniel & Whitteridge, 1961; Van Essen, Newsome & Maunsell, 1984). Thus it may be conjectured that the local pattern discrimination strategy operates within individual cortical modules, while the cortical measurement process determines the distance between stimulated modules. Calculations by Klein and Levi (1987) also support this observation.

Two further points concerning pattern discrimination should be mentioned. First, the visual system seems to employ the smallest, most precisely localized filters responding to a stimulus to perform pattern discrimination. The larger filters play little role in pattern discrimination except when the stimulus contains only low frequency information (Wilson & Richards, 1989). Thus coarse-to-fine processing strategies are apparently not employed in spatial pattern discrimination. Second, although the visual system contains a range of filters tuned to different spatial frequency ranges, spatial frequency discrimination mainly involves a spatial measurement process. Thus, it may be more appropriate to speak of spatial wavelength discrimination than spatial frequency discrimination.

The suggestion that both the local mechanism analysis and the global measurement process in pattern discrimination are limited by the spatial irregularity in the cone mosaic is unique to this study. Hirsch and Hylton (1982) have suggested that spatial interval discrimination is limited by the spacing of the cones, but they did not consider the effects of position uncertainty. Levi, et al. (1988) proposed that the spatial measurement process was limited by the coarseness or spatial irregularity of the cortical representation of the visual periphery. As new data have indicated that the cortical magnification factor may be directly related to the variation of ganglion cell density at different eccentricities (Wässle et al., 1989), it appears that the cortical measurement process is limited by the accuracy of the ganglion cell positioning, which in turn is limited by cone position irregularity.

Many previous studies have suggested that various discrimination tasks involving large separations required some form of cortical measurement strategy (Burbeck, 1987; Heeley, 1987; Hirsch & Hylton, 1982; Klein & Levi, 1987; Morgan & Regan, 1987; Watt & Morgan, 1985). The synthesis developed here suggests that local filter responses are always used for local analysis of the stimulus in the fashion previously suggested by Wilson and Gelb (1984) and Wilson (1986). The measurement process then serves to determine distances between responding filters separated by more than 8 to 10 min arc. The observation that mechanism responses increase as a power function of contrast whereas the measurement process is contrast independent provides a natural explanation for the fact that some discrimination processes improve with contrast (e.g., vernier acuity), while others are largely contrast independent (e.g., spatial frequency discrimination). Thus, it is predicted that all discrimination thresholds that improve with contrast are limited by local mechanism responses, while contrast independent thresholds are limited by the measurement process. It remains a challenge to determine whether this provides a general framework for understanding spatial pattern discrimination.

Acknowledgment

This research was supported in part by NIH grant no. EY02158.

References

Bouman, M. A. & Walraven, P. L. (1972). Color discrimination data. In D. Jameson & L. M. Hurvich (Eds.), *Handbook of sensory physiology: VII/4: Visual psychophysics* (pp. 484–516). New York: Springer-Verlag.

Bowne, S. F. (1990). Contrast discrimination cannot explain spatial frequency, orientation, or temporal frequency discrimination. *Vision Research, 30,* 449–461.

Burbeck, C. A. (1987). Position and spatial frequency in large scale localization judgments. *Vision Research, 27,* 417–427.

Campbell, F. W., Nachmias, J. & Jukes, J. (1970). Spatial frequency discrimination in human vision. *Journal of the Optical Society of America, 60,* 555–559.

Daniel, P. M. & Whitteridge, D. (1961). The representation of the visual field on the cerebral cortex in monkeys. *Journal of Physiology, 159,* 203–221.

DeValois, R. L., Albrecht, D. G. & Thorell, L. G. (1982). Spatial frequency selectivity of cells in macaque visual cortex. *Vision Research, 22,* 545–559.

French, A. S., Snyder, A. W. & Stavenga, D. G. (1977). Image degradation by an irregular retinal mosaic. *Biological Cybernetics, 27,* 229–233.

Heeley, D. W. (1987). Spatial frequency discrimination for sine wave gratings with random, bandpass frequency modulation: Evidence for averaging in spatial acuity. *Spatial Vision, 2,* 317–335.

Heeley, D. W. & Thompson, R. J. (1989). The effect of stationary, random phase discontinuities on spatial frequency discrimination. *Vision Research, 29,* 497–504.

Hirsch, J. & Hylton, R. (1982). Limits of spatial frequency discrimination as evidence of neural interpolation. *Journal of the Optical Society of America, 72,* 1367–1374.

Hirsch, J. & Miller, W. H. (1987). Does cone positional disorder limit resolution? *Journal of the Optical Society of America A, 4,* 1481–1492.

Hirsch, J. & Curcio, C. A. (1989). The spatial resolution capacity of human foveal retina. *Vision Research, 29,* 1095–1101.

Klein, S. A. & Levi, D. M. (1985). Hyperacuity thresholds of 1.0 second: Theoretical predictions and empirical validation. *Journal of the Optical Society of America A, 2,* 1170–1190.

Klein, S. A. & Levi, D. M. (1987). Position sense of the peripheral retina. *Journal of the Optical Society of America A, 4,* 1543–1553.

Legge, G. E. & Foley, J. M. (1980). Contrast masking in human vision. *Journal of the Optical Society of America, 70,* 1458–1470.

Levi, D. M., Klein, S. A. & Aitsebaomo, A. P. (1985). Vernier acuity, crowding and cortical magnification. *Vision Research, 25,* 963–977.

Levi, D. M., Klein, S. A. & Yap, Y. L. (1988). "Weber's law" for position: Unconfounding the role of separation and eccentricity. *Vision Research, 28,* 597–603.

Mayer, M. J. & Kim, C. B. Y. (1986). Smooth frequency discrimination functions for foveal, high-contrast, mid spatial frequencies. *Journal of the Optical Society of America A, 3,* 1957–1969.

Morgan, M. J. & Regan, D. (1987). Opponent model for line interval discrimination: Interval and vernier performance compared. *Vision Research, 27,* 107–118.

Movshon, J. A., Thompson, I. D. & Tolhurst, D. J. (1978). Spatial summation in the receptive fields of simple cells in the cat's striate cortex. *Journal of Physiology, 283,* 53–77.

Nachmias, J. & Sansbury, R. V. (1974). Grating contrast: Discrimination may be better than detection. *Vision Research, 14,* 1039–1042.

Nielsen, K. R. K., Watson, A. B. & Ahumada, A. J. (1985). Application of a computable model of human spatial vision to phase discrimination. *Journal of the Optical Society of America A, 2,* 1600–1606.

Parker, A. J. & Hawken, M. J. (1988). Two-dimensional spatial structure of receptive fields in monkey striate cortex. *Journal of the Optical Society of America A, 5,* 598–605.

Phillips, G. C. & Wilson, H. R. (1984). Orientation bandwidths of spatial mechanisms measured by masking. *Journal of the Optical Society of America A, 1,* 226–232.

Rovamo, J., Virsu, V. & Näsänen, R. (1978). Cortical magnification factor predicts the photopic contrast sensitivity of peripheral vision. *Nature, 271,* 54–56.

Steinman, R. M., Cunitz, R. J., Timberlake, G. T. & Herman, M. (1967). Voluntary control of microsaccades during maintained monocular fixation. *Science, 155,* 1577–1579.

Swanson, W. H. & Wilson, H. R. (1985). Eccentricity dependence of contrast matching and oblique masking. *Vision Research, 25,* 1285–1295.

Tyler, C. W. (1973). Periodic vernier acuity. *Journal of Physiology, 228,* 637–647.

Van Essen, D. C., Newsome, W. T. & Maunsell, J. H. R. (1984). The visual field representation in striate cortex of the macaque monkey: Asymmetries, anisotropies, and individual variability. *Vision Research, 24,* 429–448.

Wässle, H., Grünert, U., Röhrenbeck, J. & Boycott, B. B. (1989). Cortical magnification factor and the ganglion cell density of the primate retina. *Nature, 341,* 643–646.

Watson, A. B. & Robson, J. G. (1981). Discrimination at threshold: Labelled detectors in human vision. *Vision Research, 21,* 1115–1122.

Watt, R. J. & Andrews, D. P. (1982). Contour curvature analysis: Hyperacuities in the discrimination of detailed shape. *Vision Research, 22,* 449–460.

Watt, R. J. & Morgan, M. J. (1983). The recognition and representation of edge blur: Evidence for spatial primitives in human vision. *Vision Research, 23,* 1465–1477.

Watt, R. J. & Morgan, M. J. (1985). A theory of the primitive spatial code in human vision. *Vision Research, 25,* 1661–1674.

Westheimer, G. (1979). Spatial sense of the eye. *Investigative Ophthalmology and Visual Science, 18,* 893–912.

Westheimer, G. (1982). The spatial grain of the perifoveal visual field. *Vision Research, 22,* 157–162.

Westheimer, G. (1984). Line-separation discrimination curve in the human fovea: Smooth or segmented? *Journal of the Optical Society of America A, 1,* 683–684.

Westheimer, G. & Hauske, G. (1975). Temporal and spatial interference with vernier acuity. *Vision Research, 15,* 1137–1141.

Westheimer, G. & McKee, S. P. (1977). Spatial configurations for visual hyperacuity. *Vision Research, 17,* 941–947.

Wilson, H. R. (1985). Discrimination of contour curvature: Data and theory. *Journal of the Optical Society of America A, 2,* 1191–1199.

Wilson, H. R. (1986). Responses of spatial mechanisms can explain hyperacuity. *Vision Research, 26,* 453–469.

Wilson, H. R. (1991a). Psychophysical models of spatial vision and hyperacuity. In D. Regan (Ed.), *Spatial Vision* (Vol. 10 of *Vision and Visual Dysfunction*). New York: MacMillan.

Wilson, H. R. (1991b). Model of peripheral and amblyopic hyperacuity. *Vision Research, 31,* 967–982.

Wilson, H. R., McFarlane, D. K. & Phillips, G. C. (1983). Spatial frequency tuning of orientation selective units estimated by oblique masking. *Vision Research, 23,* 873–882.

Wilson, H. R. & Gelb, D. J. (1984). Modified line element theory for spatial frequency and width discrimination. *Journal of the Optical Society of America A, 1,* 124–131.

Wilson, H. R., Levi, D., Maffei, L., Rovamo, J. & DeValois, R. L. (1990). The perception of form: Retina to striate cortex. In L. Spillmann and J. S. Werner (Eds.), *Visual perception: The neurophysiological foundations* (pp. 231–272). New York: Academic Press.

Wilson, H. R. & Richards, W. A. (1989). Mechanisms of contour curvature discrimination. *Journal of the Optical Society of America A, 6,* 106–115.

Part V

Color and Shading

The plenoptic view of Adelson and Bergen (chapter 1) described the dimensions of information available in an image while deliberately setting aside the question of the "meaningfulness" of the information. To model the function of the visual system, it is essential also to understand the way in which visual images are generated, so that sources of meaningful information in the image can be deduced. This involves an analysis of the physics of imaging: light sources, surface and lighting geometry, the behavior of reflecting surfaces, and the like. The results of such analysis are useful for generating rich stimuli for experimental work (for example, the "computer graphics psychophysics" described in Bülthoff's chapter in part VII). At the same time, this approach is fruitful for modeling.

Perhaps the best known case concerns "color constancy." Because the role of the visual system is to establish the nature of objects, and because the appearance of objects depends both on the properties of their surfaces and on the light that illuminates them, it has long been known that the visual system must (and does) contain a mechanism capable of "discounting the illuminant" (Helmholtz, 1896). Because the contributions of the illumination and the surface properties to the spectral and spatial distribution of light in the image of an object are intrinsically indistinguishable, this problem cannot be solved for arbitrary combinations of illumination and object. It has recently become clear, however, that by modeling the surface spectral reflectance functions and illuminant spectral power distributions drawn from linear models with a small number of basis functions, this intractable problem can be reduced to a manageable form. The pairwise products of the simple (and not very numerous) basis functions, given the physics of reflection, form the basis for most useful color signals. By using a sufficient number of samples in color space (for example, those provided by the three classes of cones in the retina) at a sufficient number of spatial locations over which the illuminant changes slowly, it is often possible to deduce the illuminant, and hence derive the reflectance functions of the surfaces in the scene.

This section contains three chapters drawn from this approach. The chapter by Brainard and Wandell takes its motivation from the work of Maloney and Wandell (1986) and attempts to model the color appearance judgments of human observers across different simulated illumination conditions by reference to linear models of the illuminants and surfaces in a complex scene. D'Zmura introduces the mathematics of spherical harmonics, which turn out to be convenient and illuminating tools for understanding the geometric aspects of illuminance and reflectance functions that characterize real objects. Kersten models an even more complex world in which surfaces may be transparent as well as opaque, and the object of his model is to parse the visual scene into components due to overlapping transparent surfaces and components due to reflectance changes within a single surface. Each of these chapters represents a valuable complement and enhancement to the plenoptic view, by showing how particular aspects of the nature of the real world constrain the information available to the observer and by showing how that information may be used to solve the complex problems that arise in making inferences about the world from the visual image.

References

Helmholtz, H. (1896). J. P. C. Southall (Trans.), *Physiological optics.* New York: Dover.

Maloney, L. T. & Wandell, B. (1986). Color constancy: A method for recovering surface spectral reflectance. *Journal of the Optical Society of America A, 3,* 29–33.

13

A Bilinear Model of the Illuminant's Effect on Color Appearance

David H. Brainard and
Brian A. Wandell

A naive theory of color appearance might attempt to predict the color appearance of a test light from the spectral power distribution of the light. Many color appearance phenomena, including simultaneous color contrast and effects of observer adaptation, falsify this type of theory. In addition to the spectral power distribution of the test light, a theory of color appearance must incorporate some information about the context in which the test light is seen.

In natural viewing, we typically use color names to describe objects. Implicit in the statement "My car is red" is the idea that the redness is a property of the car. The spectral properties of the color signal reflected from an object to the eye are determined both by the spectral properties of the object's surface and by the spectral properties of the ambient illumination. For the sensation of color appearance to be a useful code for object surface properties, the visual system must actively adjust to variation in the illumination to stabilize object color appearance. A visual system is called color constant if it adjusts perfectly, so that the appearance of an object is invariant despite changes in illumination.

It has long been known that the human visual system exhibits imperfect color constancy (Evans, 1943; 1948; Helmholtz, 1896; Helson & Jeffers, 1940; see Boring, 1942; Wyszecki, 1986). For this reason, the goal of classic empirical studies was not to accept or reject human color constancy but rather to measure and model the effect of viewing context on color appearance (Burnham, Evans & Newhall, 1975; Helson & Jeffers, 1940; Helson, Judd & Warren, 1952; Hunt, 1953). To make the measurement problem tractable, these studies used a simple laboratory model where isolated test lights were presented against uniform backgrounds. Within this model, changing the viewing context is accomplished by changing the spectral properties of the background. The classic experiments and associated theories (Brewer, 1954; Burnham, Evans & Newhall, 1957; Jameson & Hurvich, 1964; Judd, 1940) form the basis of our current understanding of the effect of context on color appearance. Although this work provides a successful account of appearance effects within the restricted domain, it is not clear how to generalize the results to natural images.[1]

Natural images are formed when illumination is reflected to the eye from the objects in the image. To understand the difficulty in generalizing from uniform backgrounds to natural images, note that there are many physically distinct ways to vary a natural image. One is to change the spectral properties of the illumination. A second is to change the shape and spectral properties of the object surfaces that compose the image. If a visual system adjusts to changes in illumination, varying the illumination will affect color appearance. If a visual system exhibits contrast effects, perhaps for the purpose of enhancing object edges, then varying the surfaces will also have an effect. Experiments conducted using a uniform background confound these two types of variation. Changes in the spectral properties of the background are legitimately interpreted either as changes in illumination or as changes in surface reflectance.

In this chapter, we describe our recent experimental work designed to isolate the effect of varying the illuminant from the effect of varying the surfaces in the image. In our experiments, the viewing context is controlled by having the observer view a series of images, each of which is a simulation of a set of uniformly illuminated surfaces presented on a cathode ray tube (CRT) display device. The observer judges the color appearance of test lights embedded in these images. When there are multiple surfaces in an image, it is possible for a visual system to estimate the illuminant independent of the choice of surfaces (Buchsbaum, 1980; Maloney & Wandell, 1986). In any experimental condition we hold the simulated illuminant constant; the simulated surfaces are varied to counterbalance against contrast effects. We interpret our data as measuring the visual system's adjustment to the simulated illuminant. Our measurements indicate that the visual system's adjustment to simulated changes in illumination is regular and can be understood with a bilinear model that is motivated by the physics of natural image formation.

Fundamentals

Any quantitative discussion of color appearance must be based on an understanding of the physical properties of light and how the visual system measures these properties. Cornsweet (1970) provides an elementary introduction to the fundamentals of color vision. A detailed modern treatment using linear algebra can be found in Wandell (1987).

Figure 13.1 illustrates how the light that reaches the eye (**c**) arises when an illuminant (**e**) reflects from a surface (**s**). The illuminant is characterized by its spectral power distribution, which specifies how much power it contains at N_λ evenly spaced sample wavelengths λ_n in the visible spectrum. Typically the visible spectrum is sampled between approximately 370 nm and 730 nm with a wavelength spacing $\Delta\lambda$ between 1 nm and 10 nm. The illuminant spectral power distribution can be described graphically, as shown in the figure. We use the symbol **e** to denote illuminant spectral power distributions.

The illuminant reflects off a surface to form the light that reaches the eye. We call the light reaching the eye the color signal and denote it by the symbol **c**. The spectral power distribution of the color signal is determined by the spectral power distribution of the illuminant and the spectral reflectance function of the surface. The surface's reflectance function specifies the fraction of illuminant power that is reflected from the surface at each sample wavelength λ_n.[2] To compute the color signal power at any wavelength, we multiply the illuminant power at that wavelength by the corresponding value of the surface reflectance function.

Color vision begins when the color signal enters the eye and is measured by the visual system. The visual system makes three separate measurements on the color

---

1. Land's (1964; 1983; Land & McCann, 1971) theory, based on the retinex algorithm, has been popularized as a successful account of color appearance in natural images. It is, however, based on the many of the same fundamental ideas and is less closely tied to empirical data than the earlier models (see Brainard & Wandell, 1986; McLaren, 1986; Shapley, 1986; West & Brill, 1982; also Judd, 1960; Woolfson, 1959).

2. We assume that a surface's reflectance function does not depend on viewing geometry. This is true for diffuse illumination. For point illumination, an object's surface reflectance can depend on the angle at which the illuminant strikes the surface. This phenomenon is important but beyond the scope of this chapter. D'Zmura and Lennie (1986), Lee (1986), Shafer (1985), Tominaga and Wandell (1989), and chapter 14 of this volume contain analyses of the relation between the viewing geometry of an object and its surface reflectance.

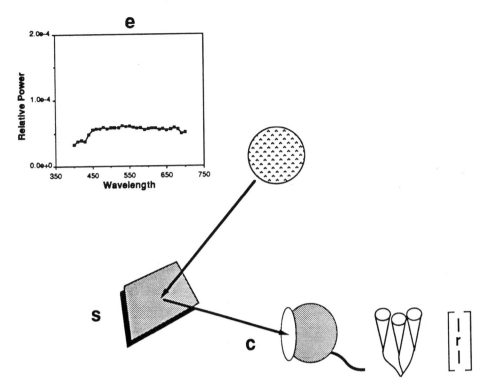

Fig. 13.1
Image formation and initial encoding. An illuminant (**e**) reflects from a surface (**s**) to form the color signal (**c**) that reaches the eye. The visual system represents the color signal by the responses of three classes of cones (**r**). (Adapted from Brainard & Wandell, 1990b.)

signal at each spatial location of an image. These measurements are the responses of three classes of light sensitive photoreceptors on the retina: the long wavelength sensitive (L) cones, the middle wavelength sensitive (M) cones, and the short wavelength sensitive (S) cones. The three cone responses generated by a color signal are called the color signal's cone coordinates.[3] They are the information available to the visual system about the color signal and about the underlying illuminant and surface.

We denote the cone coordinates of a color signal by the vector **r**, whose entries are the responses of the three cone classes. This vector is drawn in the lower right of figure 13.1. The relation between a color signal's spectral power distribution and its cone coordinates is determined by

the spectral responsivities of the three classes of cones. The spectral responsivity of a cone class specifies how strongly the cone responds to color signal power at each sample wavelength. To find a cone's quantal absorptions, we multiply the color signal power at each wavelength by the cone responsivity at that wavelength, and then sum these products over wavelength. Because the spectral responsivities of the human cones have been estimated psychophysically (Smith & Pokorny, 1975; see Boynton, 1979) and confirmed physiologically (Schnapf, Kraft & Baylor, 1987), it is possible to compute the cone coordinates to any color signal.

The relation between a color signal **c** and its cone coordinates is conveniently expressed using matrix and vector notation. We represent **c** with an N_λ dimensional column vector whose nth entry is the power at sample wavelength λ_n. Let **R** be a matrix with three rows and N_λ columns, where each row describes the responsivity of one class of cones. The first row describes the respon-

3. Strictly speaking, there can be only one photoreceptor at each spatial location. It is convenient, however, to assume that at each location the color signal is sampled by all classes of receptor. Brainard, Wandell, and Poirson (1989) discuss the implications of the fact that there can only be one receptor at each spatial location. The assumption that all three classes of receptors sample the

color signal at each location causes no difficulty as long as the color signal is constant across regions that are large compared to the spacing between photoreceptors. In addition to the cones, there is a fourth class of photoreceptor: the rods. The rods are not generally thought to play a role in color vision at the high light levels typical of daylight viewing.

sivity of the L cones: The nth entry of the first row is the responsivity of an L cone at sample wavelength λ_n. The second and third rows describe the responsivity of the M and S cones. When the cone responsivities are described by $\mathbf{R}$, the relation between a color signal's spectral power vector $\mathbf{c}$ and its cone coordinates $\mathbf{r}$ is given by

$$\mathbf{r} = \mathbf{Rc}. \qquad (1)$$

Without loss of generality, the choice of wavelength spacing $\Delta\lambda$ is incorporated into equation 1 by absorbing it in the units used to express light power.

It is useful to extend equation 1 to include the physical factors that give rise to the color signal. Let $\mathbf{e}$ be the N_λ dimensional column vector whose nth entry is the power at sample wavelength λ_n. Let $\mathbf{S}$ be the N_λ by N_λ diagonal matrix whose nth diagonal entry is the surface reflectance at sample wavelength λ_n. We then have $\mathbf{c} = \mathbf{Se}$. Combining this with equation 1 we arrive at a relation between the illuminant spectral power distribution $\mathbf{e}$ and the response vector $\mathbf{r}$ that encodes the color signal reflected from a surface:

$$\mathbf{r} = (\mathbf{RS})\mathbf{e}. \qquad (2)$$

Experimental Method

To study the visual system's adjustment, we ask what happens to the appearance of a test light when we manipulate this adjustment. Our basic experimental strategy was to use a matching paradigm. Matching paradigms have been widely used in psychophysics and offer the advantage that subjects are only required to judge identity of sensation. Such procedures are in general more reliable and less open to multiple interpretations than procedures that require subjects to name, rate, or scale sensation (see Brindley, 1970).

At the start of an experimental session, we trained the subject to remember the color appearance of a *prototype color signal*, which was presented in the context of CRT simulations of surfaces illuminated by a *standard illuminant*. During the course of an experimental session, the subject set *memory matches* to this learned appearance standard.

To set a match, the subject used a button box to adjust the spectral power distribution of a color signal emitted from a CRT. We had the subject set memory matches both in the context of CRT simulations of surfaces illuminated by the standard illuminant and in the context of CRT simulations of surfaces illuminated by a *changed illuminant*. The standard illuminant matches measured whether the subject could perform the memory matching task veridically. The changed illuminant matches defined a *matching color signal*. This color signal had the same color appearance when it was viewed in the context of the changed illuminant images as did the prototype color signal when it was viewed in the context of the standard illuminant images. The difference between the prototype and matching color signals was our measure of the effect of the visual system's adjustment on color appearance.

Figure 13.2 illustrates our experimental procedure. The upper half of the figure shows the spectral power distributions of the standard illuminant $\mathbf{e}$ and one possible changed illuminant $\mathbf{e} + \Delta\mathbf{e}$. The lower left of the figure shows the cone coordinates $\mathbf{r}$ of the prototype color signal. The lower right of the figure shows the cone coordinates $\mathbf{r} + \Delta\mathbf{r}$ of the matching color signal. The symbol "$\sim$" is used to indicate the appearance match between $\mathbf{r}$ and $\mathbf{r} + \Delta\mathbf{r}$ across the change in simulated illuminant.

We controlled the state of the visual system by having the subject judge and adjust color signals that were presented in a small region of larger *context images*. The context images were implemented as a CRT simulation of uniformly illuminated matte surfaces.[4] The spatial structure of our simulated images is shown in figure 13.3. In each image, 25 small rectangular surfaces were simulated against a background surface. The figure gives the size of the simulated surfaces in degrees of visual angle. For any given image, the simulated surfaces were chosen by random draw from the Munsell papers (Nickerson, 1957). Subjects viewed the images binocularly in an otherwise dark room. Both head and eye movements were permitted during viewing.

When we wanted the visual system to be adjusted to the standard illuminant, we simulated surfaces illuminated

---

4. To simulate an illuminated surface, we used equation 2 to compute cone coordinates $\mathbf{r}$ from the illuminant spectral power distribution $\mathbf{e}$ and surface reflectance function $\mathbf{S}$. We then used calibration measurements of our CRT monitor to compute input values for the monitor frame buffer so that the emitted color signal generated these same cone coordinates. Brainard (1989a) describes our display hardware and calibration measurements. Brainard and Wandell (1990a) describe the software that was used to implement the simulations.

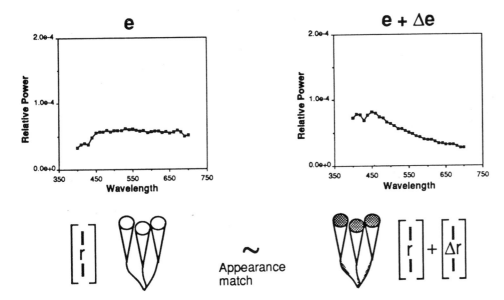

Fig. 13.2
Experimental framework. The experiment measures the cone coordinates **r** and **r** + Δ**r** of color signals that match in appearance across a change of simulated illuminant. The illuminant change is described by Δ**e**. (Adapted from Brainard & Wandell, 1990b.)

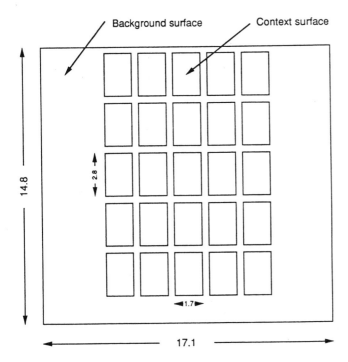

Fig. 13.3
Spatial structure of the simulated images used in the experiment. Twenty-five small rectangular surfaces were simulated against a background surface. The units of the dimensions shown in the figure are degrees of visual angle.

by the standard illuminant. When we wanted the visual system to be adjusted to the changed illuminant, we simulated surfaces illuminated by the changed illuminant. To change the subject's adjustment to the illuminant, the subject viewed a series of images where the spectral power distribution of the spatially uniform illuminant was varied slowly. The subject always viewed images characterized by a single illuminant for an extended time before setting any appearance matches.

Features of the Experimental Method

There are a number of important features about our experimental method. In this section we discuss four of these: our choice of images, how we randomize with respect to contrast effects, how we control observer adaptation, and the use of a CRT to present the images.

Choice of Images

In real world viewing, images can be quite complex: There can be multiple sources of illumination, images can contain different numbers of surfaces, the surfaces can have a huge variety of sizes and shapes, surface reflectance functions can depend on viewing geometry, and the spectral functions that describe illuminant power and surface reflectance can be nearly arbitrary. To bring all of the richness of natural images into the laboratory would make the construction, manipulation, and description of the experimental stimuli intractable. It is necessary to restrict the features of natural images that will be incorporated into the laboratory veiwing situation. Although it is desirable to keep the structure of the images as simple as possible, it is important to consider what features of natural images provide information used by the visual system to adjust to the illuminant.

It would be unreasonable, of course, to measure the visual system's adjustment using images where the relevant information about the illuminant had been removed. Over the past ten years, there has been a great deal of progress in understanding exactly what information about the illuminant is available in simple images. This understanding provides guidance to the experimentalist who wishes to choose a laboratory model that is simple but that retains this information. In particular, the work of Buchsbaum (1980) and of Maloney and Wandell (1986) shows that it is possible for the visual system to estimate the illuminant when the images consist of uniformly illuminated matte surfaces. Although the algorithms differ in detail, they share the property that their estimates of the illuminant improve with the number of surfaces in the image. To show this quantitatively, we implemented the algorithm proposed by Buchsbaum (1980) and simulated its performance on images consisting of 1, 25, and 100 surfaces. The images were created by choosing surfaces by random draw from the set of Munsell papers. We computed the location-by-location cone coordinates for each image when it was uniformly illuminated by the standard illuminant of figure 13.2. We then ran Buchsbaum's algorithm to estimate the illuminant.[5] Figure 13.4 shows the results. When there is a only a single surface in the image, the estimates of the illuminant vary wildly. As the number of surfaces in the image increases, the estimates of the illuminant improve. Clearly, an image with single surface (uniform background) does not provide enough information for the visual system to estimate the illuminant. We chose images of the form shown in figure 13.3 as a compromise between the full complexity of natural images and the simplicity of uniform backgrounds. Our images are simple compared to natural images but

contain sufficient information for the visual system to estimate the illuminant.

Contrast Effects

In the introduction we argued that when only uniform backgrounds are used, it is impossible to separate the effect of the visual system's adjustment to the illuminant from other factors such as simultaneous color contrast and color assimilation.[6] An understanding of the influence of spatial and temporal image factors that can vary within a class of images that share a common illuminant must be included in a complete theory of color appearance, but these effects are different from adjustment to the illuminant. Because we wanted to measure only the effect of changing the illuminant, we used many images throughout an experimental session. This randomized our design with respect to local spatial contrast effects. While a subject set a match, for example, the particular surfaces in the image were changed each time the subject pressed a button, as was the location of the color signal being judged. The spectral power distribution of the simulated illuminant remained constant. Because these other factors are randomized, we attribute our results to the effects of the visual system's adjustment to the simulated illuminant.

Control of Adaptation

The early experimentalists were careful to assess color appearance only after they had set the visual system's state of adaptation by having the observer view a uniform field for some minutes before any measurements were made (Burnham, Evans & Newhall, 1957; Helson & Jeffers, 1940; Helson, Judd & Warren, 1952; Hunt, 1953). Similarly, in our experiments, we were careful to adjust the visual system to the illuminant by having the observer view simulated images that shared a common illuminant for several minutes. In many recent experiments designed to study the effect of changing the illuminant on color appearance, the adjustment of the visual system was not under experimental control. Rather the illuminant

---

5. To implement the algorithm, we had to choose a reference surface and a set of basis functions for the surfaces and illuminants. For the reference surface we used the mean reflectance of the Munsell paper data set. For the surface basis functions, we used the first three prinicipal components of this data set. For the illuminant basis functions, we used the first three principal components of daylight reported by Judd, MacAdam, and Wyszecki (1964). The standard

illuminant could be expressed exactly as a linear combination of these illuminant basis functions.

6. Wyszecki (1986) provides a thorough review of such phenomena. Excellent color plates demonstrating color contrast and color assimilation can be found in Evans (1948) and Albers (1975).

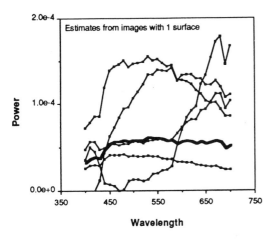

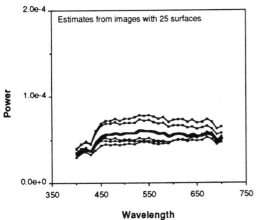

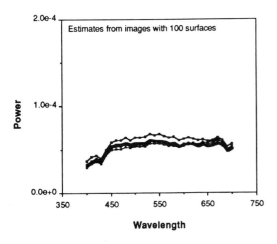

Fig. 13.4
Effect of number of surfaces on estimate of illuminant. *Top,* Illuminant estimates for five randomly chosen images consisting of a single surface. *Middle,* Illuminant estimates for five randomly chosen images consisting of 25 surfaces. *Bottom,* Illuminant estimates for five randomly chosen images consisting of 100 surfaces. In each panel, the heavy solid line shows the actual illuminant.

changed every few seconds as the subject freely compared the appearance of color signals presented in images seen either side-by-side or in quick succession (Arend & Reeves, 1986; Benzschawel, Walraven & Rogowitz, 1987; Blackwell & Buchsbaum, 1988; Hurlbert, Lee & Bülthoff, 1989; McCann, McKee & Taylor, 1976; Valberg & Lange-Malecki, 1987; Walraven, Benzschawel & Rogowitz, 1988). Although there have been some claims that adjustment to the illuminant happens almost instantaneously (Land & Daw, 1962), careful measurements (Ahn & MacLeod, 1990; Fairchild, 1990; Hunt, 1950; Jameson, Hurvich & Varner, 1979) indicate that the adjustment can take from tens of seconds to several minutes. We believe that the results of experimental work on the visual system's adjustment that permits and controls adaptation should be distinguished from the results of experiments that do not.

Use of CRT to Present Images

The use of a computer-controlled CRT to present stimuli offers great advantages in terms of stimulus control. For example, it would be technically difficult to randomize against contrast effects without software control over the images. But the use of a CRT also raises the issue of whether the visual system processes the simulated images in the same way it would have processed reflectance implementations of the same images. We believe that our current understanding of the initial encoding of light by the visual system provides a firm theoretical foundation for the use of CRT simulations: The simulated images are designed to provide the same stimulation of the retinal cone mosaic as the reflectance images. Although variation in the color matching functions between observers and with eccentricity, as well as limitations of CRT resolution and calibration accuracy, require that this match is only approximate, we believe that the simulations provide a reasonable visual match to the reflectance images they are designed to simulate. Presently it is an open empirical question as to whether the quality of simulation obtainable with a CRT is sufficient to cause the visual system to process the simulated images in the same way as it would have processed reflectance images. In adaptation experiments using uniform fields, Fairchild (1990) compared results obtained using a CRT to control adaptation and results obtained using a light booth. He found little difference between the two conditions. On the other hand, Gorzynski and Berns (1990), using a different experimental paradigm, report differences in performance when simulated and reflectance images are used.

As with any scientific research, the question of whether the results obtained in the laboratory generalize must be addressed empirically. Clearly, the use of CRT simulations to display our images is but one of many laboratory simplifications. The images we chose to simulate are themselves much simpler than natural images. In addition to validating the use of a CRT, it is important to validate these underlying simplifications. Indeed, we view the present experiments as serving this role with respect to the earlier experiments conducted with an even simpler laboratory model.

Basic Experimental Results

The measurement conditions for a single session are summarized by two vectors: the prototype color signal's cone coordinates **r** and the illuminant change Δ**e**. Implicit in this summary are the standard illuminant spectral power distribution, the spatial structure of the context images, and the surface reflectance functions used in the images. These were held fixed throughout the experiments reported here. Two subjects, one of the authors (D.B.) and a paid undergraduate (S.E.), observed in the experiments reported here. Both had normal color vision as tested with the Ishihara color plates (Ishihara, 1977). Subject D.B. was an experienced psychophysical observer and was aware of the design and purpose of the experiments. Subject S.E. began as a naive observer but became progressively better informed about the experiment over several months of observing.

The raw data from an experimental session are the cone coordinates of the subject's memory matches set when his visual system was adjusted to the standard illuminant and when his visual system was adjusted to the changed illuminant. A single session required approximately one hour of observing. Two sessions were always run for any measurement condition and the subject's responses from both sessions were pooled together. We summarize the data from the two sessions by the mean of 12 matches set under each illuminant.

Figure 13.5 shows the results of measurements of the effect of three illuminant changes on the color appearance of a single prototype color signal for subject D.B. The data are presented in three two-dimensional plots. The top panel shows the M cone coordinates of the matches

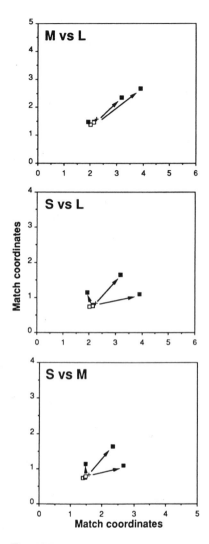

Fig. 13.5

Results of measurements for three illuminant changes. The cross indicates the cone coordinates of the prototype color signal. The open squares show the mean of the standard illuminant matches. The filled squares show the mean of the changed illuminant matches. (Prototype color signal R6_4; subject D.B.)

plotted against the L cone coordinates, the middle panel shows the S vs. the L, and the bottom shows the S vs. the M. The open symbols show the mean of the subject's standard illuminant matches. The closed symbols show the mean of the changed illuminant matches. The cross in each panel shows the cone coordinates of the prototype color signal. The arrows indicate the change in cone coordinates, Δ**r**, required to maintain constant color appearance as the illuminant was changed.

There are two important features to note about the data. First, the subject's matches set under the standard illuminant are veridical: In all three cases the open symbols lie close to the cross. Our data showed no systematic biases in subject's memory matches. Second, when the illuminant is changed there is a considerable effect on color appearance: The closed symbols are displaced from the open symbols. Each different illuminant change has a different effect on color appearance. A detailed description of our experimental method and complete tabulation of our data is given in Brainard (1989b).

Because subject's matches set under the standard illuminant were veridical, we summarize the results of an experimental condition simply by $\Delta \mathbf{r}$, the change in cone coordinates necessary to preserve color appearance. We say that $\Delta \mathbf{r}$ is the effect of the illuminant change $\Delta \mathbf{e}$ on the appearance of a prototype color signal with cone coordinates $\mathbf{r}$. To understand the visual system's adjustment to the illuminant we measure the relation between the prototype color signal's cone coordinates, $\mathbf{r}$, the illuminant change, $\Delta \mathbf{e}$, and the effect of the illuminant change on color appearance, $\Delta \mathbf{r}$.

To help interpret $\Delta \mathbf{r}$, note that if the visual system made no adjustment to the illuminant change, then $\Delta \mathbf{r}$ would be $\mathbf{0}$. Another possibility is that $\Delta \mathbf{r}$ corresponds to color constant performance. Equation 2, $\mathbf{r} = (\mathbf{RS})\mathbf{e}$, shows how the prototype color signal can be interpreted as a simulation of an illuminated surface. When this same surface is illuminated by $\mathbf{e} + \Delta \mathbf{e}$, the cone coordinates are given by $\mathbf{r} + \Delta \mathbf{r} = (\mathbf{RS})(\mathbf{e} + \Delta \mathbf{e})$. Subtracting these two expressions yields the change that corresponds to color constant performance[7]:

$$\Delta \mathbf{r} = (\mathbf{RS})\Delta \mathbf{e}. \tag{3}$$

A Bilinear Model

Overview

Our experimental method can be used to measure the effect $\Delta \mathbf{r}$ of any illuminant change $\Delta \mathbf{e}$ on the color appearance of any prototype color signal $\mathbf{r}$. Because there are

many possible pairs of $\Delta \mathbf{e}$ and $\mathbf{r}$, it is not feasible to make direct measurements for all of them. We need to find some way to organize and understand the effect of illuminant change.

To simplify the modeling task, we begin by considering the effects of the two indpendent variables separately. First we hold the cone coordinates of the prototype color signal constant and consider the effect of varying the illuminant. Then we hold the illuminant change constant and consider the effect of varying the prototype color signal. After we consider each of the variables separately, we can turn to the question of understanding how they interact with each other.

Illuminant Change Linearity

Shepard (1987) has suggested that psychological relations are often internalizations of external physical laws. Recall that equation 3 gives the physical relation between the illuminant change and the change in cone coordinates of a surface as the illuminant is changed. If the visual system were color constant, our measured relation between illuminant change $\Delta \mathbf{e}$ and measured change $\Delta \mathbf{r}$ would be predicted by equation 3. Even though we know the equation 3 will not hold exactly, it still suggests a model for performance.

Equation 3 expresses a linear relation. The linearity of equation 3 stems from the linear relation between illuminants and the cone responses of the reflected color signal, when the prototype color signal (and hence the implicit prototype surface reflectance characterized by $\mathbf{S}$) is held fixed. Because the linearity is fundamental to the physics of lights and surfaces, we might expect to find it in the psychology of color appearance. That is, the linearity of equation 3 suggests a relation between $\Delta \mathbf{r}$ and $\Delta \mathbf{e}$ that ought to hold if the visual system has internalized the physics of reflectance. We can look for a relation between these two measurable quantities of the form

$$\Delta \mathbf{r} = \mathbf{M_r}\Delta \mathbf{e}, \tag{4}$$

where $\mathbf{M_r}$ is a matrix that depends on the prototype color signal but not on the illuminant change $\Delta \mathbf{e}$. The empirical relation expressed by equation 4 can be tested by measur-

---

7. Because of surface metamerism under the standard illuminant (see Wyszecki & Stiles, 1982) there will be many different surfaces that satisfy $\mathbf{r} = (\mathbf{RS})\mathbf{e}$. Each choice of $\mathbf{S}$ leads to a different color constant $\Delta \mathbf{r}$. In this sense there is not a

unique prediction for the behavior of a color constant system. In practice, we handle this ambiguity by examining the color constant prediction for a surface whose reflectance is typical of natural surfaces.

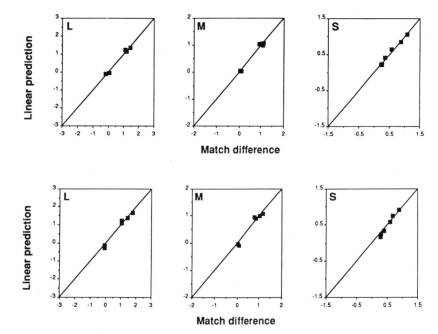

Fig. 13.6

Illuminant change linearity. The figure plots the predicted difference between the changed and standard illuminant matches against the measured difference for the L, M, and S cone components of $\Delta\mathbf{r}$. (*Top*, Prototype color signal N6; subject S.E. *Bottom*, Prototype color signal R6_4; subject D.B.) (Adapted from Brainard & Wandell, 1990b.)

ing the effect of a number of illuminant changes that are a linear combination of a small number of illuminant changes.

Suppose we fix two illuminant changes, $\Delta\mathbf{e}_1$ and $\Delta\mathbf{e}_2$ and measure their effect on color appearance, summarized by $\Delta\mathbf{r}_1$ and $\Delta\mathbf{r}_2$. Now consider any other illuminant change that is physically a linear combinaton of $\Delta\mathbf{e}_1$ and $\Delta\mathbf{e}_2$. That is, consider illuminant changes of the form $\Delta\mathbf{e} = \alpha_1 \times \Delta\mathbf{e}_1 + \alpha_2 \times \Delta\mathbf{e}_2$. If equation 4 describes behavior, then we expect that corresponding to each such $\Delta\mathbf{e}$ we will measure $\Delta\mathbf{r} = \alpha_1 \times \Delta\mathbf{r}_1 + \alpha_2 \times \Delta\mathbf{r}_2$. There is nothing special, of course, about having chosen only two basis illuminant changes. The general implication of a measurement system that obeys equation 4 is that once we measure the effect of a finite number of illuminant changes, we can predict the results for measurements for any linear combination of these illuminant changes. This is of particular interest because Judd, MacAdam, and Wyszecki measured approximately 600 daylight spectral power distributions and concluded that, within their measurement error, all of the variation in daylight could be

accounted for by a linear combination of just four basis illuminant changes.

To test whether equation 4 describes performance, we pick two basis illuminant changes, $\Delta\mathbf{e}_1$ and $\Delta\mathbf{e}_2$, and measure the effect of changing the illuminant for many linear combinations of them. We use linear regression to find the best fit to the measured data consistent with equation 4. If equation 4 describes performance, the prediction will be close to the measured data. Figure 13.6 plots, for two subjects, results for six illuminant changes that were all linear combinations of two basis illuminant changes. The plots show the linear prediction plotted against the data. For each panel, the x-axis plots one component (L, M, or S) of the measured change $\Delta\mathbf{r}$, while the y-axis plots the corresponding linear prediction. If illuminant change linearity held perfectly, then these data would fall right along the diagonal. The data support using an equation of the form of 4 to model performance.

The six illuminant changes used to test equation 4 are typical of the spectral variation of daylight. Figure 13.7 shows the CIE chromaticity coordinates of the experimental illuminants and of four CIE illumination standards. The hatched square shows the CIE chromaticity coordinates of the standard illuminant. The filled squares show the CIE chromaticity coordinates of the six changed illuminants. (Two pairs of changed illuminants differ only in intensity and thus have identical CIE coordinates.) The open squares show the chromaticities of four CIE stan-

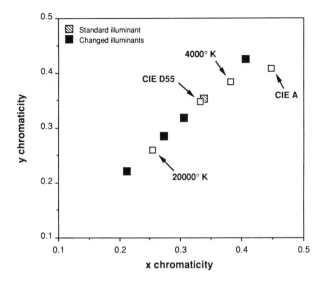

Fig. 13.7
Experimental illuminant chromaticities. The hatched square shows the
CIE chromaticity coordinates of the standard illuminant. The four
filled squares show the CIE chromaticity coordinates of the six
changed illuminants. The open squares show the chromaticities of
four CIE standard illuminants, as marked.

dard illuminants, as marked. The standard illuminant is
close to CIE standard daylight D55. The changed illuminants clearly span the range of daylight variation between
4000°K and 20,000°K equivalent blackbody radiators.
This range is typical of the range between direct sun-
light and blue skylight (see Wyszecki and Stiles, 1982,
pp. 6–7, p. 761). CIE illuminant A, which is representative
of incandescent illumination, lies outside of the range
tested. A third basis illuminant change would have to be
added to represent the spectral power distribution of CIE
illuminant A.

Prototype Linearity

A second part of understanding the effect of the illuminant change is to understand what happens as we vary
the test light's cone coordinates. We study this by reversing the roles of Δe and r in the analysis. We fix the
illuminant change and then make measurements of Δr for
several different test surfaces with different cone coordinates r_1, r_2, etc. Again, we look for a linear relation, this

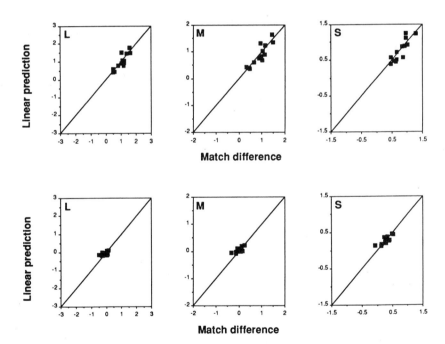

Fig. 13.8
Prototype linearity. The figure plots the predicted difference between
the changed and standard illuminant matches against the measured
difference for the L, M, and S cone components of Δr. (*Top*, Changed
illuminant 12; subject S.E. *Bottom*, Changed illuminant 1; subject D.B.)
(Adapted from Brainard & Wandell, 1990b.)

time between the cone coordinates **r** and the measured change Δ**r**. In analogy to equation 4, we look for a relation of the form:

$$\Delta \mathbf{r} = \mathbf{M}_{\Delta e} \mathbf{r}. \tag{5}$$

The use of equation 5 is also motivated by the linearity of the physics of reflection. We can test this relation in exactly the same way as we tested equation 4. Figure 13.8 shows the linear model prediction $\mathbf{M}_{\Delta e}\mathbf{r}$ plotted against the measured Δ**r** for data from two subjects. The left panels show the L cone coordinates of the two vectors, the middle panels the M cone coordinates, and the right panels the S cone coordinates. If a linear function perfectly modeled performance, the data in each panel of the two plots would fall on the diagonal lines with unit slope. The data support using an equation of the form of 5 to model performance.[8]

Bilinearity

The results presented above show that Δ**r** is a linear function of both Δ**e** and **r** when the other variable is held fixed. When a function with two inputs is a linear function for each, it is said to be bilinear (Hungerford, 1974, p. 211). The fact that the relation between Δ**r**, Δ**e**, and **r** is bilinear means that the two experimental variables Δ**e** and **r** interact in a very constrained manner.

One way to understand about the constraint imposed by the bilinearity is as follows. Let P be the dimension of **r** and M be the dimension of Δ**e**. (Here $P = 3$ and $M = 2$.) Denote the entries of **r** by r_i, $i = 1, \ldots, P$ and the entries of Δ**e** by Δe_j, $j = 1, \ldots, M$. Given **r** and Δ**e** we can construct a PM dimensional vector, **x**, where the entries of **x** are all of the products $r_i \Delta e_j$, $i = 1, \ldots, P$, $j = 1, \ldots, M$, ordered lexicographically in i and j. Brainard (1989b) shows that the relation between Δ**r**, Δ**e**, and **r** is bilinear if and only if we can write

$$\Delta \mathbf{r} = \mathbf{F}(\mathbf{r}, \Delta \mathbf{e}) = \mathbf{M}\mathbf{x}, \tag{6}$$

where the matrix **M** has dimensions 3 by PM. That is, we can re-express the bilinear relation as a simple linear relation using the constructed variable **x**. Equation 6 makes it

clear that a bilinear model has the same advantages as a linear model. Once we make measurements of the effect of a small number of illuminant changes ($\Delta \mathbf{e}_j, j = 1, \ldots, M$) on the appearance of a small number of prototype color signals ($\mathbf{r}_i, i = 1, \ldots, P$), we can predict the effect of any illuminant change Δ**e** that is a linear combination of the $\Delta \mathbf{e}_j$ on the appearance of any prototype color signal whose cone coordinates **r** are a linear combination of the $\mathbf{r}_i$.

Although we have already tested both illuminant change linearity and prototype linearity individually, we can also test bilinearity directly using equation 6. To produce enough measurement conditions for a reasonable test, we pooled the data from our two subjects. There was good consistency between the subjects for the their common measurement conditions. Since pooling the data can only reduce the quality of the bilinear fit, doing so also provides a test of how well a single model can characterize the behavior of multiple subjects. Figure 13.9 shows plots of the bilinear function prediction **Mx** against the measured Δ**r** for the entire data set. The figure shows the results of 45 measurements from 37 distinct measurement conditions. (Some conditions are measured for both subjects and subject S.E. replicated measurements for a few conditions). Since each measurement is a three-dimensional vector, there are $3 \times 45 = 135$ degrees of freedom in the data set. The bilinear model has only $3 \times (3 \times 2) = 18$ free parameters and describes the data well.

Discussion

Summary

This chapter has addressed the problem of understanding the visual system's adjustment to changes in illumination. We began by introducing the problem of understanding the effect of the visual system's adjustment. We then reviewed the fundamentals of color vision discussion of color appearance and presented our experimental method.

There were three important features of the experimental method. First, the images used to define the illuminant

---

8. When evaluating three-dimensional data, it is important to bear in mind that for any given condition, the effects may occur on only one of the three dimensions. This does not mean that the effects are any smaller. For the illuminant change Δ**e** used for subject D.B., the measured effect of illuminant change Δ**r** occurs almost entirely along the S cone coordinate dimension. For this reason, the left and center bottom panels of figure 13.8 do not show much of an effect of illuminant change.

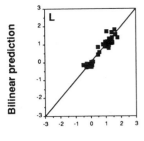
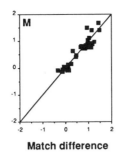
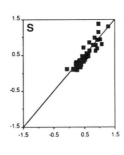

Fig. 13.9
Bilinearity. The figure plots the predicted difference between the changed and standard illuminant matches against the measured difference. (All conditions; subjects D.B., S.E.) (Adapted from Brainard & Wandell, 1990b.)

contained enough information for the visual system to estimate the illuminant. Second, for any illuminant condition we randomized our design with respect to local spatial contrast effects by using many different images that shared a common simulated illuminant. Third, our use of a memory matching paradigm allowed us to control the visual system's adjustment. The subject always viewed images that were simulations of uniformly illuminated surfaces and we assessed color appearance only after the subject had adjusted to the simulated illuminant.

We developed and tested a bilinear model for understanding the visual system's adjustment to the illuminant. The parameters of the bilinear model are determined by a small number of measurements. Once determined, the model allows us to predict the effect of the adjustment to any illuminant.

Color Constancy

The data presented in this chapter may be analyzed to address the question How color constant is performance for our laboratory model? Given a prototype color signal with cone coordinates r, we can find a surface described by S such that equation 2 holds: $r = (RS)e$. We can then ask what *equivalent illuminant change* $\Delta\hat{e}$ would we have had to have made such that measured change Δr corresponded to the behavior of a color constant visual system. That is, we can find $\Delta\hat{e}$ such that the measured Δr satisfies

$$\Delta r = (RS)\Delta\hat{e}. \qquad (7)$$

The equivalent illuminant change $\Delta\hat{e}$ is interpreted as the portion of the illuminant change to which the visual system actually adjusted.[9]

Figure 13.10 plots two illuminant changes and the corresponding equivalent illuminant changes computed from the data. If the visual system were color constant, the actual and equivalent illuminant changes would be identical. In both cases, we see that the visual system is compensating for approximately the correct relative spectral power distributon of the illuminant change, but that the magnitude of the adjustment is only about half of color constant performance. Figure 13.11 shows this quantitatively. For each of our 45 measurement conditions, we computed the equivalent illuminant change. We then found the scale factor which, when multiplied by the actual illuminant change Δe, produced the best fit to the equivalent illuminant change $\Delta\hat{e}$. Figure 13.11 plots a histogram of these 45 scale factors, which are distributed around a mean value of 0.48.

Laboratory Model

The concept of the equivalent illuminant change is useful for understanding how the results of the present experiments might be applied to natural images. From our bilinear model of performance, we can compute the equivalent illuminant change from a description of how much the illuminant in a natural scene differs from our standard illuminant. This equivalent illuminant change is a description of how much adjustment the visual system will undergo when it views this natural image, and it can be used to predict the color appearance of surfaces in the image.

---

9. As noted in note 7, because of metamerism, there is no unique prediction for a color constant system. To compute $\Delta\hat{e}$, we required that both s and $\Delta\hat{e}$ lie within three-dimensional linear models of natural surfaces and illuminants. The actual illuminant changes were described by the linear model for illuminants used in the computations.

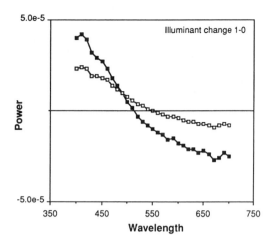

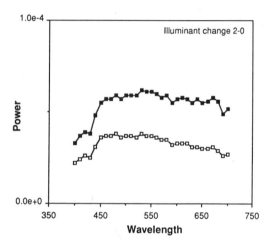

Fig. 13.10
Equivalent illuminant analysis. The closed symbols show two experimental illuminant changes. The open symbols show the corresponding equivalent illuminant changes. Because of metamerism, the computation of equivalent illuminant change from the data is not unique. We constrained our computations by requiring that both **s** and $\Delta\hat{\mathbf{e}}$ lie within three-dimensional linear models of natural surfaces and illuminants. (Prototype color signal R6_4; subject D.B.)

As we discussed in the description of our method, however, the laboratory model used in the experiments does not incorporate many aspects of natural viewing. This means that there is reason for caution in interpreting our results in terms of human performance in the real world. Because the images were presented using a CRT, they were necessarily small and of low luminance. Both of these factors may have had an effect on the magnitude of the measured adjustment, as may have the fact that the images were simulations. And it is possible that the visual system normally relies on image cues not incorporated

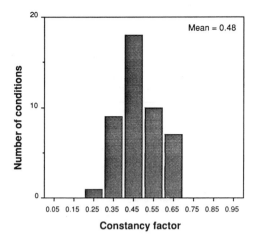

Fig. 13.11
Degree of color constancy. Histogram of the scale factor relating the actual illuminant change to the equivalent illuminant change for all 45 measurement conditions.

in our laboratory model to estimate the illuminant (see D'Zmura & Lennie, 1986; Funt & Drew, 1988; Funt & Ho, 1988; Klinker, Shafer & Kanade, 1988; Lee, 1986). One of the attractive features of the method developed here is that it can be extended to more complex laboratory models. It is possible to vary aspects of the laboratory model to see which ones have an influence on the visual system's adjustment and which ones do not.

Although there is some chance that magnitude of the visual system's adjustment to illuminant changes may depend on the laboratory model, we think it is useful to entertain the hypothesis that the bilinear nature of this adjustment, shown by the present experiments, is a consequence of the mechanisms applied by the visual system to adjust for the illuminant. While incorporating additional factors into the laboratory model may affect the parametric operation of these mechanisms, the basic structure of the adjustment may well remain bilinear.

Acknowledgments

The research reported in this chapter was supported by grant no. 2 RO1 EY03164 from the National Eye Institute, grant no. NCC 2-307 from the NASA-Ames Research Center, a National Science Foundation Graduate Fellowship, and grant no. 204E from the Cowper Institute. We thank M. Landy and A. Movshon for organizing the Cold Spring Harbor Laboratory Workshop on Computational Models of Visual Processing, where we presented this work. We also thank A. Ahumada, M. D'Zmura, L. Maloney, J. Nachmias, J. Palmer, M. Pavel, A. Poirson, D. Rumelhart, R. Shepard, and D. Varner for useful discussions. S. Ewedemi observed diligently in the experiments. Portions of the text and figures 1, 2, 6, 8, and 9 are adapted from Brainard and Wandell (1990b).

References

Ahn, S. J. & MacLeod, D. I. A. (1990). Adaptation in the chromatic and luminance channels. *Investigative Ophthalmology and Visual Science, Supplement, 31,* 109.

Albers, J. (1975). *Interaction of color.* New Haven: Yale University Press.

Arend, L. & Reeves, A. (1986). Simultaneous color constancy. *Journal of the Optical Society of America, 3,* 1743–1751.

Benzschawel, T., Walraven, J. & Rogowitz, B. (1987). Studies of color constancy. *Investigative Ophthalmology and Visual Science, Supplement, 28,* 92.

Blackwell, K. T. & Buchsbaum, G. (1988). Quantitative studies of color constancy. *Journal of the Optical Society of America A, 5,* 1772–1780.

Boring, E. G. (1942). *Sensation and perception in the history of experimental psychology.* New York: D. Appleton Century.

Boynton, R. M. (1979). *Human color vision.* New York: Holt, Rinehart & Winston.

Brainard, D. H. (1989a). Calibration of a computer controlled color monitor. *Color Research and Application, 14,* 23–34.

Brainard, D. H. (1989b). *Understanding the illuminant's effect on color appearance.* Unpublished Doctoral Dissertation, Stanford University.

Brainard, D. H. & Wandell, B. A. (1986). An analysis of the retinex theory of color vision. *Journal of the Optical Society of America A, 3,* 1651–1661.

Brainard, D. H. & Wandell, B. A. (1990a). Calibrated processing of image color. *Color Research and Application, 15,* 266–271.

Brainard, D. H. & Wandell, B. A. (1990b), The effect of the illuminant on color appearance. *Proceedings of the SPIE, 1250,* 119–130.

Brainard, D. H., Wandell, B. A. & Poirson, A. B. (1989). Discrete analysis of spatial and spectral aliasing. *Investigative Ophthalmology and Visual Science, Supplement, 30,* 53.

Brewer, W. L. (1954). Fundamental response functions and binocular color matching. *Journal of the Optical Society of America, 44,* 207–212.

Brindley, G. S. (1970). *Physiology of the retina and visual pathway.* Baltimore: Williams & Wilkins.

Buchsbaum, G. (1980). A spatial processer model for object color perception. *Journal of the Franklin Institute, 310,* 1–26.

Burnham, R. W., Evans, R. M. & Newhall, S. M. (1957). Prediction of color appearance with different adaptation illuminations. *Journal of the Optical Society of America, 47,* 35–42.

Cornsweet, T. N. (1970). *Visual perception,* New York: Academic Press.

D'Zmura, M. & Lennie, P. (1986). Mechanisms of color constancy. *Journal of the Optical Society of America A, 3,* 1662–1672.

Evans, R. M. (1943). Visual processes and color photography. *Journal of the Optical Society of America, 33,* 579–614.

Evans, R. M. (1948). *An introduction to color.* New York: Wiley.

Fairchild, M. D. (1990). *Chromatic adaptation and color appearance.* Unpublished doctoral dissertation, University of Rochester.

Funt, B. V. & Drew, M. S. (1988). Color constancy computation in near-Mondrian scenes using a finite dimensional linear model. *IEEE Computer Vision and Pattern Recognition,* pp. 544–549.

Funt, B. V. & Ho, J. (1988). Color from black and white. *Proceedings of the 2nd ICCV,* pp. 2–8.

Gorzynski, M. E. & Berns, R. S. (1990). The effect of ambient illumination color and image color balance on the perception of neutral in hybrid image display systems. *Proceedings of the SPIE/SPSE Symposium on Electronic Imaging Science and Technology.*

Helmholtz, H. (1896). In J. P. C. Southall (Ed.), *Physiological optics.* New York: Dover.

Helson, H. & Jeffers, V. B. (1940). Fundamental problems in color vision. II. Hue, lightness, and saturation of selective samples in chromatic illumination. *Journal of Experimental Psychology, 26,* 1–27.

Helson, H., Judd, D. & Warren, M. (1952). Object-color changes from daylight to incandescent filament illumination. *Illumination Engineering, 47,* 221–233.

Hungerford, T. W. (1974). *Algebra.* New York: Springer-Verlag.

Hunt, R. W. G. (1950). The effects of daylight and tungsten light-adaptation on color perception. *Journal of the Optical Society of America, 40,* 336–371.

Hunt, R. W. G. (1953). The perception of color in 1 degree fields for different states of adaptation. *Journal of the Optical Society of America, 43,* 479–484.

Hurlbert, A. C., Lee, H. & Bülthoff, H. H. (1989). Cues to the color of the illuminant. *Investigative Ophthalmology and Visual Science, Supplement, 30,* 221.

Ishihara, S. (1977). *Tests for colour-blindness.* Tokyo, Japan: Kanehara Shuppen Company, Ltd..

Jameson, D. & Hurvich, L. M. (1964). Theory of brightness and color contrast in human vision. *Vision Research, 4,* 135–154.

Jameson, D., Hurvich, L. M. & Varner, F. D. (1979). Receptoral and postreceptoral visual processes in recovery from chromatic adaptation. *Proceedings of the National Academy of Science USA, 76,* 3034–3038.

Judd, D. B. (1940). Hue, saturation and lightness of surface colors with chromatic illumination. *Journal of the Optical Society of America, 30*, 2–32.

Judd, D. B. (1960). Appraisal of Land's work on two-primary color projections. *Journal of the Optical Society of America, 50, 3*, 254–268.

Judd, D. B., MacAdam, D. L. & Wyszecki, G. W. (1964). Spectral distribution of typical daylight as a function of correlated color temperature. *Journal of the Optical Society of America, 54*, 1031.

Klinker, G. J., Shafer, S. A. & Kanade, T. (1988). The measurement of highlights in color images. *International Journal of Computer Vision, 2*, 7–32.

Land, E. H. (1964). The retinex. In A. V. S. de Reuck & J. Knight (Eds.), *CIBA Foundation Symposium on Color Vision* (pp. 217–227). Boston: Little, Brown.

Land, E. H. (1983). Recent advances in retinex theory and some implications for cortical computations: Color vision and the natural image. *Proceedings of the National Academy of Science USA, 80*, 5163–5169.

Land, E. H. & Daw, N. W. (1962), Colors seen in a flash of light. *Proceedings of the National Academy of Science USA, 48*, 1000–1008.

Land, E. H. & McCann, J. J. (1971). Lightness and retinex theory. *Journal of the Optical Society of America, 61*, 1–11.

Lee, H. (1986). Method for computing the scene-illuminant chromaticity from specular highlights. *Journal of the Optical Society of America A, 3*, 1694–1699.

Maloney, L. T. & Wandell, B. (1986). Color constancy: A method for recovering surface spectral reflectance. *Journal of the Optical Society of America A, 1*, 29–33.

McCann, J. J., McKee, S. P. & Taylor, T. H. (1976). Quantitative studies in retinex theory: A comparison between theoretical predictions and observer responses to the color Mondrian experiments. *Vision Research, 16*, 445–448.

McLaren, K. (1986). Edwin H. Land's contributions to colour science. *JDSC Proceedings, 102*, 378–383.

Nickerson, D. (1957). *Spectrophotometric data for a collection of Munsell samples.* Washington D.C.: U.S. Department of Agriculture.

Schnapf, J. L., Kraft, T. W. & Baylor, D. A. (1987). Spectral sensitivity of human cone photoreceptors. *Nature, 325*, 439–441.

Shafer, S. A. (1985). Using color to separate reflection components. *Color Research and Application, 10*, 210–218.

Shapley, R. M. (1986). The importance of contrast for the activity of single neurons, the VEP and perception. *Vision Research, 26*, 45–62.

Shepard, R. N. (1987). Toward a universal law of generalization for psychological science. *Science, 237*, 1317–1323.

Smith, V. & Pokorny, J. (1975). Spectral sensitivity of the foveal cone photopigments between 400 and 500 nm. *Vision Research, 15*, 161–171.

Tominaga, S. & Wandell, B. A. (1989). The standard surface reflectance model and illuminant estimation. *Journal of the Optical Society of America A, 6*, 576–584.

Valberg, A. & Lange-Malecki, B. (1987). Mondrian complexity does not improve "color constancy." *Investigative Ophthalmology and Visual Science, Supplement, 28*, 92.

Walraven, J., Benzschawel, T. & Rogowitz, B. (1988). Chromatic induction: a misdirected attempt at color constancy? *OSA Annual Meeting Technical Digest*, 103.

Wandell, B. A. (1987). The synthesis and analysis of color images. *IEEE PAMI, PAMI-9*, 2–13.

West, G. & Brill, M. H. (1982). Necessary and sufficient conditions for von Kries chromatic adaptation to give color constancy. *Journal of Theoretical Biology, 15*, 249.

Woolfson, M. M. (1959). Some new aspects of color perception. *IBM Journal Research Developments, 3*, 313.

Wyszecki, G. (1986). Color appearance. In K. Boff, L. Kaufman & J. P. Thomas (Eds.), *Handbook of Perception* (pp. 9-1–9-57). New York: Wiley.

Wyszecki, G. & Stiles, W. S. (1982). *Color science.* New York: Wiley.

14

Shading Ambiguity: Reflectance and Illumination

Michael D'Zmura

An object's shading is determined by its shape and position, by its surface reflectance properties, and by the pattern of illumination. Many studies of shading focus on the recovery of one of these factors by introducing constraints on the other two; one might, for instance, constrain reflectances to be Lambertian and lights to be point sources in a shape-from-shading scheme (Horn, 1975, 1986; Pentland, 1982, 1984, 1988). Yet such constraints are not met in the daily operation of the human visual system. For example, while a point source might suffice as a first-order model of illumination for outdoor viewing on sunny days, it is inadequate to describe spatially extended patterns of illumination under forest canopies, on overcast, wintry days, or within almost any indoor scene. Likewise, we encounter surfaces with many varieties of gloss in daily viewing, so that it is unreasonable to suppose that surfaces are Lambertian or that they have some fixed degree of specularity.

It could be the case that each pattern of shading comes from one specific combination of shape, reflectance, and lighting. In this event, we would find little fault with a visual system that places great stock in quantitative estimates of shape, surface gloss, and lighting from shading information. Yet patterns of shading are not uniquely determined by physical factors, rather infinitely many combinations of shape, reflectance, and lighting give rise to the same shading. This allows photographic reproduction: The reflectance of a print or the light reaching a screen from a slide are modulated to mimic the shading of objects viewed from the position of a camera.

The present concern is with a more constrained situation, namely with the shading of objects of uniform reflectance under more natural lighting conditions. To see intuitively that shading can be ambiguous under these circumstances, consider the shading of a shiny yellow sphere. When lit by a distant point source, the sphere provides a shading pattern with a spatially concentrated highlight. We can blur the highlight by diffusing the point source. We can also blur the highlight by reducing the gloss of the surface or by reducing the surface curvature in the area of the highlight. The pattern of shading associated with the blurred highlight is physically ambiguous: It can be caused by diffusing the point source, decreasing the degree of surface specularity, or reducing the surface curvature, or some combination of the three.

I present in this chapter a study of the trade-off between the spatial properties of a surface's reflectance and the spatial pattern of its illumination. Two intuitions about highlights suggest that this form of shading ambiguity is most easily characterized in the Fourier domain. The first is that a shiny surface transfers high-frequency components in a pattern of incident illumination better than a dull surface. For instance, details in an incident light pattern can be seen in the light reflected by a mirror but not in the light reflected by a matte surface. The second intuition is that surfaces act as lowpass filters of patterns of incident illumination (Cabral, Max & Springmeyer, 1987): With the exception of mirrors, surfaces blur point sources of incident illumination, and there is no "ringing" in the resulting highlights.

Reflectance functions are formally similar to "transfer" functions that one finds in much of the vision literature; they differ in that their operation on an incident light pattern to produce a reflected light pattern is described using spherical coordinates rather than a time coordinate or Cartesian coordinates on the plane. Fourier analysis on the sphere involves the spherical harmonics; these functions play a role similar to that of sinusoids in frequency-domain analysis on the line or on the plane. By expressing reflectance functions and light patterns in terms of the spherical harmonics, we can describe reflection in a way that captures the frequency-domain intuitions. The analysis reveals the structures of different kinds of reflectances, shows how to handle gracefully the reflection of spatially extended light sources, and leads readily to several results on shading ambiguity. These include solutions to problems of (1) determining the set of illumination patterns that, for a given surface, give rise to identical reflected light patterns; (2) characterizing illumination patterns in terms of their ability to reveal the spatial properties of reflectance functions; (3) finding pairs of reflectances and illuminants that give rise to identical reflected light patterns, and (4) choosing the lighting of an arbitrary collection of surfaces, seen from a given viewpoint, so that the resulting visual image matches some given image as well as possible.

After briefly reviewing the space-domain properties of lights and surface reflectances, I introduce the basic tools in linear systems analysis on the sphere, namely rotations and the spherical harmonics, in a way that I hope is useful to the reader. I then examine the reflection of light from surfaces in the Fourier domain and point out results on shading ambiguity that follow from this particular representation of the problem.

Reflectance and Illumination

Space Domain

The spatial properties of a surface's reflectance are represented by a bidirectional reflectance function (Horn & Sjoberg, 1979; Nicodemus et al., 1977). This function states what fraction of light at some wavelength, incident on a differential area from some given direction relative to the surface normal, is reflected towards some particular exitant direction. The reflectance depends not only on surface roughness (Bennett & Mattsson, 1989), which is affected by processes such as polishing, but also on surface material so that, for instance, the reflectances of dielectrics such as plastic have a form distinct from those for metals. Reflectance models have been introduced for use in computer graphics that appear to capture well the spatial properties of many materials' reflectance functions (Blinn, 1977/1988; Cook & Torrance, 1982/1987; Phong, 1975). The following brief review of reflectance in the space domain identifies those properties of reflectances that make them amenable to analysis in the frequency domain.

Spherical Coordinate System

To quantify reflectance, let us erect a spherical coordinate system about the normal to some differential area of the surface. As shown in figure 14.1a, we identify the directions of incident and exitant lights with points on the hemisphere whose equator matches the plane tangent to the surface and whose north pole matches the direction of the normal. A direction is specified by its elevation θ, $0 \leq \theta \leq \pi$, and its azimuth ϕ, $0 \leq \phi < 2\pi$. Such directions stand in one-to-one correspondence with unit vectors defined in a Cartesian coordinate system in which the z-axis is aligned with the normal and the x- and y-axes lie in the plane tangent to the surface; a direction specified by a unit vector with Cartesian coordinates $(u_x u_y u_z)$ has spherical coordinates $(\theta\,\phi) = (\arccos(u_z)\ \arctan(u_y/u_x))$.

We form a flat representation of the surface of a sphere familiar as the Mercator projection by directly mapping the parameters θ and ϕ onto the plane. As shown in figure 14.1b, the north pole or surface normal direction ($\theta = 0$) is represented along the top of the map; the equator or surface horizon ($\theta = \pi/2$, variable ϕ) is represented by the line across the middle, while the underside of the opaque surface is represented by all directions that lie below the surface horizon ($\pi/2 < \theta \leqslant \pi$).

Incident Lights: Intensity and Irradiance

Taking incident lights to be unpolarized and incoherent, we can describe a pattern of incident light intensity using a real-valued function $I(\theta, \phi)$ of the spherical coordinates set up about the surface normal (the dependence of the intensity on wavelength is suppressed). A bidirectional reflectance function operates on incident irradiance, a function of the incident intensity, to produce the reflected light (Horn & Sjoberg, 1979; Nicodemus et al., 1977). To calculate an irradiance from an intensity, note that a light source of fixed intensity provides energy to the differential area of surface in a way that falls off as $\cos(\theta)$, as shown in figure 14.2. For an opaque surface, furthermore, incident intensities at directions below the surface horizon must be set to zero, so that incident irradiance $I'(\theta, \phi)$ is given in terms of incident intensity as follows:

$$I'(\theta, \phi) = \max(\cos(\theta), 0)I(\theta, \phi). \tag{1}$$

Reflectance Properties

A reflectance operates on an incident pattern of irradiance $I'(\theta, \phi)$ to produce an exitant pattern of radiance, namely a real-valued function $E(\theta, \phi)$ that describes the amount of light returned towards a viewer at all possible directions.

The results of reflecting an incident light with three types of reflectance are shown in figure 14.3 using the Mercator projection. The top left panel shows the pattern of incident irradiance: a blurred point source that is rotationally symmetric about the direction $(\theta\,\phi) = (\pi/4\ \pi/4)$. The bottom left panel shows the radiance exiting from a perfect mirror that simply rotates the incident irradiance about the normal by π radians: $E(\theta, \phi) = I'(\theta, \phi + \pi)$. The

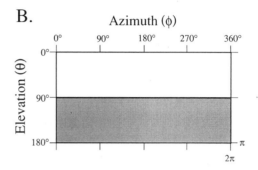

A.

B.

Azimuth (ϕ)

Elevation (θ)

Fig. 14.1
(A) Spherical coordinate system for describing lights and reflectances. (B) Mercator projection for depicting functions of direction about the origin.

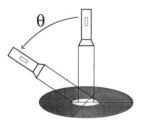

θ

Fig. 14.2
Cosine dependence of irradiance on intensity. The light energy reaching an area from a source of fixed intensity (shown as a flashlight) falls off as the cosine of the angle θ between the surface normal and the source; intensities behind an opaque surface provide zero irradiance.

perfect mirror is evidently an "all pass" filter, because all details of the incident irradiance are represented faithfully in the exitant light. The middle panel shows the light reflected by a perfectly matte surface, which suppresses all spatial detail in the incident irradiance: $E(\theta, \phi) = c$, a constant. The right panel, finally, shows the radiance pattern provided by a "mixed" reflectance with both specular and diffuse properties.

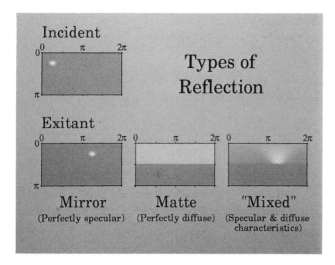

Fig. 14.3
Types of reflectance. Mercator projections of a pattern of irradiance (*top left*) and the exitant radiances from a perfect mirror (*bottom left*), a perfectly matte surface (*bottom middle*) and a surface with both specular and diffuse characteristics modeled by a Cook and Torrance (1982/1987) reflectance function.

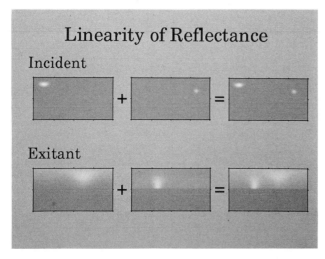

Fig. 14.4
Linearity of reflectance. On the left are shown in Mercator projection an incident pattern of irradiance and the resulting exitant radiance found with a Cook and Torrance (1982/1987) reflectance. In the middle are shown another pattern of irradiance and the resulting exitant radiance from the same surface. The radiance exiting the surface when lit by the sum of the two incident irradiances (*bottom right*) can be found either by adding the two component exitant radiances (*bottom left* and *middle*) or by reflecting directly the sum of the incident irradiances (*top right*).

Linearity

All real surface reflectances are like the "mixed" reflectance of figure 14.3 in that they lie between the extreme mirror and matte cases. We can more easily understand how they filter incident light patterns by relying on their linearity. Illustrated in figure 14.4, this property has the formal statement:

$$E_1 = R(I'_1) \text{ implies } sE_1 = R(sI'_1), \text{ and} \tag{2a}$$

$$E_1 = R(I'_1) \text{ and } E_2 = R(I'_2) \text{ imply that} \\ E_1 + E_2 = R(I'_1 + I'_2), \tag{2b}$$

for all incident irradiances I', exitant radiances E, scalars s, and reflectance functions R. As a consequence of linearity, we can express the operator R as a function of the coordinates $(\theta_i \phi_i)$ and $(\theta_e \phi_e)$ of the incident and exitant directions, respectively:

$$E(\theta_e, \phi_e) = R(\theta_e, \phi_e, \theta_i, \phi_i)I'(\theta_i, \phi_i). \tag{3}$$

Symmetry

A second property of surface reflectances is that they satisfy the Helmholtz reciprocity law, which relies on the reversibility of light paths to impose a spatial symmetry on incident and exitant directions. This symmetry is illustrated in figure 14.5; formally, we have for any pair of incident $(\theta_i \phi_i)$ and exitant $(\theta_e \phi_e)$ directions

$$R(\theta_i, \phi_i, \theta_e, \phi_e) = R(\theta_e, \phi_e, \theta_i, \phi_i). \tag{4}$$

That reflectances are symmetric may seem an innocuous property at the moment, yet real symmetric linear operators have real eigenvalues, and this helps considerably in the analysis below.

Shift variation

A third property of many reflectances is that the pattern of reflected light depends on the position of the incident light. The most common manifestation of this shift variation is shown in figure 14.6; if we take an incident light and rotate it in a way that alters its elevation, then the reflected light will change not only in its positioning but also in its pattern. However, many such reflectances are *azimuthally* isotropic (figure 14.7): If the shift (rotation) changes the azimuth but not the elevation of the incident light source, then the exitant light changes its position in azimuth but not in its pattern.

Symmetry of Reflectance

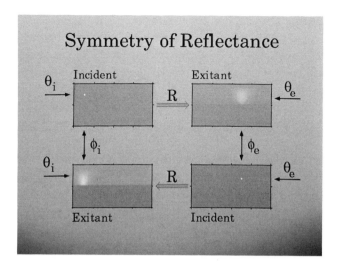

Fig. 14.5

Symmetry of reflectance. At top left is shown a point source irradiance in direction $(\theta_i \phi_i)$ which, when reflected, produces the exitant radiance at top right. At bottom right is shown a point source irradiance in direction $(\theta_e \phi_e)$ that produces an exitant radiance at bottom left. The number $R(\theta_e, \phi_e, \theta_i, \phi_i)$ that describes how much light exits in direction $(\theta_e \phi_e)$ when the surface is lit by the point source at $(\theta_i \phi_i)$ (*top panels*) is identical to the number $R(\theta_i, \phi_i, \theta_e, \phi_e)$ that describes how much light exits in direction $(\theta_i \phi_i)$ when the surface is lit by the point source at $(\theta_e \phi_e)$ (*bottom panels*).

Shift Variation in Elevation

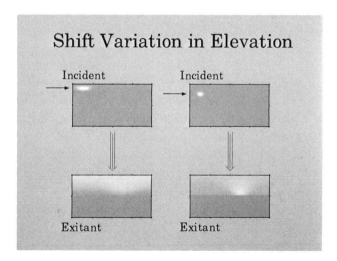

Fig. 14.6

Shift variation in elevation. Two patterns of incident light (*top*) that differ only in their elevation may, when reflected, produce patterns of exitant radiance (*bottom*) that differ in both position *and* pattern.

Shift Invariance in Azimuth

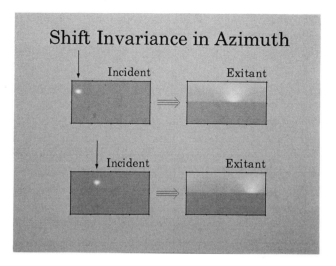

Fig. 14.7

Azimuthally isotropic reflectances. Two patterns of incident light that differ only in their azimuthal position (*top*) often produce patterns of exitant radiance that differ only in their azimuthal direction (*bottom*).

The reflectance model used in computer graphics to mimic reflectances of this sort is Cook and Torrance's (1982/1987). This model's shift variation in elevation, based on the physical model of Torrance and Sparrow (1967), (1) allows the reflectance to provide peak specularity towards a direction with an elevation (measured away from the surface normal) that is greater than that of the perfect specular direction (Cook & Torrance, 1982/1987), and (2) allows the surface to possess "sheen" (Hunter, 1975). These effects are most noticeable for lights with near-grazing angles of incidence.

Reflectances modelled by Cook and Torrance fall into a class midway between the simplest type of reflectance, a fully shift-invariant system, and the most general sort of reflectance, which is isotropic in neither elevation nor azimuth. The simplest type of reflectance often appears in computer graphics under the guise of the Phong model (Blinn, 1977/1988; Phong, 1975). The most general reflectances are "directional" (Hunter, 1975) and are typical of scored surfaces; these have not yet found widespread use in graphics. This three-way classification of reflectances according to shift variation finds a ready expression in the Fourier domain.

Fourier Domain

Because reflectance functions are linear, it is natural to examine them in the Fourier domain which, on the sphere, involves expressing spatially extended lights and reflectance functions in terms of surface spherical harmonics. The surface spherical harmonics are special functions that arise naturally in physical problems with spherical symmetry. Their study in the nineteenth century was based largely on detailed analysis initiated by Legendre and Laplace in work on gravitation; Hobson (1965), MacRobert (1967), and Walker (1988) follow this approach in their texts. It was recognized in the first half of the twentieth century that almost all special functions arise naturally in the study of continuous groups of transformations (Lie groups). The link between spherical harmonics and rotation groups is developed in many books; several such texts, accessible to nonmathematicians, are those of Gel'Fand, Minlos, and Shapiro (1963), Talman (1968), and Terras (1985). This modern approach stresses matrix representations of operators; Hoffman and Kunze (1961) provide one of many good introductions to linear algebra. More closely related to the present topic is work in computer graphics by Cabral and colleagues (1987), who transformed lights and reflectances into the Fourier domain to derive reflectance functions from surface bump maps. Press and coworkers (1988) and Swarztrauber (1979) present relevant numerical methods.

Spherical Harmonics

The surface spherical harmonics play a role similar to that played by sinusoids in Fourier series expansions of periodic functions. In particular, the surface spherical harmonics provide a complete orthonormal basis with which to express a function defined on the surface of the sphere. While surface spherical harmonics are complex-valued functions of direction about some origin, the present concern is with real-valued functions, so I follow Cabral and colleagues (1987) by using related functions called the real surface spherical harmonics (hereafter spherical harmonics or simply harmonics).

The spherical harmonics $Y_{\ell m}(\theta, \phi)$ vary according to their "frequency" ℓ, a nonnegative integer, and their "moment" m, an integer that ranges for some given frequency ℓ between $-\ell$ and ℓ. The harmonics are defined in terms of the associated Legendre functions $P_{\ell m}(x)$ as follows:

$$Y_{\ell m}(\theta, \phi) = \begin{cases} M_{\ell m} P_{\ell m}(\cos \theta) \cos m\phi, & \text{for } m \geq 0 \\ M_{\ell |m|} P_{\ell |m|}(\cos \theta) \sin |m|\phi, & \text{for } m < 0, \end{cases} \quad (5a)$$

where the normalization constants $M_{\ell m}$ are given by

$$M_{\ell m} = \begin{cases} \sqrt{\dfrac{(2\ell + 1)}{2\pi} \dfrac{(\ell - |m|)!}{(\ell + |m|)!}}, & \text{for } m \neq 0 \\ \sqrt{\dfrac{(2\ell + 1)}{4\pi}}, & \text{for } m = 0. \end{cases} \quad (5b)$$

The spherical harmonics are separable functions of elevation and azimuth: an associated Legendre function that takes $\cos \theta$ as its argument describes variation in elevation, while a sinusoid of frequency m describes variation in azimuth. In table 14.1 are listed the formulae for the first several associated Legendre functions and the corresponding spherical harmonics.

The spherical harmonics with moments m equal to zero are called zonal harmonics; they do not vary in azimuth. Figure 14.8 shows six zonal harmonics at frequencies ℓ of 0, 1, 2, 4, 8, and 16. Values brighter than the figure's background represent positive numbers, darker values

Table 14.1
Formulae for the associated Legendre functions $P_{\ell m}(x)$ and the real surface spherical harmonics $Y_{\ell m}(\theta, \phi)$ at positive moments

Frequency, moment	$P_{\ell m}(x)$	$Y_{\ell m}(\theta, \phi)$
$\ell = 0, m = 0(z)^*$	1	$(1/4\pi)^{1/2}$
$\ell = 1, m = 0(z)$	x	$(3/4\pi)^{1/2} \cos \theta$
$\ell = 1, m = 1(s)$	$-(1 - x^2)^{1/2}$	$-(3/4\pi)^{1/2} \sin \theta \cos \phi$
$\ell = 2, m = 0(z)$	$1/2(3x^2 - 1)$	$(5/16\pi)^{1/2}(3 \cos^2 \theta - 1)$
$\ell = 2, m = 1(t)$	$-3(1 - x^2)^{1/2}x$	$-(15/4\pi)^{1/2} \cos \theta \sin \theta \cos \phi$
$\ell = 2, m = 2(s)$	$3(1 - x^2)$	$(15/16\pi)^{1/2} \sin^2 \theta \cos 2\phi$
$\ell = 3, m = 0(z)$	$1/2(5x^3 - 3x)$	$(7/16\pi)^{1/2}(5 \cos^3 \theta - 3 \cos \theta)$
$\ell = 3, m = 1(t)$	$-(3/2)(1 - x^2)^{1/2}(5x^2 - 1)$	$-(21/32\pi)^{1/2}(5 \cos^2 \theta - 1) \sin \theta \cos \phi$
$\ell = 3, m = 2(t)$	$15(1 - x^2)x$	$(105/16\pi)^{1/2} \sin^2 \theta \cos \theta \cos 2\phi$
$\ell = 3, m = 3(s)$	$-15(1 - x^2)^{3/2}$	$-(35/32\pi)^{1/2} \sin^3 \theta \cos 3\phi$

*The spherical harmonics $Y_{\ell m}(\theta, \phi)$ are zonal (z), sectoral (s) or tesseral (t).

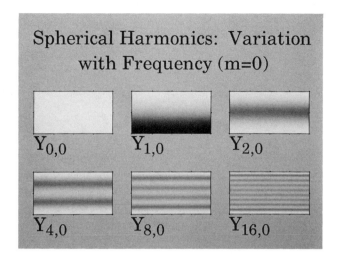

Fig. 14.8
Zonal harmonics at frequencies 0 (*top left*), 1 (*top middle*), 2 (*top right*), 4 (*bottom left*), 8 (*bottom middle*), and 16 (*bottom right*). Points brighter than the background indicate directions where the harmonic takes a positive value; points darker than the background indicate directions where a function has a negative value.

negative. The figure shows that the harmonic with frequency zero is simply a constant function of direction and that the number of cycles across the surface of the sphere increases with frequency. More precisely, the number of zeroes in a zonal harmonic that one encounters in traversing a great circle from the north to the south pole is identical to its frequency.

The number of harmonics with distinct moments increases with increasing frequency: $-\ell \leqslant m \leqslant \ell$. While there is only one harmonic at $\ell = 0$, there are three distinct harmonics at $\ell = 1$ at moments -1, 0, and 1, as shown in figure 14.9. When $|m| = \ell$, the harmonic (a) varies in azimuth as a sinusoidal function with frequency equal to the moment m, and (b) varies in elevation as the (spherical) frequency-dependent function $(\sin\theta)^{\ell}$. These harmonics divide the sphere into longitudinal sectors and are called sectoral harmonics.

Why three distinct functions are required to represent fully the frequency ℓ of one is best understood by considering what is meant by frequency. Frequency labels a subspace invariant under a group of transformations. On the line, translating a sinusoid alters its phase but not its frequency, so that frequency is preserved under actions by the group of translations. A sine and a cosine at a particular frequency provide a basis for the invariant subspace. On the sphere, frequency labels a subspace in-

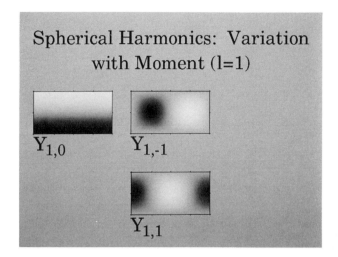

Fig. 14.9
The three harmonics $Y_{1,0}$ (*top left*), $Y_{1,-1}$ (*top middle*), and $Y_{1,1}$ (*bottom middle*).

variant under transformations by the group of rotations. The single, constant function $Y_{0,0}(\theta, \phi)$ occupies the subspace at frequency zero; an arbitrary rotation of this function about the origin returns the same function, so that the subspace at frequency zero is invariant under rotations. That this is the case for the subspace spanned by the three harmonics at a frequency of one (see figure 14.9) is seen intuitively by noting that these harmonics are "dipoles" oriented along the x-axis ($Y_{1,1}$), the y-axis ($Y_{1,-1}$), and the z-axis ($Y_{1,0}$). It turns out that such a dipole, oriented along an *arbitrary* axis, is a linear combination of the three basic dipoles. Rotating a dipole given by some particular linear combination of the three basis functions produces another dipole, given again by some combination of these basis functions, so that the subspace spanned by the three functions is invariant under rotation.

That frequency is preserved under rotation is perhaps more difficult to intuit (but nevertheless true) for the five harmonics that represent the frequency ℓ of two, shown in figure 14.10. This set includes two tesseral harmonics ($Y_{2,-1}$ and $Y_{2,1}$); these are neither zonal ($m = 0$) nor sectoral ($|m| = \ell$) and, again, vary separably in both elevation and azimuth.

Spherical Harmonic Transform

The (real surface) spherical harmonics form a complete orthonormal set of real-valued functions on the surface of the sphere, so that any incident or exitant light may be

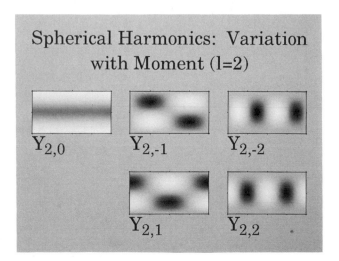

Spherical Harmonics: Variation with Moment (l=2)

$Y_{2,0}$ $Y_{2,-1}$ $Y_{2,-2}$

$Y_{2,1}$ $Y_{2,2}$

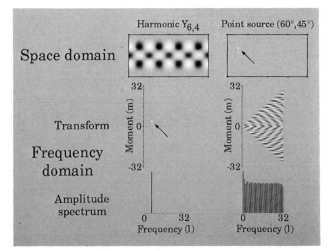

Space domain

Harmonic $Y_{6,4}$ Point source (60°, 45°)

Transform

Frequency domain

Amplitude spectrum

Moment (m)   32   0   -32
Moment (m)   32   0   -32

0   32   Frequency (l)
0   32   Frequency (l)

Fig. 14.10
The five harmonics $Y_{2,0}$ (*left*), $Y_{2,-1}$ and $Y_{2,1}$ (*middle top* and *bottom*, respectively), and $Y_{2,-2}$ and $Y_{2,2}$ (*right top* and *bottom*, respectively).

expressed in the Fourier domain as an appropriate linear combination of harmonics. In the case of an incident irradiance we have the series expansion

$$I'(\theta_i, \phi_i) = \sum_{\ell=0}^{\infty} \sum_{m=-\ell}^{\ell} a'_{\ell m} Y_{\ell m}(\theta_i, \phi_i), \tag{6a}$$

where

$$a'_{\ell m} = \int_0^{2\pi} \int_0^{\pi} I'(\theta_i, \phi_i) Y_{\ell m}(\theta_i, \phi_i) \sin\theta_i \, d\theta_i \, d\phi_i. \tag{6b}$$

In words, one determines the coefficients $a'_{\ell m}$ of the transform of the incident irradiance by integrating the product of the function I' and each individual spherical harmonic $Y_{\ell m}$ over the surface of the sphere.[1] In numerical applications, this spherical harmonic transform is carried out for frequencies ℓ up to some finite cutoff frequency L_{max}. Swarztrauber (1979) discusses methods and sampling grids with which one can more rapidly transform functions than suggested by equation 6; in particular, one can rely on the separability of the harmonics in elevation and azimuth to use an FFT algorithm to transform variations in azimuth.

I show two transforms in figure 14.11. The spherical harmonic $Y_{6,4}$ is depicted at the top middle in the space

Fig. 14.11
Spherical harmonic transform. *Left*, Transform of a harmonic. At top is depicted the harmonic $Y_{6,4}$ in the space domain. Immediately below is its transform, shown as a function of frequency (increasing from 0 at left to 32 at right) and moment (increasing from -32 at bottom to 32 at top). Positive-valued coefficients are shown using pixels brighter than the background, while negative-valued coefficients are shown using pixels darker than the background. The harmonic has energy only at $(\ell \, m) = (6 \, 4)$. At the bottom is shown the amplitude as a function of frequency (increasing from 0 at left to 32 at right). *Right*, Transform of a point source. Shown are the point source in the space domain (*top*), its full transform (*middle*), and its amplitude spectrum (*bottom*).

domain. Below are its full transform and its amplitude spectrum, both of which are discrete; frequency is represented along the abscissa in these latter plots. The ordinate for the plot of the full transform is the moment and, as expected, there is only one nonzero term (represented by the white dot at $\ell = 6, m = 4$) in the linear combination of harmonics that sums to the harmonic at the top. The amplitude spectrum (calculated in a way that I describe just below) shows that there is energy only at a frequency ℓ of six. At the top right is a point source in the space domain. The figure shows that nonzero terms at all frequencies and at many moments are needed to represent the point source in the frequency domain.

To define the "amplitude" of a function $f(\theta, \phi)$ at a particular frequency ℓ', we must take into account the number of moments at that frequency. Let $f_{\ell' m}$ be the

---

1. Note that a differential area on the surface of the sphere is $\sin\theta \, d\theta \, d\phi$, not simply $d\theta \, d\phi$. This dooms the attempt to generate a basis for analysis on the sphere by replacing the associated Legendre functions in equation 5 with sinusoidal functions of elevation: The resulting functions are not orthogonal to one another.

set of transform coefficients at frequency ℓ'. There are $2\ell' + 1$ of these coefficients, so that the amplitude $A_{\ell'}$ is defined as follows:

$$A_{\ell'} = \frac{1}{\sqrt{2\ell' + 1}} \sqrt{\sum_{m=-\ell'}^{\ell'} f_{\ell'm}^2}. \tag{7}$$

We can represent the "phase" of the function at frequency ℓ' by the vector of coefficients $f_{\ell'm}/\|f_{\ell'm}\|$, which is normalized to unit length.

Shift-Invariant Filters and Point-Spread Functions

On the line we most easily filter a function by passing it through a shift-invariant filter. The filter is represented either by a point-spread function (PSF) in the space domain (more generally an impulse response) with which an input function is convolved, or by a transfer function in the Fourier domain, namely the transform of the PSF, which acts multiplicatively on the transform of the input function (Bracewell, 1978). Shift-invariant filtering on the sphere is very similar. Figure 14.12 shows a noisy pattern in the left column; on the right is shown the result of filtering the noise with a shift-invariant filter whose multiplicative attenuation at each frequency is described by a (discrete) Gaussian function. The spectral properties of the filter are shown as an amplitude at the bottom of the middle column and as a (rotationally symmetric) PSF centered on the north pole at the top of the middle column. While the amplitude at each frequency is attenuated according to the Gaussian, the phase at each frequency is unchanged, so that the filtering blurs the input but preserves its position.

Shift-Invariant Reflectances

The simplest sort of reflectance, typified by Phong's (1975) model, closely resembles a shift-invariant filter: In response to a point-source irradiance, the reflectance produces an exitant radiance pattern (impulse response) that does not depend on incident direction. However, the reflectance does not blur the incident irradiance but blurs the result of using a perfect mirror to reflect the incident irradiance. To calculate the exitant radiance, we rotate the incident irradiance pattern about the surface normal by π radians and apply a shift-invariant filter to the result.

We can readily compute such an exitant radiance in the Fourier domain. A first step is to make the incident irra-

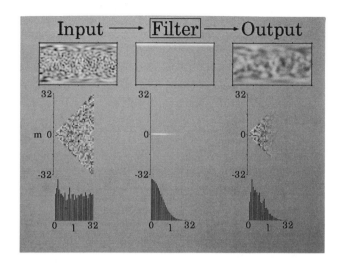

Fig. 14.12
Shift-invariant filtering. A noisy pattern (*left column*) is filtered by a shift-invariant filter (*middle column*) to produce a blurred noisy pattern (*right column*). The patterns at left and right are shown as space-varying functions (*top*), as spherical harmonic transforms (*middle*), and as amplitude spectra (*bottom*). The shift-invariant filter (*middle column*) is described by a (discrete) Gaussian function in the transform domain. To the spectrum representing the shift-invariant filter (*bottom middle*) corresponds a spherical harmonic transform (*middle middle*) with no energy at nonzero moments. The corresponding point-spread function in the space domain (*top middle*) is a linear combination of zonal harmonics and is symmetric about the z-axis (surface normal).

diance transform coefficients $a'_{\ell m}$ into a (column) vector $\mathbf{a}'$. A natural way to order the coefficients is to order by frequency ℓ: $(a'_{0,0}\ a'_{1,-1}\ a'_{1,0}\ a'_{1,1}\ a'_{2,-2}\ a'_{2,-1}\ a'_{2,0}\ a'_{2,1}\ a'_{2,2}\ \ldots)^{\mathrm{T}}$. The second step is to represent with matrices the linear operations to be performed on $\mathbf{a}'$. To construct the "perfect reflection" matrix, note that (see figures 14.8 to 14.10): (1) rotating a spherical harmonic with an even moment m by π radians about the z-axis returns unscathed the same harmonic, and (2) rotating a harmonic with an odd moment changes its sign. The matrix $\mathbf{P}$ that represents perfect reflection is thus a diagonal matrix (entries off the diagonal are equal to 0) with entries along the diagonal $+1$ or -1 according to whether the harmonic has even or odd moment, respectively. The matrix $\mathbf{P}$ is its own inverse (idempotent).

To construct the matrix $\mathbf{R}$ that represents the shift-invariant filtering by the reflectance, recall that such filters attenuate each spherical harmonic in a way that depends on its frequency ℓ alone. Such a reflectance is completely characterized by a set of numbers $\rho(\ell)$ that describe the attenuation of harmonic components at each frequency. The corresponding matrix is diagonal; its components along the diagonal are the frequency-dependent attenuations specific to the reflectance, each appearing $2\ell + 1$ times.

Reflecting the incident irradiance $I'(\theta_i, \phi_i)$ is thus represented by

$$\mathbf{b} = \mathbf{RPa}', \tag{8}$$

in which $\mathbf{b}$ is a column vector, ordered by frequency ℓ, whose entries are the coefficients of the transform of the exitant radiance $E(\theta_e, \phi_e)$:

$$E(\theta_e, \phi_e) = \sum_{\ell=0}^{\infty} \sum_{m=-\ell}^{\ell} b_{\ell m} Y_{\ell m}(\theta_e, \phi_e), \tag{9a}$$

where

$$b_{\ell m} = \int_0^{2\pi} \int_0^{\pi} E(\theta_e, \phi_e) Y_{\ell m}(\theta_e, \phi_e) \sin \theta_e \, d\theta_e d\phi_e. \tag{9b}$$

One sets a frequency limit when doing numerical calculations based on these equations; the vectors and matrices in equation 8 are then finite-dimensional. The minimal frequency limit (which allows the most efficient computation) is set by the particular cutoff frequency $\ell_{\max}(\mathbf{R})$ of a reflectance $\mathbf{R}$; beyond its cutoff frequency, the reflectance transfers numerically insignificant amounts of incident energy.

Azimuthally Isotropic Reflectances

Reflectance functions that are azimuthally isotropic are a more general class than that discussed above; reflectances modelled by Cook and Torrance (1982/1987) fall into this category. It is possible to represent their action on an irradiance in a form like that of equation 8.

To determine the form that an azimuthally isotropic reflectance takes in the Fourier domain, note that rotating harmonics about the surface normal does not alter the frequencies of the sinusoids that describe variation in azimuth: the absolute value of the moment, $|m|$, is preserved under rotations about the z-axis (see equation 5a and figures 14.8 to 14.10). Azimuthally isotropic reflectances must preserve the absolute value $|m|$ of the moment of an incident harmonic in the reflected pattern of light. Reflectances modeled by Cook and Torrance also preserve the *sign* of the moment: Factoring out the per-

fect reflection $\mathbf{P}$, these reflectances preserve the azimuthal phase of an incident harmonic. The reflectances preserve subspaces labeled by moment m.

Because these reflectances may vary with shift in elevation, they are not generally represented by diagonal matrices, rather they transform linearly terms with varying ℓ but fixed m. In addition, these linear transformations labelled by m must be symmetric in incident and exitant indices because the symmetry of reflectances (equation 4) is unaltered by a linear transformation such as the spherical harmonic transform. Finally, note that the reflectance is insensitive to the phase of the sinusoid that describes a harmonic's variation in azimuth: The linear transformation at some non-negative moment m (cosine phase) must be identical to the transformation at $-m$ (sine phase).

The matrix that represents an azimuthally isotropic reflectance is, therefore, a symmetric block-diagonal matrix in which the blocks are labelled by m with identical blocks at $\pm m$ (figure 14.13). One can order by moment m the components $a'_{\ell m}$ within the vector $\mathbf{a}'$ that represents the incident irradiance to maintain consistency with this block structure. The most general type of reflectance, a directional reflectance typical of scored surfaces, need be isotropic in neither elevation nor azimuth and so is represented in the Fourier domain by a symmetric but otherwise unstructured matrix.

Intensity to Irradiance Revisited

A final ingredient is needed to round out the Fourier-domain description of light reflected by some differential area, namely a representation for the cosine-windowing operator $\max(\cos(\theta), 0)x$ of equation 1 that turns an intensity I into an irradiance I'. An intensity I and an irradiance I' related in this fashion may be transformed into the Fourier domain, in which they are described by a vector $\mathbf{a}$ and a vector $\mathbf{a}'$, respectively. To determine the Fourier-domain structure of the cosine-windowing operator taking $\mathbf{a}$ to $\mathbf{a}'$, note that (1) the operator is linear and symmetric, and that (2) while the operator varies with elevation, it is azimuthally isotropic. The transformation of intensity to irradiance is thus represented by a symmetric block-diagonal matrix that I will call $\mathbf{C}$ with blocks labelled by moment $|m|$ (figure 14.14, right):

$$\mathbf{a}' = \mathbf{Ca}. \tag{10}$$

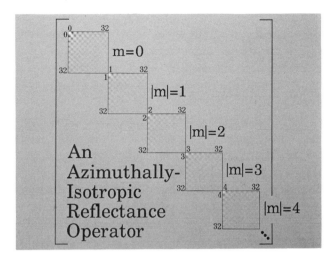

Fig. 14.13
Matrix representation of an azimuthally isotropic reflectance $\mathbf{R}^m$. The reflectance is calculated from Cook and Torrance's model (1982/1987) for a specular reflectance ($s = 1.0$) with coefficient m set to 0.4. Shown are terms in the block-diagonal matrix for blocks labeled by the first several moments. Blocks with the same absolute moment $|m|$ are identical. Positive-valued matrix entries are shown using pixels brighter than the background, while negative-valued coefficients are shown using pixels darker than the background.

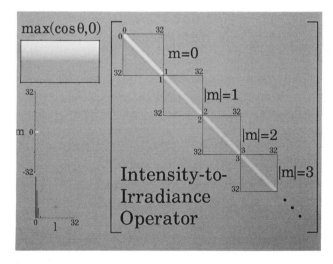

Fig. 14.14
Matrix representation of the intensity-to-irradiance operator. *Left,* The function $\max(\cos\theta, 0)$ in the space (*top*) and transform (*middle* and *bottom*) domains. *Right,* Terms in the block-diagonal matrix representing the corresponding multiplicative operator $\mathbf{C}^m$ for blocks labelled by the first several moments. Blocks with the same absolute moment $|m|$ are identical.

Preserved-Subspace Notation

To distinguish in notation between the structures of various operators in the Fourier domain I shall use superscripts to refer to preserved subspaces. A shift-invariant reflectance preserves both the frequency ℓ and the moment m of an incident harmonic, so the matrices for these operators are written $\mathbf{R}^{\ell m}$. An azimuthally isotropic reflectance preserves moment m but transforms linearly components at moment m with varying frequency ℓ, so that these are written $\mathbf{R}^m$. The set of azimuthally isotropic reflectances includes the shift-invariant reflectances as special cases. The most general sort of reflectance (a class that includes the previous two) need preserve neither frequency nor moment, so that it is written $\mathbf{R}$.

Following this convention, the perfect reflection matrix is $\mathbf{P}^{\ell m}$, while the cosine-windowing operator of equation 10 is written $\mathbf{C}^m$. Note also that reflectances of the form $\mathbf{R}^{\ell m}$ or $\mathbf{R}^m$ commute with the perfect reflection matrix $\mathbf{P}^{\ell m}$:

$$\mathbf{R}^{\ell m}\mathbf{P}^{\ell m} = \mathbf{P}^{\ell m}\mathbf{R}^{\ell m}, \tag{11a}$$

and

$$\mathbf{R}^m\mathbf{P}^{\ell m} = \mathbf{P}^{\ell m}\mathbf{R}^m. \tag{11b}$$

This is not necessarily true for some directional reflectance $\mathbf{R}$; in this case one can always determine the matrix $\mathbf{R}'$ that satisfies

$$\mathbf{R}'\mathbf{P}^{\ell m} = \mathbf{P}^{\ell m}\mathbf{R}. \tag{11c}$$

To formulate the reflection of a pattern of intensity that is expressed as a vector $\mathbf{a}$ in the frequency domain, we combine equation 8 (exitant radiance from incident irradiance) and equation 10 (incident irradiance from incident intensity). This combination takes three forms:

(a) For shift-invariant reflectances:

$$\mathbf{b} = \mathbf{R}^{\ell m}\mathbf{P}^{\ell m}\mathbf{C}^m\mathbf{a} = \mathbf{P}^{\ell m}\mathbf{R}^{\ell m}\mathbf{C}^m\mathbf{a}, \tag{12a}$$

(b) For azimuthally isotropic reflectances:

$$\mathbf{b} = \mathbf{R}^m\mathbf{P}^{\ell m}\mathbf{C}^m\mathbf{a} = \mathbf{P}^{\ell m}\mathbf{R}^m\mathbf{C}^m\mathbf{a}, \tag{12b}$$

(c) For directional reflectances:

$$\mathbf{b} = \mathbf{R}'\mathbf{P}^{\ell m}\mathbf{C}^m\mathbf{a} = \mathbf{P}^{\ell m}\mathbf{R}\mathbf{C}^m\mathbf{a}. \tag{12c}$$

The decomposition of surface reflection separates non-varying,[2] geometrical components of reflection, represented by $\mathbf{C}^m$ (which takes into account surface orientation) and $\mathbf{P}^{\ell m}$ (which represents perfect reflection), from those components represented by $\mathbf{R}$ that vary from surface to surface in a way that depends on surface roughness and material properties.

Ambiguity

Arbitrary Views of Flat Surfaces

I turn now to the question of how reflectances and illuminants may be traded off against one another to produce identical reflected light patterns. The trade-offs described below involve determining the inverses of the reflectances used in equation 12 to find exitant radiances; the properties of these inverses are found by studying eigenilluminants.

Eigenilluminants and Kernels

An eigenfunction of a linear operator W is a function G that passes unscathed through the operation except for multiplication by its corresponding eigenvalue ω, which is some scalar:

$$WG = \omega G. \tag{13}$$

Because reflectances are real symmetric linear operators (equation 4), the eigenvalues of a reflectance are real-valued; furthermore, the (normalized) eigenfunctions of a reflectance form a complete orthonormal basis for the space of all possible lights on which the reflectance acts. I call the eigenfunctions of a reflectance eigenilluminants and distinguish, when the need arises, between eigenirradiances, which are the eigenfunctions of a reflectance represented by a matrix $\mathbf{R}$, and eigenintensities, which I take to be the eigenfunctions of an operator represented by a matrix $\mathbf{RC}^m$ (see equation 12).

The eigenirradiances of a shift-invariant reflectance $\mathbf{R}^{\ell m}$ are the spherical harmonics themselves; the corresponding eigenvalues are the frequency-dependent attenuations $\rho(\ell)$ particular to that reflectance. Such an eigenirradiance can be represented by a vector on which $\mathbf{R}^{\ell m}$ acts: The spherical harmonic transform provides a one-to-one correspondence between eigenfunctions of a reflectance and eigenvectors of its matrix representation. The set of eigenirradiances of a shift-invariant reflectance is represented in the Fourier domain by the set of vectors $\{(1\,0\,0\,0\ldots)^{\mathsf{T}}, (0\,1\,0\,0\ldots)^{\mathsf{T}}, (0\,0\,1\,0\ldots)^{\mathsf{T}}, \ldots\}$.

Note that spherical harmonics at frequencies beyond the cutoff $\ell_{\max}(\mathbf{R}^{\ell m})$ of a particular shift-invariant reflectance are eigenirradiances with eigenvalue zero: $\rho(\ell) = 0$ for $\ell > \ell_{\max}(\mathbf{R}^{\ell m})$. Eigenirradiances of eigenvalue zero provide a basis for a subspace of incident irradiance patterns characterized by having no impact whatsoever on exitant light patterns. Such a subspace is called an operator's kernel and can be written $\ker(W)$ for arbitrary operator W. As applied to reflectances, we have, for example: if

$$K(\theta, \phi) = \sum_{\ell = \ell_{\max}(\mathbf{R}^{\ell m})+1}^{\infty} \sum_{m=-\ell}^{\ell} k_{\ell m} Y_{\ell m}(\theta, \phi), \tag{14a}$$

for some arbitrary real coefficients $k_{\ell m}$ and some shift-invariant reflectance $\mathbf{R}^{\ell m}$, then the transform $\mathbf{k}$ of $K(\theta, \phi)$ satisfies

$$\mathbf{k} \in \ker(\mathbf{R}^{\ell m}), \tag{14b}$$

so that

$$\mathbf{R}^{\ell m}\mathbf{k} = 0. \tag{14c}$$

The eigenvectors of a block-diagonal matrix are the eigenvectors of the individual blocks, so that an eigenirradiance of an azimuthally-isotropic reflectance $\mathbf{R}^m$ combines linearly terms at some particular moment m that vary in frequency ℓ. Matrices $\mathbf{R}^{\ell m}\mathbf{C}^m$ and $\mathbf{R}^m\mathbf{C}^m$ have the same structure as $\mathbf{R}^m$, namely block-diagonal in moment m, so that their eigenintensities also combine linearly terms at some particular moment m that vary in frequency ℓ. Figure 14.15 shows the spectral decomposition of the azimuthally isotropic operator $\mathbf{R}^m\mathbf{C}^m$ in terms of its eigenintensities and eigenvalues, where $\mathbf{R}^m$ is the reflectance depicted in figure 14.13. The eigenintensities at low values of m are exhibited as (column) eigenvectors at the top left of figure 14.15; corresponding eigenvalues are exhibited in the spectrum at the bottom left. The particular eigenintensity marked by the vertical dotted line with

---

2. This decomposition is suitable for most opaque surfaces. By suitably altering the operators it can be extended to handle thin translucent surfaces.

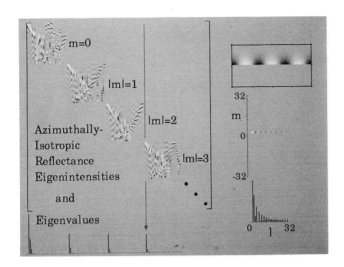

Fig. 14.15
Eigenintensities of the azimuthally isotropic reflectance R^m depicted in figure 14.13. At left are blocks labelled by moment that contain column vectors, each of which is an eigenvector of matrix R^mC^m. Beneath these eigenvectors in corresponding columns are the corresponding eigenvalues, shown as a spectrum. The eigenvectors in the right halves of each block correspond to eigenfunctions (of eigenvalue zero) that are nonzero only behind the surface. The eigenvector marked by the vertical dotted line (with eigenvalue marked by the arrow at the bottom) is shown as an eigenfunction at the right; it has energy only at terms with moments equal to three.

eigenvalue marked by the arrowhead at the bottom is exhibited as an eigenfunction to the right. Note that all intensities that take nonzero values only in the lower hemisphere ($\pi/2 \leqslant \theta \leqslant \pi$) are eigenintensities of eigenvalue zero and so lie in the kernel of all matrices RC^m.

Black Light Patterns

The simplest example of shading ambiguity due to the confounding of illumination and reflectance follows readily. The example is analogous to an ambiguity studied in color vision (Wyszecki & Stiles, 1982): Lights that lie in the kernel of some chromatic operator (e.g., trichromatic transduction) may be added to any transferred (e.g., visible) light to produce a metameric light. In analogy, eigenilluminants of a particular reflectance that have an eigenvalue of zero may be added to an incident light pattern to produce a set of "metameric" illuminants for

that reflectance; lights reflected *toward all viewpoints* are identical. Following terminology in color research on metamerism (Brainard, Wandell & Cowan, 1989), I call these eigenilluminants, within the kernel of a reflectance, black light patterns.

This notion applies in a straightforward way to flat, extended surfaces of uniform reflectance if one supposes that light sources are sufficiently distant so that intensities expressed about local normals to the surface are the same. More formally, if $k \in \ker(RC^m)$, then for any incident intensity a we may rely on linearity and equation 12 to write

$$b = P^{\ell m}RC^m a = P^{\ell m}RC^m(a + k).^3 \qquad (15)$$

A viewer of such a surface who has prior knowledge of its reflectance properties can thus recover the pattern of illumination from the reflected light only up to an equivalence class of reflectance-dependent metamers.

Adequate Illumination

Can a viewer of a flat, extended surface with prior knowlege of its position and pattern of illumination (due to sufficiently distant sources) determine the spatial properties of its reflectance function? In the simplest case the reflectance is represented in the transform domain by a diagonal matrix with frequency-dependent entries; evidently the only requirement for complete recovery is that the illuminant have nonzero energy at all frequencies passed by the reflectance. The more generally stated requirement—that an illuminant have nonzero projections along all of a reflectance's significant eigenilluminants—is one of *adequate illumination*. By significant eigenilluminants are meant those with nonzero eigenvalues. This requirement may be weakened in the simplest case if the viewer has prior knowledge of the general form of the reflectance[4]; in this case, interpolation and extrapolation can be used to provide an accurate estimate of reflectance despite inadequate illumination. Point sources, environments that present edges in the illumination, and white, brown, etc. noise are prototypical adequate illuminants. The prototypical inadequate illuminant is spatially uniform lighting.

---

3. In practice we must, of course, meet the constraint that incident intensities are non-negative.

4. The specular component in the Phong model, for instance, is drawn from the family of point-spread functions $[\cos \theta]^n$.

Inadequate Illumination

It is through inadequate illumination that further instances of confounding are most easily devised. Intuitively, one makes the light reflected from a shiny surface like that from a dull surface by lighting the former with patterns limited to low frequencies. Conversely, one can attempt to make the light reflected from a dull surface like that from a shiny surface by lighting the former with patterns with greater energy at high frequencies.

To make identical exitant lights from two flat surfaces with different reflectances, one need but choose an illuminant for one of the surfaces that lies in the intersection of the subspaces spanned by the two surfaces' significant eigenilluminants; the illuminant for the other surface is calculated by matrix inversion. A wide variety of possibilities corresponding to this choice of the first surface's illuminant are then generated by adding patterns to each surface's illuminant that are black light patterns for the respective reflectances.

I shall work this through in detail for two flat surfaces with shift-invariant reflectances $\mathbf{R}_1^{\ell m}$ and $\mathbf{R}_2^{\ell m}$. Supposing that the first surface has incident intensity $\mathbf{a}_1$, the task is to find, if possible, an incident intensity $\mathbf{a}_2$ for the second surface so that the exitant radiance patterns from the two surfaces are identical towards all viewpoints. Using equation 12a, the desired state of affairs can be written

$$\mathbf{b} = \mathbf{P}^{\ell m}\mathbf{R}_2^{\ell m}\mathbf{C}^m\mathbf{a}_2 = \mathbf{P}^{\ell m}\mathbf{R}_1^{\ell m}\mathbf{C}^m\mathbf{a}_1. \tag{16a}$$

By multiplying the three parts of this equation on the left by the inverse $[\mathbf{P}^{\ell m}]^{-1}$ of $\mathbf{P}^{\ell m}$ (namely $\mathbf{P}^{\ell m}$ itself) and by converting intensities $\mathbf{a}_i$ into irradiances $\mathbf{a}_i'$, we find the following condition for equality:

$$\mathbf{R}_2^{\ell m}\mathbf{a}_2' = \mathbf{R}_1^{\ell m}\mathbf{a}_1'. \tag{16b}$$

The two reflectances share the same eigenfunctions, namely the spherical harmonics. $\mathbf{R}_1^{\ell m}$ and $\mathbf{R}_2^{\ell m}$ differ in their transfer functions, which are described by the two sets of eigenvalues $\rho_1(\ell)$ and $\rho_2(\ell)$, respectively (see under Shift-Invariant Reflectances). We can define the inverse $[\mathbf{R}_2^{\ell m}]^{-1}$ of $\mathbf{R}_2^{\ell m}$ to be the transfer function $1/\rho_2(\ell)$ for those frequencies ℓ at which $\rho_2(\ell) > 0$. With this restricted inverse we can solve equation 16b for $\mathbf{a}_2'$ using

$$\mathbf{a}_2' = [\mathbf{R}_2^{\ell m}]^{-1}\mathbf{R}_1^{\ell m}\mathbf{a}_1', \tag{16c}$$

if we simultaneously impose the restriction that the exitant radiance $\mathbf{R}_1^{\ell m}\mathbf{a}_1'$ have no energy at frequencies ℓ at

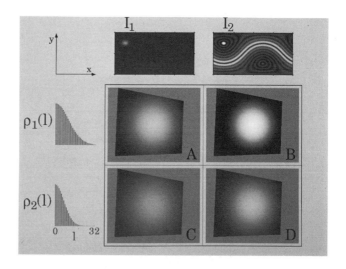

Fig. 14.16

Images of two surfaces with distinct reflectances. Flat surfaces with distinct shift-invariant reflectances shown at the left are lit by two distinct illuminants with intensities shown at the top. The 2 by 2 matrix of simulated reflected lights shows that distinct combinations of reflectance and illumination can produce identical reflected lights (A and D). *Left*, two distinct shift-invariant reflectances represented by their (discrete) Gaussian eigenvalues $\rho_1(\ell)$ and $\rho_2(\ell)$, respectively. *Top*, patterns of intensity I_1 and I_2. I_1 is a Gaussian-blurred point source at $(\theta\,\phi) = (45°\ 45°)$ to which has been added some spatially uniform illumination. The x- and y-axes lie in the page (see *top left*); the z-axis points out towards the viewer. The pattern I_2 was determined by (1) transforming I_1 into an irradiance; (2) convolving the result with $\rho_1(\ell)/\rho_2(\ell)$ (boosting the high frequencies), and (3) transforming the resulting irradiance into the intensity I_2. The shinier surface lit by the diffuse source (A) produces a highlight identical to that produced by the duller surface lit by the "sharp" source (D).

which $\rho_2(\ell) = 0$. The incident intensity $\mathbf{a}_2$ on the upper hemisphere is then found by multiplying the space-domain function represented by $\mathbf{a}_2'$ by the inverse $1/\cos(\theta)$ of the cosine-windowing operator over the restricted domain $\theta \in [0, \pi/2]$.

Figure 14.16 shows two simulated flat surfaces distinguished by their (shift-invariant) reflectance functions; these functions are represented to the left by their eigenvalues $\rho_1(\ell)$ and $\rho_2(\ell)$ given, in this example, by (discrete) Gaussian functions of frequency. The surfaces are lit by two distant light source patterns shown at the top; these are chosen so that the surface with reflectance described by $\rho_1(\ell)$ under the first light provides an exitant radiance pattern identical to that of the surface with reflectance $\rho_2(\ell)$ under the second light found using equation 16c. Adding black light patterns to these incident lights will not alter the exitant radiances.

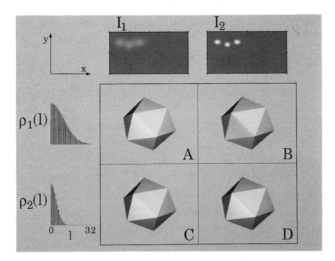

Fig. 14.17
Similar images of two icosahedral surfaces with distinct reflectances. Icosahedra with distinct shift-invariant reflectances shown at the left are lit by two distinct illuminants with intensities shown at the top. Intensity I_1 is found from intensity I_2 by convolving I_2 with $\rho_2(\ell)/\rho_1(\ell)$ (lowpass filtering); the shading patterns in (A) and (D) are indistinguishable.

If one supposes that the amplitudes of natural patterns of incident illumination fall off with frequency, on average, then patterns with a high-frequency boost needed to make a dull surface resemble a shiny surface are, on the whole, unlikely. Surfaces with exitant radiance patterns limited to low frequencies are far more ambiguous under this natural lighting supposition.

Arbitrary View of Convex Surfaces

In the attempt to extend from flat surfaces to identically shaped convex surfaces this way to generate physically distinct pairs of surfaces that appear identical *from all viewpoints*, we find two results: (1) almost all such matches can be shown to be physically imperfect, but (2) one can often find patterns of illumination that can make two convex[5] objects with distinct reflectances differ negligibly in their appearance. The evidence for the latter assertion is best seen; I show in figure 14.17 two icosahedra with the same shape but with distinct (shift-invariant) reflectance functions that nevertheless look very much the same when lights are chosen in accordance with equation 16.

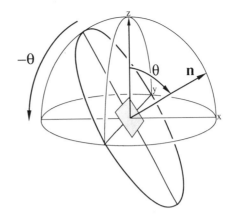

Fig. 14.18
Rotating the pattern of intensity to match surface orientation. The light reaching a piece of surface with unit normal **n** comes from directions lying in the hemisphere aligned about the normal. To reflect this pattern of light using equation 12, we must rotate the pattern of light intensity so that the hemisphere of lights incident on the oriented surface is aligned with the (northern) hemisphere in which we have represented the reflectance operators. If, as shown in this figure, the surface normal is described by an elevation θ in some global coordinate system, then we must rotate the pattern of light intensity through $-\theta$ to perform this alignment.

To see why the reflected light patterns (at all viewpoints) are not completely identical, we can construct an equation similar to equation 16a that takes into account the additional fact that incident light patterns, drawn from some "global" pattern of distant light sources, vary with surface orientation. With this equation we find that the pattern of intensity that compensates for a change in reflectance depends on surface orientation, so that there is no one global pattern of light sources that compensates correctly at all surface orientations for all viewpoints.

Rotations

To describe the light exiting a convex surface at a location with some particular surface orientation, we must first describe the relationship between incident irradiance, a local quantity, and the global pattern of illumination. Figure 14.18 shows a tilted piece of surface within the global coordinate system in which are described the distant light sources that form the illumination pattern

---

5. By limiting ourselves to convex objects we can ignore problems that arise with self-interreflection. Kajiya (1986) reviews methods for treating reflected light under circumstances in which interreflection plays a role.

$I(\theta_g, \phi_g)$. If the surface normal were aligned with this global coordinate system, then we could simply use equation 12 to determine the exitant radiance. Yet the tilted surface does not "see" the northern hemisphere of illumination but the hemisphere of illumination centered on the surface normal. To reflect the lights in this tilted hemisphere, we must first rotate the global pattern of illumination so that the hemisphere of illumination impinging on the tilted surface becomes the northern hemisphere of illumination (which we know how to reflect). If we rotate the illumination appropriately, then the exitant radiance found using equation 12 will have the proper pattern.[6]

Let us express this use of rotations more formally by letting $\mathbf{D}(\mathbf{n})$ stand for the rotation that takes the hemisphere of illumination impinging on the piece of surface with unit normal $\mathbf{n}$ into the northern hemisphere. The exitant radiance $\mathbf{b}(\mathbf{n})$, which depends on the surface normal, is then given by

$$\mathbf{b}(\mathbf{n}) = \mathbf{P}'^m \mathbf{R} \mathbf{C}^m \mathbf{D}(\mathbf{n}) \mathbf{a}. \tag{17}$$

The form of the rotation matrix $\mathbf{D}$ used in equation 17 has been discussed above (see especially under Spherical Harmonics and Azimuthally Isotropic Reflectances). Rotations leave invariant subspaces labelled by frequency ℓ but transform linearly terms at each frequency that vary in moment. Rotations are thus represented by block-diagonal matrices $\mathbf{D}^\ell$. The entries of these matrices depend on the particular rotation under consideration; these are most often parameterized by the three Euler angles.[7] I shall continue, however, to parameterize the rotations by the unit surface normal as in equation 17.

In analogy to equation 16a, the equation that expresses the desired identity between the lights reflected by two identically shaped convex surfaces with distinct reflectances is

$$\mathbf{b}(\mathbf{n}) = \mathbf{P}'^m \mathbf{R}_2 \mathbf{C}^m \mathbf{D}'(\mathbf{n}) \mathbf{a}_2(\mathbf{n}) = \mathbf{P}'^m \mathbf{R}_1 \mathbf{C}^m \mathbf{D}'(\mathbf{n}) \mathbf{a}_1. \tag{18a}$$

This equation expresses the sought pattern of intensity $\mathbf{a}_2(\mathbf{n})$ for the second surface as a function of surface orientation: It is not clear that there exists *a* pattern of

intensity for this second surface, given a pattern of intensity $\mathbf{a}_1$ and reflectances $\mathbf{R}_1$ and $\mathbf{R}_2$, that makes the reflected lights identical at all viewpoints.

To solve for $\mathbf{a}_2(\mathbf{n})$, we first rid equation 18a of the perfect reflection $\mathbf{P}'^m$ by multiplying both sides by its inverse. We can then use restricted inverses $[\mathbf{R}_2]^{-1}$ and $[\mathbf{C}^m]^{-1}$ and the inverse $[\mathbf{D}'(\mathbf{n})]^{-1}$ of the rotation $\mathbf{D}'(\mathbf{n})$ to write

$$\mathbf{a}_2(\mathbf{n}) = [\mathbf{D}'(\mathbf{n})]^{-1} [\mathbf{C}^m]^{-1} [\mathbf{R}_2]^{-1} \mathbf{R}_1 \mathbf{C}^m \mathbf{D}'(\mathbf{n}) \mathbf{a}_1. \tag{18b}$$

Recall from the discussion in Inadequate Illumination that the restricted inverse $[\mathbf{C}^m]^{-1}$ is a multiplication by $1/\cos(\theta)$ and has the restricted domain $\theta \in [0, \pi/2]$. The intensity $\mathbf{a}_2(\mathbf{n})$ recovered by equation 18b thus takes values only within the hemisphere centered on the surface normal. Two distinct surface normals $\mathbf{n}_1$ and $\mathbf{n}_2$ will provide two hemispheric intensities $\mathbf{a}_2(\mathbf{n}_1)$ and $\mathbf{a}_2(\mathbf{n}_2)$, and the question is whether it is possible for these intensities to agree at those directions where the hemispheres overlap.

Commutativity

The question can be answered by considering the commutativity of the various operators used in equation 18b. We know, for instance, that a shift-invariant reflectance commutes with an arbitrary rotation: the order in which we apply reflectance $\mathbf{R}'^m$ and rotation $\mathbf{D}'(\mathbf{n})$ does not matter. More formally,

$$\mathbf{R}'^m \mathbf{D}'(\mathbf{n}) = \mathbf{D}'(\mathbf{n}) \mathbf{R}'^m. \tag{19}$$

This commutativity is handily expressed in terms of the commutator $[\mathbf{A}, \mathbf{B}] = \mathbf{A}\mathbf{B} - \mathbf{B}\mathbf{A}$. With this notation, the commutativity expressed by equation 19 is equivalent to saying that the commutator $[\mathbf{R}'^m, \mathbf{D}'(\mathbf{n})]$ is equal to $\mathbf{0}$. Note that neither azimuthally isotropic reflectances nor general reflectances commute with all rotations (particularly those rotations *not* about the surface normal), so that *in general*

$$[\mathbf{R}'^m, \mathbf{D}'(\mathbf{n})] = \mathbf{0}, \tag{20a}$$

$$[\mathbf{R}^m, \mathbf{D}'(\mathbf{n})] \neq \mathbf{0}, \tag{20b}$$

---

6. The exitant radiance found this way (equation 17) will not generally have the correct position: It is aligned with the northern hemisphere. If we want the exitant light to have both the proper pattern and the proper position in global coordinates, then we must rotate it back to the position determined by the surface normal using the rotation that is the inverse of the initial rotation.

7. While the formula for these entries (e.g., Talman (1968) equations 9.19 and 9.20) is somewhat forbidding (and must be altered to apply to real-valued rather than to complex-valued harmonics), the entries are readily computed.

and

$$[\mathbf{R}, \mathbf{D}^{\ell}(\mathbf{n})] \neq \mathbf{0}. \tag{20c}$$

By examining equation 18b for shift-invariant reflectances, we see that *if* rotations commute with the intensity-to-irradiance operator $\mathbf{C}^m$ then we can shift $\mathbf{D}^{\ell}(\mathbf{n})$ over to a position in the right-hand side of the equation beside its inverse $[\mathbf{D}^{\ell}(\mathbf{n})]^{-1}$. The rotations would then cancel, as would the dependence of intensity $\mathbf{a}_2$ on surface orientation. Yet the intensity-to-irradiance operator does not commute with arbitrary rotations:

$$[\mathbf{C}^m, \mathbf{D}^{\ell}(\mathbf{n})] \neq \mathbf{0}. \tag{21}$$

This is intuitively evident in the space domain and follows in the Fourier domain from the distinct structures of the matrices that represent the operators.

We could still succeed in cancelling the rotations (and the dependence on surface orientation) if reflectances commuted with the intensity-to-irradiance operator. If, in equation 18b, we could pass $\mathbf{C}^m$ through the reflectances so that it came to rest beside its inverse, then we could cancel the operators with which rotations do not commute. We could then rid the equation of its dependence on surface normal if the reflectances were shift-invariant (equation 20a). Shift-invariant reflectances do *not* commute with the intensity-to-irradiance operator, however:

$$[\mathbf{R}^{\ell m}, \mathbf{C}^m] \neq \mathbf{0}. \tag{22}$$

Finally, while it is theoretically possible for an azimuthally isotropic reflectance $\mathbf{R}^m$ to commute with $\mathbf{C}^m$, we still cannot remove the dependence on surface normal from equation 18b because such reflectances do not commute with arbitrary rotations (equation 20b).

It is generally impossible to make the lights from identically shaped convex surfaces with distinct reflectances identical towards all viewpoints. For shift-invariant reflectances, the trade-off between reflectance and illumination can be accomplished in an approximate fashion if the known illumination pattern $\mathbf{a}_1$ and the reflectances $\mathbf{R}_1$ and $\mathbf{R}_2$ are chosen to minimize the result of applying the commutator $[[\mathbf{R}_2^{\ell m}]^{-1}\mathbf{R}_1^{\ell m}, \mathbf{C}^m]$ to the local intensities $\mathbf{D}^{\ell}(\mathbf{n})\mathbf{a}_1$.

Single Views

Ambiguity increases as the number of views decreases. Let us now turn from the extreme case of infinitely many views considered above to the other extreme, namely the case in which the viewer is allowed just a single view. We can use a more general strategy to study ambiguity in this case: Make identical the images of surfaces with distinct reflectances *and* shapes.

Two tactics present themselves. In the first we carefully examine image ambiguity under strong constraints on surfaces, for instance, the constraint that shapes be convex (thereby forbidding self-interreflection). It is under such constraints that our intuitions are strongest. For instance, we know that we can create almost any image shading pattern by adjusting the illumination of a convex surface with a mirrorlike reflectance; likewise, the set of shading patterns that we can create using a matte surface is far more limited (for results of this sort with point sources see Horn, Szeliski & Yuille, 1989).

The second tactic is to rely solely on the constraints that we have used throughout, namely that light sources be distant from the viewed surfaces and that observation by the viewer does not interfere with the system. In tandem with the linearity of reflectance, we can use these constraints to provide a general way to choose the lighting of a particular surface or collection of surfaces so that the pattern of shading matches, as well as possible, some given pattern of shading.

Fourier-Domain Representation of the Linear Rendering Operator

Let us suppose that our lights are distant and that we are viewing an arbitrarily complex set of surfaces with known shapes, positions, and reflectances. We can render such a scene (i.e., calculate the light returned towards the viewer from each image location) either by (1) reflecting some sum of point sources at each position and then using this point-wise information to make a spatially extended image, or (2) calculating the spatially extended image due to each point source and then making the final image by summing over images from each point source. Either method can be employed if one uses a ray tracing procedure to render the scene. The latter method works also with more sophisticated rendering procedures such as radiosity (Cohen et al., 1988; Goral et al., 1984; Kajiya, 1986), in which interreflections among surfaces are taken into account.

Rather than compute the images that result from individual point sources and then sum over these to find the final image, we can form the images that arise from each spherical harmonic component in the illumination and then sum over these. Let us call S the linear operator that, for some given scene and choice of viewpoint, transforms a pattern of illumination $I(\theta_g, \phi_g)$ into its corresponding continuous image $J(x, y)$:

$$J(x, y) = S(I(\theta_g, \phi_g)). \tag{23}$$

The images $J_{\ell m}(x, y)$ that arise from spherical harmonic patterns of illumination are then given by

$$J_{\ell m}(x, y) = S(Y_{\ell m}(\theta_g, \phi_g)), \tag{24}$$

so that the image $J(x, y)$ that arises from illumination pattern $I(\theta_g, \phi_g)$ with vector representation $\mathbf{a}$ is

$$
\begin{aligned}
J(x, y) &= \sum_{\ell=0}^{\infty} \sum_{m=-\ell}^{\ell} a_{\ell m} J_{\ell m}(x, y) \\
&= \sum_{\ell=0}^{\infty} \sum_{m=-\ell}^{\ell} a_{\ell m} S(Y_{\ell m}(\theta_g, \phi_g)) \\
&= \sum_{\ell=0}^{\infty} \sum_{m=-\ell}^{\ell} S(a_{\ell m} Y_{\ell m}(\theta_g, \phi_g)) \\
&= S\left(\sum_{\ell=0}^{\infty} \sum_{m=-\ell}^{\ell} a_{\ell m} Y_{\ell m}(\theta_g, \phi_g) \right) \\
&= S(I(\theta_g, \phi_g)). \tag{25}
\end{aligned}
$$

We must discretize not only the illumination but also the spatially continuous image to put this decomposition to use. The latter is done most simply using the discrete Fourier transform (Bracewell, 1978), which assigns to a continuous image $J(x, y)$ with rectangular domain a vector $\mathbf{j}$ with complex components j_{uv}. The (space-domain) operator S is then represented in the Fourier domain by a matrix $\mathbf{S}$ that takes as input an illumination vector $\mathbf{a}$ and provides as output the transform $\mathbf{j}$ of the resulting image:

$$\mathbf{j} = \mathbf{S}\mathbf{a}. \tag{26a}$$

In terms of the discrete Fourier transform indices u and v for the image and the spherical harmonic transform indices ℓ and m for the illumination, we have

$$j_{uv} = \sum_{\ell=0}^{\infty} \sum_{m=-\ell}^{\ell} S_{uv, \ell m} a_{\ell m}. \tag{26b}$$

Least-Squares Lighting

Determining the entries $S_{uv, \ell m}$ in the matrix $\mathbf{S}$ is clearly a laborious procedure. One must first render a scene for each individual spherical harmonic $Y_{\ell m}(\theta_g, \phi_g)$ to find the corresponding continuous image $J_{\ell m}(x, y)$. Each of these images must then be Fourier transformed to provide, for each choice of ℓ and m, the entries $S_{uv, \ell m}$.[8] Having computed these entries, however, we can rapidly find the discrete Fourier transform of an image arising from an arbitrary pattern of illumination. With the entries we can, furthermore, invert the rendering process.

The matrix $\mathbf{S}$ has both a range, namely the subspace of image transforms that can arise from the scene, and a kernel, namely the transforms of the set of illumination patterns that are mapped by S to the zero image $J(x, y) = 0$. If some particular image transform lies within the range of the matrix $\mathbf{S}$, then $\mathbf{S}$ may be inverted to determine the spherical harmonic transform of the pattern of illumination that gives rise to that image. If, on the other hand, the image lies outside of the range of $\mathbf{S}$, then there is no pattern of illumination for the scene and viewpoint represented by $\mathbf{S}$ that will produce the image. Under these circumstances it is nevertheless possible to find the pattern of illumination that produces an image that is the best possible fit in the least-squares sense to the given image. This approximation is found by performing a singular value decomposition of $\mathbf{S}$, which is a standard numerical procedure (Press et al., 1988) for "inverting" singular matrices. The procedure provides not only a restricted inverse $\mathbf{S}^{-1}$ but also a basis for the range of images that could arise from the scene and a basis for the illumination patterns that lie in the scene's kernel.

With the restricted inverse $\mathbf{S}^{-1}$ we can find the pattern of illumination $\mathbf{a}$ for the scene[9] that provides an image that is the best possible fit to an arbitrary image $\mathbf{j}$:

$$\mathbf{a} = \mathbf{S}^{-1}\mathbf{j}. \tag{27}$$

This is a very general result, as befits the tactic of placing constraints on neither surface shapes nor reflectances. It rests on the fact that the map between illumination and image is linear; the particular representation

---

8. If the image in the space domain is already discrete, then this step may obviously be skipped; the transformed images would be preferred, in this case, only if the image has negligible energy at high spatial frequencies, allowing one to truncate the representation.

9. As noted earlier, the inverse transform $I(\theta_g, \phi_g)$ of $\mathbf{a}$ must be a non-negative function in practice.

for the map used here relies on the constraint that the illumination be distant. It is more difficult to find such a representation if we loosen the constraints by allowing arbitrary light source positions.

Discussion

By representing lights and reflectances in the Fourier domain, we have found several results on shading ambiguity. The first is that a reflectance has an infinite number of black light patterns, so that a viewer who knows a surface's reflectance properties can recover the pattern of illumination from the reflected light only up to an equivalence class of reflectance-dependent metamers. The second is that a pattern of illumination must be adequate if the viewer is to recover the spatial properties of reflectance from the shading of a surface. Third, we can use inadequate illumination to make surfaces with distinct reflectances look alike, although such matches are almost always imperfect in the case of closed surfaces potentially viewed from all directions. Fourth, we have found a way to choose the lighting of an arbitrary collection of surfaces, seen from a particular viewpoint, so that the resulting visual image matches some given image as well as possible. Finally, this approach makes evident the linear relationship between illumination and image for complex scenes.

The constraint that illumination be distant and unperturbed by the viewer disallows translation-varying intensity, shadows cast by the viewer, and interreflections between surfaces and the viewer. While these features of more realistic scenes are readily synthesized in computer graphics applications, their analysis appears far more difficult. With the constraints, we can analyze for *extended surfaces* the intuition that surface reflectances blur incident light patterns and study lights reflected towards all viewpoints as well as towards single viewpoints.

The analysis shows that the *spatial* trade-offs between reflectance and illumination are formally similar to the *chromatic* trade-offs between reflectance and illumination so important in studies of surface color appearance. The chromatic spectrum of the light from a small area of (optically inactive) surface is given by the wavelength-by-wavelength product of the surface's reflectance function and the illuminant's spectral power distribution: $E(\lambda) = R(\lambda)I(\lambda)$. The action of a reflectance can be represented by a simple multiplication in the wavelength domain because light incident at a particular wavelength gives rise only to exitant light at the same wavelength: Monochromatic lights are eigenfunctions for the chromatic component of reflectances.

While the "blurring" action of a reflectance on spatial patterns of incident light seems far more complex than the simple multiplication in the wavelength domain, this is so only because point sources of light are not eigenfunctions for the spatial component of physically realizable reflectances. The simplest type of reflectance has spherical harmonic patterns of light as its eigenfunctions; such a reflectance acts on incident light patterns in the space domain by convolution and in the Fourier domain by simple multiplication. The present results on black light patterns, on the adequacy of illumination and on ambiguity in cases of inadequate illumination are wholly analogous to corresponding results in the chromatic domain.

Extending this work on shading ambiguity to the simultaneous consideration of spatial and chromatic properties of reflectance is straightforward, particularly so for reflectances with "specular" components that have separable spatial and chromatic properties. While this separability is known not to hold in some cases (e.g., for materials like red metals with refractive indices that vary substantially with wavelength; see Cook & Torrance, 1982/1987), Healey (1989) has recently shown that many of these inseparable specular reflectances are approximated well by separable functions. Under the condition that the specular component of a reflectance is spatiochromatically separable, the standard models of reflectance used in the vision literature (see, e.g., D'Zmura & Lennie, 1986; Healey, 1989; Klinker, Shafer & Kanade, 1988; Shafer, 1984; Tominaga & Wandell, 1989) are translated readily from the space domain into the Fourier domain. The reflection of spatiochromatically inhomogeneous illuminants by colored surfaces may be analyzed in a way similar to that presented here.

Patterns of shading, highlights in particular, are very sensitive to the precise details of surface material and roughness and to the spatial pattern of illumination. While these details can be controlled in a manufacturing inspection setting in which, for instance, specularity can be used as a cue to shape (e.g., Healey & Binford, 1988; Sanderson, Weiss & Nayar, 1988), this control is not present in the normal, everyday viewing of scenes. If we are to infer precise shape from shading patterns, we need accurate estimates of both lighting and reflectance.

One thus cannot find fault with the human visual system for using shading information to estimate shape in such a half-hearted fashion. For instance, Barrow and Tenenbaum (1981) showed that contour generally overrides shading information in determining perceived shape (see also Witkin & Tenenbaum, 1983). Mingolla and Todd (1986; see also Todd & Mingolla, 1983) have shown that shading provides a weak input to the perception of variations in depth, in that observers consistently underestimate depth variation from shading information alone. Bülthoff and Mallot (1988) have shown that human shape-from-shading mechanisms perform better in stereo, where shading disparity can cue degree of convexity or concavity (Blake, 1985), but that edges nevertheless override shading disparity.

We must likewise know surface shape and pattern of illumination if we are to infer correctly surface reflectance properties. While the pattern of inference from shading to the spatial properties of reflectance is incompletely understood, there is one well-known inference illustrated by Beck (1972). Beck made two pictures of a vase under known illumination that are identical except for the presence or the (artificial) absence of a highlight. The vase with the highlight appears shiny across its entire surface, while the picture of the same vase with highlight removed appears completely matte. The visual system seems to infer automatically that a surface is glossy from the presence of a highlight. We know that this is a robust inference because a highlight is seen by the viewer only if several conditions are met: (1) the surface must be glossy; (2) the illumination must be adequate, and (3) the viewer must occupy a viewpoint at which the highlight is visible. The failure to see a highlight, on the other hand, can be caused by a matte reflectance, by inadequate illumination, or by poor choice of viewpoint, so that the viewer must have further knowledge of these factors if the correct inference about surface reflectance is to be drawn.

I have invoked a lot of machinery to make a simple point, namely that variation in the spatial properties of reflectances and illuminants leads to ambiguity in shaded images. Yet the machinery and the intuitions behind its use are similar to those belonging to linear systems analysis on the line or on the plane. Furthermore, spherical harmonic transforms, rotation matrices, and the like are readily implemented numerically on a personal computer,[10] albeit at a low resolution. I hope that the methods presented here will prove useful in psychophysical studies; taking shading ambiguity into account is an important ingredient in conducting controlled psychophysical experiments on the perception of shape, reflectance, and illumination.

Acknowledgments

I thank Al Ahumada, Dave Brainard, Geoff Iverson, Mike Landy, and Per Møller for helpful discussions and comments. This work was supported by NEI grants EY04440, EY01319, and RR03825 and by funds from the School of Social Sciences at UC Irvine.

References

Barrow, H. G. & Tenenbann, J. M. (1981). Computational vision. *Proceedings of the IEEE, 69*, 572–595.

Beck, J. (1972). *Surface color perception.* Ithaca, NY: Cornell.

Bennett, J. M. & Mattsson, L. (1989). *Introduction to surface roughness and scattering.* Washington, D.C.: Optical Society of America.

Blake, A. (1985). Specular stereo. *Proceedings of the 9th Intentional Joint Conference on Artificial Intelligence,* Los Angeles, 973–976.

Blinn, J. F. (1977/1988). Models of light reflection for computer synthesized pictures. In W. Richards (Ed.), *Natural computation* (pp. 214–223). Cambridge, MA: MIT.

Bracewell, R. N. (1978). *The Fourier transform and its applications* (2nd ed.). New York: McGraw-Hill.

Brainard, D. H., Wandell, B. A. & Cowan, W. B. (1989). Black light: How sensors filter spectral variation of the illuminant. *IEEE Transactions in Biomedical Engineering, 36*, 140–149.

Bülthoff, H. H. & Mallot, H. A. (1988). Integration of depth modules: Stereo and shading. *Journal of the Optical Society of America A, 5,* 1749–1758.

---

10. Rendering complex surfaces using equation 17 on a computer such as an Apple Macintosh II can readily tax one's patience, however; even more demanding are equations 26 and 27, which should be avoided completely on such a platform.

Cabral, B., Max, N. & Springmeyer, R. (1987). Bidirectional reflection functions from surface bump maps. *ACM Computer Graphics, 21,* 273–281.

Cohen, M. F., Chen, S. E., Wallace, J. R. & Greenberg, D. P. (1988). A progressive refinement approach to fast radiosity image generation. *ACM Computer Graphics, 22,* 75–84.

Cook, R. L. & Torrance, K. E. (1982/1987). A reflectance model for computer graphics. In W. Richards & S. Ullman (Eds.), *Image Understanding 1985–86* (pp. 1–19). Norwood, New Jersey: Ablex.

D'Zmura, M. & Lennie, P. (1986). Mechanisms of color constancy. *Journal of the Optical Society of America A, 3,* 1662–1672.

Gel'Fand, I. M., Minlos, R. A. & Shapiro, Z. (1963). *Representations of the rotation and Lorentz groups and their applications.* Oxford: Pergamon.

Goral, C. M., Torrance, K. E., Greenberg, D. P. & Battaile, B. (1984). Modeling the interaction of light between diffuse surfaces. *ACM Computer Graphics, 18,* 213–222.

Healey, G. (1989). Using color for geometry-insensitive segmentation. *Journal of the Optical Society of America A, 6,* 920–937.

Healey, G. & Binford, T. O. (1988). Local shape from specularity. *Computer Vision, Graphics, and Image Processing, 42,* 62–88.

Hobson, E. W. (1965). *The theory of spherical and ellipsoidal harmonics.* New York: Chelsea.

Hoffman, K. & Kunze, R. (1961). *Linear algebra.* Englewood Cliffs, NJ: Prentice-Hall.

Horn, B. K. P. (1975). Obtaining shape from shading information. In P. H. Winston (Ed.), *The Psychology of machine vision* (pp. 115–155). New York: McGraw-Hill.

Horn, B. K. P. (1986). *Robot vision.* New York: McGraw-Hill.

Horn, B. K. P. & Sjoberg, R. W. (1979). Calculating the reflectance map. *Applied Optics, 18,* 1770–1779.

Horn, B. K. P., Szeliski, R. S. & Yuille, A. L. (1989). Impossible shaded images. *MIT AI Lab TR.*

Hunter, R. S. (1975). *The measurement of appearance,* New York: Wiley.

Kajiya, J. T. (1986). The rendering equation. *ACM Computer Graphics, 20,* 143–150.

Klinker, G. J., Shafer, S. A. & Kanade, T. (1988). The measurement of highlights in color images. *International Journal of Computer Vision, 2,* 7–32.

MacRobert, T. M. (1967). *Spherical harmonics. An elementary treatise on harmonic functions with applications* (3rd ed.). New York: Pergamon.

Mingolla, E. & Todd, J. T. (1986). Perception of solid shape from shading. *Biological Cybernetics, 53,* 137–151.

Nicodemus, F. E., Richmond, J. C., Hsia, J. J., Ginsberg, I. W. & Limperis, T. (1977). Geometrical considerations and nomenclature for reflectance. *NBS Monograph 160.* Washington, D.C.: National Bureau of Standards.

Pentland, A. P. (1982). Finding the illuminant direction. *Journal of the Optical Society of America, 72,* 448–455.

Pentland, A. P. (1984). Local shading analysis. *IEEE Transactions on Pattern Analysis and Machine Intelligence, 6,* 170–187.

Pentland, A. P. (1988). Shape information from shading: a theory about human perception, *MIT Media Lab Visual Science TR,* 103.

Phong, B. T. (1975). Illumination for computer generated pictures. *Communications of the ACM, 18,* 311–317.

Press, W. H., Flannery, B. P., Teukolsky, S. A. & Vetterling, W. T. (1988). *Numerical recipes in C. The art of scientific computing.* New York: Cambridge.

Sanderson, A. C., Weiss, L. E. & Nayar, S. K. (1988). Structured highlight inspection of specular surfaces. *IEEE Transactions on Pattern Analysis and Machine Intelligence, 10,* 44–55.

Shafer, S. A. (1984). Using color to separate reflection components. *Department of Computer Science TR, 136.* New York: University of Rochester.

Swarztrauber, P. N. (1979). On the spectral approximation of discrete scalar and vector functions on the sphere. *SIAM Journal of Numerical Analysis, 16,* 934–949.

Talman, J. D. (1968). *Special functions: A group theoretic approach.* New York: W. A. Benjamin.

Terras, A. (1985). *Harmonic analysis on symmetric spaces and applications I.* New York: Springer.

Todd, J. T. & Mingolla, E. (1983). Perception of surface curvature and direction of illumination from patterns of shading. *Journal of Experimental Psychology: Human Perception and Performance, 9,* 583–595.

Tominaga, S. & Wandell, B. A. (1989). The standard surface reflectance model and illuminant estimation. *Journal of the Optical Society of America A, 6,* 576–584.

Torrance, K. E. & Sparrow, E. M. (1967). Theory for off-specular reflection from roughened surfaces. *Journal of the Optical Society of America, 57,* 1105–1114.

Walker, J. S. (1988). *Fourier analysis.* New York: Oxford.

Witkin, A. P. & Tenenbaum, J. M. (1983). On the role of structure in vision. In J. Beck, B. Hope & A. Rosenfeld (Eds.), *Human and machine vision* (pp. 481–543). New York: Academic.

Wyszecki, G. & Stiles, W. S. (1982). *Color science. Concepts and methods, quantitative data and formulae* (2nd ed.). New York: Wiley.

15

Transparency and the Cooperative Computation of Scene Attributes

Daniel Kersten

Cooperativity and Integration

A major goal of vision research is to understand how the brain constructs a perceptual model of the visual environment from the pattern of changing retinal light intensities. Even in the absence of motion, a pattern of intensities in a natural image is interpreted as due to changes in material, illumination, depth, or viewpoint with no apparent effort. How is this done and what are the computational principles involved? It will be argued that an essential component of perception under natural viewing conditions is the process of finding multiple representations of scene characteristics that must be consistent with each other. The perception of transparency provides a simple example of computing multiple and consistent representations and is the focus of the rest of this chapter.

In general, computational vision research has modularized the problem of computing perceptual scene models from image data. Examples include surface-color-from-radiance (Land, 1959), shape-from-shading (Horn, 1975), and structure-from-motion (Ullman, 1979). A primary result of computational analysis is that scene reconstruction from image data is often underconstrained—there are many solutions that satisfy the data provided by the image. Prior constraints, such as assuming that surfaces or reflectances are smooth, then have to be sought to find a unique interpretation of the environment from the image intensities. Although strong constraints may be required for impoverished viewing conditions, in general one would like to relax prior assumptions without losing uniqueness. It is useful to distinguish two strategies—*integration* and *cooperativity*—that become useful when the image content becomes complex as under natural viewing conditions.

Integration refers to the combination of input information or cues pertaining to a particular scene attribute, such as depth at a point, from a variety of sources such as motion, stereo, and shading as shown in the top of figure 15.1 (Bülthoff & Mallot, 1987; Chou & Brown, 1988; Terzopoulos, 1986). In cooperative computation, the estimates of two or more scene attributes (such as depth and transparency) are required to be consistent with each other and with constraints on natural imaging (bottom of figure 15.1). A scene attribute can be represented as a spatially indexed map or "intrinsic image" (Barrow & Tenenbaum, 1978). One approach to computing scene attribute maps is to label edges in an image according to the cause in the scene (Poggio, Gamble & Little, 1988). The computer detection of useful edges in natural images has turned out to be more problematic than at first anticipated. In addition to coping with multiple spatial scales and image noise, a useful edge detection must ultimately label edges according to the source in the scene. Changes in image intensity can be due to scene discontinuities such as shadows, surface self-occlusion, occlusion of one surface by another, reflectance change, and texture change. For example, if one primary goal of vision is object recognition, the explicit representation of surface boundaries and orientation discontinuities may be particularly critical (Biederman, 1987). But there are many changes of intensity in natural images that are not useful for finding object boundaries. Examine a good line drawing made by an artist—almost all the edges represent object or material boundaries, and very few represent shadows. An artist makes complex inferences in order to filter out uninformative edges while sketching.

A classic example of cooperative computation that may involve edge detection and labeling is the problem of lightness constancy. One approach is to classify edges according to whether they are reflectance or illumination changes (Gilchrist, Delman & Jacobsen, 1983). Although we now have a good understanding of the kinds of algorithms that can filter out slow illumination changes from sharp reflectance changes (Grossberg & Todorović, 1988; Horn, 1973; Land, 1959), the problem of image factoring, when both intrinsic images have discontinuities, is unsolved. There is very little difference in the human estimation of reflectance in complex Mondrians when they are behind a fuzzy shadow vs. a sharp transparency (Plummer & Kersten, 1988). This suggests that at some level, there may be common principles underlying splitting an image into representations of reflectance and illumination, or reflectance and transmittance. Understanding the interaction between two such maps is only a start. Perceptual observations have shown that just two such interacting maps are in general insufficient to account for lightness perception. Ernst Mach showed over a century ago that the perceived surface lightness of a simple folded gray card, placed on a table, depends on the interaction between perceived light source direction, and the bistably perceived geometry of the card, that is, whether it appears convex or concave (Mach, 1886). One needs to take into account the cooperative interaction of shape, illumination, and material reflectance to arrive at a complete account of lightness phenomena.

Studies of lightness perception have been plagued to some extent by ambiguity in both definition and psychophysical results (Beck, 1972). The root of the problem may be that perception of lightness and brightness depends on the extent to which there is an accompanying unambiguous perception of a real surface. This depends on the state of the observer and the naturalness of the image. One way of getting around this problem is to require reflectance estimates, rather than lightness judgments (Arend & Goldstein, 1987). This raises objections that reflectance judgments tap into inferential mechanisms

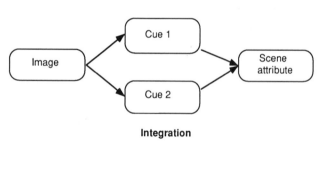

Integration

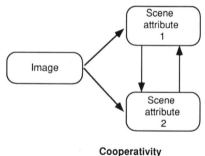

Cooperativity

Fig. 15.1
The distinction between integration of cues to compute a single scene attribute representation, and cooperativity—the computation of several scene attribute representations that interact.

that are more part of cognition than perception. In this chapter I attempt to circumvent these issues by investigating the perception of surface transparency. Phenomenal transparency may be a less ambiguous percept than lightness by virtue of the fact that it is more tightly coupled to surface perception.

The next two sections of this chapter will treat first the perception and then the computation of transparency. The first section provides perceptual evidence that the problem of transparency, or "seeing through" one cause of image intensity to another, involves cooperative computation. There are several components that interact. These include the various surface representations that have opaque or transparent attributes, the depth of these surfaces derived from other sources, and the relation of the contour shapes to the values of the regions they enclose. The problem of surface transparency, even in its simplest form, poses a number of unsolved computational and perceptual problems. In particular, it shows the power of human vision to incorporate global constraints, even when solving what may be an a priori local problem.

The second section provides a computational analysis of a simplified model of transparency in which the goal of the computation is to arrive at two distinct spatial maps, one representing opaque reflectance values, and one the transmittances corresponding to a transparent component. Here cooperative computation is analyzed in terms of an "ideal image understander." The intention is not to provide a theory of human transparency perception, but to illustrate the role of the statistical approach as a "quantitative computational theory" that encompasses a wide family of possible algorithms. This enables one to distinguish, at least in principle, between the correctness of the statistical model and the correctness of algorithms used to solve it. Purely local constraints are used to specify the statistical problem. Despite the inherent local nature of the constraints, purely local algorithms for computing transparency are inadequate.

Perception of Transparency

Transparency has received relatively little attention compared to other problems of image understanding. This probably reflects both the observation that simple surface transparency is rare in nature, and the anticipation that the computation of transparency is hard. From a general perspective, the problem of transparency may not be all that esoteric. For the purposes of this paper, the word transparency will be used to refer to the "seeing through" of one cause of image intensity to another at the same point. This is phenomenal, as distinct from physical, transparency. Seeing through one cause to another is a general problem that arises continually in everyday viewing. Here are a few examples that can be distinguished on the basis of the physical origins.

Specular transparency is a form of transparency in which a shiny or mirrorlike surface reflects some of the incident light with little diffusion, as with a polished apple. It is usually modeled as a component added to the matte reflectance of surface luminance. It is also commonly seen when looking through a window in which reflections off the glass add to the light coming through the window pane. Identifying specular transparency may be important to infer depth—either by discounting it in establishing stereo correspondence (Marr, 1982), or by using it to infer relative depth (Bülthoff & Blake, 1989).

Film transparency is the familiar form of multiplicative transparency where a clear surface absorbs some fraction of the light without scattering it. This darkens the image of the surfaces beneath it (figure 15.2, left panel). Film transparency will be the prototypical example returned to below in the computational section. Multiplicative trans-

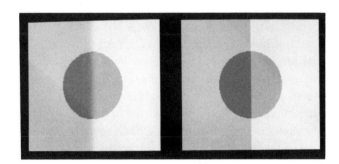

Fig. 15.2

Left, A circular transparent patch over a vertical line. The circular patch is usually seen as transparent. This is an example of multiplicative transparency. Because the image formation constraint is symmetrical, there is no local information at X junctions to bias the edge labeling. Thus a computation based on local information should provide an alternative solution—the circular patch is opaque and behind two abutting transparent rectangles. This interpretation can be seen at times, and demonstrates the multistability of transparency perception. *Right*, Shadow transparency can be seen by the introduction of blur to the vertical edge. This changes the assignment of surface attribute to the circular patch.

Transparency and the Cooperative Computation of Scene Attributes

parency is a good example of the inherent ambiguity that can arise when two images are combined with a symmetric operation. Although the circular patch in the left panel of figure 15.2 can be seen as transparent and the rectangular regions opaque, sometimes the surface attribute assignments are reversed. In fact, sometimes the four regions appear as they really are—all opaque.

A strong impression of a *depth-induced transparency* can result when two random dot patterns move over each other in different directions. The visual system segregates the dots into two different depth planes, the nearer one appearing to be a perfectly clear, but dotted, transparent surface. An analogous effect can also be produced with a random dot stereogram. The brain seems to interpolate a surface between points of similar depths based on disparity or motion directions and, to be consistent with seeing through the plane, gives the near surface the attribute of transparency. From a physical point of view, this is a form of multiplicative transparency, with only binary valued reflectances and transmittances, which requires depth to be seen.

Diaphanous transparency, or gauzy or sheer transparency corresponds to the case where the holes in a perforated occluder are below the viewer's spatial resolution limit, contributing an additive component to the light shining through. Under everyday viewing, one can have various combinations of film and diaphanous transparency. These combinations should be distinguished from translucency, where scattering hides the spatial structure of the stuff shining through. In a formal sense, additive transparency exists in any low-pass filtered representation of an image of multiple objects. For example, imagine viewing an object through a leafless bush. At low spatial frequencies the object intensities add to those of the bush. Another instance of additive transparency arises because of our limited depth of field. Borders of the images of close objects get smeared over distant objects that are in focus.

For flat surfaces, sharp shadow boundaries are locally identical to multiplicative transparency induced by a dark film overlay (Metelli, 1975). We call this *shadow transparency* to underscore this similarity. Although these cases appear phenomenally quite different—a shadow is an intensity change perceptually attributed to illumination and a dark film is attributed to a surface—some aspects of the underlying computational problems are similar. The simple addition of a fuzzy penumbra to an apparent sur-

face transparency is often sufficient to change the perception to a shadow (figure 15.2). With a more general model of shading where intensity is the vector product of surface normal and illumination direction, computing shadows is quite different from the problem of transparency and requires splitting or factoring the image into vector rather than scalar fields.

From a formal point of view, *occlusion* is the limiting case of zero transparency. There is increasing evidence that occlusion information may be represented fairly early in the visual system (Nakayama, Shimojo & Silverman, 1989). There is also evidence that depth relations inferred from surface transparency must be represented at least at the same level as depth from motion (Kersten, Bülthoff & Furuya, 1989).

Finally, we can see phenomenal transparency even when there is no real or simulated physical cause. We frequently have unfused binocular images when disparity gradients are outside our fusional limits. Most of the time, we do not notice that two different surfaces are actually visible at the same cyclopean point. This *binocular transparency* may be seen when a near surface occludes part of each eye's view. These two surfaces can at various times appear to combine leading to perception of transparency, or to compete for dominance, depending on the circumstances.

Transparency Formation

All of the above cases (except for binocular transparency) can be considered to result from the combination of at least two independent physical processes; for simplicity, we will consider opaque, $R(x, y)$, and transparent, $I(x, y)$ components. For film transparency, $R(x, y)$ and $I(x, y)$ are proportional to reflectance and transmittance, respectively. The image $L(x, y)$ is a function of these two:

$$L(x, y) = f(R(x, y), I(x, y)).$$

This function provides an image *formation constraint*. In general, the image formation constraint is quite complex and requires a complete model of rendering and projection of objects (Magnenat-Thalmann & Thalmann, 1987). An analysis of transparency formation is found in Richards and Witkin (1979). For multiplicative film transparency, the function is the pointwise product of the opaque and transparent components. It is easy to see that in the case of multiplication, the image formation constraint will not necessarily produce an image that looks transparent to us. Any image can be considered the product of an arbitrary nonzero image, and a suitably chosen cofactor. Phenomenal transparency assumes additional nonpointwise constraints on the nature of the substances that produce it. These are *a priori statistical constraints*. One example follows from the cohesiveness of matter. Clumpiness of similar material often produces smooth self-occluding contours. With a multiplicative image formation function, this assumption would produce "X" junctions at the crossings of the clump boundaries in R and I. The crossing of the two X edges will in general produce four intensities. The relations among these four intensities that give rise to the perception of transparency have been studied by Metelli (1974) and Beck, Prazdny, and Ivry (1984).

One simplification made here, and in the computational analysis below is to assume one transparent and one opaque component. Even a simple image could be composed of two transparencies and an opaque surface. For example, two overlapping squares seen in the bottom of figure 15.7 could both be transparent. The human visual system seems to make the default assumption of opaqueness unless there is evidence to the contrary. Even when the transparency is bistable, the dominant percepts alternate between two cases: If one edge of an X junction is seen as transparent, the other is opaque, and vice versa. It is rare to see both edges as transparent. The conditions under which observers report multiple transparencies have yet to be systematically studied.

Transparency Detection

A first and basic level problem is, given an image, does the evidence favor the hypothesis of a transparent surface? The crossing of two boundaries provides one form of evidence for transparency, and has been the only one considered until recently. Given the right figural relations, to a first approximation transparency is seen if the intensities at X junctions satisfy the constraint that the image was caused by multiplicative and/or additive combination of two source images (Richards & Witkin, 1979). More exact models take into account the observation that the visual system is not sensitive to exact metric relations of intensities: rather, it respects the inequality relations derived from such a constraint (Metelli, 1974). Further, under certain conditions, these relations need to be adjusted to allow for compressive nonlinearity be-

tween subjective lightness and physical luminance (Beck et al., 1984)

Can there be local depth information at an X transparency crossing? It is useful to categorize one of the edges in an X junction with respect to qualitative changes of the intensities at the boundary of the other edge (Adelson, personal communication). For concreteness, imagine using a transparent film with a horizontal edge to cover the bottom half of two regions that are separated by a vertical boundary. The horizontal edge is attached to, or "intrinsic" to the bottom region of the image (Nakayama, et al., 1989). One can imagine this bottom film as either preserving or reversing the contrast polarity of the two regions separated by the vertical edge. A contrast-reversing surface does not in general tend to appear transparent, although it is physically realizable by a refractive element. Suppose the horizontal edge is contrast preserving. Then it can either lighten or darken the underling regions, or it could reduce or enhance the contrast at the vertical edge. For example, when the horizontal edge of a neutral density filter crosses the vertical boundary, it darkens the intensity on both sides of this edge. A purely additive transparency lightens both regions that it covers. Of particular interest is an edge that reduces contrast. Specifically, define a contrast-reducing edge to be one that lightens the darker of the two regions it covers, and darkens the lighter without reversing the contrast polarity. If the horizontal edge reduces contrast, there must be a vertical edge that darkens both regions while reversing contrast. Further, the horizontal edge, if considered attached to the top region, is contrast enhancing. This is defined as darkening the darker of two regions it covers, and lightening the lighter without changing contrast polarity. Surfaces attached to contrast-enhancing edges are not likely to be seen as transparent surface discontinuities. This provides a cue to edge attachment. These observations also suggest an ordering cue. In fact, the surfaces attached to contrast-reducing edges, if seen as transparent, tend to be seen in front in a monocular view (see figure 15.7). The above analysis is consistent with how a contrast-reducing edge may be realized physically. The nearer surface may contribute both diaphanous and multiplicative components. Contrast-reducing edges cannot be produced by a simple binary multiplicative or additive operation, but require a combination of both.

In the computational section below, it will be assumed that the combination function is a binary reversible operation as one would find with a purely multiplicative or additive interaction. This leaves ambiguity at X junctions, and places more demands on global computation to decide which edge is in front. If all junctions had a contrast-reducing edge, the computational problem of simple transparencies would be much easier. As pointed out above, the contrast-reducing edge would be a local sign identifying it with the nearer or transparent surface.

Are sharp edges in an X junction necessary to see transparency? Figure 15.3 shows that surface transparency can be seen when a sharp edged figure is overlayed on a smoothly shaded object. X junctions are eliminated altogether in figure 15.4, where depth information from stereo indicates transparency. Transparency can also be seen, if rather than X junctions, we have ψ junctions. in which there is a discontinuity in the derivative of one of the crossing lines. This can be seen in the bottom two panels of figure 15.8 when the center "book" is seen with its outside edges receding from the viewer.

Is an X junction even sufficient for transparency to be seen? Figure 15.5 shows that transparency is not seen if there is only one X junction. If the same X junction is repeated and arranged appropriately, it provides a consistent interpretation of a square transparent surface demonstrating the global nature of transparency perception.

In the computational analysis, the fact that X junctions are not necessary for the perception of transparency will be ignored. It will be assumed that local scene processes produce X junctions. This is not entirely unreasonable, in that occlusion may be treated as a special case of transparency. It will also be assumed that shapes are flat. Factoring out general shape and orientation representations is part of the problem of splitting images into scene attribute maps. Solving the problem of splitting images into two flat components is a first step. The observation that X junctions are neither necessary nor sufficient for the perception of transparency emphasizes the importance of understanding the global factors that cooperate to compute transparency. Even with X junction information locally available, simple local computations do not work to compute transparency.

Contour Binding

A second problem is how to integrate the local evidence to arrive at a global description of each of the multiple

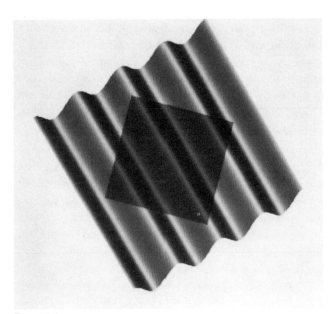

Fig. 15.3
Transparency can still be seen when sharp edges overlap smooth intensity variations.

sources. This can be viewed as a process of perceptual organization in which one tries to globally bind pieces of the image that belong to one object based on a surface attribute. One important factor that contributes to binding is the contour shape. Figure 15.6 shows some examples adapted from Kanizsa (1979) in which the organization into transparent and opaque parts depends on how we segregate contours. A model has to take into account statistical knowledge of how contours typically bend to arrive at an account of the likelihood of the various stable percepts. Of particular importance is the tendency, at an X junction, to assume that a discontinuity in a single physical cause is more likely to be straight than curved. Minimizing an integrated measure of curvature is one way to express this constraint (Kass, Witkin & Terzopoulos, 1987). One problem that arises immediately is deciding whether to bind the four segments at an X junction together, at the cost of high curvature, or to bind pairs of segments (e.g., reflectance and transmittance changes) into lines of low or zero curvature. In the computational section below, curvatures are assigned discrete local probabilities on a fixed lattice using Markov random fields. Multiple lines at a point are allowed only if they have different causes and are thus represented in different intrinsic images. This problem underscores the need to per-

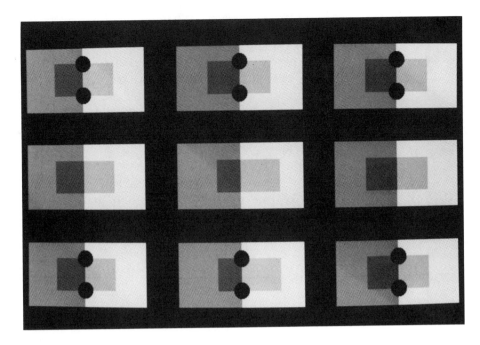

Fig. 15.4
Depth from stereo is sufficient to induce perception of transparency
even when the X crossings are covered by dark patches.

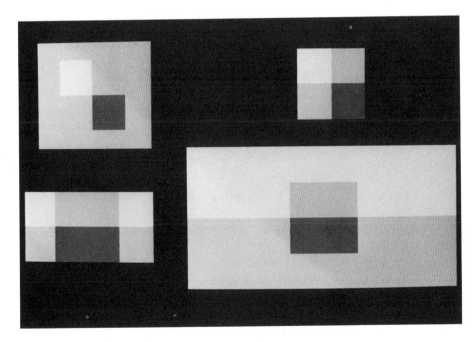

Fig. 15.5
One X junction does not necessarily induce phenomenal
transparency. If a single X junction is repeated and arranged
appropriately, an interpretation of a square transparent surface
emerges. This illustrates the global nature of transparency perception.

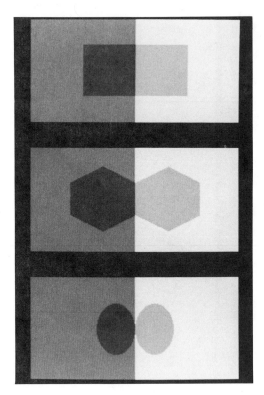

Fig. 15.6
Contours have a perceptual orientation momentum that determines
how they bind across junctions. These demonstrations, adapted from
Kanizsa (1979), show how the strength of apparent transparency
in the presence of these grouping factors. There may also be an effect
of symmetry.

mit multiple edge directions at a point in models of early
edge detection (Zucker et al., 1988).

Attribute Attachment

A third problem is to attach the attribute of opaqueness
or transparency to the surface components factored out.
Sometimes the evidence at an X junction is informative;
for example, contrast-reducing edges tend to be seen as
transparent. If the combination resulted from a symmetric
or commutative operation, and if the local evidence favors transparency, one has a more ambiguous choice. We
have already seen in figure 15.2 that the perception of
transparency can be multistable. Observers report seeing
either the circle as transparent and the two rectangles as
opaque, or the reverse, although there is a strong bias to
seeing the circle as transparent. Observers sometimes see
the entire pattern as it really is—an opaque figure in
fairly uniform illumination—but seldom, if ever, see both
circle and rectangles as transparent at the same time.
When shadow transparency is introduced by simply blurring the vertical edge, the contour of the circle is seen as
an opaque reflectance change on the background, rather
than as a film transparency. A computational model must
take into account both attribute assignment and its multistability. In the computational section, the opaque and
transparent components are represented by distinct spatial maps. The ambiguity is represented by a symmetric
image formation equation.

Depth and Transparency

Perceived depth affects surface attribute attachment. Similar to Mach's observations of the dependence of lightness
on depth, perceived transparency depends on depth. If X
junctions are covered, surface transparency can be seen
with a stereo cue to depth (see figure 15.4). This suggests
that depth, rather than intensity changes, should be the
input to transparency computation; however, figure 15.7
shows that intensity relations can also affect the ability to
see depth from stereo. In a monocular view, the light
rectangular ring is invariably seen in front of the darker
ring due to the presence of a contrast reducing edge.[1] If
disparity cues are used to force the dark ring in front
(seen by fusing the two right-hand panels with crossed
eyes), observers report either rivalry or the rectangles
marking the intersections as appearing opaque. Reaction
times for seeing correct depth relations between two
planes are longer if the observer initially perceives depth
from transparency to be inconsistent with subsequent
depth from motion or stereo (Kersten et al., 1989). Additional evidence of the importance of early transparency
assignment is its apparent affect on motion coherence
(Ramachandran, 1989). Two superimposed square-wave
gratings moving in different directions tend to be seen as
moving in one coherent direction if the superposition is
not seen as transparent.

1. A monocular version of this figure was designed by Edward Adelson and
demonstrated informally at the Cold Spring Harbor Workshop.

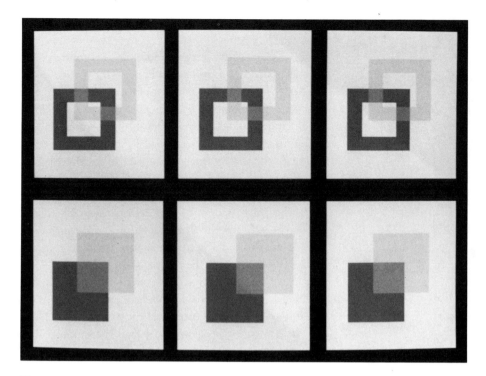

Fig. 15.7

Top, Intensity relations can affect the ability to see depth from stereo. In a monocular view, the light rectangular ring is invariably seen in front of the darker ring. If disparity cues are used to force the dark ring in front (seen by fusing the two right hand panels with crossed eyes, or the left two with uncrossed), one either sees rivalry or the rectangles marking the intersections as opaque. For some observers, the transparency information overrides the disparity information. The effect is not as easily seen in the bottom panel, in part due to the observation that the depth relation between the surfaces is more ambiguous in the monocular view.

Another example of how perceived depth affects attribute attachment is seen in figure 15.8. In the top panel, the central rectangle is easily seen as transparent. The same luminance values when arranged so that they appear to derive from a folded card give rise to an alternative interpretation in the second panel from the top. Here, all the edges seem to be reflectance edges, except for the central vertical edge, which now appears to be due to a change in orientation. Note too how the apparent contrast of the two central regions differs in the two top panels. The apparent contrast is much less for the folded than for the flat card. This is another example of how the estimation of one scene attribute affects the perception of another. The bottom two panels show that if the X crossings are changed to ψ crossings, the central "book like" smaller patches can appear to be either behind transparent larger rectangles, or as an opaque book coming out from the page.

Computation of Transparency

In this section, we will look at the computational problems involved in computing the simplest transparency case—multiplicative combination of just two piece-wise constant components. The goal is to understand computational requirements for estimating the opaque and transparent factors from a single image. It has been argued previously that the Bayesian approach to computing scene descriptions from images provides a quantitative "computational theory" (Kersten, 1987; Marroquin, 1985). The Bayesian estimator can be thought of as an "Ideal Image Understander." It is an extension of the Ideal Observer for detection and discrimination used in early vision (Geisler, 1989) to scene estimation. The Ideal Image Understander makes optimal use of both hard constraints on image formation and soft constraints on the prior likelihoods of scene characteristics.

Bayesian estimation requires three steps: One must specify (1) *the posterior* (or a posteriori) probability of a scene representation conditional on the image data, (2) a statistic representing what one would like to estimate

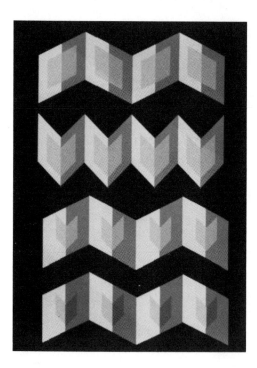

Fig. 15.8
In the top panel, the central rectangle can be seen as transparent. The same luminance values when arranged so that they appear to derive from a folded card give rise to an alternative interpretation in the second panel. Here, all the edges appear as reflectance edges, except for the central vertical edge, which now appears to be due to a change in orientation. This is another example of how the estimation of one scene attribute affects the perception of another, thereby affecting the edge labeling. The third and fourth panels show that the result is not simply a matter of changing the X to ψ crossings. The central patches can be seen as going behind larger transparent rectangles, or as open opaque books.

(e.g., mode or mean) on this distribution, and (3) an algorithm to find this estimate. The posterior probability function embodies statistical knowledge about the world, and the model of how the image was caused. The model will tell us how probable any particular solution is. In particular, it should give low values to those scene interpretations we never see and high and similar values to the (possibly multiple) perceptual interpretations we do see. In our case, we want to find probable scenes, that is, opaque and transparent components, conditional on the image luminance. Below, the largest mode or peak of the posterior distribution is estimated. This is called *maximum a posteriori* or MAP estimation. MAP estimation is optimal in the sense that it minimizes the probability of error. The Ideal Image Understander developed below is defined

to be a MAP estimator of a scene representation conditional on the image.

What is an Ideal Image Understander good for? In general, questions of optimality have to take into account functional goals of the animal or machine, biological or hardware constraints, and processing time. The Ideal Image Understander is only limited by the uncertainty in the information provided and by the simple goal of minimizing classification error without regard for time. It provides an upper bound on the estimation performance of observers or algorithms attempting to achieve the same goal. The Ideal Image Understander makes the useful distinction between the *statistical model* and the *algorithm*. The statistical model is a quantitative statement of the constraints and goal of the computation (parts 1 and 2). In principle, the statistical model can be evaluated as to whether it is right or wrong independent of the specifics of the algorithm. The algorithm is the particular technique used to compute the answer based on the model. There are, in general, many algorithms that can find the MAP estimate for a given problem. But there are countless other algorithms that are suboptimal in the sense that their probability of error is higher. In principle one could make algorithm-independent predictions regarding what are the likely human interpretations of a scene given image data. Modes of the posterior probability should correspond to stable perceptual states. If they do not, then either the brain's algorithm does not locate these modes, or its perceptual model of the scene properties is different from the ideal's statistical model.

The first step of specifying the posterior probability is handled more conveniently if Bayes' rule is used to split the probability into two parts: $p(image|scene)$ represents the image formation constraint discussed above, and $p(scene)$ specifies the *prior* (or a priori) conditions on the scene parameters that we would like to estimate. *Scene* and *image* can be thought of as two very long vectors with the parameters describing a potential scene and its image. The posterior probability is

$$p(scene|image) = \frac{p(image|scene)p(scene)}{p(image)}.$$

The probability also depends on $p(image)$, but this is constant for a given image. One can think of the prior probability model as a procedure that draws sample scene descriptions with the likelihoods specified by the model.

In principle, one could independently try to verify the prior model based on a sample population drawn from the real world. In practice, this may be difficult. Statistical models of scene parameters from real-world data have been sought in only a few cases (e.g., spectral reflectances, Maloney & Wandell, 1986). Suitable mathematical modeling tools are needed to specify the prior model. Markov random fields (MRFs) provide one such tool for specifying prior probabilities of scene parameters represented on a spatial lattice. One of the strengths (and limitations) of MRFs is that they are defined in terms of local, and thus manageable constraints. An MRF is defined in terms of local conditional probabilities on neighborhoods. A neighborhood, N_i, of a site i, is a set of sites not containing the point itself and, further, if the point i is a member of some neighborhood N_j, j must be in the neighborhood of i. An MRF is defined by the rules that (1) the probability of any field (e.g., reflectance map) is positive, and (2) the probability of a site value (e.g., reflectance) conditional on all the other values is equal to the probability conditional on only those values in its neighborhood. Bayesian estimation on MRFs provides a general statistical framework for regularization (Poggio, Torre & Koch, 1985). Many neural net algorithms are doing MAP estimation over MRFs (Golden, 1988). Their limitations are essentially those of regular grammars (Miller, Roysam, Smith & Udding, 1990).

The posterior probability, over an MRF, can be expressed in terms of an energy or cost function E_G:

$$p(scene \,|\, image) \propto e^{-E_G/T},$$

where the energy, E_G, is the sum of terms corresponding to the prior and image constraints (Besag, 1972). The energy is the sum of small local interactions or potentials. Finding modes is equivalent to finding minima of E_G. The T, or temperature, parameter is useful in some applications for expanding and compressing the distribution in a search for modes.

Consider the following energy function for splitting an image into just two components, a transparent and an opaque part:

$$E_G = V_I(\mathbf{I}, \mathbf{l}^I) + V_R(\mathbf{R}, \mathbf{l}^R)$$
$$+ \, \lambda_1 V_L(\mathbf{L}, \mathbf{R}, \mathbf{I}) + \lambda_2 V_E(\mathbf{l}^L, \mathbf{l}^R, \mathbf{l}^I, \mathbf{l}^D).$$

The first two energy terms capture prior statistical assumptions about the cohesiveness of like matter, and include specific terms to constrain contour binding. Only the second two terms depend on the data. The energies can be summed because the probabilities, expressed as exponentials, are independent, and thus multiply. V_R and V_I represent energies for the prior statistical models of the opaque $\mathbf{R}$ and transparent $\mathbf{I}$ vectors, respectively. The opaque and transparent vectors contain the reflectance and the transmittance of the corresponding components. $\mathbf{l}^R$ and $\mathbf{l}^I$ represent *line processes* and are binary vectors representing the discontinuities in the opaque and transparent factors (Geman & Geman, 1984). In the implementation below, horizontal and vertical line processes are placed between vertical and horizontal pixel pairs, respectively. A value of one indicates the presence of a line, and zero its absence. Knowing V_R means that we can assign a global probability to any sample two-dimensional opaque map in our model.

V_L represents the luminance or image constraint. The image luminance vector, $\mathbf{L}$ is a function of $\mathbf{R}$ and $\mathbf{I}$. Each luminance value is determined by the point wise application of the image formation equation. Minimizing V_L encourages the estimate of the image, which is in turn a function of the estimates of the transparent and opaque components, to agree with the measured image data. The exponential of its negative is proportional to the probability of a given image conditional on a scene vector. V_E is an edge data constraint that allows conditional probabilities relating scene discontinuities to image discontinuities (Poggio et al., 1988), and cooperatively couples scene discontinuity estimates from other modules, such as depth. $\mathbf{l}^L$ and $\mathbf{l}^D$ are line process vectors marking image and depth continuities.

λ_1 controls the weight given to the multiplicative image constraint. If $\lambda_1 = 0$, then the product of opaque and transparent components does not have to equal the image luminance to produce a low energy. The noise level in the imaging process determines λ_1. In the simulations, it is assumed that there is no imaging noise, and λ_1 is used for constraint relaxation, and as such it is not a free parameter, but starts small and tends to infinity. λ_2 controls the weight given to the interaction between the discontinuities. In the simulations, it is set to either one or zero, depending on whether the constraint is used or not.

Let us return to the modeling of the prior terms, V_R and V_I. The opaque component is modeled in terms of local conditional probabilities of reflectance values and the invisible line processes between them. Recall that by the definition of an MRF, the conditional probability of a reflectance value, R_i at site i depends only on the values, R_j, of its neighbors, where j is a site in the neighborhood of i. A neighborhood system where each site i has as its neighbors the four nearest pixels is shown in figure 15.9. In particular, the clumpiness of "like matter" would require the central reflectance to have a value near its neighbors. The neighborhood can be broken if a discontinuity, marked by a line process being on, exists between two sites. In simulations, the neighborhood consisted of the four nearest neighbors when there are no line processes turned on.

The prior energy term for the reflectance is determined by the sum of local potentials which are in turn determined by the local conditional probabilities

$$\mathbf{V_R}(\mathbf{R}, \mathbf{l^R}) = \sum_{i,j \in N_i} V_R(R_i, R_j)(1 - l_{ij}^R) + \sum_{C_l} V_{l^R}(l_{ij}^R, l_{kl}^R).$$

l_{ij}^R represents the binary line process between pixels i and j. If equal to one, it knocks out the contribution of the jth neighbor. N_i is the four nearest neighbors of i. In general, a global prior potential is determined by summing local energies for each *clique*. A clique, C, is a single site or a set of sites such that each member is a neighbor of the others. For the four nearest neighborhood system, cliques are either single sites, or nearest vertical or horizontal pairs.

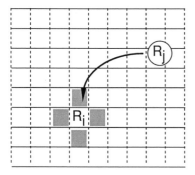

Fig. 15.9
Site i in a Markov random field. Its four neighbors are shown shaded and make up the neighborhood N_i. A smoothness constraint assumes that the probability of the value, R_i, conditional on the four nearest neighbors is higher when it is close to the values of its neighbors. An example of a clique is the pair of sites i and j.

The first sum above is over pairwise cliques. The second sum represents the cost of various contour arrangements. The cliques for line processes (C_l), are slightly more complicated than those for the field (i.e., reflectance or transmittance) values and are discussed below.

The form of the prior potential is based on heuristic judgement. One convenient form is the quadratic potential which encourages smoothness by giving increasingly low probabilities to large differences of reflectance between neighbors[2]:

$$V_R(R_i, R_j) = (R_i - R_j)^2/\sigma^2.$$

For the simulations, the transparency problem is approximately symmetric in both image formation and priors, so the transparent component is similar to the opaque reflectance term

$$\mathbf{V_I}(\mathbf{I}, \mathbf{l^I}) = \sum_{i,j \in N_i} V_I(I_i, I_j)(1 - l_{ij}^I) + \sum_{C_l} V_{l^I}(l_{ij}^I, l_{kl}^I).$$

$V_I(I_i, I_j)$ is also a quadratic potential which, together with the line processes, captures the piecewise smooth characteristic of transparent overlays. In the simulations, $\sigma = 1$ for both reflectance and transmittance potentials.

The line processes represent physical discontinuities in the reflectance (or transparency) function and break the neighborhood determining the local potential as one goes from one type of clump to another. Line processes are also modeled as MRFs. In the simulations here, there are only vertical lines and horizontal lines. Each line has six neighbors. Each line site has a neighborhood structure that enables one to characterize the probabilities of various contour configurations in terms of just local interactions (figure 15.10). For example, two lines of the same orientation are more likely than ones at right angles. One can discourage "T" junctions for transparencies, but not for opaque functions, and so forth. For the clique cases: no lines, a collinear pair, one line, a pair at right angles, three lines and four lines, the values of the potential, V_{l^R}, used for the reflectance line processes were determined from configuration energies: 0.0, 0.0, 2.0, 1.8, 1.8, and 2.0 respectively. The values for the configuration energies of the transmittances, V_{l^I} were: 0.0, 0.0, 3.0, 1.8, 3.7, 3.7. The

---

2. Another example of a local potential is a "smoothed Ising potential"

$$V_R(R_i, R_j) = \frac{-\beta}{1 + (R_i - R_j)^2/\alpha}$$

which, like the quadratic potential, gives high probabilities to similar intensities, but on the other hand, gives nonvanishing probabilities to very large differences in intensity between two neighboring reflectances. It encourages piecewise constant patterns even without line processes.

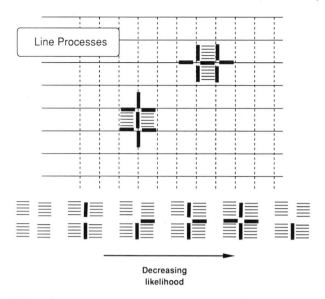

Fig. 15.10

The line processes represent physical discontinuities in the modeled surface property. They have binary values and, when turned on, mark the break in the neighborhood as one goes from one value of surface property to another. Line processes are modeled as Markov random fields with their own prior probability structure. The bottom of the figure shows decreasingly likely configurations as one goes from left (no lines) to right (an isolated line).

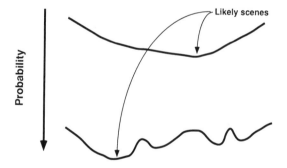

Fig. 15.11

Examples of hypothetical one-dimensional energy functions that are inversely related to some corresponding posterior probability. The horizontal axis indexes the scene attribute map under consideration. *Top,* A convex energy function. Gradient or other descent methods could find the bottom and thus the most likely scene interpretation. *Bottom,* An example with local minima. Each minimum represents either one of several stable perceptual interpretations, or states that may never be "seen" by our hypothetical visual system if the particular algorithm chosen never settles there.

exact values are not critical. The relative weighting is more important. The additional energy for three and four line configurations penalized this sort of junction more heavily for the transparent than for the opaque surface and provided the only asymmetry in the simulations described below.

An additional advantage of making the scene discontinuities explicit is that one can model the interactions between image and scene discontinuities expressed in V_E. Image edges can be coupled to the scene discontinuity estimates and to each other. Shadow edges are transparent and intersect with each other less frequently than occlusion edges. Edges due to shadows or transparency rarely coincide with the other types of discontinuity. On the other hand, edges due to occlusion often coincide with reflectance or texture change. Weights given to these constraints can be embodied in V_E (see tables 15.1 and 15.2).

For multiplicative transparency, the following image formation energy function enforces the constraint that the image be the product of the estimates of the opaque and transparent parts

$$\mathbf{V_L(L, R, I)} = \sum_i (L_i - R_i I_i)^2.$$

It is straightforward to put in alternative image formation constraints.

At this point, one could pause and ask whether the statistical model is any good in the sense that if one plugged in answers, inferred from human perception studies, would these answers be at the global energy minimum? Although one could plug in the solutions that some observer has produced, the remaining problem is to compare these probabilities (or energies) with the Ideal Image Understander's. Unfortunately, it is not always clear when one is at the global minimum. Just because we have an energy function does not mean we understand how to solve the problem (Yuille, 1987). An algorithm is required to find minima.

The Algorithm and Results

To get an intuitive understanding for the nature of the algorithmic problem, figure 15.11 shows hypothetical one-dimensional energy functions to illustrate the kind of problems one encounters when seeking a global minimum. If lucky, the energy function would be like the top panel of figure 15.11, that is, convex. Gradient or other descent methods could get one to the bottom and thus to the most likely scene interpretation. For the transparency problem as formulated here, we have a problem somewhat akin to trying to find the bottom of the curve in the lower panel of figure 15.11, in which there are multiple minima. On the one hand, we do not want to eliminate multiple minima, which are required to represent multistable perceptions; on the other hand, there may be numerous false solutions that are never seen. Two possible approaches are either to try new representations that do not lead to craggy energy functions, or to find brute force algorithmic techniques that work with the existing statistical model. The easier, but less satisfactory, brute force approach will be taken here. The positive lesson will be an understanding of the limitation of local algorithms to deal with a local statistical model. There are several tricks that can be used to search for both global minima, and ones close to it.

Gibbs Sampler with Gradient Descent and Image Edge Constraint

The Gibbs Sampler was originally developed by Geman and Geman (1981). Initially, all the scene estimates are chosen at random. The idea is to draw a sample from the local conditional posterior probability (calculated from the global posterior distribution) at a randomly chosen site. The local probabilities at site i depend on the image intensity, reflectance, and transmittance at that location and the neighborhood values of the reflectance and transmittance. The sampled values of reflectance and transmittance replace the previous values. The order in which the sites are visited does not matter as long as each one is visited "often enough." In the simulation results shown below, the pixels were visited in a raster order. Figure 15.12 illustrates the local sampling part of the algorithm. If the sampling is done with temperature set to zero, the procedure corresponds to gradient descent on the energy function. Zero temperature compresses the distribution around a single point approaching the mode. Figure 15.13 illustrates some results using gradient descent. The top panel of figure 15.13A represents the input data (thickened lines indicate image edge markings). The bottom left and right panels are the initially randomized representations of the opaque reflectance, and transmittance respectively. The thick gray lines between square pixels indicate line processes that are turned on. Figure 15.13B shows

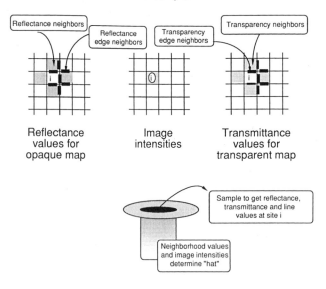

Fig. 15.12
The Gibbs sampling procedure used in the simulations to estimate reflectance and transmittance maps from the data. The opaque and transparent maps are initialized with random values. A site is then selected, a sample is drawn from an appropriate "hat," and used to replace the previous value. Each site is visited in a raster fashion (random asynchronous updating can be used). In general, the algorithm gradually converges to a stable state representing the estimate of reflectance and transmittance consistent with the image intensities. See the text for more details.

how gradient descent quickly leads to a local energy minimum satisfying the image formation constraint. In this example, $\lambda_2 = 0$; that is, there is no image edge constraint.

One problem with this solution is that lines show up in the solution that do not have support from lines in the image. Intensity changes in the image can usefully constrain the search for opaque and transparency edges. If there is an edge in the image, this increases the likelihood that there is either an edge in the opaque component, or one in the transparent component. Further, it is unlikely that both types of edge coexist at a site. The potential for this constraint is

$$\mathbf{V}_E(\mathbf{l}^L, \mathbf{l}^R, \mathbf{l}^I) = \sum V_E(l^L, l^R, l^I).$$

Table 15.1 shows values used for V_E. Figure 15.13C shows the local minimum arrived at using gradient descent with this image edge data potential. Although coming closer to being reasonable, the solution is clearly unsatisfactory as a perceptual interpretation. The solution

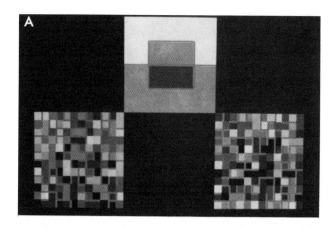

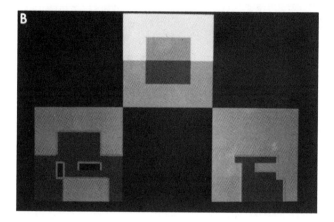

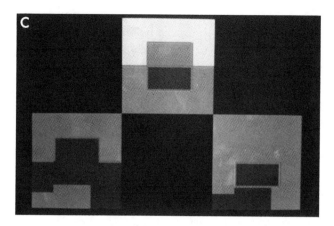

Fig. 15.13
Each of the three panels consists of a triad. The picture at the top of each triad represents the input image data. The original input picture was 12 by 12 pixels, with 64 possible graylevels. The reflectance and transmittance scene maps had 8 levels each. Thick gray lines indicate line processes that are turned on. The bottom left and right pictures of each triad indicate the current estimate of reflectance and transmittance, respectively. (A) The starting configuration for a simulation. (B) The local minimum after 24 iterations of gradient descent. One iteration is completed after all sites have been visited once. (C) A local minimum after 20 iterations, but here scene edges are constrained to have support in the image edges and to not overlap.

Table 15.1
Values of the edge potential (inversely related to probability) for various configurations of edge labels

Image edge	Reflectance edge	Transmittance edge	Potential V_E
1	0	0	1
1	1	0	0
1	0	1	0
1	1	1	1
0	0	0	0
0	1	0	1
0	0	1	1
0	1	1	1

Note: High energies are assigned to unlikely combinations.

again corresponds to a perceptual interpretation that is never seen. Because the input image was constructed by multiplying a known reflectance and a known transmittance, the correct answer is known, and the energy can be calculated. Note that this correct answer may not necessarily correspond to the global minimum of the posterior probability. If the statistical model is wrong, then the global minimum of the posterior probability does not correspond to the correct answer. So even a "perfect" algorithm, such as one capable of an exhaustive search, would find the wrong answer. The energy for the two solutions shown so far is much higher than the correct energy. If the statistical model is correct, this would indicate a local minimum. Additional techniques are needed to avoid monotonic descent of the energy landscape.

Bag of Tricks Search

Even for simple transparencies, reasonable solutions in a few iterations have only been obtained by using a combination of techniques to avoid local minima. These tricks include image edge data (from above), simulated annealing, constraint relaxation, and neighborhood relaxation. The power of each of these techniques was evaluated separately, and none of them provided consistent solutions to the simple transparency shown in the top panel of figure 15.13. The best solutions were obtained when all four techniques are combined into a "bag of tricks." In *simulated annealing*, the temperature parameter, T, is initially set high. For high temperatures, the Gibbs sampler samples from a local distribution with a large variance. This means that sometimes parameters of the scene estimate are chosen that are locally unlikely, but allow escapes from local energy minima. The temperature is gradually lowered until one is doing strict descent on the energy function. In theory, a sufficiently gradual annealing schedule is guaranteed to find the global minimum, but in practice it is too slow (Geman & Geman, 1984). In *constraint relaxation*, one starts off with small values of λ_1, initially ignoring the image formation constraint to find independent samples of opaque and transparent components. This helps to lower extremely high barriers in the energy function caused by hard constraints. λ_1 is gradually raised until the data constraint eventually dominates the energy function.

The principal difficulty is trying to find a global minimum with only local propagation of constraints. The local conditional prior probabilities may in fact be the right ones, from the point of view of the statistical model, but the algorithm is bad because it fails to propagate these local constraints over a wide region, especially with the multiplicity of local rninima in the transparency problem. One empirical trick devised for this problem is *neighborhood* relaxation to initially construct the conditional probability for the Gibbs sampler using an expanded neighborhood. In these simulations, the same number of neighbors are maintained (i.e., four field neighbors and six line neighbors), but in the first iterations they are at distant points. As the iterations proceed, the neighborhood size is contracted. Neighborhood relaxation sketches in a global

solution, and then fine tunes it. It is in the spirit of coarse to fine multigrid techniques (Terzopoulos, 1984).

Figure 15.14 shows results using the Bag of Tricks descent.[3] Part A shows an intermediate stage in the convergence in which the distance between neighbors is two rather than one pixel. Part B shows a solution corresponding to a common perceptual interpretation—a square transparent film overlaying two opaque rectangles. A less common interpretation is to see the pattern as it is—all the edges are reflectance changes, and there is no transparency. The algorithm also finds this solution, shown in part C. With different random starting configurations and the parameters chosen, the algorithm finds four major interpretations. In addition to the two shown, it also tends to converge to the symmetric solutions, namely, in which all the edges are transmittance changes, or where only the central square is a transparent surface.

Even the bag of tricks does not work well for more complicated transparencies such as the one shown in figure 15.15. After many iterations (figure 15.15B), the descent has traveled down a slope distant to any reasonable perceptual interpretation. One, however, can achieve reasonable solutions by incorporating additional sources of depth information. For example, if an independent stereo process has labeled the edges simply according to whether they are at the same depth plane or not, an improved solution is obtained. This constraint is incorporated into a potential term

$$\mathbf{V}_E(\mathbf{l}^L, \mathbf{l}^R, \mathbf{l}^I, \mathbf{l}^D) = \sum V_E(l^L, l^R, l^I, l^D).$$

Table 15.2 shows values of V_E used in the simulations. Figure 15.15C shows results (after 818 iterations) using the Bag of Tricks with an additional depth constraint. The added complexity of a depth constraint may seem premature in that *we* can see the transparent plane in a monocular view, even if the model has difficulty. Eventually, stereo information has to be incorporated into models of transparency, even when X junctions are visible. Figure 15.16 shows a stereo pair of many overlapping

---

3. The constraint relaxation schedule was:

$\lambda_1 = \log(2 + i)/\lambda_0,$

and the annealing schedule was:

$T = T_0/\log(2 + i),$

where i is the iteraction number. Typical values of λ_0 and T_0 were 2 and 4. The neighborhood relaxation started off at a diameter of 12 pixels, and was reduced by one after every four iterations.

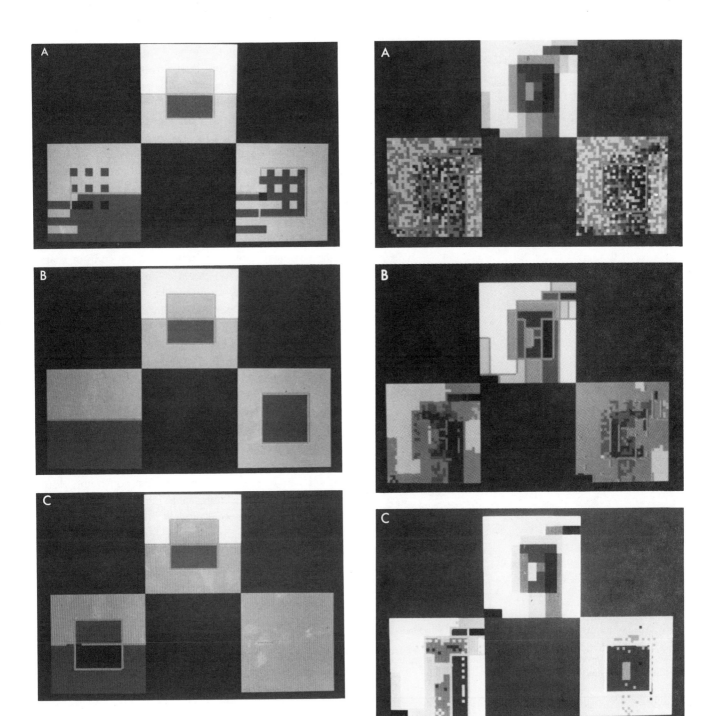

Fig. 15.14
The results of a simulation combining image edge data constraint, an annealing schedule, constraint relaxation, and neighborhood relaxation. (A) The progress of the simulation after 18 iterations. The checkerboard appearance is a consequence of the neighborhood relaxation. Convergence to reasonable solutions is fairly rapid, 20 and 23 iterations for (B), and (C), respectively. Other details are as for figure 15.13.

Fig. 15.15
(A) The starting configuration for a more complicated transparency problem. The transparent surface is a square as in the previous example, but the opaque background is Mondrian-like. (B) Results using the "bag of tricks" after 54 iterations. This simulation never recovered after over 1000 iterations steering down a valley distant from anything remotely resembling what we perceive. A considerable improvement obtains when in addition to the bag of tricks, an edge constraint (see table 15.2) is used to group line elements that are in the same depth. (C) The state of the convergence after 818 iterations.

Table 15.2
Values of the edge potential when depth labels are assigned to line locations

Image edge	Reflectance edge	Transmittance edge	Depth index	Potential V_E
1	0	0	0	1
1	1	0	0	0
1	0	1	0	0
1	1	1	0	1
0	0	0	0	0
0	1	0	0	1
0	0	1	0	1
0	1	1	0	1
1	0	0	1	1
1	1	0	1	0
1	0	1	1	0
1	1	1	1	0
0	0	0	1	1
0	1	0	1	1
0	0	1	1	1
0	1	1	1	1

Note: The depth index serves solely to indicate that line segments are at the same depth plane and not their relative depth.

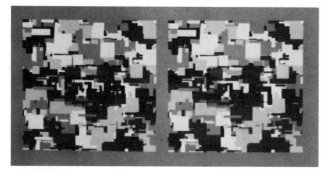

Fig. 15.16
A stereo pair of many overlapping rectangles, some of which are transparent and some opaque. The transparency of many of the rectangles is only apparent when viewed stereoscopically, despite the visibility of X junctions.

rectangles. The observation that some rectangular patches are transparent is only apparent in the stereo view.

Summary

Several new perceptual observations were made that theories of transparency must ultimately have to deal with. The central argument is that perceived transparency is determined by the cooperative computation of distinct scene attributes including depth from stereo, motion or perspective, and the opacity of the surfaces behind. One piece of evidence is the multistability of the perception of the attachment of opacity and transparency attributes to surfaces. A second line of evidence is that not only does the perception of depth affect the perception of transparency, but that perceived transparency can affect depth. The fact that an X junction is neither necessary nor sufficient for the perception of transparency indicates the importance of global computation (depth from stereo is sufficient for the perception of transparency in the absence of X crossings). The prior statistics of the contour shape have a strong affect on the attachment of surface attributes and is explicitly represented in the computation.

The computation section outlined a simplified Ideal Image Understander or Bayesian approach to computing surface transparency. The model was simplified in that it only dealt with multiplicative transparency of flat Mondrian-like surfaces. It was pointed out that a major strength of the Bayesian approach is the separation of the statistical model from the algorithm. Markov random fields provide tools for the statistical modeling of scene attributes that may be useful in the long term. However, because the posterior energy landscape for transparency is extremely rugged when set up in terms of local constraints, local algorithms based on Gibbs sampling may be less useful for computing perceptual models from images—that is, for finding modes of the posterior distribution. Neighborhood relaxation was one new useful technique that helped to overcome this limitation. Incorporating information on depth relations between edges, derived from other sources (e.g., stereo) was another trick that improved the search for modes. There remains a big discrepancy between the Bag of Tricks descent used and human computation of transparency. This gap is left for future research to resolve.

Acknowledgments

This work was supported by NSF grant BNS-8708532 to Daniel Kersten. This research began thanks to time at the Center for Biological Information Processing at MIT, which is supported in part by the Office of Naval Research, Cognitive and Neural Sciences Division, Contract No. N00014-88-K-0164, and in part by the National Science Foundation, Contract No. IRI-8719394. The author would like to thank Norberto Grzywacz, Edward Adelson, Michael Landy, David Knill, and Heinrich Bülthoff for many useful comments and suggestions.

References

Arend, L. E. & Goldstein, R. (1987). Simultaneous constancy, lightness and brightness. *Journal of the Optical Society of America A, 4,* 2281–2285.

Barrow, H. G. & Tenenbaum, J. M. (1978). Recovering intrinsic scene characteristics from images. In A. R. Hanson & E. M. Riseman (Eds.), *Computer Vision System* (pp. 3–26). New York: Academic Press.

Beck, J. (1972). *Surface color perception.* Ithaca, NY: Cornell University Press.

Beck, J. Prazdny, K. & Ivry, R. (1984). The perception of transparency with achromatic colors. *Perception & Psychophysics, 35,* 407–422.

Besag, J. (1972), Spatial interaction and the statistical analysis of lattice systems. *Journal of the Royal Statistical Society B, 34,* 75–83.

Biederman, I. (1987). Recognition-by-components: A theory of human image understanding. *Psychological Review, 94,* 115–147.

Bülthoff, H. H. & Blake, A. (1989). Does the seeing brain know physics? *Supplement to Investigative Ophthalmology and Visual Science, 30,* 262.

Bülthoff, H. H. & Mallot, H. A. (1987). Interaction of different modules in depth perception. *Proceedings of the International Conference on Computer Vision* (pp. 295–305). Washington, DC: IEEE.

Chou, P. B. & Brown, C. M. (1988). Multimodal reconstruction and segmentation with Markov Random Fields and HCF optimization. *Proceedings Image Understanding Workshop,* pp. 214–221. Cambridge, MA: Morgan Kaufmann, San Mateo, CA.

Geisler, W. (1989). Sequential Ideal-Observer analysis of visual discriminations. *Psychological Reveiw, 96,* 267–314.

Geman, S. & Geman, D. (1984). Stochastic relaxation, Gibbs distributions, and the Bayesian restoration of images. *IEEE Transactions or Pattern Analysis and Machine Intelligence, PAMI-6,* 721–741.

Gilchrist, A. L., Delman, S. & Jacobsen, A. (1983). The classification and integration of edges as critical to the perception of reflectance and illumination. *Perception & Psychophysics, 33,* 426–436.

Golden, R. (1988). A unified framework for connectionist systems. *Biological Cybernetics, 59,* 109–120.

Grossberg, S. & Todorović, D. (1988). Neural dynamics of 1-C and 2-D brightness perception: A unified model of classical and recent phemomena. In S. Grossberg (Ed.), *Neural Networks and Natural Intelligence.* Cambridge, MA: MIT Press.

Horn, B. K. P. (1973). On lightness. *MIT Artificial Intelligence Memo,* 295.

Horn, B. K. P. (1975). Obtaining shape from shading information. In P. H. Winston (Ed.), *The psychology of computer vision* (pp. 115–155). New York: McGraw-Hill.

Kanizsa, G. (1979). *Organization of vision.* New York: Praeger.

Kass, M., Witkin, A. & Terzopoulos, D. (1987). Snakes: Active contour models. *International Conference on Computer Vision,* London.

Kersten, D. (1987). Statistical limits to image understanding. Symposium on "Vision: Coding and Efficiency" Cambridge, England. To appear in C. Blakemore (Ed.), *Vision: Coding and Efficiency,* 1990. Cambridge: Cambridge University Press.

Kersten, D., Bülthoff, H. H. & Furuya, M. (1989). Apparent opacity affects perception of structure from motion and stereo. *Supplement to Investigative Ophthalmology and Visual Science, 30,* 264.

Land, E. H. (1959). Color vision and the natural image. Parts I & II. *Proceedings of the National Academy of Sciences, 45,* 115–129, 636–644.

Mach, E. (1886). *The analysis of sensations.* Translated by S. Waterlow from the 5th German edition. New York: Dover.

Maloney, L. T. & Wandell, B. A. (1986). Color constancy: A method for recovering surface spectral reflectance. *Journal of the Optical Society of America A, 3,* 29–33.

Magnenat-Thalmann, N. & Thalmann, D. (1987). *Image synthesis: Theory and practice.* Tokyo: Springer-Verlag.

Marr, D. (1982). *Vision: A computational investigation into the human representation and processing of visual information.* San Francisco: W. H. Freeman.

Marroquin, J. L. (1985). *Probabilistic solution of inverse problems* (A. I. Technical Report 860). Cambridge, MA: MIT.

Metelli, F. (1974). The perception of transparency. *Scientific American, 230,* 91–98.

Metelli, F. (1975). Shadows without penumbra. In S. Ertel, L. Kemmler & L. Stadler (Eds.), *Gestaltentheorie in der modernen psychologie* (pp. 200–209). Darmstadt: Dietrich Steinkopff.

Miller, M. I., Roysam, B., Smith, K. & Udding, J. T. (1990). On the equivalence of regular grammars and stochastic constraints: Applications to image processing on massively parallel processors. AMS-IMS-SIAM Joint Conference on Spatial Statistics and Imaging (A. Possolo, Ed.). American Mathematical Society.

Nakayama, K., Shimojo, S. & Silverman, G. H. (1989). Depth: Its relation to image segmentation, grouping, and the recognition of occluded objects. *Perception, 18,* 55–68.

Plummer, D. J. & Kersten, D. (1988). Estimating reflectance in the presence of shadows and transparent overlays. *Technical Digest, 11,* Optical Society of America, Washington, DC., pp. WQ3.

Poggio, T., Gamble, E. B. & Little, J. J. (1988). Parallel integration of vision modules. *Science, 242,* 436–440.

Poggio, T., Torre, V. & Koch, C. (1985). Computational vision and regularization theory. *Nature, 317,* 314–319.

Ramachandran, V. (1989). Constraints imposed by occlusion and image segmentation. Conference on *Vision and Three-dimensional Representation*, May 24–26, Minneapolis, MN.

Richards, W. & Witkin, A. P. (1979). *Efficient computations and representations of visible surfaces* (AFOSR Report, Contract Number AFOSR-79-0020). Cambridge, MA: MIT.

Terzopoulos, D. (1984). Multigrid relaxation methods and the analysis of lightness, shading and flow. MIT *Artificial Intelligence Memo, 803*.

Terzopoulos, D. (1986). Integrating visual information from multiple sources. In A. Pentland (Ed.), *From pixels to predicates* (pp. 111–142). Norwood, NH: Ablex.

Ullman, S. (1979). The interpretation of structure from motion. *Proceedings of the Royal Society London B, 203*, 405–426.

Yuille, A. L. (1987). Energy functions for early vision and analog networks. *MIT Artificial Intelligence Memo, 987*.

Zucker, S. W., David, C., Dobbins, A. & Iverson, L. (1988). The organization of curve detection: Coarse tangent fields and fine spline coverings. Proceedings 2nd International Conference on Computer Vision. Tarpon Springs, FL.

Part VI

Motion and Texture

Objects of interest in the world almost always move, and even when they do not their images on the retina do, because the head and eyes are never entirely still. It is therefore not surprising that the visual system contains special mechanisms for the analysis of visual motion. These mechanisms have recently been the subject of much study. Adelson and Bergen (1985) described the computation of the *motion energy* content of a spatio-temporal signal, and their formulation has proved to be a very satisfactory way of capturing the behavior of a number of models, and of the early analysis of motion itself.

Surfaces in the world often differ in their "texture," or local average spatial structure, and it has long been known that the analysis of texture is of fundamental importance to the processes by which the visual system segregates objects, and learns about the spatial relationships among objects and their visual surroundings. Though at first blush the analysis of visual texture might not seem to have a great deal in common with the analysis of motion, the formal structure of recent models of texture segregation has a great deal in common with Adelson and Bergen's formal analysis of motion energy. Indeed, this similarity falls simply out of a consideration of these two problems in the plenoptic view, where they emerge as similar problems arrayed along different dimensions: motion in space-time (x-t), texture in two-dimensional space (x-y).

The analysis of visual texture segregation can be accomplished in a fashion similar to motion. It seems that the same machinery used in the initial representation of visual information in multiple spatial channels can also serve as the front end for texture analysis. The essential basis for texture discrimination is a computation of average local spatial structure. The suitably pooled outputs of a family of spatial channels can be used to compute a "texture energy" quantity in a manner almost identical to that used in motion energy formulations.

Each of the chapters in this section describes recent work along these same lines. Grzywacz and Yuille review their work in motion analysis. They are interested in the problem of how multiple motion energy measurements may be combined in order to detect coherent stimulus motion. The chapters by Graham and by Bergen and Landy both elaborate the basic texture energy model in order to account for psychophysical data. Finally, the chapter by Chubb and Landy describes a technique for analyzing the nonlinearity used in the energy computation for spatial texture segregation.

In aggregate, these chapters represent a large step in the direction of unifying the formal treatment of seemingly dissimilar visual problems in a manner foreshadowed in chapter 1 by the presentation of the plenoptic framework for representing visual information.

Reference

Adelson, E. H. & Bergen, J. R. (1985). Spatiotemporal energy models for the perception of motion. *Journal of the Optical Society of America A, 2,* 284–299.

16

Theories for the Visual Perception of Local Velocity and Coherent Motion

Norberto M. Grzywacz and
Alan L. Yuille

Humans can measure local visual velocity with high accuracy. Their error in this measurement is about 5% for velocities ranging from 2°/sec to at least 15°/sec (McKee, 1981; McKee & Welch, 1985). Assuming a 2°/sec velocity and an 80 to 100 msec integration time for accurate velocity discrimination (McKee & Welch, 1985), one can estimate that precise velocity measurements can be made for motions spanning less than 10 min arc. Such short-span discriminations may have at least two advantages from a computational perspective. First, local (and instantaneous) velocity is the most basic information one can extract from any motion. Second, the more localized the measurements are, the better the estimates of motion discontinuities can be. Because local computation of velocity is such a basic function of the visual system, it is tempting to hypothesize that this computation is performed in the primary visual cortex. However, its cells do not seem to detect velocities. Rather, motion-sensitive cells in the primary visual cortex are directionally selective and tuned to spatiotemporal frequencies (Holub & Morton-Gibson, 1981; Ikeda & Wright, 1975; Tolhurst & Movshon, 1975).

But human motion processing is not limited to local computations; the visual system also combines, to its advantage, motion signals from different spatial regions. In particular, the Gestaltists proposed the law of shared common fate. In it, features tend to be perceived as moving coherently (Koffka, 1935). This law is supported by recent psychophysical findings such as motion capture (Ramachandran & Anstis, 1983) and the cooperativity of the motion system (Williams, Phillips & Sekuler, 1986; Williams & Sekuler 1984). Furthermore, these percepts of coherent motion can be justified on two computational grounds. First, if two features are close, then they probably belong to the same object, and thus tend to move together. (Work by Yuille and Ullman [1987] suggests that there is a statistical relation between the smoothness of motion in the image plane and the rigidity of the object in three-dimensional space.) Second, measurements of local motion are not completely accurate, and an integration of motion information over large areas may help to improve the performance.

This chapter summarizes our research on computational theories for the biological measurement of local velocity and for the spatial integration that produces the perception of coherent motion. To make this summary, the chapter condenses the material of papers published elsewhere (Grzywacz, Smith & Yuille, 1989; Grzywacz & Yuille, 1990; Yuille & Grzywacz, 1988a,b, 1989a) with the addition of new illustrations. The chapter keeps some of the essential mathematics of these papers for illustrating the techniques involved. But in many points of the text, the chapter substitutes the mathematical language of these papers by a more physical, intuitive one. We refer the reader to these papers for more detail on the mathematics and on the theoretical interpretations, and for more illustrations.

There are two main sections in this chapter: one dealing with local velocity and the other with coherent motion. The first section introduces a model for the estimation of local velocity that is correct for any pure translation. That section describes theorems on the velocity estimates and shows that the model is generally consistent with cortical physiology. The second section deals with the problem of how to obtain coherent motion information from local velocity measurements, as for example, of the type described in the first section. We present our theory for the perception of coherent motion and prove a number of theoretical results. It is shown that, without further assumptions, the theory provides a solution for problems related to the aperture problem (discussed in the first section). Moreover, the theory agrees with experiments by Nakayama and Silverman (1988a,b) that investigate variations of the aperture problem.

Local Velocity

Models of velocity perception must face the following problem: Motion-sensitive cells in the primary visual cortex do not detect velocities but rather are directionally selective and tuned to spatiotemporal frequencies (for reviews on cortical motion analysis see Andersen & Siegel, 1990; Maunsell & Newsome, 1987; Nakayama, 1985). One can roughly decompose these cell's spatiotemporal

tuning curves into the product of separate spatial and temporal frequency responses (Holub & Morton-Gibson, 1981; Ikeda & Wright, 1975; Tolhurst & Movshon, 1975), although this decomposition does not hold in the cat's area 18 (Bisti et al., 1985; Galli et al., 1988). Further evidence against velocity selectivity and for frequency tuning (Movshon, Davis & Adelson, 1980) is the dependency of single cell's directional tuning on stimulus shape (Hammond, 1979, 1981) and speed (Hammond & Reck, 1981).

Accordingly, physiologically motivated theories use directionally selective frequency tuned filters (Adelson & Bergen, 1985; Poggio & Reichardt, 1976; Watson & Ahumada, 1985) of which the most relevant for this chapter are spatiotemporally oriented (motion energy filters, Adelson & Bergen, 1985). The main computational motivation underlying the use of spatiotemporally oriented filters is that image motion is characterized by orientation in space-time (Fahle & Poggio, 1981; Adelson & Bergen, 1985). There is evidence that cells in the primary visual cortex detect such orientation (Emerson, Bergen & Adelson, 1987a; Emerson, et al., 1987b; McLean & Palmer, 1989).

We introduce a model for the estimate of local velocity from the outputs of motion-energy filters that is correct for any pure translation (see also Fleet & Jepson, 1989; Heeger, 1987). This section describes theorems on the velocity estimates, shows that the model is generally consistent with cortical physiology, and compares the model with that of Heeger (1987). The neural circuitries proposed by the model use to their advantage the wide bandwidth of the primary cortex temporal tuning curves (wide compared to the relatively well-tuned spatial tuning curves). Also, the circuitries profit from the inverse relationship between the optimal spatial frequencies and receptive field size.

The Model's First Stage

The model has two stages: The first measures motion energies (the output of motion energy filters), and the second estimates velocity from these energies. This section describes the first stage.

The starting point for the model is illustrated in figure 16.1 and is the observation that image motion is characterized by orientation in space-time (Adelson & Bergen, 1985; Fahle & Poggio, 1981).

Adelson and Bergen (1985) suggested that one can detect this orientation with spatiotemporally oriented filters. An example of such a filter is the Gabor filter (Daugman, 1985; Gabor, 1946). (This filter comes from the multiplication of a Gaussian function by a cosine or a sine function. The Gabor filter can be thought of as a series of damped oscillations oriented in space or space-time; figure 16.1.) By using complex exponentials to write the sine and the cosine functions ($\exp(ix) = \cos(x) + i\sin(x)$), this filter is

$$F(\mathbf{r}, t : \Omega_r, \mathbf{n}, \Omega_t, \sigma_r, \sigma_t) = \frac{1}{(2\pi)^{3/2}(\sigma_r)^2(\sigma_t)} \exp\left(-\frac{|\mathbf{r}|^2}{2\sigma_r^2}\right)$$
$$\times \exp(-i\Omega_r \mathbf{n}\cdot\mathbf{r})\exp\left(-\frac{t^2}{2\sigma_t^2}\right)$$
$$\times \exp(-i\Omega_t t), \qquad (1)$$

where $\mathbf{r}$ and t are a spatial location in the image and time respectively, $\sigma_r > 0$, $\sigma_t > 0$, Ω_r, and Ω_t are scalar parameters, and $\mathbf{n} = (\cos\theta, \sin\theta)$ is a unit vector parameter. For convenience, we will sometimes combine the spatial magnitude Ω_r and direction $\mathbf{n}$ into the vector $\boldsymbol{\Omega}_r = (\Omega_x, \Omega_y) = \Omega_r \mathbf{n}$.

From equation 1, we model the responses, N, of directionally selective cells in primary cortex to an arbitrary image, $I(\mathbf{r}, t)$. The responses are the absolute value squared of the image convolved with the filter F. (To understand convolution, think of the function F as being the response to a dot of light flashed quickly in position $\mathbf{r}$ at time t. Next, think of the stimulus, $I(\mathbf{r}, t)$, as an infinite set of quickly flashed dots. Then, the total response—the convolution of F and I—is the sum of F an infinite number of times, each time shifted and delayed, and suitably scaled by $I(\mathbf{r}, t)$. In our model, the absolute values of the convolution are squared to give the cells' response.) Formally, these responses are

$$N(\mathbf{r}, t : \Omega_r, \mathbf{n}, \Omega_t, \sigma_r, \sigma_t) = |F(\mathbf{r}, t : \Omega_r, \mathbf{n}, \Omega_t, \sigma_r, \sigma_t) * I(\mathbf{r}, t)|^2, \qquad (2)$$

where * stands for convolution. The definition of response is similar to the one proposed by Adelson and Bergen (1985) who call it motion energy.

To understand to what aspects of the signal such filters are tuned, it is useful to remember that Gabor filters perform something like a localized Fourier transform. While the Fourier transform properties come from the sine and cosine parts of the filter, the localization comes from the

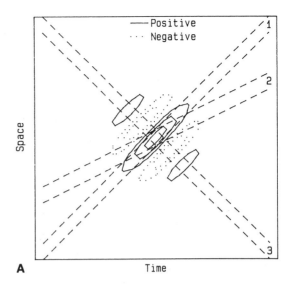

A

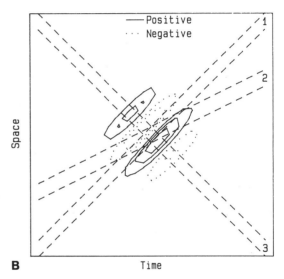

B

Fig. 16.1
Image translation as space-time orientation and its detection by spatiotemporally oriented filters. The figure illustrates the contour plot of the real part (cosine) of a Gabor filter (A) and of its imaginary part (sine—B), and three velocities of a slit of light. The output of the system is the sum of the squares of the filters convolved with the image. Velocity 1 would elicit the maximal output, since it crosses the central positive portion of the cosine filter. On the other hand, velocity 2 is too slow and thus crosses both positive and negative portions of the filters. Finally, velocity 3 has the right speed but the wrong direction, thus again crossing positive and negative portions of the filters.

Gaussian. Thus, the nonlinear filter defined in equation 2 is best tuned to sinusoidal gratings that have: (1) spatial frequency Ω_r; (2) motion direction $\mathbf{n}$; (3) temporal frequency Ω_t. The parameters σ_r and σ_t determine the sharpness of the tunings. Also, it can be shown that these tunings are separable in $\mathbf{n}$, Ω_r, and Ω_t (see for example, Grzywacz & Yuille, 1990).

We suggest a physiological interpretation for the model as follows. The variable N is the response at time t of a primary visual cortex cell, whose center of receptive field lies at position $\mathbf{r}$ in the image. Alternatively, one may interpret N as the sum of the responses of two cells with same preferred direction, but whose spatiotemporal profile is $90°$ out of phase, that is, a quadrature pair (Pollen & Ronner, 1981). The sizes of the receptive field and its temporal window are σ_r and σ_t, respectively. The direction, spatial frequency, and temporal frequency of the sinusoidal stimulus eliciting the maximal response are $\mathbf{n}$, Ω_r, and Ω_t, respectively. Following these interpretations, the analyses below do not assume that σ_r and σ_t are constant for all cells. Cells with large optimal spatial frequency have small receptive field size and vice versa (Andrews & Pollen, 1979; Hochstein & Shapley, 1976; Maffei & Fiorentini, 1977). For generality, and from data appearance (Bisti et al., 1985), we also allow the cells' optimal temporal frequency to increase as the temporal window decreases. Finally, at some stages, the analyses use the assumption that the bandwidth of the temporal frequency tuning curves is relatively wide compared to the spatial bandwidth. More precisely, the assumption states that the speeds are much smaller than the ratio between the spatial and the temporal bandwidths. Informally, it was verified by literature inspection that typically $3 \leqslant (\sigma_r/(|\mathbf{U}|\sigma_t))^2 \leqslant 60$, where $\mathbf{U}$ is velocity.

Because, as discussed above, the tuning of the responses to sinusoidal gratings is separable in $\mathbf{n}$, Ω_r, and Ω_t, it strongly suggests that for moving images the filter (equation 2) is not tuned to any particular velocity.

One filter cannot estimate the velocity, but, as we will show in the next section, the set of filters responding most vigorously can.

Velocity Estimate

This section shows that the largest responses of the motion energy filters as a function of their optimal spatial frequency, optimal temporal frequency, and optimal direction of motion can determine velocity uniquely.

To do so, three theorems and two corollaries are described. The starting point of these mathematical results is the observation that the spatiotemporal power spectrum of a translating image lies on the plane $\boldsymbol{\omega}_r \cdot \mathbf{U} + \omega_t = 0$ in the frequency domain, where $\boldsymbol{\omega}_r$ is spatial frequency and ω_t is temporal frequency (Daugman, 1988; Heeger, 1987; Watson & Ahumada, 1985). This suggests using the combination of the outputs of cells tuned to specific spatiotemporal frequencies to detect this plane. Our results show how to combine these cells' responses in a computationally sensible way.

In words, theorem 1 says: "If one defines primary visual cortical cells by their optimal temporal frequency and two optimal spatial frequencies (the horizontal and vertical components of the optimal spatial-frequency vector), then in this three-dimensional space, for translations, the maximal responses lie on a known plane." (More precisely, the equation describing the plane is $\Omega\mathbf{n} \cdot \mathbf{U} + \Omega_t = 0$.) This result does *not* follow trivially from the knowledge that the spatiotemporal power spectrum of a translating image lies on a plane (Daugman, 1988; Heeger, 1987; Watson & Ahumada, 1985), because this result depends on the filtering properties of the cells. The plane that the theorem refers to is a plane in the space of the cells' parameters. Actually, one can show that filters other than Gabor filters do not have the same property (this is related to the scale-space theorems; Yuille & Poggio, 1986). The theorem is strictly correct only when the receptive field sizes and temporal windows are constant for all cells. However, in theorem 3 and its corollary, we show that this constancy requirement can be relaxed under physiological conditions.

Theorem 2 provides the response distribution in the three-dimensional space defined by the cells' optimal spatial and temporal frequencies. An important corollary of this theorem (corollary 1) shows that if the receptive field sizes and temporal windows are constant, then the responses follow a known Gaussian distribution centered on the plane of theorem 1. (Thus, the claim in theorem 1 follows from this corollary.)

A problem with the above theorems and corollary is that they assume that receptive field sizes and temporal windows do not depend on the cells' optimal frequencies. Fortunately, the following theorem does not suffer from this problem.

Theorem 3 asserts: "If the temporal tuning curves' bandwidths are wide relative to the spatial ones, then irrespective of the receptive field sizes and temporal windows being constant, the response distribution in the optimal-frequency space is of a simple form. This form consists of the product of two functions. The first function depends only on the distance to the plane defined in theorem 1. The second function is completely independent of the optimal temporal frequencies of the cells. It absorbs the spatial characteristics of the image and is independent of velocity." Let us state theorem 3 formally:

Theorem 3.   Given the approximation $|\mathbf{U}|^2 \ll (\sigma_r/\sigma_t)^2$ (see The Model's First Stage for justification), and possibly allowing for arbitrary dependences of σ_t on Ω_t and of σ_r on Ω_r, we find that the response $N(\mathbf{r}, t : \Omega_r, \Omega_t, \sigma_r, \sigma_t)$ is weakly separable in the sense that there exists a function q, independent of Ω_t and σ_t, such that $N(\mathbf{r}, t : \Omega_r, \Omega_t, \sigma_r, \sigma_t) \approx q(\mathbf{r}, t : \Omega_r, \sigma_r) \times \exp\{-\sigma_t^2(\Omega_t + (\Omega_r \cdot \mathbf{U}))^2/2\}$.

A corollary of theorem 3 (corollary 2) shows that under the assumptions of this theorem, in the three-dimensional space of optimal frequencies, the response distributions as a function of temporal frequency have maxima on the plane defined in theorem 1. This means that the overall distribution has a maximal ridge on the plane.

The Model's Second Stage

The previous section suggests that although primary visual cortical cells are not velocity selective, their population responses may be so. We think of these cells as forming a three-dimensional space defined by their optimal temporal frequency and two optimal spatial frequencies (the Ω_r components). If these parameters span sufficiently large ranges, then the cells' strongest responses lie close to the plane $\Omega_r \mathbf{n} \cdot \mathbf{U} + \Omega_t = 0$ for an image translating with velocity $\mathbf{U}$. In cat, these ranges are five to six octaves large (Holub & Morton-Gibson, 1981).

The problem is how to estimate velocity from the combination of the outputs of motion-energy cells (quadrature pairs of directionally selective frequency tuned cells), whose center of receptive field lie in a single spatial location. This locality may be critical for the system's ability to detect motion boundaries in a natural way. (For a broader discussion on some computational, psychophysical, and implementational aspects of this problem see Grzywacz & Yuille, 1990.)

There are many possible strategies for computing the velocities given the results of the previous section, and in this chapter, we discuss three closely related examples.

The Ridge Strategy

This strategy uses corollary 2 as a starting point and proposes to make excitatory connections from each motion-energy cell to the velocity selective cells most consistent with it (figure 16.2). These connections should weakly prefer velocities with small components perpendicular to the preferred direction, so as to give a unique answer for *the aperture problem in the large*. That is to say, if the image motion is consistent with an infinite set of possible velocities, then the smallest velocity is perceived.

Suppose we have a set of M motion-energy cells $(\Omega_r^\mu, \Omega_t^\mu, \sigma_r^\mu, \sigma_t^\mu)$ with $\mu = 1, \ldots, M$. A possible implementation is to define the response, $R(\mathbf{r}, t : \mathbf{U})$, at time t of a velocity selective cell tuned to velocity $\mathbf{U}$, and whose receptive field is centered at position $\mathbf{r}$, by

$$R(\mathbf{r}, t : \mathbf{U}) = A \sum_\mu N(\mathbf{r}, t : \Omega_r^\mu, \Omega_t^\mu, \sigma_r^\mu, \sigma_t^\mu) e^{-(\sigma_t^\mu)^2(\Omega_t^\mu + (\Omega_r^\mu \cdot \mathbf{U}))^2/2}$$

$$\times \; e^{-(\mathbf{U} \cdot \Omega_r^{\mu*}/k)^2}, \tag{3}$$

where Ω_r^* is orthogonal to Ω_r, and A and k are constant parameters.

This equation suggests that the strength of the connection between cell $(\Omega_r^\mu, \Omega_t^\mu, \sigma_r^\mu, \sigma_t^\mu)$ and the velocity selective cell tuned to the velocity $\mathbf{U}$ should be $\exp\{-(\sigma_t^\mu)^2(\Omega_t^\mu + (\Omega_r^\mu \cdot \mathbf{U}))^2/2\}\exp\{-(\mathbf{U} \cdot \Omega_r^{\mu*}/k)^2\}$.

This method is similar to correlation and template matching methods in computer vision. If we fix Ω_r and let Ω_t vary, then from theorem 3, we know that the form of the variation of the filtered response is $\exp\{-\sigma_t^2(\Omega_t + (\Omega_r \cdot \mathbf{U}))^2/2\}$; this defines our template. The largest value of the correlation of this template with $N(\mathbf{r}, t : \Omega_r^\mu, \Omega_t^\mu)$, as we vary the value of $\mathbf{U}$ while fixing Ω_r, gives an estimate for the velocity. To combine the results as Ω_r varies, we simply add the magnitude of the responses for each Ω_r. The factor $\exp\{-(\mathbf{U} \cdot \Omega_r^{\mu*}/k)^2\}$ is designed to prevent the aperture problem in the large (if the image motion is consistent with an infinite set of possible velocities, then the smallest velocity is perceived). The parameter k should be sufficiently large to maintain the validity of the results of the previous section.

A number of velocity selective cells will be excited and the one with the largest response corresponds to the

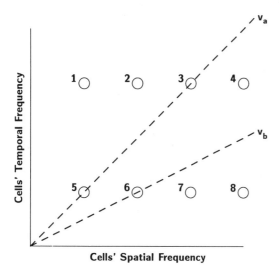

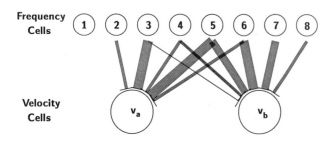

Fig. 16.2
The Ridge strategy. *Top,* The eight open circles represent some sampling locations in the space of the cells' optimal frequencies. Here, the diameters of the circles are not bandwidth. The cross-sections of two velocity planes (corresponding to velocities v_a and v_b) are shown. *Bottom,* How each of the eight cells make excitatory connections to cells tuned to the velocities v_a and v_b. The number of lines in each connection is roughly proportional to the connection's strength. Motion-energy cells, whose parameters are close to a velocity plane make strong connections to the corresponding velocity cells. Otherwise, if the motion-energy cells are far from the plane, then the connections are weak. A part of the model not illustrated here is a winner-take-all mechanism to choose the strongest velocity cell. Also, we do not show the implementation of the solution to the aperture problem in the large (equation 3). As it will be illustrated by the simulation in figure 16.4, only two temporal frequencies are, in principle, necessary.

velocity estimate. A winner-take-all mechanism (Feldman & Ballard, 1982; Koch & Ullman, 1985; Yuille & Grzy-wacz, 1989b) may then select the maximally responding cell.

This method is local, parallel, and instantaneous, gives the right answer for arbitrarily dense sampling, and degrades well as the sampling becomes more sparse.

The Estimation Strategy

This strategy is only sketched here. The strategy attempts to estimate the image's spatial characteristics and compute the velocity simultaneously by minimizing a goodness-of-fit criterion. Theorem 3 underlies this strategy, by providing the form of the variation of the motion-energy cells' response distribution in the Ω_t direction. If one places several cells on the same line in this direction, then one can estimate the distribution on this line obtaining measurements for velocity computations. Without such an alignment the problem would be ill posed, since with only a finite number of cells, there would be insufficient information to estimate the signal and the velocity.

This method is local, can be implemented in parallel, is instantaneous, gives the correct answer even for a finite number of cells (in principle), and should degrade well with noise.

The Extra Information Strategy

This strategy uses the outputs of purely spatial frequency tuned cells to calculate the spatial characteristics of the image. This information can then be used to modify the estimation strategy by giving estimates for the form of $q(\Omega_r)$.

Comparison with Heeger's Method

This section compares our model to the elegant method presented by Heeger (1987).

In general, Heeger's method gives accurate velocity estimates for translating textured patterns, some sine-grating plaid patterns, and natural textures, and appears to simulate psychophysical data on the coherence of sine-grating plaids (Adelson & Movshon 1982).

However, we see three main problems with Heeger's model.

The first problem is that it assumes, and works best with, images with a flat power spectrum. This assumption will lead to incorrect velocity estimates for several images. Our method, however, does not suffer from this assumption and estimates velocity correctly for a greater variety of stimuli (see Velocity Estimate).

A second problem with Heeger's method has to do with his spatiotemporal integration of motion energies. The range of his spatial integration is not limited to the cells' receptive field size but also spans across cells whose centers of receptive field lie in different spatial locations. A manifestation of this problem is the smoothing that occurs when the integration windows straddle motion boundaries (Heeger, 1987). As we have shown, this type of integration is unnecessary to compute velocities. We argue that there is no computational rationale to integrate motion energies over space as his method does. In contrast, our method computes local velocity estimates (for example, equation 3), and thus allows for integration methods that have explicit computational rationale (see Coherent Motion, below, and also, Bülthoff, Little & Poggio, 1989; Hildreth, 1984).

Finally, our weakest objection to Heeger's method is to the suggestion that his proposed parallel implementation of his method is a model for MT (middle temporal visual area) cells. The method uses mathematical operations that may not be easy to implement biologically (Grzywacz & Koch, 1987; Grzywacz & Poggio, 1989; Ratliff, 1965; compare to The Model's Second Stage).

Comparison with Primary Visual Cortex

The behavior of the new model accounts qualitatively for some of the data obtained from directionally selective cells of the primary visual cortex. Elsewhere (Grzywacz & Yuille, 1990), we show that the model may explain the rough decomposition of these cells' spatiotemporal tuning curves into the product of separate spatial and temporal frequency responses (Holub & Morton-Gibson, 1981; Ikeda & Wright, 1975; Tolhurst & Movhon, 1975). Also, in that same paper, we show that the model accounts for the facilitation and suppression for responses to apparent motions in the preferred and null directions respectively (Emerson et al., 1987a,b).

In this section, we discuss an example that illustrates the qualitative agreement between the model and primary visual cortical data: the dependence of the directional tuning on the stimulus shape and speed.

The directional tuning of directionally selective complex cells tends to be unimodal when stimulated with bars or low speed dot textures but bimodal for high speed dot textures (Hammond, 1979, 1981; Hammond & Reck, 1981). Whenever this tuning is bimodal, the two preferred directions are distributed symmetrically about the bar's preferred direction.

This section shows that the model accounts for these observations. Our results confirm the arguments of Movshon and colleagues (1980) that these phenomena are consistent with spatiotemporal frequency tuned cells. Their idea starts with the observation that dots have Fourier components in all directions. Furthermore, the speed of a given component for a moving dot decreases with this component's angle with the direction of motion. Thus, if a dot moves fast, then to elicit maximal response from a given spatiotemporal filter, the dot should not move in parallel to the filter's best direction. This is because in that case, the optimal Fourier component for the filter can move at the optimal speed. However, if a dot moves slowly, then it should move in the best direction of the filter, so that the optimal Fourier component has the best possible, though not optimal, speed. A potential problem with these arguments is that they do not take into account the contributions of nonoptimal Fourier components. Our results show that this problem can be neglected.

For the sake of simplicity, we use sine gratings instead of bars and single dots instead of dot textures. Also, the results below assume that σ_r and σ_t are constants.

Direct calculations demonstrate that the best direction for the sine grating is approximately the direction of the filter's orientation, $\mathbf{n}$ (figure 16.3).

Consider now a dot travelling with constant speed. (The "shape" of the dot is conveniently represented by $\delta(x)$, the Dirac delta function. This function is the limit of the Gaussian distribution when its standard deviation goes to zero. One can think of the delta function as an infinitesimally narrow function with infinitely high amplitude. The narrowness and the amplitude compensate each other such that the function's integral is equal to unity. This function is ideal to represent a dot, because ideal dots are infinitesimally narrow and because they need nonzero total amount of light contrast to be visible.)

$$I(\mathbf{r} - \mathbf{U}t) = I_1 \delta(\mathbf{r} - \mathbf{U}t). \tag{4}$$

For simplicity, we give the response of the cells for which the dot passes through the center of their receptive field,

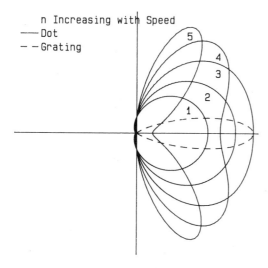

n Increasing with Speed
——Dot
– –Grating

Fig. 16.3

Dependence of single cells' directional tuning on stimulus shape and speed. These polar plots are directional-tuning curves of the responses of a motion-energy cell to translating sinusoidal gratings (Grzywacz & Yuille, 1990) and dots (equation 5). The plots are such that the cell response and stimulus direction correspond to the distance from the origin and angle, respectively. The optimal direction for the grating and the dots moving slowly is identical. However, when the dots move fast the directional tuning curves become bimodal with their lobes being symmetrical about the grating's best direction.

and for the time t at which the dot is at this center

$$N(\Omega_r, \mathbf{n}, \Omega_t, \sigma_r, \sigma_t)$$

$$= \frac{\sigma_r^2 \sigma_t^2}{\sigma_r^2 + \sigma_t^2 \mathbf{U}^2} e^{-(\sigma_r \sigma_t)^2 (\mathbf{U} \cdot \mathbf{n} \Omega_r + \Omega_t)^2 / (\sigma_r^2 + \sigma_t^2 \mathbf{U}^2)}. \quad (5)$$

One can show that for other trajectories and times this section's conclusions will be the same. By differentiating this equation with respect to the direction of motion, one finds that the extrema of $N(\Omega_r, \mathbf{n}, \Omega_t)$ occur when

$$(\mathbf{U} \cdot \mathbf{n} \Omega_r + \Omega_t) \mathbf{U}^* \cdot \mathbf{n} \Omega_r = 0, \quad (6)$$

where $\mathbf{U} = |\mathbf{U}|(\cos \phi, \sin \phi)$ and $\mathbf{U}^* = |\mathbf{U}|(-\sin \phi, \cos \phi)$. By substituting back into equation 5, one can determine that these extrema are maxima.

Thus, the dot's and sine's best directions are similar when the dot moves slowly, but the dot's tuning is bimodal for high speeds (figure 16.3). If $|\mathbf{U}| \leqslant |\Omega_t/\Omega_r|$, then only $\mathbf{U}^* \cdot n = 0$ satisfies equation 6, implying that $\mathbf{U}$ is in the direction $\mathbf{n}$. However, if $|\mathbf{U}| \geqslant |\Omega_t/\Omega_r|$, there exist two preferred directions symmetrical about $\mathbf{n}$ satisfying $\mathbf{U} \cdot \mathbf{n} \Omega_r + \Omega_t = 0$, with $\mathbf{U}^* \cdot n = 0$ now determining a minimum.

Comparison with the Middle Temporal Visual Area

We now discuss how the new model may account for the detection of velocity in the middle temporal visual area (MT). The results of this section use the complete model, including the outputs of the motion energy filters (equation 2) and the combination of these outputs (see The Model's Second Stage). This is different from what was done in Comparison with Primary Visual Cortex (see earlier), which only required the motion energy filters.

Movshon, Adelson, Gizzi and Newsome (1985) distinguished between two classes of directionally selective cells in monkey's MT: component cells and pattern cells (see also Rodman & Albright, 1989).

The component cells respond to the motion direction of single oriented contours but not of complex patterns. For these patterns, these cells only respond when an oriented portion of the patterns moves perpendicularly to the cell's preferred orientation. All primary visual cortical cells are of the component type and about 40 percent of MT cells appear to belong to this class.

The pattern cells respond both to the direction of motion of single oriented contours and of complex patterns. These cells appear to represent about 25 percent of MT cells. The other 35 percent of MT cells cannot be clearly classified as either component or pattern cells. Movshon and coworkers (1985) argue that this ambiguity is mostly due to the statistical insensitivity of their methods. However, it is possible that other classes of cell exist.

To distinguish between these cell types, researchers (Movshon et al., 1985; Rodman & Albright, 1989) measured the difference in response to moving sinusoidal grating and sinusoidal plaid stimuli. (The latter is the sum of a pair of crossed sinusoidal gratings.) The component cells' directional tuning was bimodal for the plaids. The optimal directions roughly occurred when the plaid gratings were perpendicular to the cells' preferred direction as determined by single gratings. On the other hand, the optimal direction of the pattern cells for the plaid were approximately coincident with that of the single gratings.

We now show that the motion energy filters (equation 2) behave like component cells, while the filters' combination by one of the strategies presented earlier behave like pattern cells.

We use plaids that are the superposition of two orthogonal sine wave gratings travelling with the same velocity $\mathbf{U}$:

$$I(\mathbf{r} - \mathbf{U}t) = I_1 \sin(\Lambda\xi \cdot (\mathbf{r} - \mathbf{U}t)) + I_1 \sin(\Lambda\xi^* \cdot (\mathbf{r} - \mathbf{U}t)),$$
(7)

where Λ is the gratings' spatial frequency, and ξ and ξ^* are the gratings' directions. The time-averaged response is is a linear combination of Gaussians centered on $(\Omega_r, \Omega_t) = (\Lambda\xi, -\Lambda\mathbf{U} \cdot \xi) = (-\Lambda\xi, \Lambda\mathbf{U} \cdot \xi) = (\Lambda\xi^*, -\Lambda\mathbf{U} \cdot \xi^*) = (-\Lambda\xi^*, \Lambda\mathbf{U} \cdot \xi^*)$. Because these Gaussians are centered on the plane $\Omega_r \cdot \mathbf{U} + \Omega_t = 0$, any of the strategies discussed earlier will yield the true velocity.

Figure 16.4 plots the directional tuning curve to the plaid (equation 7) of a component and a pattern cell assuming the Ridge strategy. The optimal directions in these tuning curves agree with those recorded in MT (Movshon et al., 1985; Rodman & Albright, 1989). The directional tuning is sharper for component than for pattern cells coinciding with the sharper tuning in the primary visual cortex when compared to MT. This raises the possibility that primary visual cortical cells feed directly into pattern cells without using as intermediate the MT component cells (like scheme A in figure 9 of Rodman & Albright, 1989). Also, the tuning difference in figure 16.4 might be reduced by a mutual inhibitory network implementing a partial winner-take-all mechanism (Yuille & Grzywacz, 1989b).

Finally, the model also appears to be consistent with the finding that type II cells in Albright's classification of MT cells (Albright, 1984) correspond to the pattern cells (Rodman & Albright, 1989). The property characterizing type II cells is that their preferred direction for moving spots and preferred orientation for stationary slits are parallel. Our model accounts for the correspondence between type II and pattern cells as follows. Because the slits are stationary, they would activate pattern cells in MT through motion-energy cells tuned to low temporal frequencies. The only such cells consistent with a given velocity vector are those tuned to gratings parallel to it. This is because these are the only gratings not expected to move. Thus the best stationary slits are those whose Fourier components are parallel to the pattern cell's preferred direction. This explanation is essentially the same one that was provided by Rodman and Albright (1989).

Discussion: Local Velocity

We presented a model for cortical motion computation which provides a new interpretation for MT cells: They might be trying to compute velocity rather than trying

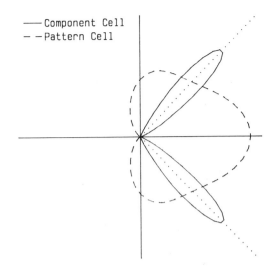

— Component Cell
- - Pattern Cell

Fig. 16.4

The directional tuning curve of the responses to the plaid of a component and a pattern cell. These polar plots have the same convention as in figure 16.3. The component cells respond mainly when one of the gratings composing the plaid moves in parallel to the cell's preferred direction (to the right; Grzywacz & Yuille, 1990). This occurs when the plaid moves parallel to the dotted lines. The pattern cells' responses were simulated by using the Ridge strategy without a winner-take-all mechanism and with only two temporal frequencies (see The Model's Second Stage). The directional tuning is sharper for component than for pattern cells, coinciding with the sharper tuning in the primary visual cortex when compared to MT. This tuning difference might be reduced by a mutual inhibitory network implementing a partial winner-take-all mechanism (Yuille & Grzywacz, 1989b).

to solve the aperture problem (see discussion below), as commonly thought. The model, which is qualitatively consistent with physiology, postulates two stages for cortical velocity estimation. The first stage measures motion energies (Adelson & Bergen, 1985) from the moving stimulus, and the second estimates velocity from these energies. Primary visual cortex cells or MT component cells might implement the first stage (Movshon et al., 1985; Rodman & Albright, 1989). The intuition for how the second stage combines the first stage outputs is similar to that suggested by McKee, Silverman, and Nakayama (1986). The model would yield arbitrarily correct velocity if the sampling of spatiotemporal frequencies by the first stage was arbitrarily dense. Evidence for high density measurements for spatial frequencies has been provided (Silverman, Grosof, De Valois & Elfar, 1989).

The model's second stage computes velocity *locally* from the motion-energy distribution across first stage cells, and thus may explain (see also Adelson, 1987; Fleet & Jepson, 1989) the perhaps related phenomena of motion transparency (Adelson & Movshon, 1982) and discontinuities (Anstis, 1970). The computation uses only motion-energy cells whose receptive field centers lie in a single spatial location. It two different motion fields are adjacent, then a bimodal distribution of motion energies is generated, implying two velocities (figure 16.5). Bimodal distributions would also occur in motion transparency (figure 16.5). To detect two velocities from these bimodal distributions, the Ridge strategy (see above) might use a *local* winner-take-all mechanism. (Such a mechanism is consistent with the inhibition of pattern cells when stimulated with a motion not parallel to their preferred direction; Movshon, personal communication.) However, it is possible that the brain uses a *global* winner-take-all strategy. In this case, with no winner in MT, another visual pathway might compute velocities directly from the primary visual cortex. An alternative is that with a global winner-take-all mechanism the winners would switch transiently between themselves as the image changes leading to the perception of transparency. Schemes that integrate velocity signals (see Coherent motion, below; Bülthoff et al., 1989; Hildreth, 1984) may have to do so by segregating velocities that differ locally.

Why do we say that the model works locally despite the theorems' assumption that the velocity is constant over the whole image? The reason is that in practice this assumption can be greatly relaxed for the following reason: Because the cells have essentially a limited spatio-temporal range, determined by σ_r and σ_t, the velocity only needs to be constant over this range. Thus the model provides good velocity estimate almost everywhere for classes of motion, such as rotation or expansion, that can be locally approximated as translation.

We will now discuss one assumption of the model's first stage that is probably incorrect in physiological details: Gabor filtering (equation 1). This incorrect assumption follows from the modeling of cell responses by simple mathematics instead of realistic biophysics (Grzywacz & Poggio, 1989). However, our main idea, the combination of motion-energy filters, seems to be conveniently modeled by this chapter's methods.

The Gabor function is, strictly speaking, the only filter for which we can guarantee that the extrema of responses in the cells' optimal-frequency space lie on a ridge (unpublished calculations). This is due to the fact that the

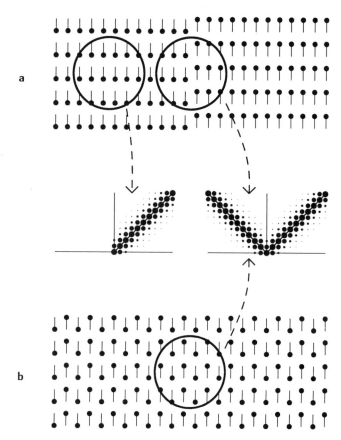

Fig. 16.5

Transparency and motion discontinuities. (A) Two adjacent fields of dots moving in opposite directions, thus forming a boundary of motion discontinuity. (B) Two superimposed fields of dots moving in opposite directions, thus forming a region of motion transparency. The diameters of the circles represent the receptive field sizes of motion-energy cells. If such cells are near the discontinuity or are seeing motion transparency, then the motion-energy distribution for these cells lie around two planes (the graphs are cross-sections of the motion-energy distributions). Otherwise, if there is only one motion field on these cells' receptive fields, then the motion energies lie around a single plane. To detect two velocities from the above bimodal distributions, the Ridge strategy (see The Model's Second Stage) might use a local winner-take-all mechanism. Schemes that integrate velocity signals may have to do so by segregating velocities that differ locally.

Gaussian is the only separable rotationally invariant function. If, however, the filters are similar, but not exactly, like Gabors, then we expect the results described in the Model's First Stage to be true most of the time. This expectation is confirmed by the velocity computation in real images with filters that were built by a self-organizing developmental model, and which resemble Gabor functions only roughly (Yuille & Cohen, 1989).

To what extent are Gabor functions good models of the properties of primary visual cortex cells? Some researchers suggest that these functions model well the receptive field structure in cat (Jones & Palmer, 1987). Also, physiologically plausible models that resemble spatiotemporal Gabor filters have been advanced (Adelson & Bergen, 1985). However, there are at least three problems with Gabor models. First, they predict that the cells' spatial tuning curves follow a Gaussian function. However, the data show that these tuning curves often follow a lognormal function (Gaussian when plotted on a logarithmic scale; Gaddum, 1945; Holub & Morton-Gibson, 1981), with typically more than 85 percent of the area under the curves being for spatial frequencies higher than optimal. Such lognormal behavior might be significant, since it would naturally provide the scaling properties necessary for good velocity estimates. If tuning curves are lognormal, the frequency range of a cell is proportional to its optimal frequency. An alternative to Gabor models that would have the same scaling property are wavelet models (Grossmann & Morlet, 1984; Mallat, 1988). Second, the Gabor filter temporal part is noncausal, that is, since it is not zero for negative times, it uses future information in its computations. A filter, whose temporal tuning curve is lognormal, as in cortical cells (Holub & Morton-Gibson, 1981), might correct this problem (typically more than 99 percent of this tuning curve occurs for temporal frequencies higher than optimal). On the other hand, the noncausality may also imply that velocity computation is not "on-line," a delay that is consistent with the temporal integration necessary to estimate velocity accurately (McKee & Welch, 1985; Nakayama & Tyler, 1981; Regan & Beverly, 1984). Third, using a Gabor filter implies an initially linear mechanism, which is not always supported by experiments (Emerson & Citron, 1988; Reid & Shapley, 1988). One neural mechanism that destroys the linearity of the cells is ON-OFF rectification. Another neural nonlinearity that may have a role in velocity computations is shunting inhibition, which seems to account for *retinal* directional selectivity (Amthor & Grzywacz, 1991; Marchiafava, 1979; Torre & Poggio, 1978).

Our final argument in this section is that biological motion perception may use at least three stages; two for velocity estimation and at least one more to deal with coherent motion (see below). The first two stages are similar to those proposed by Adelson and Movshon (1982; Movshon et al., 1985), although we suggest a

different role for these stages than they do. Direct psychophysical evidence for two stages in the computation of velocity has recently been given (Welch, 1989). Interestingly, in theory, velocity estimation requires only one stage (Verri, Girosi & Torre, 1989).

We suggest that the primary visual cortex and MT represent two stages needed to estimate velocity, and argue, contrary to Movshon and colleagues (1985), that MT is not concerned with the aperture problem. To do so, we first define what we mean by the aperture problem. It is the impossibility to measure locally velocity components other than that parallel to the luminance gradient (Marr & Ullman, 1981). Movshon and coworkers postulate that the role of the primary visual cortex is to analyze motions of one-dimensional patterns. These researchers also advance the idea that MT solves the resulting aperture problem. In particular, they propose a model assuming that primary visual cortex cells compute the *velocity normal* to one-dimensional patterns. This proposition is consistent with the finding that primary visual cortex cells are "velocity selective" for moving bars (Baker, 1988; Movshon, 1975; Orban, Kennedy & Bullier, 1986). As a curiosity, our model predicts this selectivity (unpublished calculations). However, the receptive field size of primary visual cortex cells is typically larger than regions of the visual world where significant curvature and texture exist. Thus these cells have to deal with two-dimensional patterns. Under these conditions, the assumptions of Movshon and colleagues lead to incorrect estimates of velocity. We suggest that the primary visual cortex does not assume a one-dimensional visual world. Thus we argue that the role of MT is to compute local velocity without having to deal with the aperture problem. It is tempting to identify the speed selective cells found in MT (Newsome, Gizzi & Movshon, 1983) with its pattern cells (Movshon et al., 1985; Rodman & Albright, 1989). A problem with this identification is that studies with sinusoidal gratings suggest that it applies only to a small percentage of MT cells (Movshon, personal communication). However, one must be careful in interpreting results from sinusoidal-grating experiments, since they may, for two reasons, represent poor stimuli for the pattern cells. The first reason is that sinusoidal gratings are one-dimensional and the pattern cells may not be designed to solve the aperture problem in the large (see The Model's Second Stage). The second reason is sinusoidal gratings may stimulate effectively very few of the motion-energy cells, leading to signal-to-noise problems. The facilitatory interaction between component cells (Ferrera & Wilson, 1987; Movshon, personal communication) emphasizes that a good stimulus should probably comprise several Fourier components.

At least one more motion-processing stage is needed to deal with another problem, which is related to the aperture problem. This new problem occurs when objects larger than the receptive field size of MT cells move. In this case, the cells may compute different velocities for different portions of these objects. Nevertheless, as discussed in the introduction, it is often important to assign a global motion to the objects. The solution for this coherence problem requires a motion-processing stage, which might occur in later cortical areas (Saito, Yukio, Tanaka, Hikosaka, Fukuda & Iwai, 1986; Tanaka, Hikosaka, Saito, Yukie, Fukada & Iwai, 1986) that perform spatial integration over large receptive fields. The next section discusses our computational theory for the perception of coherent motion.

Coherent Motion

The previous section dealt with the problem of how local velocity might be estimated in the visual cortex. In this section, we take one step forward and ask how the visual system might extract coherent motion information from local velocity measurements.

Until recently, coherent motion percepts were not fully accounted for by the extant theories of visual motion. These theories were limited, since they did not integrate local measurements (e.g., Adelson & Bergen, 1985), they integrated motion only when the measurements were dense (e.g., Hildreth, 1984; Horn & Schunck, 1981), or they did not reward coherence (e.g., Ullman, 1979). These limitations, however, do not exist in three new theories that emphasize motion coherence: that of Bülthoff and colleagues (1989), that of Reichardt, Egelhaaf, and Schlögl (1988), and ours (see below).

In this section, we present our theory for the perception of coherent motion, discuss the relationship with other theories, and prove a number of theoretical results. We call this theory the motion coherence theory. It is shown that, without further assumptions, the theory provides a qualitative solution for the problem of coherence discussed at the end of the last section (related to the

aperture problem). Moreover, the theory agrees with experiments by Nakayama and Silverman (1988a,b) that investigate variations of the aperture problem, and which are not easily explained by current theories.

Throughout most of this section, the theory assumes that motion discontinuities do not exist. However, in a later subsection, we discuss possible extensions of the theory that deal with motion discontinuities, including an extension consistent with the mechanism illustrated in figure 16.5. Two other extensions of the theory appeared elsewhere, one incorporating temporal integration (Grzywacz et al., 1989), and another accounting for long-range apparent motions (Yuille & Grzywacz, 1989a). These extensions provide generalizations to the minimal mapping theory for long-range apparent motions (Grzywacz & Yuille, 1988; Ullman, 1979). This theory, which is largely successful, fails to explain inertial effects of motion history (Grzywacz, 1987) and spatial interactions between neighboring motions (Grzywacz et al., 1989).

The Theory

The theory divides the computation of motion into two stages; the measuring and the smoothing stages. In the measuring stage, motion is measured locally as in any of the previous theories of visual motion. One example of such a theory is the mechanism for the measurement of local velocity described in Local Velocity. In the smoothing stage, a velocity field is constructed over the entire visual field; even where no estimates of motion have been made. It is postulated that this velocity field obeys, as strictly as possible, the restrictions found in the measuring stage and, simultaneously, is as smooth as possible. These requirements force the velocities of neighboring features to be similar, while "respecting" the restrictions of the measuring stage.

We now present the theory formally. Let the velocity measurement obtained by the measuring stage at point $\mathbf{r}_i$ be $M(\mathbf{U}_i)$, where $\mathbf{U}_i$ is the true image velocity. The measurement operator M will depend on the measurements. If for example, isolated pointlike features move, then both their velocity components may be measured. For contour motion, on the other hand, the measurements may correspond to the normal component of the velocity field along edge contours. The following sections discuss three examples of the operator M.

The motion coherence theory proposes that the smoothing stage constructs a velocity field, which we denote $\mathbf{v}(\mathbf{r})$. A way to force this field to obey the restrictions found in the measuring stage is to postulate that the differences between the measured and constructed fields are small at the points of measurement. Mathematically, it is convenient to express this requirement as the minimization of $\sum_i (M(\mathbf{v}(\mathbf{r}_i)) - M(\mathbf{U}_i))^2$. Besides obeying this motion-measurement requirement, the constructed field must also be as smooth as possible. Smoothness implies that the field should have few or no sharp changes. In mathematics, this is achieved by saying that the derivatives (of first or higher orders) are small. One may enforce such a requirement over the entire space by minimizing the integrated values of all derivatives, $\int \sum_{m=0}^{\infty} c_m (D^m \mathbf{v})^2$, where $c_m > 0$ are constants and D are two-dimensional derivatives. (More precisely, D^{2m} is the mth power of the Laplacian and D^{2m+1} is the gradient of the mth power of the Laplacian. Smoothness operators of this type correspond to Tikhonov stabilizers; Bertero, Poggio & Torre, 1987; Tikhonov & Arsenin, 1977.) The mixture of the smoothing and the measuring stages may written as

$$E(\mathbf{v}(\mathbf{r}), \mathbf{U}_i) = \sum_i (M(\mathbf{v}(\mathbf{r}_i)) - M(\mathbf{U}_i))^2$$

$$+ \lambda \int d\mathbf{r} \sum_{m=0}^{\infty} c_m (D^m \mathbf{v})^2, \qquad (8)$$

where $\lambda \geqslant 0$ is a constant.

The precise form of the smoothness operator is important. It determines the form of the interactions between measurements in different parts of the visual field and, in particular, the way these interactions fall off with distance.

The parameter λ sets the strength of the smoothing and the c_m ($c_m \geqslant 0$) determine its form. There are many possible forms for the smoothing function. Next, we discuss several conditions that this function must satisfy. Also, we argue that a good choice is a smoothness function that yields an interaction that has the spatial behavior of a Gaussian function.

We impose two criteria on our smoothness function: (i) It must impose enough smoothness to make the problem well posed, and (ii) the interactions between different measurements must fall off to zero at large distances. This second criterion is important for images without boundaries (see Grzywacz et al., 1989, for psychophysical evidence). But it is also important for images with boundaries. One example that illustrates the importance of the

locality of smoothness even in the presence of boundaries was presented by Grzywacz and colleagues (1989). If an object moves in a nonrigid way, then regions near different portions of its boundary move with different velocities. The locality of the smoothing operation would ensure that regions moving with the different velocities would interact little. (See the sections Extensions to Motion Discontinuity and Transparency and Discussion: Coherent Motion for further consideration of the case where boundary conditions are used.)

We now state two theorems that give necessary and sufficient conditions for (i) and (ii). The first theorem is proven by Duchon (1979).

Theorem 4. *A necessary and sufficient condition for (i) is that derivatives of higher than first order exist in the smoothing operator.*

This condition applies regardless of whether there are boundaries in the image.

Intuitively, the amount of smoothness required depends on the dimensionality of the space and the dimensionality of the data. For isolated data points (such as features) in two dimensions, an operator with only first-order derivatives does not supply enough smoothness. This would correspond to fitting a membrane surface to isolated data points. The human visual system, however, obtains coherent percepts even for discrete features.

Theorem 5. *A necessary and sufficient condition for the interaction to fall faster than $1/r$, where r is the distance from a motion measurement site, is that $c_0 > 0$.*

(In practice, if $c_0 = 0$, the interaction does not fall at all. Also, for the total contribution of a data point to the computed velocity field to be finite, it is critical that the interaction falls faster than $1/r$.)

An important corollary of these theorems (corollary 3) is that smoothing operators involving only first-order derivatives do not satisfy either of the conditions (i) and (ii). Theorem 4 requires the existence of high-order derivatives and theorem 5 requires a zero-order derivative.

This corollary is important, since previous theories that integrated motion over space (Hildreth, 1984; Horn & Schunck, 1981) used a similar mathematical structure as in equation 8 with only first-order derivatives (although Horn and Schunck suggested the possibility of using Laplacians). Thus any attempts to extend these theories directly to deal with sparse data will encounter difficulties. It can also be shown (Yuille & Grzywacz, 1989a) that these difficulties will start to occur even for dense data.

The two theorems say that to satisfy our criteria, the smoothing operator must have positive c_0 and one or more derivatives higher than first order.

For this chapter, we choose the smoothing so that the interaction is a Gaussian. This form of interaction was chosen for four reasons: First, it meets the criteria above; second, it generates analytic solutions; third, it has a natural spatial scale; and fourth, it may be an optimal smoothing filter (Marr & Hildreth, 1980; Witkin, 1983; Yuille & Poggio, 1986). Moreover, variations of the higher-order terms, c_m for $m \geqslant 2$, seem to have little effect on the interaction, which thus usually resembles a Gaussian (Poggio, Vorhees & Yuille, 1985). To obtain a Gaussian interaction we set $c_m = \sigma^{2m}/(m!2^m)$.

Smoothing has been traditionally justified in vision as a method for dealing with noise or filling in sparse data. We would like to stress that smoothing also gives rise to computational efficiency. If computation is done at a coarse scale, then the interpolated result can be used to reduce significantly the complexity of calculation at finer scales.

Isolated Features and Motion Cooperativity

This section deals with the simplest form of motion: that of isolated features undergoing short-range motions. The example that we present here shows that the motion coherence theory may account for the cooperativity of the motion system (Williams & Sekuler 1984; Williams et al., 1986). This cooperativity is demonstrated by an experiment as follows. The stimulus consists of random-dot patterns in which the dots make a random walk, with their direction of motion at each step taken from some distribution. If the distribution is uniform over all directions, one sees dynamic noise. However, only a slight bias of the range of motion directions may lead to a percept of global motion in the direction of the bias. The theory predicts this behavior, because the small variance of the constructed velocity field may enable the mean motion to be detected.

We assume that in this case, the velocity measurements are the velocities of the dots. Suppose that the dots are at points $\mathbf{r}_i$ with velocities $\mathbf{U}_i$. The motion coherence theory suggests minimizing

$$E(\mathbf{v}(\mathbf{r}), \mathbf{U}_i) = \sum_i ((\mathbf{v}(\mathbf{r}_i)) - (\mathbf{U}_i))^2$$

$$+ \lambda \int d\mathbf{r} \sum_{m=0}^{\infty} c_m (D^m \mathbf{v})^2. \qquad (9)$$

To minimize equation 9, we use the standard techniques of the calculus of variations. (Equation 9 depends not only on a variable, but actually on an entire function, that is, $\mathbf{v}(\mathbf{r})$. Expressions that depend on functions rather than on variables are called functionals. To minimize functionals, we must use the branch of mathematics called calculus of variations.) The minimum of equation 9 has the form:

$$\mathbf{v}(\mathbf{r}) = \sum_i \frac{\beta_i}{2\pi\sigma^2} \exp \frac{-(\mathbf{r} - \mathbf{r}_i)^2}{2\sigma^2}, \qquad (10)$$

where the β_i are the solutions of the following system of linear equations:

$$\sum_j (\lambda \delta_{ij} + G_{ij}) \beta_j = \mathbf{U}_i, \qquad (11)$$

where δ_{ij} is the Kronecker delta ($\delta_{ij} = 1$ if $i = j$ and $\delta_{ij} = 0$ if $i \neq j$) and where

$$G_{ij} = \frac{1}{2\pi\sigma^2} \exp \frac{-(\mathbf{r}_j - \mathbf{r}_i)^2}{2\sigma^2}. \qquad (12)$$

The solution will depend on the values of σ and λ. To understand these dependencies, we took two approaches. First, simulations were made of motion cooperativity examples, by solving equation 11, with fixed values of λ and changing values of σ (figure 16.6), and also, with fixed σ and changing λ (figure 16.7). Second, we performed analytical calculations with a simplified version of the motion cooperativity paradigms.

If we fix λ (figure 16.6) and make σ large, then the magnitude of the velocity vectors in the constructed field is small. This is as if the interactions drag empty space, which slows the motions down. On the other limit, that is, for small σ, there is no interaction and the constructed field coincides with the data in the measurement sites. However, over a large intermediate range of σ, the solution is close to the data bias.

If σ is fixed (figure 16.7) and λ is large, the constructed field is again small. This is due to the c_0 of equation 9, which enforces the interactions' locality and leads to small velocities. On the other hand, if λ is small, the solution is noisy, because with little smoothing the problem of minimizing equation 9 becomes ill-conditioned. Once again,

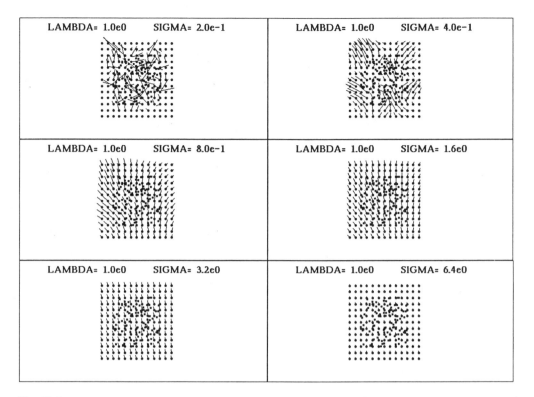

Fig. 16.6
Motion cooperativity and the spatial extent of the interactions. One hundred dots were randomly placed inside a square region of unit sides; the dot positions are indicated by the small solid squares. Each of these dots was assumed to be moving. The horizontal components of their velocity were obtained from a homogeneous random distribution whose values ranged from −1 to 1. The vertical components had the same distribution plus a constant bias upwards of 0.25. The dots' velocities are not shown but are close to those shown in the upper left panel. The figure shows the velocity field computed by the motion coherence theory by minimizing equation 9 with fixed λ and six values of σ. The computed field is shown as lines attached to small circles positioned in a grid. (However, the solution is continuous, because it is computed analytically as in equation 10; the grid is shown for purposes of illustration.) For small σ, no interactons occur and the output is similar to the input. On the other hand, for large σ, the computed motion is small due to interactions with empty space. However, in a wide range of σ, the computed field at the position of the dots is close to the 0.25 bias. The output coherence in this range is similar to the psychophysical phemomenon of motion cooperativity (Williams & Sekuler, 1984; Williams et al., 1986).

for a large intermediate range of λ, a solution that is close to the data bias is obtained. We also verified that these close-to-bias solutions are maintained if σ and λ are varied simultaneously, provided that they are in their correct range.

We performed a complete mathematical analysis of a simplified version of the motion cooperativity paradigm. In that version, the dots are randomly and homogeneously distributed all over the space, that is, they are not constrained to a small region as in figures 16.6 and 16.7. We analyze how the mean and the variance of the output velocity field depend on the statistics of the input and its dot density. It was found that the constructed field's mean velocity is smaller than the input's mean. But if λ is sufficiently small as compared to the dot density, then these means are arbitrarily close. (This provides a first guiding rule for the choice of λ in a given computation.) Also, the analysis showed that not surprisingly the output variance falls with smoothing, λ, and the range of interactions, σ. Furthermore, the variance increases unbounded as the smoothing decreases.

Our model may need to be modified to estimate λ and σ from the image dynamically (adaptation) by a process that decides how much smoothing is necessary and how

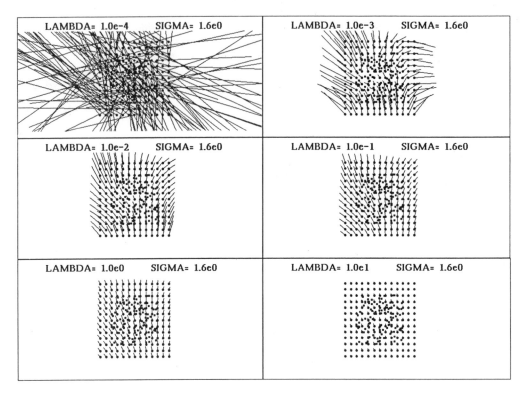

Fig. 16.7
Motion cooperativity and smoothness. This figure is identical to figure 16.6, except that this time we fixed σ and varied λ. For small λ, the computed field is noisy, because with little smoothing the problem of minimizing equation 9 becomes ill-conditioned. However, if λ is large, the motion is small. This is due to c_0 of Equation 9, which enforces the interactions' locality and leads to small velocities. Once again, for a large intermediate range of λ, a solution that is close to the input's bias is obtained.

wide the range of interaction should be. This adaptation may be fooled in experiments by quick changes of dot density.

Relations with the Theories of Hildreth, and Horn and Schunck

We now discuss how the theory compares to two previous theories for short-range motion, one that deals with contour motion (Hildreth, 1984) and another that deals with optical flow (Horn and Schunck, 1981).

Hildreth assumes that contours have been extracted from the image by a previous process, for example, by edge detection. In this case, the velocity information is known only along a contour. Moreover, only the normal component of the velocity field can be measured directly without further assumptions. Hildreth proposes determin-

ing the velocity field by minimizing a functional defined on the contour C

$$E_H(\mathbf{v}(s)) = \int_C ds(\mathbf{v}(s) \cdot \mathbf{n}_C(s) - u(s))^2$$
$$+ \lambda \int_C ds \frac{\partial \mathbf{v}(s)}{\partial s} \cdot \frac{\partial \mathbf{v}(s)}{\partial s}, \tag{13}$$

with respect to $\mathbf{v}(s)$, where $\mathbf{n}_C(s)$ is the normal vector to the curve and $u(s)$ is the measured normal velocity field as functions of the arc-length s. (Unlike equations 8 and 9, whose integrals are over the entire space, the integrals in equation 13 are along contours. We denote this contour integration by the symbol C appearing below the integral sign.)

For our purposes, the important thing about Hildreth's formulation is that the velocity is only smoothed along the contour.

The motion coherence theory can also deal with contour motion. However, this theory does it differently than the way that Hildreth's theory deals with the problem. In both theories, the measurement of the velocity field is the component of velocity perpendicular to the contour, $M(\mathbf{v}(s)) = \mathbf{v}(s) \cdot \mathbf{n}_C(s)$. However, while the smoothing part of the motion coherence theory is over all space, the smoothing part of Hildreth's theory is only over the contour (figure 16.8). Compare Hildreth's formulation (equation 13) with ours, which is

$$E(\mathbf{v}(s)) = \int_C ds (\mathbf{v}(s) \cdot \mathbf{n}_C(s) - u(s))^2$$

$$+ \lambda \int d\mathbf{r} \sum_{m=0}^{\infty} c_m (D^m \mathbf{v})^2. \tag{14}$$

The motion coherence theory allows for the motions on nearby objects to affect the perception of the motion on the contour. A demonstration of this effect by Nakayama and Silverman (1988a,b) will be discussed in the next section.

Another example of motion measurement that the motion coherence theory can deal with is that considered by Horn and Schunck (1981). They propose measuring motion directly from the intensity field. Their basic measurement is based on constraints imposed by intensity gradients and by temporal derivatives of the intensity. From these measurements, only one component of the velocity field is available locally, namely, the component in the direction of the image gradient. Horn and Schunck proposed to obtain the other component by smoothing the velocity field. Our theory works in a similar way on intensity gradient measurements of the type defined by Horn and Schunck. However, the smoothing operator of the motion coherence theory is more general, including Horn and Schunck's as a particular case. Also, their smoothing operator, which in their simulations is based only on first order derivatives, does not satisfy our criteria (i) and (ii) defined immediately before theorem 4. This does not matter for their application, becasue they are considering dense data. But these criteria are important when only sparse data are available; a situation relevant for human perception.

The Aperture Problem and Motion Capture

There are two important problems in motion perception that the motion coherence theory can deal with, and which are the topics of this section: the problem of coherence (related to the aperture problem) and motion capture.

An example of the aperture problem consists of finding the motion of a large contour; local motion detectors can only detect motion that is perpendicular to the contour.

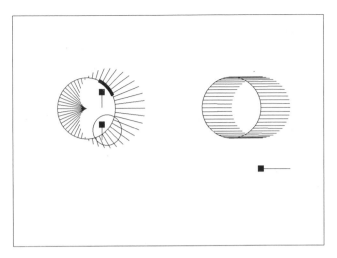

Fig. 16.8
The aperture problem. A circle of unit radius was assumed to be moving to the right with a velocity of 1.0. If the motion is measured with local detectors, then only the components of the motion perpendicular to the contour can be measured. This is an example of the aperture problem, and in the left figure, these perpendicular components are shown. The velocity field along the contour, as predicted by the motion coherence theory, is shown in the right figure. This field was computed by solving equation 14 with $\lambda = 0.001$ and $\sigma = 3$. The isolated dot moving at the bottom of the right figure has the correct velocity of the circle, implying that the aperture problem has been solved. The average speed of the computed velocity field along the contour was 0.996, which is incorrect by only 0.4 percent. The motion coherence theory solves the aperture problem in a different way than Hildreth proposed (Hildreth, 1984). She suggested that the visual system integrates motion information along contours, as illustrated in the left figure by the contour's highlight. In this case, the contour motion does not interact with off-the-contour information. The motion coherence theory, on the other hand, integrates motion over space (left figure's small circle). Thus this theory predicts that the solution of the aperture problem may interact with off-the-contour motion.

The motion coherence theory for contour motion appears in equation 14. We obtain the smoothest velocity field in two-dimensional space, in contrast to Hildreth, who obtains the smoothest velocity field along the contour (figure 16.8).

For the present solutions, the computed speed is smaller than the true one (Yuille & Grzywacz, 1989a). This is due to the term c_0, which forces the overall speed down, but is necessary to ensure that spatial interactions drop off at infinity. If $c_0 = 0$, we can prove that the correct solution may be obtained for a certain class of stimuli, and in particular, the correct answer is always obtained for translational motion. Similar results hold for Hildreth's method

(Yuille, 1984). Psychophysical experiments, such as the rotating-ellipse illusion (Hildreth, 1984), show that humans may not estimate the correct velocity fields for other stimuli. In a number of examples, Hildreth showed that when her method gave the incorrect velocity field, it was often close to the perceived motion.

The motion coherence theory also agrees with experiments by Nakayama and Silverman (1988a,b) that investigated variations of the aperture problem that are not easily explained by current theories. These experiments displayed curves translating over time (figure 16.9) and showed that the correct motion is not always perceived even when the curves are moving rigidly, that terminators in the curves enhance the rigid percepts, and that terminators near the curves may also lead to this enhancement. The motion coherence theory accounts for the nonrigidity (figure 16.9), because if $c_0 \neq 0$ the aperture problem is not completely solved (Yuille & Grzywacz, 1989a). However, if the display includes terminators, then they provide extra information that helps to improve the solution.

The theory gives a possible explanation for motion capture (Ramachandran & Anstis, 1983). In this phenomenon, randomly moving dots are captured and move coherently with a superimposed grating or a surrounding contour. The motion coherence theory simultaneously solves the aperture problem of the surrounding contour and captures the internal dots. The theory also predicts that capture may happen when only a few dots move. An example of this occurs when a central ambiguous motion is captured by a peripheral unambiguous motion. Psychophysical experiments with such paradigms were performed. The results were consistent with the motion coherence theory and inconsistent with minimal mapping theory (Grzywacz et al., 1989).

Extensions to Motion Discontinuity and Transparency

There are several possible ways to extend this work to deal with motion discontinuities. These include the following three alternatives: First, using line processors to break the smoothing (Gamble & Poggio, 1987; Hutchinson et al., 1988; Yuille, 1987); second, detecting edges in the velocity field (see Discussion: Local Velocity and figure 16.5) and then smoothing inside the edge region again (see the next section); and third, using estimation of the

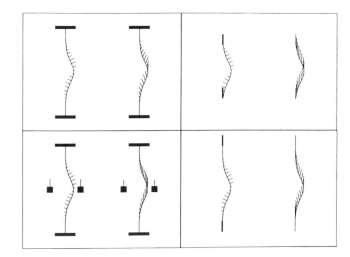

Fig. 16.9
Variations on the aperture problem. In this figure, Gaussians move upward with the speed highlighted in the right panels. In all panels, the left and the right displays show the motion with the aperture problem and the predictions of the motion coherence theory, respectively. Nakayama and Silverman (1988a, b) studied these paradigms, and their results are consistent with the theory. In the left panels, the Gaussian's extremities were occluded. In this case, the theory predicts a nonrigid percept (*upper left*). However, when features that move with the same velocity as the curve flank it, they capture it and make it look rigid (*lower left*). This is consistent with the motion coherence theory but not with Hildreth's theory (Hildreth, 1984; see figure 16.8). Furthermore, if we break the curve, then the information from the extremities helps to solve the aperture problem (*upper right*). It is solved less well if the extremities are far from the center (*lower right*).

velocity field whereby neighboring elements support each other if they are similar, but do not if they are dissimilar.

There seem two possible, and maybe complementary, hypotheses to explain transparency effects. In the first, if the motions are too dissimilar, then no interaction between them occurs (see Discussion: Local Velocity and figure 16.5). In the second, motion effects over time are included: If the estimate of velocity changes too quickly with time, then this may be due to integrating over different surfaces and two or more regions are created. (However, this hypothesis cannot explain all transparency phenomena, because they may occur when the moving features are short-lived; Siegel & Andersen, 1988.)

Discussion: Coherent Motion

In conclusion, we propose a motion coherence theory that deals simultaneously with the problem of coherence (see Discussion: Local Velocity), and the phenomena of motion capture and motion cooperativity.

The exact choice of the theory's smoothing filter is an important experimental question. We have chosen the Gaussian because of its many fine properties, but there are many alternatives. The situation is slightly analogous of action-at-a-distance theories of physics, such as Newton's theory of gravity, where the force between two points falls off inversely proportional to the square of the distance. For the motion coherence theory, using the Gaussian filter, we have an interaction between features that falls off as the negative exponential of the square of the distance. This decreases rapidly with distance. Psychophysical experiments to determine what the exact fall off law is, and in particular, if it is a Gaussian, can be done.

We have emphasized the importance of requiring that the interaction falls off with distance. If this condition is not satisfied then the velocity field will become arbitrarily large the further away we are from the data. Perhaps more seriously, a feature is more likely to be captured by an object that is far way from it, rather than by an object close by. In our theory the interaction is controlled by the c_0 term of the cost function.

An alternative way to prevent the velocity field from blowing up at infinity is to impose boundary conditions on the field. However, in this case, the resulting velocity field will depend strongly on the choice of the boundary. In some situations a boundary may be found naturally (for example, by image segmentation through brightness, texture, color, or motion; see the previous section) and natural boundary conditions on the velocity field would occur. In this case, capture may only occur inside the object.

Thus, if the boundaries can be found reliably, then the c_0 term can be dropped. (One can show that if c_0 is dropped, then the correct velocity field would always be computed for two-dimensional translations.) In this case the boundary conditions would have a stronger effect on the velocity field than if $c_0 \neq 0$. It is an open experimental question to see if this occurs.

However, if the boundaries cannot be found reliably and are set arbitrarily, then if the c_0 term is dropped, the resulting velocity field will depend strongly on this arbitrary choice (unless the data are dense everywhere). *The boundary terms behave like measurement sources that influence (and sometimes capture) the motion of the internal features.*

This theory is specified at an abstract level in terms of minimizing a cost functional. We stress that the minimiza-tion of such a cost functional is inherently a parallel process and could be performed on a parallel computer or a neural network. Elsewhere (Grzywacz & Yuille, 1988), we describe a parallel network that implements our long-range theory (Yuille & Grzywacz, 1989a) under certain conditions.

Acknowledgments

We thank Lyle Borg-Graham, Dave Heeger, Ellen Hildreth, Tommy Poggio, Jeff Schall, Tai Sing, and Jim Smith for critically reading the section on local velocity. Also, comments from Ted Adelson, Jim Clark, Dave Heeger, Ellen Hildreth, Dan Kersten, Tommy Poggio and Jim Smith helped clarifying the section on coherent motion. We would also like to acknowledge Consuelita Correa-Grzywacz, Ivan Correa, and Michelle Borde for inspiration and encouragement. This work was undertaken while N. M. G. was at the Center for Biological Information Processing, Department of Brain and Cognitive Sciences, Massachusetts Institute of Technology, and was supported by the grant BNS-8809528 from the National Science Foundation, by the Sloan Foundation, by a grant to Tomaso Poggio, Ellen Hildreth, and Peter Schiller from the Office of Naval Research, Cognitive and Neural Systems Division, and by the grant IRI-8719394 to Tomaso Poggio, Ellen Hildreth, and Edward Adelson from the National Science Foundation. A. L. Y. was supported by the Brown-Harvard-MIT Center for Intelligent Control Systems with the United States Army Research Office grant DAALO3-86-K-0171.

References

Adelson, E. H. (1987). Transparency in motion perception. *Investigative Ophthalmology and Visual Science, 28, 232.*

Adelson, E. H. & Bergen, J. (1985). Spatiotemporal energy models for the perception of motion. *Journal of the Optical Society of America A, 2, 284–299.*

Adelson, E. H. & Movshon, J. A. (1982). Phenomenal coherence of moving visual patterns. *Nature, 300, 523–525.*

Albright, T. D. (1984). Direction and orientation selectivity of neurons in visual area MT of the macaque. *Journal of Neurophysiology, 52, 1106–1130.*

Amthor, F. R. & Grzywacz, N. M. (1991). Nonlinearity of the inhibition underlying retinal directional selectivity. *Visual Neuroscience, 6, 197–206.*

Andersen, R. A. & Siegel, R. M. (1990). Motion processing in primate cortex. In G. M. Edelman, W. E. Gall & W. M. Cowan (Eds.), *Signal and sense: Local and global order in perceptual maps* (pp. 143–184). New York, NY: Wiley.

Andrews, B. W. & Pollen, D. A. (1979). Relationship between spatial frequency selectivity and receptive field profile of simple cells. *Journal of Physiology, 287,* 163–176.

Anstis, S. (1970). Phi movement as a subtraction process. *Vision Research, 10,* 1411–1430.

Baker, C. L. Jr. (1988). Spatial and temporal determinants of directionally selective velocity preference in cat striate cortex neurons. *Journal of Neurophysiology, 59,* 1557–1574.

Bertero, M., Poggio, T. & Torre, V. (1987). Regularization of ill-posed problems. *MIT Artificial Intelligence Memo, 924.*

Bisti, S., Carmignoto, L., Galli, L. & Maffei, L. (1985). Spatial-frequency characteristics of neurones of area 18 in the cat: Dependence on the velocity of the visual stimulus. *Journal of Physiology, 359,* 259–268.

Bülthoff, H., Little, J. & Poggio, T. (1989). A parallel algorithm for real-time computation of optical flow. *Nature, 337,* 549–553.

Daugman, J. G. (1985). Uncertainty relation for resolution in space, spatial frequency, and orientation optimized by two dimensional visual cortical filters. *Journal of the Optical Society of America A, 2,* 1160–1169.

Daugman, J. G. (1988). Pattern and motion vision without Laplacian zero-crossings. *Journal of the Optical Society of America A, 5,* 1142–1148.

Duchon, J. (1979). Splines minimizing rotation-invariant semi-norms in Sobolev spaces. In W. Schempp & K. Zeller (Eds.), *Lecture notes in mathematics* (vol. 571; pp. 85–100). Berlin: Springer-Verlag.

Emerson, R. C., Bergen, J. R. & Adelson, E. H. (1987a). Movement models and directionally selective neurons in the cat's visual cortex. *Neuroscience Abstracts, 13,* 1623.

Emerson, R. C. & Citron, M. C. (1988). How linear and nonlinear mechanisms contribute to directional selectivity in simple cells of cat striate cortex. *Investigative Ophthalmology and Visual Science, 29,* 23.

Emerson, R. C., Citron, M. C., Vaughn, W. J. & Klein, S. A. (1987b). Nonlinear directionally sensitive subunits in complex cells of cat striate cortex. *Journal of Neurophysiology, 58,* 33–65.

Fahle, M. & Poggio, T (1981). Visual hyperacuity: Spatio-temporal interpolation in human vision. *Proceedings of the Royal Society, London, B, 213,* 451–477.

Feldman, J. A. & Ballard, D. H. (1982). Connectionist models and their properties. *Cognitive Science, 6,* 205–254.

Ferrera, V. P. & Wilson, H. R. (1987). Direction specific masking and the analysis of motions in two dimensions. *Vision Research, 27,* 1783–1796.

Fleet, D. J. & Jepson, A. D. (1989). Computation of normal velocity from local phase information. *Technical Reports on Research on Biological and Computational Vision, RBCV-TR-89-27,* Department of Computer Science, University of Toronto, Toronto, Canada.

Gabor, D. (1946). Theory of communication. *Journal of the Institute of Electrical Engineering, 93,* 429–457.

Gaddum, J. H. (1945). Lognormal distributions. *Nature, 156,* 463–466.

Galli, L. Chalupa, L., Maffei, L. & Bisti, S. (1988). The organization of receptive fields in area 18 neurones of the cat varies with the spatio-temporal characteristics of the visual stimulus. *Experimental Brain Research, 71,* 1–7.

Gamble, E. & Poggio, T. (1987). Visual integration and detection of discontinuities: The keys role of intensity edges. *MIT Artificial Intelligence Memo, 970.*

Grossmann, A. & Morlet, J. (1984). Decomposition of Hardy functions into square integrable wavelets of constant shape. *SIAM Journal of Mathematics, 15,* 723–736.

Grzywacz, N. M. (1987). Interactions betweem minimal mapping and inertia in long-range apparent motion. *Investigative Ophthalmology and Visual Science, 28,* 300.

Grzywacz, N. M. & Koch, C. (1987). Functional properties of models for direction selectivity in the retina. *Synapse, 1,* 417–434.

Grzywacz, N. M. & Poggio, T. (1989). Computation of motion by real neurons. In S. F. Zornetzer, J. L. Davis & C. Lau (Eds.), *An introduction to neural and electronic networks* (pp. 379–403). Orlando, FL: Academic Press.

Grzywacz, N. M., Smith, J. A. & Yuille, A. L. (1989). A common theoretical framework for visual motion's spatial and temporal coherence. In *Proceedings of the IEEE Workshop on Visual Motion* (pp. 148–155). Washington, DC: IEEE Computer Society Press.

Grzywacz, N. M. & Yuille, A. L. (1988). Massively parallel implementations of theories for apparent motion. *Spatial Vision, 3,* 15–44.

Grzywacz, N. M. & Yuille, A. L. (1990). A model for the estimate of local image velocity by cells in the visual cortex. *Proceedings of the Royal Society, London, B, 239,* 129–161.

Hammond, P. (1979). Stimulus-dependence of ocular dominance and directional tuning of complex cells in area 17 of the feline visual cortex. *Experimental Brain Research, 35,* 583–589.

Hammond, P. (1981). Simultaneous determination of directional tuning of complex cells in cat striate cortex for bar and for texture motion. *Experimental Brain Research, 41,* 364–369.

Hammond, P. & Reck, J. (1981). Influence of velocity on directional tuning of complex cells in cat striate cortex for texture motion. *Neuroscience Letters, 19,* 309–314.

Heeger, D. (1987). A model for the extraction of image flow. *Journal of the Optical Society of America A, 4,* 1455–1471.

Hildreth, E. C. (1984). *The measurement of visual motion*. Cambridge, MA: MIT Press.

Hochstein, S. & Shapley, R. M. (1976). Quantitative analysis of retinal ganglion cell classifications. *Journal of Physiology, 262*, 237–264.

Holub, R. A. & Morton-Gibson, M. (1981). Response of visual cortical neurons of the cat to moving sinusoidal gratings: Response-contrast functions and spatiotemporal integration. *Journal of Neurophysiology, 46*, 1244–1259.

Horn, B. K. P. & Schunck, B. G. (1981). Determining optical flow. *Artificial Intelligence, 17*, 185–203.

Hutchinson, J., Koch, C., Luo, J. & Mead, C. (1988). Computing motion using analog and binary resistive networks. *Computer, 21*, 52–63.

Ikeda, H. & Wright, M. J. (1975). Spatial and temporal properties of "sustained" and "transient" neurones in area 17 of the cat's visual cortex. *Experimental Brain Research, 22*, 363–383.

Jones, J. P. & Palmer, L. A. (1987). An evaluation of the two-dimensional Gabor filter model of simple receptive fields in cat striate cortex. *Journal of Neurophysiology, 58*, 1233–1258.

Koch, C. & Ullman, S. (1985). Shifts in selective visual attention: Towards the underlying neural circuitry. *Human Neurobiology, 4*, 219–227.

Koffka, K. (1935). *Principles of gestalt psychology*. New York: Harcourt, Brace and Wood.

Maffei, L. & Fiorentini, A. (1977). Spatial frequency rows in the striate visual cortex. *Vision Research, 17*, 257–264.

Mallat, S. G. (1988). *Review of multifrequency channel decompositions of images and wavelet models* (Robotics Research Technical Report 412). New York: Computer Science Division, New York Univeristy.

Marchiafava, P. L. (1979). The responses of retinal ganglion cells to stationary and moving visual stimuli. *Vision Research, 19*, 1203–1211.

Marr, D. & Hildreth, E. C. (1980). Theory of edge detection. *Proceedings of the Royal Society, London, B, 207*, 187–217.

Marr, D. & Ullman, S. (1981). Directional selectivity and its use in early visual processing. *Proceedings of the Royal Society, London, B, 211*, 151–180.

Maunsell, J. H. R. & Newsome, W. T. (1987). Visual processing in monkey extrastriate cortex. In W. M. Cowan, E. M. Shooter, C. F. Stevens & R. F. Thompson (Eds.), *Annual reviews of neuroscience* (vol. 10, pp. 363–401). Palo Alto, CA: Annual Reviews Inc.

McKee, S. P. (1981). A local mechanism for differential velocity detection. *Vision Research, 21*, 491–500.

McKee, S. P., Silverman, G. H. & Nakayama, K. (1986). Precise velocity discrimination despite random variations in the temporal frequency and contrast. *Vision Research, 26*, 609–619.

McKee, S. P. & Welch, L. (1985). Sequential recruitment in the discrimination of velocity. *Journal of the Optical Society of America A, 2*, 243–251.

McLean, J. & Palmer, L. (1989). Contribution of linear spatiotemporal receptive field structure to velocity selectivity of simple cells in area 17 of cat. *Vision Research, 29*, 675–679.

Movshon, J. A. (1975). The velocity tuning of single units in cat striate cortex. *Journal of Physiology, 249*, 445–468.

Movshon, J. A., Adelson, E. H., Gizzi, M. S. & Newsome, W. T. (1985). The analysis of moving visual patterns. In C. Chagas, R. Gattas & C. G. Gross (Eds.), *Pattern recognition mechanisms* (pp. 117–151). Rome: Vatican Press.

Movshon, J. A., Davis, E. T. & Adelson, E. H. (1980). Directional movement selectivity in cortical complex cells. *Neuroscience Abstracts, 6*, 230.

Nakayama, K. (1985). Biological motion processing: A review. *Vision Research, 25*, 625–660.

Nakayama, K. & Silverman, G. H. (1988a). The aperture problem—I. Perception of nonrigidity and motion direction in translating sinusoidal lines. *Vision Research, 28*, 739–746.

Nakayama, K. & Silverman, G. H. (1988b). The aperture problem—II. Spatial integration of velocity information along contours. *Vision Research, 28*, 747–753.

Nakayama, K. & Tyler, C. W. (1981). Psychophysical isolation of movement sensitivity by removal of familiar position cues. *Vision Research, 21*, 427–433.

Newsome, W. T., Gizzi, M. S. & Movshon, J. A. (1983). Spatial and temporal properties of neurons in macaque MT. *Investigative Ophthalmology and Visual Science, 24*, 106.

Orban, G. A., Kennedy, H. & Bullier, J. (1986). Velocity sensitivity and direction selectivity of neurons in areas V1 and V2 of the monkey: Influence of eccentricity. *Journal of Neurophysiology, 56*, 462–480.

Poggio, T. & Reichardt, W. E. (1976). Visual control of orientation behaviour in the fly: Part II: Towards the underlying neural interactions. *Quarterly Review of Biophysics, 9*, 377–438.

Poggio, T., Vorhees, H. & Yuille, A. L. (1985). A regularized approach to edge detection. *MIT Artificial Intelligence Memo, 833*.

Pollen, D. & Ronner, S. (1981). Phase relationships between adjacent simple cells in the visual cortex. *Science, 212*, 1409–1411.

Ramachandran, V. S. & Anstis, S. M. (1983). Displacement thresholds for coherent apparent motion random dot-patterns. *Vision Research, 24*, 1719–1724.

Ratliff, F. (1965). *Mach bands: Quantitative studies on neural networks in the retina*. San Francisco: Holden-Day.

Regan, D. & Beverley, K. I. (1984). Figure ground segregation by motion contrast and by luminance contrast. *Journal of the Optical Society of America A, 1*, 433–442.

Reichardt, W., Egelhaaf, M. & Schlögl, R. W. (1988). Movement detectors provide sufficient information for local computation of 2-D velocity field. *Die Naturwissenschaften, 75*, 313–315.

Reid, R. C. & Shapley, R. M. (1988). Complex temporal stimuli increase relative sensitivity of cat striate cortical neurons to high temporal frequencies. *Investigative Ophthalmology and Visual Science, 27*, 142.

Rodman, H. R. & Albright, T. D. (1989). Single-unit analysis of pattern-motion selective properties in the middle temporal visual area (MT). *Experimental Brain Research, 75*, 53–64.

Saito, H., Yukio, M., Tanaka, K., Hikosaka, D., Fukuda, Y. & Iwai, E. (1986). Integration of direction signals of image motion in the superior temporal sulcus of the macaque monkey. *Journal of Neuroscience, 6*, 145–157.

Siegel, R. M. & Andersen, R. A. (1988). Perception of three-dimensional structure from motion in monkey and man. *Nature, 331*, 259–261.

Silverman, M. S., Grosof, D. H., De Valois, R. L. & Elfar, S. D. (1989). Spatial-frequency organization in primate striate cortex. *Proceedings of the National Academy of Science USA, 86*, 711–715.

Tanaka, K., Hikosaka, K., Saito, H., Yukie, M., Fukada, Y. & Iwai, E. (1986). Analysis of local and wide-field movements in the superior temporal visual areas of the macaque monkey. *Journal of Neuroscience, 6*, 134–144.

Tikhonov, A. N. & Arsenin, V. Y. (1977). *Solutions of ill-posed problems*. Washington, DC: Winston and Sons.

Tolhurst, D. J. & Movshon, J. A. (1975). Spatial and temporal contrast sensitivity of striate cortical neurons. *Nature, 257*, 674–675.

Torre, V. & Poggio, T. (1978). A synaptic mechanism possibly underlying directional selectivity to motion. *Proceedings of the Royal Society of London, B, 202*, 409–416.

Ullman, S. (1979). *The interpretation of visual motion*. Cambridge, MA: MIT Press.

Verri, A., Girosi, F. & Torre, V. (1989). Mathematical properties of the 2D motion field: From singular points to motion parameters. In *Proceedings of the IEEE Workshop on Visual Motion* (pp. 190–200). Washington, DC: IEEE Computer Society Press.

Watson, A. B. & Ahumada, A. J. (1985). Model of human visual-motion sensing. *Journal of the Optical Society of America A, 2*, 322–341.

Welch, L. (1989). The perception of moving plaids reveals two motion-processing stages. *Nature, 337*, 734–736.

Williams, D. W., Phillips, G. C. & Sekuler, R. (1986). Hysteresis in the perception of motion direction: evidence for neural cooperativity. *Nature, 324*, 253–255.

Williams, D. W. & Sekuler, R. (1984). Coherent global motion percepts from stochastic local motions. *Vision Research, 24*, 55–62.

Witkin, A. (1983). Scale-space filtering. In *Proceedings of the International Joint Conference on Artificial Intelligence* (pp. 1019–1021). Karlsruhe, West Germany.

Yuille, A. L. (1984). The smoothest velocity field and token matching schemes. *MIT Artificial Intelligence Memo, 724*.

Yuille, A. L. (1987). Energy functions and analog networks. *MIT Artificial Intelligence Memo, 987*.

Yuille, A. L. & Cohen, D. S. (1989). *The development and training of motion and velocity sensitive cells* (Harvard Robotics Laboratory Technical Report, 89–9).

Yuille, A. L. & Grzywacz, N. M. (1988a). A computational theory for the perception of coherent visual motion. *Nature, 333*, 71–74.

Yuille, A. L. & Grzywacz, N. M. (1988b). The motion coherence theory. In *Proceedings of the Second International Conference of Computer Vision* (pp. 344–353). Washington, DC: IEEE Computer Society Press.

Yuille, A. L. & Grzywacz, N. M. (1989a). A mathematical analysis of the motion coherence theory. *International Journal of Computer Vision, 3*, 155–175.

Yuille, A. L. & Grzywacz, N. M. (1989b). A winner-take-all mechanism based on presynaptic inhibition feedback. *Neural Computation, 1*, 334–347.

Yuille, A. L. & Poggio, T. (1986). Scaling theorems for zero-crossings. *IEEE Transactions on Pattern Analysis and Machine Intelligence, PAMI-8*, 15–25.

Yuille, A. L. & Ullman, S. (1987). Rigidity and smoothness. *MIT Artificial Intelligence Memo, 989*.

17

Computational Modeling of Visual Texture Segregation

James R. Bergen and
Michael S. Landy

Why Study Texture?

Visual texture segregation is the perceptual phenomenon illustrated in figure 17.1. In this image a rectangular area composed of small X-shaped patterns appears as a distinct region against a background of L-shaped patterns. This segregation occurs rapidly and unconsciously, without effort or search. The rectangular area composed of T-shaped patterns, however, does not appear as a distinct region in this sense. It is very easy to *discriminate* among all three patterns, but only the X and L regions display spontaneous segregation. This distinction between pattern discrimination and perceptual segregation gives particular interest to the study of this aspect of visual texture perception. Other aspects of texture perception include the role of texture in the perception of surface orientation and shape and the influence of surface texture in determining color appearance. In this paper we limit consideration to the phenomenon of segregation.

Pure texture-based *segregation* is not a very important phenomenon in everyday visual experience. Objects are not usually distinguished from their backgrounds purely by textural differences. In this respect, the study of pure texture differences (in the absence of differences in brightness, color, depth, or other properties) is analogous to the study of isoluminant color differences, which also are not very common in natural scenes. The relative rarity of isoluminant color discrimination in the real world does not imply that color perception is an unimportant component of seeing. Similarly, the rarity of pure texture differences does not reduce the potential importance of texture perception, especially in the visual processing of complex scenes.

Background

The study of texture segregation has been greatly influenced by theoretical considerations. The primary issue

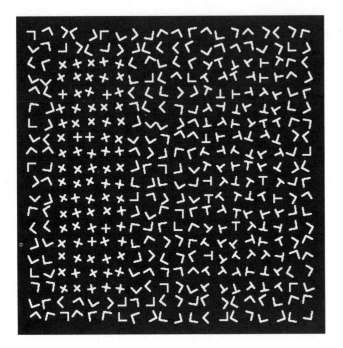

Fig. 17.1
Demonstration of texture-based segregation. The region on the left composed of X-shaped figures appears as a distinct area against the background of L-shaped figures. The region on the right composed of T-shaped figures does not.

is the level of processing at which texture segregation phenomena are determined. Accompanying this question is the associated distinction between the view of texture segregation as an *analytic* process by means of which two regions are distinguished and the view that it is a *synthetic* process by means of which elements group together to form a whole (or fail to do so). Readers interested in the development of these ideas are referred to a previous review (Bergen, 1991). In this chapter we concentrate on the relationship between texture segregation and early visual processes. In particular, we consider the consequences of spatial filtering.

Origins of this approach can be found in the early work of Julesz (Julesz, 1962), although his later work took a somewhat different approach. The earliest explicit treatment of texture in the context of early visual processing is the work of Richards and Polit (1974) on texture matching. Here and in a later paper (Richards, 1979), the authors adapt the matching paradigm used to obtain information about the spectral sensitivities of color mechanisms. As in the case of color, the goal is to infer the early representa-

tion of information through analysis of metamerism. These studies used textures composed of sums of sinusoidal gratings. A few years later a number of papers appeared relating texture perception phenomena to the properties of psychophysically identified spatial mechanisms (Caelli, 1982; Harvey & Gervais, 1978, 1981). Harvey and Gervais used similarity grouping and scaling methods, also with textures composed of sums of sinusoidal gratings. A multidimensional scaling analysis of these data showed them to be consistent with a representation of spatial information based on a family of 1.5 to 2 octave wide quasibandpass linear filters similar to those identified by previous studies (Mostafavi & Sakrison, 1976; Richards & Polit, 1974; Wilson & Bergen, 1979). Caelli (1982) performed an experiment to specify the two-dimensional properties of a class of oriented bandpass linear filters, and then showed that two interval same-different discrimination performance for a set of natural texture images was consistent with the hypothesis that the outputs of these filters formed the image representation.

More recent work in this vein has been done by Caelli (1985, 1986) and Bergen and Adelson (1986, 1988). These studies present more explicit computational descriptions of the ideas developed in the earlier work. They also emphasize the necessary *nonlinear* characteristics of the texture extraction process.

Modeling Strategy

In this paper we describe a computational model of human texture segregation performance. Because it is a computational model, it starts with the actual stimulus images as input. Because it is a model of human performance, it has predictions of experimental outcomes as output. In between, we attempt to have as little as possible that is specifically concerned with texture. Instead, we concentrate on operations that seem to be involved in general early visual processing. In this respect, the style of modeling is closely related to that found in the studies mentioned in the previous section. Our goal is to investigate the extent to which texture segregation phenomena are consequences of the structure of early visual processes and the representations computed by them. We do not intend to imply that visual texture segregation is epiphenomenal. Rather, we wish to explore the influence of early visual processing in determining the characteristics of these phenomena.

The model proposed has three parts. The first computes a generic image representation that resembles in a very crude way the spatial processing characteristics of the early visual cortical areas. This representation consists of simple cell-like linear mechanisms as well as complex cell-like energy mechanisms. This first part is proposed as a general early representation, computed in a way which is not task specific. The second part of the model concerns the computation of more specific properties that may need to be computed differently for different tasks. The example developed is somewhat specialized for the analysis of orientation differences. The representation computed at this level consists of normalized opponent measures. The third part of the model computes predictions of human performance in a particular type of discrimination task.

The two salient characteristics of early visual representation of spatial information are size and orientation tuning. This is supported both by physiological studies of visual cortex (De Valois, Albrecht & Thorell, 1982a; De Valois, Yund & Hepler, 1982b; Hubel & Wiesel, 1968) and by psychophysical evidence including masking (Phillips & Wilson, 1984; Stromeyer & Julesz, 1972) and subthreshold summation data (Wilson & Bergen, 1979). These characteristics of early visual mechanisms have led to the view of early visual representation as a set of parallel channels or mechanisms, varying in their orientation and size (or spatial frequency) selectivities. A caricature of this type of representation can be constructed by having a family of similar orientation tuned filters at each of a range of spatial scales. This type of idealized representation has been described by Watson (1983, 1987). One of the convenient properties of such a representation is that it can be made approximately symmetrical with respect to scale and orientation. This means that changes in the scale or orientation of the input pattern shift the activity in the representation from one region to another but do not greatly change the pattern of activity in other ways. This is a useful property because many textural phenomena are not very sensitive to overall scale and orientation changes, such as those produced by changes in viewing distance and head position. Another useful property of such a representation is that it can be computed very efficiently, as is described below.

Computational Model

Generic Early Representation

The model that we propose is based on the representation shown in figure 17.2. An input image is first represented at a range of different spatial resolutions. Each of these resolution levels is then divided into a set of four orientation tuned components. Since these two transformations both involve linear operations, their order of application is arbitrary. It is also equivalent (though grotesquely inefficient) to compute a single filter representing the result of each of these cascades and apply these individually to the input image. None of these implementation options has any effect on the behavior of the model since they all compute exactly the same thing. However, one obtains a better sense of the level of complexity of this computation by considering an efficient algorithm for computing it.

Pyramids

The first operation represents the input image at a range of spatial resolutions. This involves low-pass filtering (i.e., blurring) the image and subsampling (i.e., reducing the size of the image by deleting samples). (We restrict our consideration in this paper to spatial scales differing by factors of 2, although this is not an essential limitation.) Low-pass filtering an image requires larger and larger convolution kernels as the desired cut-off frequency of the filter decreases. However, these large convolutions can be factored into a cascaded sequence of linear filtering operations and thereby be performed much more efficiently. In other words, rather than generating a very low resolution version of an image by massive blurring (which is expensive to do because each blurred image point depends on a large area of the input image) followed by massive subsampling, it is much more efficient to generate it by repeatedly blurring slightly (which is cheap) followed by a small amount of subsampling. This is especially the case if the desired output is a family of *progressively* low-pass filtered versions of the input image such as we require for our modeling. An efficient algorithm incorporating this type of cascaded processing is the Gaussian pyramid algorithm of Burt (1981). The sequence of outputs is shown in figure 17.3. The input image is filtered with a small

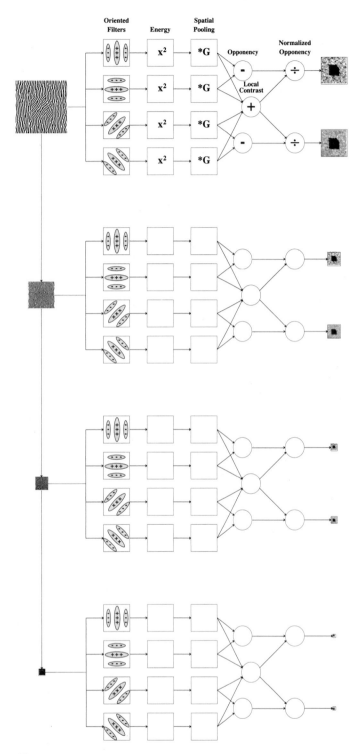

Fig. 17.2

Basic image representation to be used for texture analysis. The image
at each scale is decomposed into a set of four oriented components
and a local pooled energy is computed for each. Orthogonal
orientations are put in opponency. Finally, the system is made
contrast independent by a normalization that uses the local oriented
energy summed over all orientations.

Gaussian-like filter *G*, and subsampled by a factor of 2 in each direction. This produces the first reduced resolution version of the image. This operation is repeated, using the same filter *G*, but taking the previous output as input, to produce the second reduced resolution version. This process is continued until the lowest desired resolution is obtained. Using this method, a reduction of resolution by a factor of 16, for example, can be achieved by four applications of the same filter used to reduce resolution by a factor of 2. Direct reduction of resolution by a factor of 16 would require a filter approximately 8 times as large in each direction. For all of the computations shown in this paper, *G* is taken to be the Cartesian separable filter with values (.05, .25, .4, .25, .05). This means that the effective two-dimensional filter kernel or weighting function is the "multiplication table" product of the weights of the one-dimensional filter *G* placed vertically and horizontally. A Cartesian separable filter is used for reasons of computational efficiency; it allows the spatial filtering operations involved in pyramid construction to be performed as a two-pass cascade of one-dimensional filtering steps. The particular weights chosen produce a pyramid representation with Gaussian-like properties, that is the result of the repeated applications involved in pyramid construction is a Gaussian-like filter (Burt, 1981).

Directional Derivatives

In order to construct a representation with orientation selective elements, we now pass each resolution level through a bank of four small orientation selective filters. These filters approximate the second directional derivatives of the corresponding resolution level in the vertical, horizontal and right and left diagonal directions. In order to obtain diagonal filters that have frequency responses that are as similar as possible (except for orientation) to those for the vertical and horizontal filters, we rotated the vertical filter, truncated it to a 5 by 5 kernel size, and then adjusted its weights using PRAXIS (Brent, 1973; Powell, 1964) to minimize the difference between its frequency response and that of the vertical filter. The weights for these filters are given in tables 17.1 and 17.2.

This choice of orientation selective filters is not critical; first derivatives also suffice for many purposes (Bergen, 1988, 1991; Landy & Bergen, 1988). However, the use of second derivatives yields frequency and orientation band-

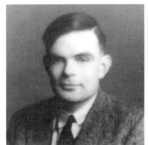

Fig. 17.3
Gaussian pyramid computation illustrated using a picture of Alan Turing. Each picture is produced by applying a small Gaussian-like filter to the previous output, followed by subsampling by a factor of two in each direction.

Table 17.1
Vertical second derivative mask ("V")

0	−1	2	−1	0
0	−4	8	−4	0
0	−6	12	−6	0
0	−4	8	−4	0
0	−1	2	−1	0

Table 17.2
Up and left second derivative mask ("L")

−.163	−.075	−3.610	1.112	1.700
−.075	5.662	−.047	−7.612	1.112
−3.610	−.047	11.301	−.0468	−3.610
1.112	−7.612	−.047	5.662	−.0746
1.700	1.112	−3.610	−.075	−.163

widths that are in reasonable agreement with physiological and psychophysical estimates. The full frequency bandwidth at half height is approximately 1.6 octaves, and the orientation bandwidth is approximately 40° for the filter that we used. Both of these values are consistent with physiological measurements of the properties of cortical cells in monkeys (De Valois et al., 1982a, b; see also Watson, 1983, 1987). The two-dimensional frequency response of two of the filters is shown in figure 17.4. One consequence of this relatively broad tuning is that filters tuned to neighboring orientations and sizes have quite a lot of overlap in sensitivity. It is therefore quite inappropriate to think of this representation as a local frequency analysis. The outputs of the entire bank of filters for all orientations and scales are shown in figure 17.5.

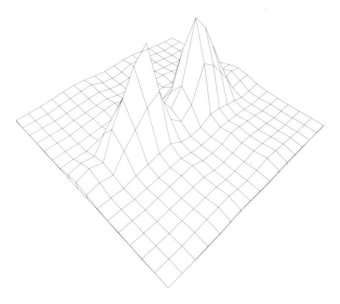

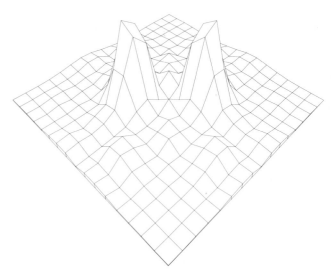

Fig. 17.4
Two-dimensional spatial frequency spectra of two of the filters used to generate the oriented representation.

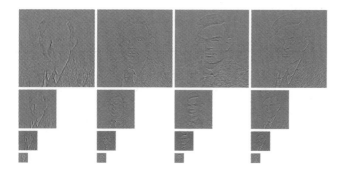

Fig. 17.5
Oriented filter outputs at each scale. The left panels show the vertical filter ouputs (*V*), those immediately to their right show the orientation 45° counterclockwise from vertical (*L*), followed by horizontal (*H*) and 45° counterclockwise from horizontal (*R*).

Energy

The actual representation upon which we base our texture analyses is not the linear output of oriented bandpass filters, but rather the *local energy* in these outputs. The reason for relating textural properties to an energy measure comes from the idea that textural characteristics derive from the nature of local spatial structure within an image region, rather than from the exact placement of features within that region. What energy measures indicate is the total amount of a particular type of spatial structure within their region of pooling. They are insensitive to the spatial distribution of that structure within the region. We are using the word "energy" very loosely to refer to the result of applying some rectifying nonlinearity to the outputs of the linear filters, and then pooling the transformed responses over some region of space. If the representation shown in figure 17.5 is a caricature of the responses of simple cells in visual cortex, then these energy measures correspond to complex cell responses.

We compute energy by squaring the output of the linear units and then taking a weighted average over a small region. This weighted average is achieved by reducing resolution by a factor of 4 using the same Gaussian pyramid algorithm used to construct the linear filters. The result of this operation is shown in figure 17.6.

Opponency

The next stage in the computation of orientation measures involves constructing opponent signals by subtracting the vertical energy response from the horizontal, and the right diagonal from the left diagonal. The physiological and psychophysical justification for this stage is weak, although *qualitatively* orientation opponency seems to be a reasonable thing from a perceptual standpoint. Computationally it serves two purposes: It makes the orientation tuning of the resulting opponent mechanisms somewhat insensitive to the orientation tuning of the underlying linear filters, and it produces responses "in quadrature" with respect to the orientation of image structure. This is

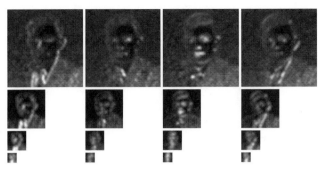

Fig. 17.6
Oriented energy outputs. These are the oriented pyramid filter outputs, squared and averaged locally.

because regardless of the actual orientation bandwidths of the linear filters, the opponent responses must have a zero response where their respective input responses are equal. By symmetry, the $H-V$ mechanism must have maximum absolute responses at $0°$ and $90°$ and have 0 response at $45°$ and $135°$. Similarly, the $R-L$ mechanism must peak at $45°$ and $135°$ and have a null response at $0°$ and $90°$. This is independent of the orientation bandwidths of the linear filters. This is a desirable property if we want to interpret the outputs of the mechanisms as an orientation measure.

Normalization

The responses that have been computed thus far all increase monotonically with input contrast. Therefore, it is impossible to look at a single unit and determine how closely the local image structure matches that unit's preference. A particular level of response could indicate appropriate structure at moderate contrast or inappropriate structure at high contrast. In order to obtain more direct information about local structure not confounded with contrast, we need to introduce a form of contrast gain control (Shapley & Enroth-Cugell, 1984; Shapley & Victor, 1978). This kind of interaction has been inferred from physiological experiments (Bonds, 1989; Heeger & Adelson, 1989; Ohzawa, Sclar & Freeman, 1985; Robson, 1988) and recently invoked to explain some psychophysical phenomena (Wilson & Ferrera, 1989). We model this interaction by computing a sum of all of the energy responses (i.e., a sum across orientations) at a particular resolution level and dividing each oriented energy response by this sum. If we denote the energy response at

resolution level ρ and orientation θ by $E(\rho, \theta)$ then the normalized response of the $H-V$ mechanism is:

$$N(\rho, \theta) = \frac{E(\rho, 0) - E(\rho, 90)}{\sum_{i=0}^{3} E(\rho, \phi_i)}.$$

Note that in performing this normalization we have lost all information about actual stimulus contrast. Clearly, humans can see differences in contrast as well as differences in local spatial structure. Rather than describing this normalization as a *loss* of contrast information, therefore, it is better to say that we have *separated* the contrast information from the structure information. A more complete model of visual perception would need to specify how the contrast information is represented. The point is not that we cannot see contrast differences, but that we do not generally confuse contrast differences and structure differences.

Normalized opponent outputs are shown in figure 17.7.

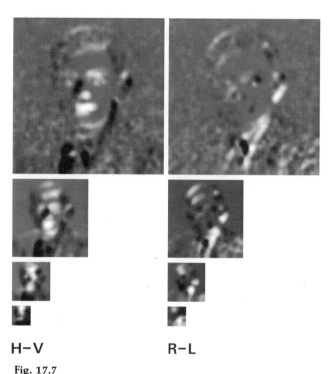

H–V   **R–L**

Fig. 17.7
Normalized opponent outputs. The oriented energy outputs at each scale are divided by the sum of all of the energies at that scale for contrast normalization, and two differences are computed: $H-V$ and $R-L$.

Orientation Analysis

As noted above, some of the analysis that this model performs is somewhat specific to the particular type of texture segregation task that we wish to model. The texture differences occurring in this task involve local orientation, so the computation described is designed to isolate these differences and to ignore differences in size, contrast, and other factors. In one of the examples described below the texture difference is based on scale differences rather than orientation. In this case the orientation opponent measure is not the appropriate one. This part of the analysis can be made more general either by making it more symmetric with respect to other image properties (as suggested by Heeger and Adelson, 1989; see also chapter 9) or by constructing a parallel set of specific image measures. Heeger and Adelson perform a normalization based on the sum of responses at all orientations and also at neighboring scales. This means that the same measure can be used to compute both orientation and scale differences. It is also possible that this level of processing is adaptive in a task-dependent mode. In many ways this adaptive approach is similar to the parallel one unless multiple types of texture differences occur simultaneously.

Modeling Performance

Thus far, we have described an image processing algorithm, that is, the output of each stage in the model has been a transformed image. In order to predict observer performance in a specific task, we need to relate the images produced by the model to performance of the task. In essence, this requires constructing an algorithm that computes the same decisions required of the human observer, using the output of the image processing part of the model as input. We postpone discussion of this part of the modeling until after the description of the texture experiments. First, we present some examples that illustrate the function of the model up to this point.

Texture Examples

Orientation-based Textures

In the first set of examples, the dominant cue for the texture difference is orientation. This is generally a rather strong component in determining texture segregation. A series of examples follow ranging from very simple arrays of lines to textures taken from natural scenes.

Oriented Lines

Figure 17.8A shows an example of a texture composed of line segments. This texture shows strong segregation. The oriented energy and normalized opponent energy outputs are shown in Figure 17.8B and C. As might be expected, the vertical and horizontal energy outputs and the $H-V$ opponent outputs do not show anything interesting. This is because the vertical and horizontal filters have the same outputs for the diagonal line segments comprising the textures. On the other hand, the diagonal energy outputs convert the texture difference between the regions into an intensity difference. In this case neither the contrast normalization or opponent processing has much further effect.

Observations of Mayhew and Frisby

A second example involving simple orientation differences is shown in figure 17.9A. This shows an example taken from an experiment of Mayhew and Frisby (1978). In the lower half of the image are two sinusoidal gratings differing in orientation by 30°. In the upper half, each panel contains the sum of three sinusoidal gratings differing in orientation by 60°. The orientations in the left and right panels differ by 30°. Mayhew and Frisby observed that the difference between the two panels on the bottom is very clear, while the difference between the two on the top is much less so. They quantified this observation with psychophysical experiments. This difference exists in spite of the fact that the differences in orientation between frequency components are exactly the same (30°) on the top and on the bottom. The normalized opponent energy outputs for this image are shown in Figure 17.9B. The normalized opponent outputs show considerably larger differences for the simple gratings, and thus are qualitatively in agreement with the Mayhew and Frisby result. The reason for this difference lies primarily with the large orientation bandwidths of the underlying filters. This means that the change in response with change in orientation for the upper patterns is smaller than that for the simple gratings.

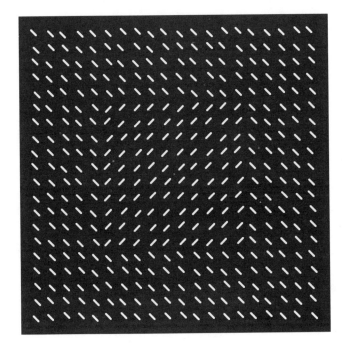

A

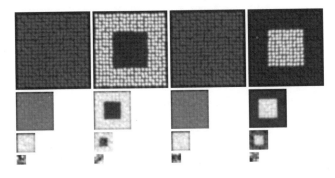

B

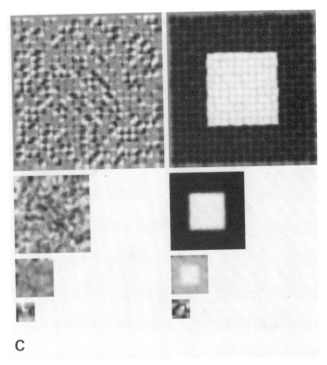

C

Fig. 17.8
(A) A texture composed of oriented line segments. (B) Oriented
energy outputs. (C) Normalized opponent energy outputs.

Natural textures

A final example of an orientation based texture difference
is shown in figure 17.10A. This image contains two natural textures taken from Brodatz (1966): one a picture of
rough bark and the other of a bundle of straw. In this case,
the individual oriented energy images show fairly little
coherent difference between the center square (straw) and
the outside region (bark), because the differences that
exist are masked by local variations in image contrast and

scale. The normalized opponent images, however, show a
very clear division. The $H-V$ and $R-L$ normalized opponent energy outputs are shown in figure 17.10B

Micropatterns

Textures such as the one shown in figure 17.1 are sometimes referred to as "micropattern" textures because they
are constructed by quasi-random placement of small shapes
or patterns. There has been a tradition in the perceptual
literature of relating these textures and their properties to
characteristics of the micropatterns, such as their sizes,
orientations or other geometrical properties (Beck, 1966a,
b; Julesz, 1981a, b). However, such analyses tacitly imply
the existence of some process that extracts these descriptions from the texture images. We can treat these images
in the same way as those discussed above and gain some
understanding of their perceptual properties. The oriented
energy outputs for the texture shown in figure 17.1 are
shown in figure 17.11. Note that at an appropriate scale,
differences appear between the segregating region and
the background, while this is not the case for the non-
segregating region. This suggests that the percept of
segregation generated in these textures may have a basis
similar to that underlying the perception of orientation
based textures.

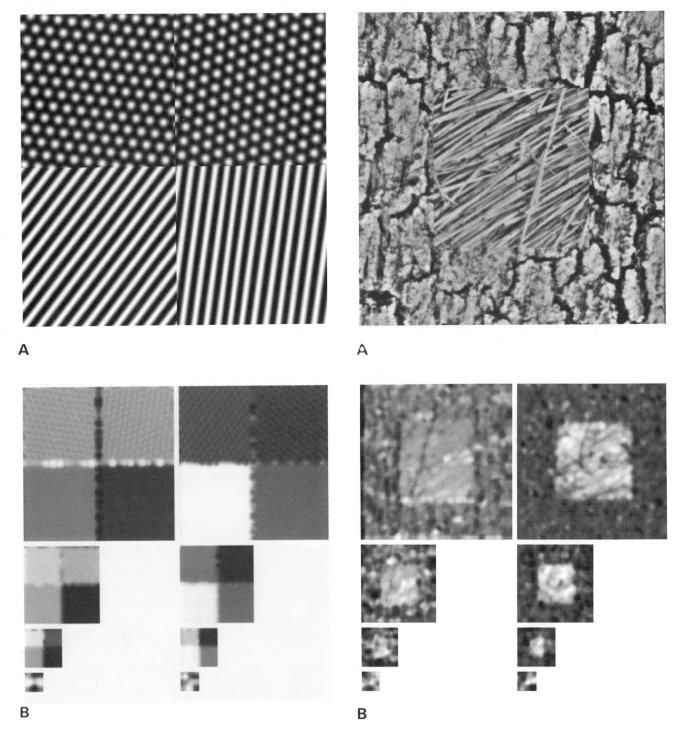

Fig. 17.9
(A) Example taken from Mayhew and Frisby (1978). (B) Normalized opponent outputs. Note that the differences between the left and right panels are generally larger for the simple gratings (*lower half*) than for the sums of gratings (*upper half*).

Fig. 17.10
(A) Synthetic image composed of two natural textures. (B) Normalized opponent outputs.

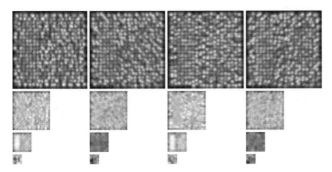

Fig. 17.11
Oriented energy outputs for the texture of figure 17.1. Note difference at low resolution between segregating region and background.

Texture Experiments

To analyze models such as the one described above, it is useful to consider stimuli that require only a portion of the full model in order to account for texture segregation performance. Consider the texture stimulus shown in figure 17.12A. The figure consists of two regions, each of which is narrowband in terms of the range of spatial frequencies and orientations present. Since the stimulus is restricted in spatial frequency content, only one spatial scale of the model will be sensitive to it. Thus, by varying the orientation content of the images, it is possible to analyze the processing of local orientation by a single scale of the model.

We have carried out a series of experiments using textures of the kind in figure 17.12 (taken from Landy and Bergen, 1991). In the next section we will describe how to account for performance in those experiments using the model we have described above, and so we present them in some detail.

The stimuli used in the experiments consist of regions of filtered noise. The noise was IID (independent pixels, identically distributed) Gaussian noise, and at each pixel location, the filter kernel (or impulse response) was in the form of a Gabor function (a sine wave windowed by a two-dimensional Gaussian). The filter kernel varied from location to location, resulting in a *nonisoplanatic* filtering operation. In figure 17.12A, for example, a vertically oriented Gabor was used in the background region, and a diagonal filter was used in the foreground. The stimuli varied in the amount of orientation difference $\Delta\theta$ between the foreground and background. For example, in figure 17.12A the orientation difference is $36°$ while in part B $\Delta\theta$

is $18°$. In addition, the change in orientation from the background to the foreground was either abrupt (the kernel rotated by an angle of $\Delta\theta$ between one pixel and its immediate neighbor across the edge between the foreground and background figures) as in figure 17.12A, or could occur across a spatial interval Δx, as in part C. In the latter case, kernels of intermediate orientation are used at the intermediate pixel locations. Another way to think about this is that when Δx is increased, the textural edge resulting from the change in *"local orientation"* is blurred. The original motivation for this experiment was to further investigate a suggestion by Nothdurft (1985) that texture segregation was a function of the gradient of a textural property (e.g., $\Delta\theta/\Delta x$). Here, we will show how the results of such experiments may be modeled.

In the experiment, a stimulus such as one of those shown in figure 17.12 was presented, followed by a blank interval, followed by a masker (a field of high contrast random dots). The foreground figure was a $16.7°$ square with a missing corner on a $32.7°$ background, and the dominant spatial frequency in the textures was 1.5 cycles/degree. The mean luminance was 53 cd/m^2, and the peak contrast was approximately 98 percent. The subject's task was to identify which of the four corners was missing. Experimental variables included $\Delta\theta$, Δx, and the stimulus onset asynchrony (SOA) between the stimulus and the postmasker. Across trials, the following were varied randomly in order to eliminate certain undesirable subject strategies: the absolute orientation used (θ), the position of the truncated square figure within the stimulus, and the time delay between the cue spot that signaled the upcoming trial and the appearance of the texture stimulus. For further details of the experimental procedure and stimulus generation, see Landy and Bergen (1991).

Figure 17.13A shows typical texture segregation performance as a function of SOA. Performance improves with increasing SOA, reaching an asymptote by 133 msec. Across different conditions, it was found that the time course of performance improvement did not vary substantially. The results are concisely summarized by the asymptotic performance values shown in figure 17.13B, which are computed by fitting a rising exponential to the performance data. The asymptotic performance levels are poorer for increasing Δx and for decreasing $\Delta\theta$ (which is consistent with Nothdurft's conjecture). Next, we show how the results shown in figure 17.13B may be modeled quantitatively using the sort of model described above.

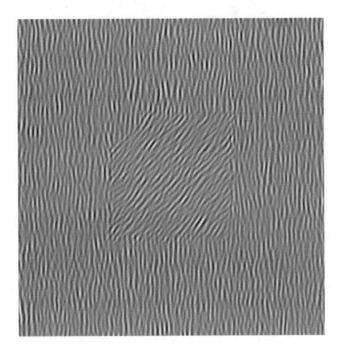

A

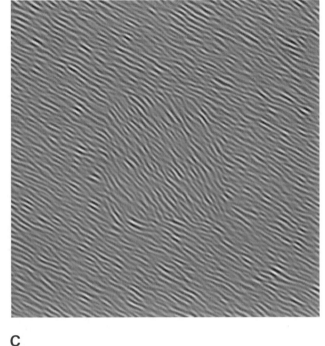

C

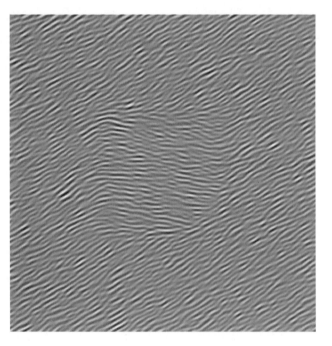

B

Fig. 17.12
Filtered noise stimuli used in discrimination experiments.
(A) $\Delta\theta = 36°$, $\Delta x = 0°$. (B) $\Delta\theta = 18°$, $\Delta x = 0°$.
(C) $\Delta\theta = 36°$, $\Delta x = 3.0°$.

Modeling Performance

The experiments described in the previous section show a systematic relationship between the characteristics of texture images and human subjects' performance in a discrimination task involving them. The computation described above produces a set of processed images for each input image. The model outputs for one of the stimuli used in the experiments are shown in figure 17.14. In order to examine quantitatively the properties of this computation as a model of human texture segregation, we must relate these processed images to predictions of performance in the discrimination task. In other words, we must construct an algorithm that maps the outputs of the computational model described above into a prediction of probability of correct discrimination for the stimuli in question. Since the model that we have described provides no description of temporal characteristics, we can analyze only the asymptotic performance levels.

A simple model of the discrimination process can be based on a cross-correlator. If we assume that the system has perfect knowledge of the shape of the four patterns (the four orientations of the truncated square) among which it is trying to discriminate, then we can compute the cross-correlation function of the model outputs with

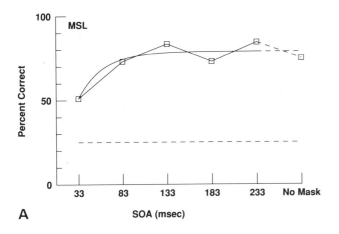

A

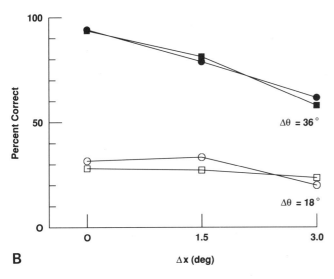

B

Fig. 17.13
Example of discrimination performance. (A) As a function of SOA.
Curve through points is described in text. (B) Asymptotic
performance levels for two subjects.

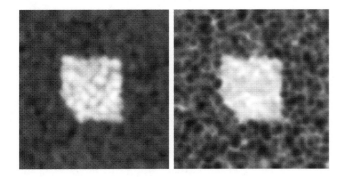

Fig. 17.14
Example of normalized opponent outputs for an experimental
stimulus.

the expected output for each of the possible orientations.
Since we have randomized the position of the square we
do not know where the peak of the cross-correlation
function will be, but we can still decide which stimulus
occurred: Whichever cross-correlation gives the highest
peak output determines the predicted choice of response.
This scheme is illustrated in figure 17.15. In order to
calculate a probability of correct discrimination, we compute the predicted responses for the same set of pseudo-
random stimuli used in the experiments. In effect, we run
the same experiment on the model that was run with the
human subjects.

For the noiseless cross-correlator shown in figure 17.15,
the prediction for all experimental conditions is perfect
performance, that is, 100 percent correct identification of
the stimulus orientation. This fact is not very surprising,
given the appearance of the model output images shown
in figure 17.14; it is very easy to decide which of the four
possible orientations is present when looking at these
images, much easier than it is to decide when looking at
the original texture images. Furthermore, the stimuli in
the experiments were presented quite briefly, so that their
effective contrast might be rather low. This might cause
effects of noise to become more significant. In order to
reflect this, we can replace the ideal cross-correlation with
a noisy one. This is equivalent to adding noise to the
input images (the outputs of the oriented energy computation) before correlating them with the templates. This
discrimination model is shown in figure 17.16A. We do
not know how much noise to add, but we can ask whether *any* noise level gives performance predictions that
match the experimental results.

Results of adding noise are shown in figure 17.16B.
The noise used was additive, Gaussian, and white, that is
the increment to each pixel was an independent sample
from a Gaussian random variable. Each prediction is the
proportion of correct model decisions over the set of 12
experimental stimuli for that condition, and over 10 "trials"
per stimulus, each using independent samples of noise.
The model no longer predicts perfect performance under
all conditions when the noise level is raised sufficiently.
Here, we have a noise level such that the signal-to-noise
ratio (i.e., $\sigma_{norm}/\sigma_{noise}$, where σ_{norm} is the standard deviation of the normalized opponent image and σ_{noise} is the
standard deviation of the added noise image) for the
easiest condition ($\Delta\theta = 36°$ and $\Delta x = 0°$) is .288. However, the results are still not satisfactory: The predicted

Computational Modeling of Visual Texture Segregation

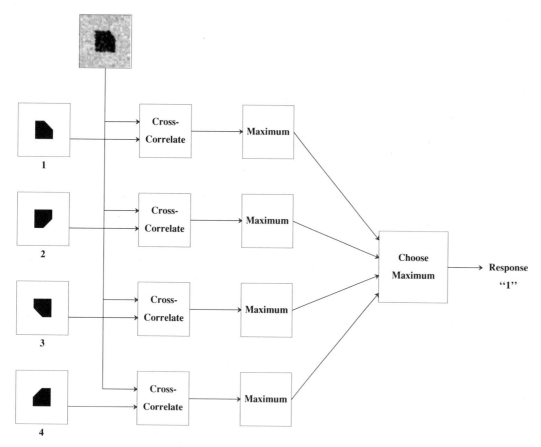

Fig. 17.15

Noiseless cross-correlator model of the discrimination process.

decline in performance with Δx is considerably smaller than that seen in the experimental results. The effect of adding more noise is simply to reduce the predicted performance roughly uniformly for all conditions.

The lack of sensitivity to changing Δx might be due to the fact that the cross-correlation makes use of information from the entire shape of the embedded figure, while increasing Δx affects only the edges of the shape. To test this idea, we introduced an edge extraction step between the normalized opponent energy computation and the noisy cross-correlator (see figure 17.17A). This is indicated by showing the inputs to the cross-correlators as outlines, rather than solid figures. Edge extraction can be thought of as a kind of nonlinear lateral inhibitory interaction. Only where the normalized opponent energy is changing rapidly will the edge response be large. This edge extraction was formulated as a Sobel operator (Gonzalez & Wintz, 1987), which is simply a discrete implementation of a gradient magnitude measure. Thus the

edge output is just the magnitude of the gradient vector at each point, or the square root of the sum of the squares of the vertical and horizontal partial derivatives. The result of performing this operation on two of the experimental stimuli is shown in figure 17.17B. In the case with $\Delta x = 0°$ (on the left) the edge is clear and distinct, while in the case with $\Delta x = 3.0°$ (on the right) the edge is somewhat fuzzy. Since we are using this modified input, we must cross-correlate with the expected output from the edge extraction stage to generate predictions.

The predicted performance is shown in figure 17.17C. Once again, the influence of Δx is insufficiently great. The effect of increasing Δx is to make the change in orientation between the two texture regions less abrupt. This causes the change in intensity in the normalized opponent energy images to become less rapid which, in turn, makes the magnitude of the spatial gradient of these images smaller. The observation that in order to fit the data the effect of noise needs to be greater for the large Δx conditions than for the small is equivalent to the condition that the noise be more effective for small values of the edge

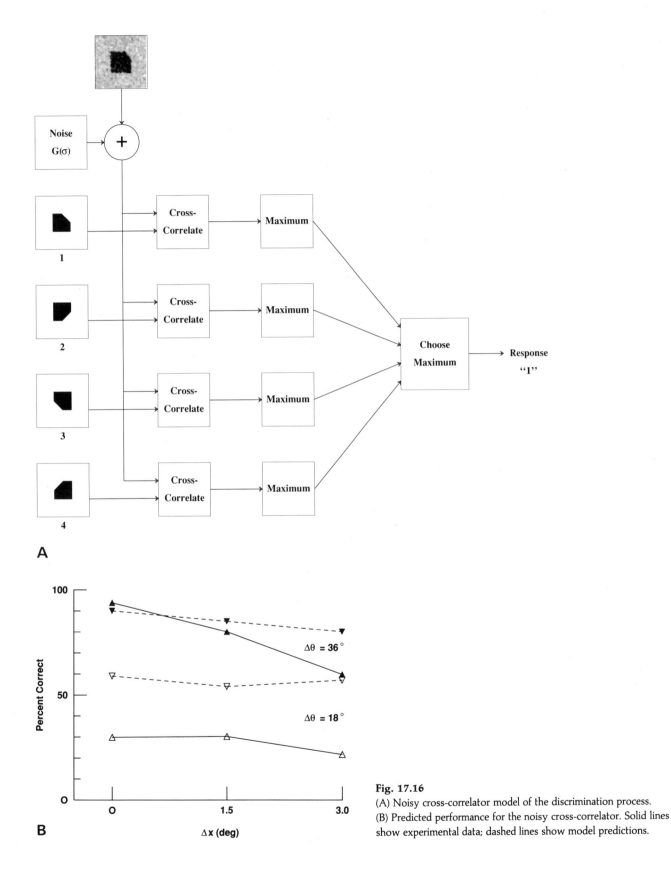

Fig. 17.16
(A) Noisy cross-correlator model of the discrimination process.
(B) Predicted performance for the noisy cross-correlator. Solid lines show experimental data; dashed lines show model predictions.

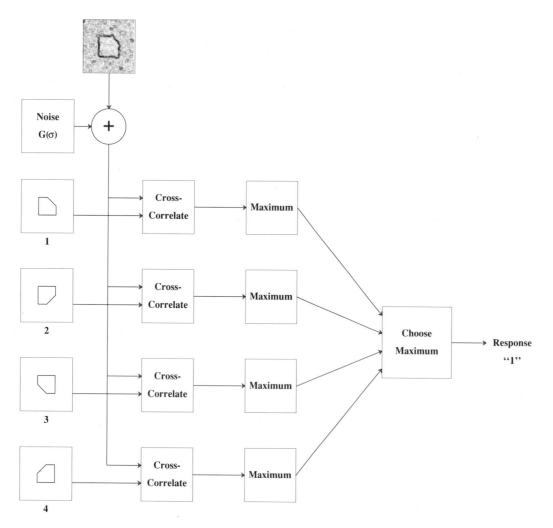

A

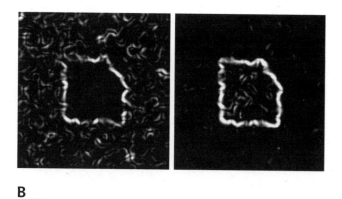

B

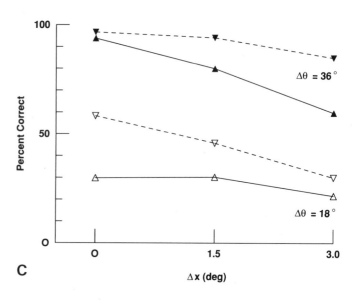

C

Fig. 17.17

(A) Noisy cross-correlator operating on edges. (B) Output of
Sobel operator applied to normalized opponent outputs (*left*,
$\Delta x = 0°$; *right*, $\Delta x = 3.0°$). (C) Predicted performance for the noisy
edge cross-correlator. Solid lines show experimental data; dashed
lines show model predictions.

strength than for large. This effect can be achieved by passing the edge strength measure through an accelerating nonlinearity prior to the noisy cross-correlation stage. Qualitatively, this is similar to setting a threshold for the edge strength values, below which they are disregarded.

The nonlinearity chosen was the fourth power of the input. The predicted performance for this fourth power of gradient magnitude decision process is shown in figure 17.18A. This model gives a good fit to the data, with respect to both the effects of increasing Δx and decreasing

$\Delta\theta$. The complete structure used in this prediction is shown in figure 17.18B.

Note that in the development of this discrimination model we have not needed to change the computation of the basic model outputs. The filter shapes, spatial pooling parameters, and contrast normalization parameters have all remained fixed. These are the factors that determine the fundamental response of the model to such stimulus characteristics as $\Delta\theta$ and Δx.

The question naturally arises as to the *necessity* of the model components that we have introduced. If we take the normalized opponent energy computation as input, we argued that the subsequent stages (gradient magnitude, noise, cross-correlation, maximum detection) are all necessary since we were unable to fit even the limited set of data described here with any subset of them. For this set of stimuli there are undoubtedly much simpler models that would provide a good account of the data. However, our purpose is to describe the process of human texture segregation, not simply to model a particular set of psychophysical measurements. For this purpose many of the features of the computation that we have described, including orientation and scale selectivity, rectifying nonlinearities and some form of contrast normalization, must be incorporated.

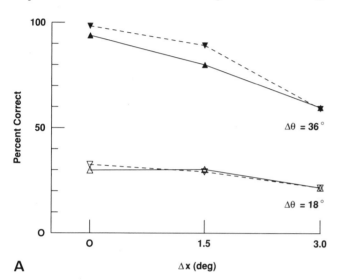

A

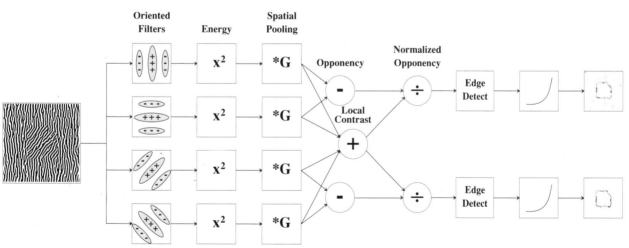

B

Fig. 17.18
(A) Predicted performance for model with added fourth power nonlinearity at the output. Solid lines show experimental data; dashed lines show model predictions. (B) Sequence of processing steps in model that successfully predicts discrimination performance.

Conclusions

We have examined the representation of visual textures within a simple multiple scale- and orientation-based model of early vision. This representation converts many conspicuous texture differences into explicit intensity differences. On this basis, the process of textural segregation can be interpreted as one of extracting structure from these intensity differences. It is not necessary to postulate sophisticated mechanisms specifically concerned with the extraction of textural information.

We have also shown that this simple representation can be related quantitatively to human performance in a texture based discrimination task using a simple pattern discrimination model. This model involves extraction of texture edges by computing the gradient of a local texture measure, followed by an accelerating nonlinearity that de-emphasizes weak edges. This edge extraction is used as input to a noisy cross-correlator that finds the best match among the set of discriminanda. The probability of correct discrimination predicted by this model matches accurately the results obtained with human observers, including the effects of varying the orientation difference or the orientation gradient.

The success of this simple procedure in predicting human performance without detailed manipulation of model parameters is somewhat surprising. However, this model has as yet had only a very limited trial. Presumably, more careful determination of model parameters based on psychophysical measurements will be required to produce a model of more general applicability.

References

Beck, J. (1966a). Effect of orientation and of shape similarity on perceptual grouping. *Perception and Psychophysics, 1,* 300–302.

Beck, J. (1966b). Perceptual grouping produced by changes in orientation and shape. *Science, 154.* 538–540.

Bergen, J. R. (1988). Visual texture segmentation and early vision. In *OSA Annual Meeting, 1988 Technical Digest,* Vol. 11, Optical Society of America, Washington, DC.

Bergen, J. R. (1991). Theories of visual texture perception. In D. M. Regan, (Ed.), *Spatial vision* (Vol. 10 of *Vision and Visual Dysfunction*) (pp. 114–134). New York: Macmillan.

Bergen, J. R. & Adelson, E. H. (1986). Visual texture segmentation based on energy measures. *Journal of the Optical Socity of America A, 3,* 98.

Bergen, J. R. & Adelson, E. H. (1988), Visual texture segmentation and early vision. *Nature, 333,* 363–364.

Bonds, A. B. (1989). Role of inhibition in the specification of orientation selectivity of cells in the cat striate cortex. *Visual Neuroscience, 2,* 41–55.

Brent, R. P. (1973). *Algorithms for minimization without derivatives.* Englewood Cliffs, NJ: Prentice Hall.

Brodatz, P. (1966). *Textures: A photographic album for artists and designers.* New York: Dover.

Burt, P. J. (1981). Fast filter transforms for image processing. *Computer Graphics and Image Processing, 16,* 20–51.

Caelli, T. M. (1982). On discriminating visual textures and images. *Perception and Psychophysics, 31,* 149–159.

Caelli, T. M. (1985). Three processing characteristics of visual texture segmentation. *Spatial Vision, 1,* 19–30.

Caelli, T. M. (1986). Three processing characteristics of texture discrimination. In *Vision interface '86* (pp. 343–348). Irvine, CA.

De Valois, R. L., Albrecht, D. G. & Thorell, L. G. (1982a). Spatial frequency selectivity of cells in macaque visual cortex. *Vision Research, 22,* 545–559.

De Valois, R. L., Yund, E. W. & Hepler, N. (1982b). The orientation and direction selectivity of cells in macaque visual cortex. *Vision Research, 22,* 531–544.

Gonzalez, R. C. & Wintz, P. (1987). *Digital image processing.* Reading, MA: Addison Wesley.

Harvey, L. O. & Gervais, M. J. (1978). Visual texture perception and fourier analysis. *Perception and Psychophysics, 24,* 534–542.

Harvey, L. O. & Gervais, M. J. (1981). Internal representation of visual texture as the basis for the judgment of similarity. *Journal of Experimental Psychology: Human Perception and Performance, 7,* 741–753.

Heeger, D. J. & Adelson, E. H. (1989). Mechanisms for extracting local orientation. *Investigative Ophthalmology and Visual Science (Suppl), 30,* 110.

Hubel, D. H. & Wiesel, T. N. (1968). Receptive fields and functional architecture of monkey striate cortex. *Journal of Physiology, 195,* 215–243.

Julesz, B. (1962). Visual pattern discrimination. *IRE Trans. Information Theory, IT-8,* 12–18.

Julesz, B. (1981a). Textons, the elements of texture perception and their interactions. *Nature, 290,* 91–97.

Julesz, B. (1981b). A theory of preattentive texture discrimination based on first-order statistics of textons. *Biological Cybernetics, 41,* 131–138.

Landy, M. S. & Bergen, J. R. (1988). Texture segregation by multiresolution energy or by structure gradient? In *OSA Annual Meeting, 1988, Technical Digest* (pp. 162–163), Washington, DC.

Landy, M. S. & Bergen, J. R. (1991). Texture segregation and orientation gradient. *Vision Research, 31,* 679–691.

Mayhew, J. E. W. & Frisby, J. P. (1978). Texture discrimination and fourier analysis in human vision. *Nature, 275,* 438–439.

Mostafavi, H. & Sakrison, D. J. (1976). Structure and properties of a single channel in the human visual system. *Vision Research, 16,* 957–968.

Nothdurft, H. C. (1985). Sensitivity for structure gradient in texture discrimination tasks. *Vision Research, 25,* 1957–1968.

Ohzawa, I., Sclar, G. & Freeman, R. D. (1985). Contrast gain control in the cat's visual system. *Journal of Neurophysiology, 54,* 651–667.

Phillips, G. C. & Wilson, H. R. (1984). Orientation bandwidths of spatial mechanisms measured by masking. *Journal of the Optical Society of America A, 1,* 226–232.

Powell, M. J. D. (1964). An efficient method for finding the minimum of a function in several variables without calculating derivatives. *Computer Journal, 7,* 155–162.

Richards, W. (1979). Quantifying sensory channels: Generalizing colorimetry to orientation and texture, touch, and tones. *Sensory Processes, 3,* 207–229.

Richards, W. & Polit, A. (1974). Texture matching. *Kybernetic, 16,* 155–162.

Robson, J. G. (1988). Linear and nonlinear operations in the visual system. *Investigative Ophthalmology and Visual Science (Suppl), 29,* 117.

Shapley, R. M. & Enroth-Cugell, C. (1984). Visual adaptation and retinal gain controls. *Progress in Retinal Research, 3,* 263–353.

Shapley, R. M. & Victor, J. D. (1978). The effect of contrast on the transfer properties of cat retinal ganglion cells. *Journal of Physiology, 285,* 275–298.

Stromeyer, C. F. & Julesz, B. (1972). Spatial-frequency masking in vision: Critical bands and spread of masking. *Journal of the Optical Society of America, 62,* 1221–1232.

Watson, A. B. (1983). Detection and recognition of simple spatial forms. In O. J. Braddick & A. C. Sleigh (Eds.), *Physical and biological processing of images* (pp. 100–114). New York: Springer-Verlag.

Watson, A. B. (1987). The cortex transform: Rapid computation of simulated neural images. *Computer Vision, Graphics, and Image Processing, 39,* 311–327.

Wilson, H. R. & Bergen, J. R. (1979). A four mechanism model for threshold spatial vision. *Vision Research, 19,* 19–31.

Wilson, H. R. & Ferrera, V. P. (1989). Nonlinear facilitation of spatial masking by orthogonal gratings. In *OSA Annual Meeting, 1989, Technical Digest*, Washington, DC.

18

Complex Channels, Early Local Nonlinearities, and Normalization in Texture Segregation

Norma Graham

Since the work of Jacob Beck and Bela Julesz and their colleagues in the 1960s and 1970s, it has been clear that two-dimensional spatial-frequency content (i.e., spatial-frequency and orientation) is a critical stimulus variable in how well differently patterned or textured regions of the visual field *segregate*, that is, how well they are perceived immediately and effortlessly as separate regions. (An excellent review of the perceived texture-segregation work can be found in Bergen, 1991.) This dependence of perceived segregation on spatial frequency and orientation —coupled with the mounting psychophysical and physiological evidence for low-level analyzers of spatial frequency and orientation in the visual system (reviewed, e.g., in Graham, 1985, 1989b)—has led a number of people to try to explain region (texture) segregation on the basis of such analyzers or sometimes, contrariwise, to try to prove that it cannot be so explained (e.g., chapter 17; Beck, Sutter & Ivry, 1987; Bovik, Clark & Geisler, 1987; Caelli, 1982, 1985, 1988; Chubb & Sperling 1988; Clark, Bovik & Geisler, 1987; Coggins & Jain, 1985; Daugman, 1987, 1988; Fogel & Sagi, 1989; Klein & Tyler, 1986; Landy & Bergen, 1988, 1989; Malik & Perona, 1989a,b; Nothdurft, 1985a,b; Turner, 1986; Victor, 1988; Victor & Conte, 1987, 1989a,b). Heavily influenced by Julesz's original conjecture about texture segregation—which was phrased in statistical language—discussions of texture segregation have often been mathematically sophisticated. (The relationship between such spatial-frequency analyzer models and Julesz's original statistical conjecture has been discussed in some detail by Klein and Tyler, 1986, and Victor, 1988. Related issues have been considered by Yellott and Iverson, 1990.) Only in the last years, however, has there been an emphasis on explicit and quantitative comparisons between psychophysical data on the one hand and predictions from computable models on the other.

Jacob Beck, Anne Sutter, and I calculated quantitative predictions from a simple spatial-frequency analyzers

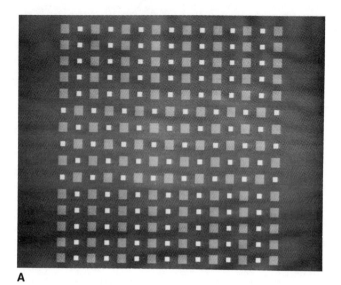

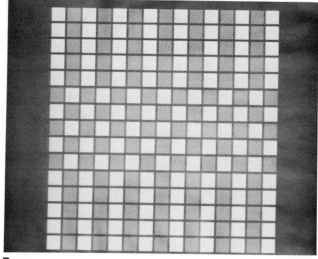

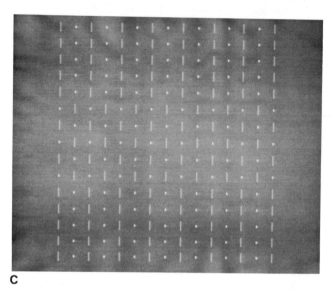

Fig. 18.1

Examples of element-arrangement textures. Identical elements are contained in all three regions but they are arranged in a checkerboard in the center region and in columns in the top and bottom regions.

model and compared these with quantitative measurements of region (texture) segregation collected for patterns like those in figure 18.1 (Graham, Beck & Sutter, 1989; Graham, Beck & Sutter, in preparation; Sutter, 1987; Sutter, Beck & Graham, 1989). These patterns are members of the class of *element-arrangement* texture patterns used originally by Beck, Prazdny, and Rosenfeld (1983) and explored further by Beck, Sutter, and Ivry (1987). They are composed of a uniform background on which

are superimposed two types of elements arranged in stripes in the bottom and top regions and arranged in a checkerboard in the middle region. The observer's task is to indicate (on a scale from 0 to 4) to what degree the whole pattern seems effortlessly and immediately to contain two different kinds of region (striped vs. checkerboard).

Our simple spatial-frequency analyzers model is closely related to the class Chubb and Landy (see chapter 19) call *back pocket* models. We already knew on the basis of previous research that the simple model would work well but probably not perfectly. Our aim was to find out what such a simple model could do and, on the basis of systematic discrepancies between it and the data, to add further visual processes (either low- or higher-level) to the model and then again test the enhanced model. As it turned out, the comparisons between the predictions of the simple spatial-frequency analyzers model and the data from experiments using patterns like those in figure 18.1 were very revealing, showing both the simple spatial-frequency analyzers model's strengths and its weaknesses. The systematic discrepancies we found suggested adding two nonlinear processes to the simple model, where both nonlinearities are presumably the result of low-level (e.g., cortical V1 and V2 or below) visual processes. The second part of this chapter briefly describes these hypothesized nonlinear processes and presents some preliminary predictions from the enhanced model for one kind of experiment (a kind for which calculating predictions is easy if one is willing to make some reasonable simplifying assumptions). These predictions are in very good agreement with the psychophysical results.

Simple Model

The simple spatial-frequency analyzers model we used consists both of assumptions about the analyzers themselves (described in Graham, 1989a, and Sutter, Beck & Graham, 1989) and assumptions relating the outputs of these analyzers to the responses produced by the observer in an experiment (described in Sutter, Beck & Graham, 1989). As in all such models, both sets of assumptions are crucial, although the second set is sometimes not explicit.

Characteristics of Simple Spatial-Frequency Channels (Linear Filters)

Each spatial-frequency channel in the model discussed first below is assumed to be a linear, translation-invariant filter. We described the spatial weighting functions characterizing each filter (the physiological substrate for which might be the receptive-field sensitivity profiles of the individual neurons) as a two-dimensional Gabor function (as used, e.g., by Bovik, Clark & Geisler, 1987; Clark, Bovik & Geisler, 1987; Daugman, 1987, 1988; Field, 1987; Fogel & Sagi, 1989; Rubenstein & Sagi, 1989; Turner, 1986; Watson, 1983), but the precise function makes little difference to these predictions (e.g., a pyramid computation like that used by Bergen and Adelson 1988 and Bergen and Landy, chapter 17, will produce similar enough filter outputs that it should make no difference to the conclusions here). The spatial-frequency and orientation half-amplitude full-bandwidths of each filter were 1 octave and 38° of rotation respectively (as in Watson, 1983) and in good agreement with results from near-threshold psychophysics (reviews in Graham, 1985, 1989b), but again, within rather a large range, the precise bandwidth makes little difference for anything said here. The filters' center spatial frequencies were separated by the squareroot of 2 over the visible range. Three orientations—vertical, horizontal, and half-way between (oblique)—were used. (These three are sufficient for the patterns under consideration here, and we used only three to save computing time; but for more general purposes one would want several more orientations.) The spatial weighting functions were all even-symmetric in the filter computations. (Given our full model, however, using mul-

tiple symmetries of weighting function at each position—that is, multiple phases—would make little or no difference to the predictions if the phases were combined as typically done by others. See discussion below.)

Figure 18.2 (middle and right panels) shows the outputs of two of these simple spatial-frequency channels (linear filters) to the pattern in the left panel. In this pattern, the two element types are squares, one had four times the area of the other, and the contrasts of the two element types were equal. The filter that is sensitive to the vertical orientation and to the fundamental spatial frequency of the striped regions (middle panel) has a spatial weighting function (i.e., receptive field) that will cover one column of squares with its center while covering the adjacent columns of squares with its inhibitory surround. This filter responds well in the top and bottom striped regions but responds little in the middle checkerboard region. A similar-sized obliquely oriented filter responds well in the checkerboard region and not at all well in the striped region. Thus these filters tuned to the fundamental frequency could easily contribute to an observer's ability to segregate the striped from the checkerboard regions.

Any filter tuned to spatial frequencies much higher than the fundamental (e.g., that producing the output in right panel of figure 18.2) has a weighting function much smaller than the period of the pattern. It will respond well (and, considering the whole of each region, about equally well) in both the checked and striped regions because: (1) its output is ample at the edges of all the individual elements (is proportional to edge contrast in fact); and (2) the total amount of element edge is the same in both

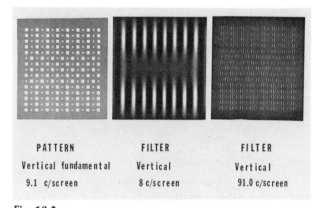

PATTERN	FILTER	FILTER
Vertical fundamental	Vertical	Vertical
9.1 c/screen	8 c/screen	91.0 c/screen

Fig. 18.2
A pattern (*left*) and the responses to it from two simple channels (*middle* and *right*).

the striped and checkerboard regions in these element-arrangement patterns. Thus simple linear channels sensitive to higher spatial frequencies can contribute little to segregation of the striped versus checked regions if any contribution depends on the difference between the total responses in the two regions (as it does in our simple model and in all models of the back pocket type).

Consider what happens, however, when the pattern in the left panel of figure 18.2 is replaced by one in which contrast of the small squares is raised to be a factor of 3 or 4 greater than the contrast of the large squares so that the product of area and contrast is approximately the same for the two sizes of squares. Now the channels sensitive to the fundamental do not respond at all well in either the checked or striped regions because excitation and inhibition balance out within each spatial weighting function (i.e, within each single neuron's receptive field). Thus these channels cannot contribute to perceived region segregation. Channels responsive to the higher spatial frequencies cannot contribute either, for the same reasons they could not for the pattern in figure 18.2. (They continue to respond well and equally well in both regions, since their response is to the edge of individual elements and the amount of and contrasts of element edges continues to be the same in both regions.) In short, neither the channels at the fundamental nor those at higher frequencies can contribute to segregation of the two regions. Thus our simple model (and all similar models) predicts that there should be a trade-off between contrast and area so that two regions differing in arrangement of elements (i.e., the striped versus the checkerboard regions) will not segregate well when the product of area and contrast is the same for the two types of elements. (Photographs illustrating the outputs of all the simple channels can be found in Graham, 1989a, and Sutter, Beck, and Graham 1989.)

From Channels' Outputs to an Observer's Responses

To turn the channel outputs into a quantitative prediction of the observer's ratings of perceived region (texture) segregation, we computed various measures of the degree to which there are gross differences in overall activity between the outputs of the filters to the checkerboard versus to the striped regions.

The first step is to compute a *spatially pooled response* from each channel in both the checked region and the striped region. Let the output at position (x, y) of the channel tuned to the ith frequency and jth orientation be called $O_{ij}(x, y)$. The spatially pooled response of the ijth channel to the checked region is taken to equal:

$$R_{ij}(ch) = \sqrt[k']{\sum_{\substack{(x,y)\ \text{in checked} \\ \text{region}}}^{N_x} \sum^{N_y} \frac{|O_{ij}(x, y) - A_{ij}|^{k'}}{N_x \cdot N_y}}, \qquad (1)$$

where N_x and N_y are the numbers of spatial positions in the x and y directions in one period of the pattern and the summing is done over one period in the checked region. A_{ij} is the average value of $O_{ij}(x, y)$ over this one period. (The construction of the patterns assures that for each filter the values of A_{ij} are very similar in both the checked and striped region, and the fact that the filters are all bandpass means that these values are all very close to zero.) When the exponent k' is set equal to 2 the above measure is equal to the *standard deviation* of the outputs at different positions in one period of the given region. By crude analogy to other situations, this measure is also sometimes described as *energy*. We used exponents $k' = 1, 2, 3, 4$, in the above formula as well as using the maximum output, the minimum output, and the maximum-minimum difference between the outputs at different positions. All conclusions given below held for all choices. The spatially pooled response in the striped region is exactly analogous to the definition in equation 1 for the checked region.

The difference between each filter's spatially pooled responses to the checked and to the striped regions is then computed yielding a *within-channel difference* for the ij[th] filter of

$$Diff_{ij} = |R_{ij}(ch) - R_{ij}(st)|. \qquad (2)$$

Finally, after weighting each within-channel difference by the observer's sensitivity to the corresponding spatial frequency and orientation, the within-channel differences are pooled across all channels to form R_{pool} given by the following definition:

$$R_{pool} = \sqrt[k]{\sum_i^{N_{freq}} \sum_j^{N_{orien}} \{Diff_{ij} \cdot S_{obs,ij}\}^k}, \qquad (3)$$

where $S_{obs,ij}$ is the observer's contrast sensitivity to the ith frequency and jth orientation, N_{freq} is the number of frequencies (usually 13—from 2 to 128 cycles/screen in steps of the square root of 2) and N_{orien} is the number of orientations (usually 3: horizontal, vertical, and oblique). With the exponent $k = 2$, R_{pool} is the root-mean-square difference between regions. We also use exponents of 1, 3, and 4 as well as infinity (taking the maximum of all the differences). All conclusions below hold for all choices. (Victor, 1988, and Chubb and Landy (chapter 19), also consider a whole family of rules, but typically calculations in the texture segregation literature have used pooling with an exponent equal to 2. An exponent of infinity corresponds to taking the channel that best discriminates the two regions which has sometimes been done in the psychophysical discrimination literature and was done in the multispatial-frequency filter model of Fogel and Sagi, 1989.)

The degree to which two regions (textures) segregate perceptually (as reflected by the observer's ratings of perceived segregation) is assumed to be *a monotonic function of R_{pool}*.

Before looking at some predictions of this model, let me briefly discuss alternatives to these assumptions relating the channels' outputs to the observer's responses.

Relationship of Our Pooling Measures to Other Approaches and Boundary Extraction

Instead of pooling across exactly one period of the pattern, which is like pooling with an abrupt-edged window exactly one period wide, one might use a gradual-edged window of about one period's width (about twice the width of the excitatory center of the corresponding filter's receptive field). With an exponent of 2, this is the local-energy measure which has been recently used in models of texture segregation and motion perception (e.g., chapter 17; Bergen, 1988; Bergen & Adelson, 1986, 1988; Landy & Bergen, 1988, 1989).

Instead of using only even-symmetric spatial weighting functions, one might use both odd-symmetric and even-symmetric ones (or any other pair having phase characteristics 90° apart) and then take the Euclidian (Pythagorean) sum of the outputs of the pair located at any internal position in the texture region (e.g., Adelson & Bergen, 1985; Bovik, Clark & Geisler, 1987; Clark, Bovik & Geisler, 1987; Fogel & Sagi, 1989, Turner, 1986). This will again produce essentially the same predictions as the pooling across a region using an exponent $k' = 2$

in the above. Either of these two alternative approaches can lead naturally into a model of how the boundaries between texture regions can actually be computed. In essence, one first computes, for each position in the pattern, the spatially pooled response or the sum of odd and even receptive fields. One then needs a process that ensures that all positions for which the set of these numbers from all channels is much the same belong to the same texture region (see, e.g., discussions in Bergen, 1991; Bovik, Clark & Geisler, 1987; Fogel & Sagi, 1989). This is an extremely interesting topic that has been discussed by a number of people (in addition to those just mentioned: Caelli, 1985, 1986, 1988; Grossberg, 1987; Grossberg & Mingolla 1985) although not explicitly studied here. Gradients at the boundary between two regions may well be important (chapter 17; Nothdurft, 1985b; Landy & Bergen, 1988, 1989). For simplicity, we currently ignore these gradients; this seems at least moderately safe for the results reviewed here since the spatial extent of the gradient in any one filter (the distance over which a local energy measure changes as one goes from the checked to the striped region, for example) is much the same for all the patterns used.

Contrast-Area Trade-off Experiments

In one series of experiments (Sutter, 1987; Sutter, Beck & Graham, 1989), we investigated the tradeoff between contrast and size of elements that is predicted by the simple spatial-frequency channels model (as discussed in connection with figure 18.2 above). The patterns all contained two element types that were the same shape but generally differed in size as in figure 18.1. The mean luminance of all the patterns in a given experiment was the same. Then the luminance (and hence contrast) of the larger element type was held constant while that of the smaller elements was varied and perceived texture segregation was measured. We did this for squares of different sizes, for different fundamental frequencies of patterns (different scalings of the overall patterns), for different duty cycles of patterns (different relationships between element size and interelement spacing), and for line-shaped elements as well as square-shaped elements. In each case, minimal segregation as rated by the observers occurred when the product of area times contrast was approximately equal for the two element types.

The predictions of the simple spatial-frequency channels model were computed for all the patterns used in all these experiments. As expected from the intuition discussed in connection with figure 18.2 above, the model always predicts minimal segregation when the product of area times contrast is approximately the same for the two element types (the exact contrast ratio producing the minimum depends on the duty-cycle of the pattern). In this respect the predictions of the model agreed with the experimental results.

However, the model did not predict all of the details of the experimental results correctly. While the contrast ratio at which the minimal segregation should occur was correctly predicted, the amount of segregation at this minimum was incorrectly predicted for many patterns. As is described briefly below and in much more detail in Sutter, Beck, and Graham (1989), we think we know how to modify the model by adding a "spatial nonlinearity" so that the enhanced model will make the correct predictions for the contrast-size tradeoff experiments.

Complex Channels: A Spatial (Rectification-type) Nonlinearity

The following modification of the simple model seems to resolve the discrepancies between our simple model and the contrast-area trade-off experimental results: Replace or supplement the totally linear spatial-frequency channels (simple channels as above) with "complex channels," as shown in figure 18.3. (The assumptions relating the channels' outputs to the observer's responses remain the same as in the simple model.) These complex channels have three stages: two stages of linear filtering with a pointwise nonlinearity (that is dramatic near zero) in between. For our purposes to date, the nonlinearity might be a full-wave rectification (that takes the absolute value of the first filter's output at each point in space), a half-wave rectification (that substitutes zero for the negative values and leaves the positive values untouched), a squarer (that squares the output at each point), or some other similar function. (See Heeger, chapter 9, for some discussion of the differences among these nonlinearities however.) These proposed complex channels are more complicated than the simple linear channels discussed earlier in much the same way that complex cells in area V1 of primate visual cortex are more complicated than

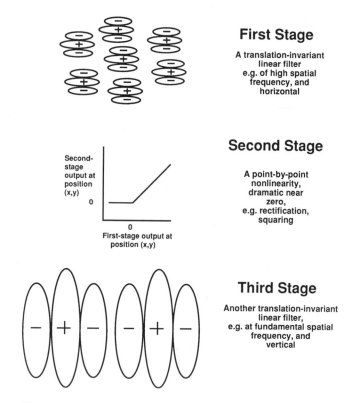

First Stage

A translation-invariant linear filter e.g. of high spatial frequency, and horizontal

Second Stage

A point-by-point nonlinearity, dramatic near zero, e.g. rectification, squaring

Third Stage

Another translation-invariant linear filter, e.g. at fundamental spatial frequency, and vertical

Fig. 18.3
Diagram of a complex channel.

simple cortical cells (e.g., Hochstein & Spitzer 1985). However, the bandpass nature of the third-stage filtering in the complex channels proposed here may not be confirmed for cortical complex cells; and, in any case, it is premature to take the possible physiological analogue of the complex channels too seriously. A number of other people have suggested the use of complex-cell-like computations in tasks like texture segregation (chapter 17; Bergen & Adelson, 1988; Chubb & Sperling, 1988; Fogel & Sagi, 1989; Grossberg & Mingolla, 1985; Robson, 1980; Sagi, 1989; Sperling, 1989; Sperling & Chubb, 1989). Some of these suggested complex-cell like computations, however, may be more like our simple model (simple linear channels followed by the nonlinear pooling operations contained in the assumptions relating channel outputs to observers' responses) than like our complex model (complex channels consisting of a linear-nonlinear-linear sandwich followed by the nonlinear pooling operations).

A qualitative description of how (i.e., insights into why) complex channels might explain all the discrepancies between the results of area-contrast trade-off experiments and the simple model's predictions can be found in

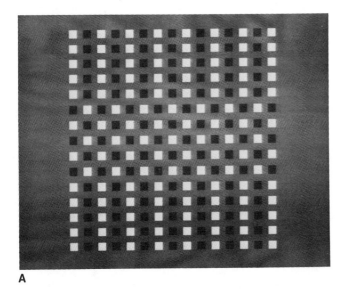

A

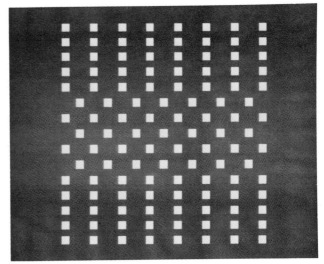

B

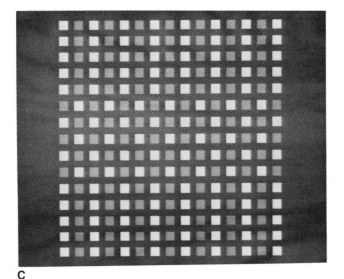

C

Fig. 18.4
Examples of element-arrangement textures used in *on-off* experiment.
(A) An opposite-sign-of-contrast pattern. (B) A one-element-only
pattern. (C) A same-sign-of-contrast pattern.

Sutter, Beck, and Graham (1989), but we have not yet
done quantitative predictions. Briefly, the intuition is this:
the kind of complex channel where the third-stage filter
responds to much lower spatial frequencies than does the
first-stage filter (as in the diagram of figure 18.3) will
respond to *low-spatial-frequency patterns composed of high-
spatial-frequency elements*. (To put it in terms of an auditory
analogue that may be helpful to some people: this kind of
complex channel is sensitive to the "missing fundamen-

tal".) Thus complex channels responding to higher harmonics can contribute to perceived segregation (although
simple channels sensitive to higher harmonics do not,
as was discussed in connection with figure 18.2). As it
turns out, this response of the complex channels to higher
harmonics can account for the discrepancies between the
area-contrast trade-off experimental results and the predictions of the original simple model.

It is important to note that although a two-stage channel—just a pointwise nonlinearity followed by a linear
filtering—works in principle to explain many previously-
noted failures of simple linear channels (e.g., Peli, 1987), it
will not work here.

On-Off Experiments

The rest of this chapter will describe another type of
experiment—which we will call an *on-off* experiment—in
somewhat more detail than were the area-contrast trade-
off experiments. The results of the on-off experiments
suggest the existence of (at least) two rather different
nonlinearities: (l) the "spatial nonlinearity" embodied in
the complex channels just described, and (2) an "intensity-
dependent nonlinearity," for which we can propose at
least two candidate processes known to occur at relatively low levels in the visual system.

For the patterns used in the on-off experiment (examples are shown in figure 18.4), the two types of elements
were always squares of the same shape and size but differing in sign of contrast (i.e., lighter or darker than the

Complex Channels, Early Local Nonlinearities, and Normalization background—hence the "on" and "off" in the name of these experiments) and/or in amount of contrast. In the experiment described here, we used the set of stimuli diagrammed in figure 18.5, where each dot represents a stimulus; that is, we used the texture patterns defined by all possible pairs of a number of different contrasts. (Equivalently, since the background luminance was kept constant, all possible pairs of a number of different luminances were used.) There is only half a matrix of possibilities shown because the other half is presumably redundant. Notice that the contrast of any individual element relative to the background was never greater than 25 percent; this value is small for the literature on texture segregation (where black/white patterns, i.e., patterns of 100 percent contrast, predominate) but large for the literature on detection and identification of near-threshold patterns (from which much of the best evidence for the properties of spatial-frequency and orientation analyzers derives). (For the results shown here, the background luminance was 16 ft-L and the fundamental frequency of the striped texture pattern was 1 cycle/degree. The squares were slightly wider than the inter-square spaces.)

Constant-Difference Series and Simple-Model Predictions

Series of patterns like that illustrated in figure 18.6 are particularly interesting. In such a series the *difference* between the luminances of the two element types is held constant. The absolute luminances of the two element types vary together. In such a *constant-difference* series, which generally contains more patterns than the five shown here, there are patterns where both element types have the *same sign of contrast* (both darker or both lighter than the background), patterns where one element type has the same luminance as the background so there is *one element type only* apparent (which can be either dark or light), and patterns where the two element types are of *opposite sign of contrast*.

In the matrix-of-stimuli diagram (figure 18.5) any such series where $L_2 - L_1$ is constant occurs along lines parallel to the positive diagonal (bottom right). Notice also (bottom left) that all patterns on a line through the origin have the same incremental luminance ratio ($\Delta L_1 / \Delta L_2$) and also the same contrast ratio. For example, the patterns on the negative diagonal have element types with opposite (but equal) contrasts and thus a ratio of -1; all patterns

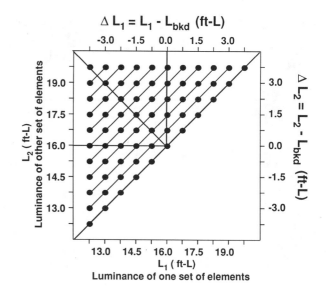

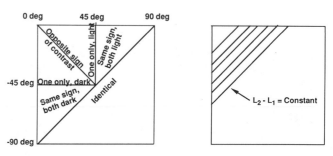

Fig. 18.5
Diagram of stimuli used in *on-off* experiment.

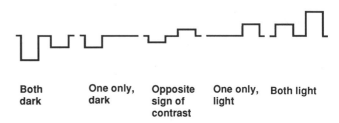

Fig. 18.6
Luminance profiles of the two element types from each of five patterns in a *constant-difference series* from an *on-off* experiment.

on the vertical ray upwards from the origin have one element type only, and that element type is bright. Rather than using L_2 and L_1 to describe a pattern, two other numbers have proved very useful: (1) the luminance difference $L_2 - L_1$, and (2) the angle, which we will call the *contrast-ratio angle*, between the negative diagonal in a plot such as figure 18.5 and the line going through the point representing a stimulus. (Some examples of contrast-ratio angles are indicated in the bottom left of figure 18.5 on the left and top edges of the square.)

The constant-difference series of patterns are of particular interest because models of texture segregation involving multiple, linear, spatial-frequency and orientation channels (like our simple model) make a particularly simple prediction for such a series. These models predict that all members of a constant-difference series of patterns should show segregation to approximately the same degree (Graham, Beck & Sutter, 1989, and in preparation). Why do these simple linear models make this prediction? According to these models, segregation is based on the degree to which the linear spatial-frequency and orientation-selective channels show differences in amount of activity in the different texture regions. In other words, segregation depends approximately on the difference between the Fourier transforms' amplitudes in the checkerboard vs. the striped regions. For element-arrangement patterns like those used here, as mentioned earlier, the only substantial difference is at the fundamental frequency of the texture regions. And the fundamental frequency's amplitude is approximately constant throughout a constant-difference series of patterns; thus segregation is predicted to be approximately constant.

In terms of receptive fields (spatial weighting functions) the above explanation goes as follows. According to the simple models, segregation in element-arrangement texture patterns such as those of figures 18.1 and 18.4 is determined primarily by the receptive fields that are just big enough so that when a column of one element type stimulates the receptive field's excitatory center, then columns of the other element type stimulate the inhibitory surround. (This is the size of weighting function associated with the filter having the output displayed in the middle panel of figure 18.2.) Since for this size of receptive field the background is stimulating both the excitatory center and inhibitory surround to approximately the same extent, the effects of the background cancel out and it is only the two element types that contribute to the response. Further, for this size of receptive field in the appropriate position (that position producing the maximal response and thereby being the largest determinant of the whole channel's spatially pooled response), one element type stimulates the excitatory center and the other element type stimulates the surround; hence this receptive field essentially subtracts the effect of one element type from that of the other. Since in the on-off

experiments the two element types have the same shape and size and differ only in luminance, this size of receptive field responds proportionally to the difference between the two element types' luminances.

In symbols, letting R_S be the pooled response of the simple channels (called R_{pool} earlier but distinguished here for reasons that will become clear later) and w_S the proportionality constant, then the following is true approximately (and the approximation is very good; Graham, Beck & Sutter, in preparation)

$$R_S = w_S \cdot |L_1 - L_2| = w_S \cdot |\Delta L_1 - \Delta L_2|. \qquad (4)$$

The absolute value sign occurs because the quantity R_S is the value pooled across all such channels of the absolute value of the difference between each channel's spatially pooled response to one region (e.g., striped) and that to the other (e.g., checkerboard). Note that R_S is essentially entirely determined by the simple channels sensitive to the fundamental frequency of the texture regions. As mentioned earlier, the pooled response is assumed to be monotonic with (but not necessarily proportional to) the observer's segregation rating.

Empirical Results

Some empirical results are shown in figure 18.7. Each curve in the figure connects points representing patterns in a constant-difference series. The size of that constant difference increases from the bottom to the top curve. The horizontal axis shows the contrast-ratio angle of each pattern. The vertical axis gives the average observer rating of segregation.

As discussed above, the simple model predicts that all members of a constant-difference series segregate to the same extent approximately. Thus the predictions of the simple model would be approximately horizontal lines on this kind of plot. The results do not look at all like the predictions: First, each curve sinks dramatically at both its ends, with different curves actually converging for same-sign-of-contrast patterns when both element types' luminances are far from the background. (Thus, for the patterns at the ends of the curves, only the ratio of the contrasts in the two element types matters for segregation; the size of the difference between the contrasts or luminances does not.) Second, there are "ears" in the curves since there is maximal segregation for the one-element-type-only patterns with somewhat less segrega-

Complex Channels, Early Local Nonlinearities, and Normalization

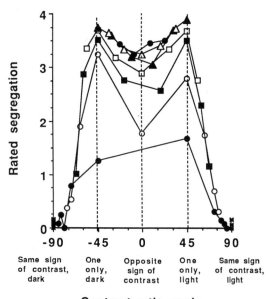

L2-L1 in ft-L

———●——— 5.25
———△——— 4.5
———▲——— 3.75
———□——— 3
———■——— 2.25
———○——— 1.5
———●——— 0.75
———✕——— 0

EXPERIMENTAL RESULTS
Square elements
Fundamental = 1 c/deg
16 ft-L mean luminance
10 Subjects

Fig. 18.7
Results from on-off experiment. The average rating from 10 observers is plotted vertically. The contrast-ratio angle is plotted horizontally. Each curve connects points representing patterns in a constant-difference series.

tion for the opposite-sign-of-contrast patterns in the middle of the curves (as well as much less segregation for the same-sign-of-contrast patterns at the ends of the curves).

Role of the Complex Channels in On-Off Experiments

Our explanation of these results rests on two different nonlinearities. The first we have already discussed. It is the *spatial nonlinearity* in the complex channels that was needed to explain the discrepancies between the simple

model's predictions and the contrast-size trade-off experiments' results. These complex channels can also account for part of the discrepancies between the simple model's predictions and the on-off experiments' results, namely, for the fact that one-element-only patterns segregate better than opposite-sign-of-contrast patterns. The remainder of this paragraph attempts to describe (in the spatial rather than the frequency domain) the intuition behind this prediction. Consider a complex channel in which the first-stage filter is at relatively high spatial-frequencies (as in the diagram of figure 18.3) and the third-stage filter is at the fundamental frequency of the pattern. (To have a name for this type of channel in the following, we will call it a *high-low complex channel*.) No matter what the pattern, the high-frequency first-stage filter of such a high-low complex channel responds well at the edges of all elements, giving little Mach-bandlike responses, both positive and negative (cf. the right panel of figure 18.2). The second-stage rectification-type nonlinearity turns these positive and negative Mach-bandlike responses at the edges of every element into entirely positive responses. What happens then at the third-stage filtering, done at the fundamental frequency of the pattern? Think of a vertical receptive field superimposed on the output from the second-stage nonlinearity in the striped region. It is tuned to the fundamental frequency of the striped region and so can be placed with its center lying on a column of rectified responses to bright elements and its surround either on empty columns (in the case of *one-element-type-only* patterns) or on columns of rectified responses to dark elements (in the case of *opposite-sign-of-contrast* patterns). Thus this receptive field (and hence the overall complex channel) will respond strongly to the one-element-only patterns (since only its excitatory center is stimulated—it is getting no inhibition from its surround). But it will not respond at all to the opposite-sign-of-contrast patterns since both its center and surround are stimulated and stimulated equally (since the second-stage's rectified responses to both the bright and the dark elements are the same)!

In fact, one can write the following equation to (approximately) describe R_C, the pooled response of the high-low complex channels (the complex channels in which the first filtering is at higher harmonics of the pattern and the second filtering is at the fundamental frequency):

$$R_C = w_C \cdot ||\Delta L_1| - |\Delta L_2||. \tag{5}$$

This is just like equation 4 for the simple channels (dominated by the simple channels at the fundamental frequency) except that $|\Delta L_i|$ has replaced ΔL_i. Why is this equation (approximately) correct? The first-stage filter of a high-low complex channel responds in proportion to the edge contrast ΔL_i, which the second-stage nonlinearity then rectifies to $|\Delta L_i|$ before sending it on as an input to the third-stage filtering done at the fundamental. Then, by an argument analogous to that given earlier for the simple channel at the fundamental frequency, the third-stage filtering in these high-low complex channels will respond in proportion to the difference between its inputs, that is to the difference between $|\Delta L_1|$ and $|\Delta L_2|$. It might be useful to consider what a plot of R_C in the format of figure 18.7 would look like. Each constant-difference curve would be flat for all same-sign-of-contrast patterns (for contrast-ratio angles greater than $+45$ or less than -45). But as the contrast-ratio angle moved in toward zero from either $+45$ or -45, the value of R_C drops steadily reaching zero at a contrast-ratio-angle of zero (zero segregation for opposite-but-equal patterns).

If the only channels that existed were these high-low complex channels (higher frequency at the first stage and fundamental frequency at the third stage), the opposite-sign-of-contrast patterns would not segregate at all. That they do segregate to some extent in figure 18.7, although not as well as the one-element-only patterns, can be explained by assuming that, in addition to high-low complex channels, there are either simple channels at the fundamental frequency or complex channels whose first filtering is at the fundamental frequency. (Such complex channels will act much like the simple channels at the fundamental, both kinds obeying equation 4.) These channels respond as much to the opposite-sign-of-contrast as to the one-element-only patterns and thus will contribute to the segregation of both.

Patterns Lacking Energy at the Fundamental

If one removes all the energy at the fundamental frequency from the pattern, however, neither the simple channels at the fundamental nor the complex channels having a first-stage filtering at the fundamental are stimulated. The high-low complex channels can segregate some patterns lacking energy at the fundamental (e.g., one-element-only patterns), but these high-low channels cannot segregate opposite-sign-of-contrast patterns at all. We used some patterns lacking energy at the fundamental; they were much like those in figures 18.1 and 18.4 but the individual elements had balanced sub-areas of positive and negative contrast and thus averaged out to the same luminance as the background. Indeed, the opposite-sign-of-contrast patterns made from such elements did not segregate at all although the one-element-only patterns segregated very well indeed; this result provides more and quite direct support for the notion of high-low complex channels (Graham, Beck, and Sutter, in preparation).

The Intensity-Dependent Nonlinearity: Two Candidate Processes

The second nonlinearity used to explain the on-off results (figure 18.7) will be called the intensity-dependent nonlinearity. This nonlinearity is needed to explain why the segregation decreases so sharply at the ends of the curves in figure 18.7. We will discuss two possible candidates for this second nonlinearity: (1) a local (pointwise) nonlinearity occurring early (before the channels), and (2) a normalization process, which might result from intracortical interaction, operating at the level of the channels themselves.

An Early Local Nonlinearity: One Possibility

Suppose, for example, that early local light adaptation processes readjust the operating range of the visual system to be centered on the recent mean luminance—the background luminance in this case—maximizing discriminability between luminances near that level, and, therefore, sacrificing discriminability for luminances far away. Figure 18.8 shows a hypothetical early local nonlinearity of this sort. ("Early" is meant only to imply that it occurs before the channels, that is, at the retina or lateral geniculate nucleus [LGN], presuming the channels are cortical; "local" is mean to imply that it is a process that is quite localized compared to the filtering done by the channels and can thus be assumed to act at each point on the stimulus.) Indicated on the horizontal axis of figure 18.8 are five pairs of luminances corresponding to five different patterns in a constant-difference series. Vertical lines

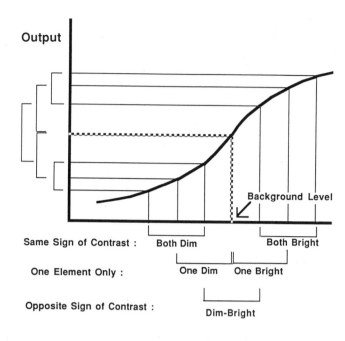

Output

Background Level

Same Sign of Contrast : | Both Dim | Both Bright

One Element Only : | One Dim | One Bright

Opposite Sign of Contrast : | Dim-Bright

Input, e.g. Luminance

Fig. 18.8
Diagram of early-local-nonlinearity explanation of on-off experiment's results.

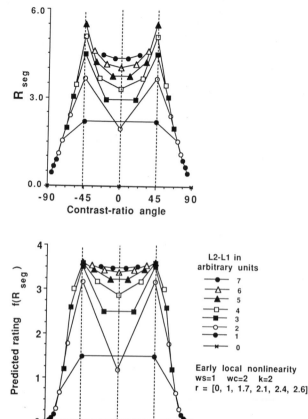

L2-L1 in arbitrary units

- ● 7
- △ 6
- ▲ 5
- □ 4
- ■ 3
- ○ 2
- ● 1
- ✻ 0

Early local nonlinearity
ws=1   wc=2   k=2
r = [0, 1, 1.7, 2.1, 2.4, 2.6]

Fig. 18.9
Predictions of on-off experiment from a model incorporating complex channels and an early local nonlinearity.

extend from these luminances up to the nonlinear curve and then horizontal lines extend over to the vertical axis to show the outputs for each pair of luminances. Note that the difference between the two outputs for the same-sign-of-contrast patterns is much smaller than that for the one-element-type-only patterns or for the opposite-sign-of-contrast patterns. In general, as the luminances get further from the background in either direction, this output difference gets smaller. (It is interesting to note that once you get fairly far from the background, the early local nonlinearity would need to be a logarithmic function of $|\Delta L|$ to make the curves for constant-difference series converge at their ends, that is, to make the amount of segregation depend only on contrast ratios and not on luminance differences, as is the tendency in the empirical results of figure 18.7.)

To calculate approximately the predictions from such an early local nonlinearity applied before the channels, one can start with equation 4 for the channels at the fundamental and equation 5 for the high-low complex channels but then substitute the outputs of the early local nonlinearity for the luminances in those equations and

combine the two pooled responses. In symbols, let R_{seg} be the pooled response over all the simple and high-low complex channels that contribute to segregation of the checkerboard versus the striped region; let k be the parameter that describes the manner in which outputs of the different channels are pooled as in equation 3. Then

$$R_{seg} = \{R_S^k + R_C^k\}^{1/k}, \tag{6}$$

where outputs from the early local nonlinearity have been substituted for luminances in equations 4 and 5. The texture-segregation ratings given by the observer are assumed to be a monotonic function of R_{seg}.

Figure 18.9 shows some predictions from equation 6 where the top panel shows the R_{seg} values themselves and the bottom panel shows R_{seg} transformed by a monotonic transformation f to produce a better fit of R_{seg} to the data of figure 18.7. (Remember that the observer's ratings are only assumed to be a monotonic function of R_{seg}.) As intended, there are ears in the prediction (due to the presence of high-low complex channels), and the ends of the curves drop and different curves converge. Indeed, as comparison of figures 18.7 and 18.9 will show, these predictions fit the data very well. (The r^2 between $f(R_{seg})$ and the average observer rating across all 66 stimuli was 0.9873.) The parameter values are given in the figure inset but should not be overinterpreted as there are strong interactions among parameters and a wide range of any one parameter can work well given the correct value of other parameters.[1]

The good fit between the predictions of figure 18.9 and the data of figure 18.7 is pleasing on the one hand. On the other hand, one needs to think carefully about just what visual process this early local nonlinearity might correspond to. The heavy solid curve in figure 18.10, which shows the early local nonlinearity that was used for figure 18.9 (the dotted curves show alternatives that were clearly less good), is already strongly compressed at 18 or 14 ft-L, which—on a background of 16 ft-L—is a contrast of 13 percent. This seems too much compression for the light adaptation processes generally talked about in the retina (see reviews in Hood & Finkelstein, 1986; Shapley & Enroth-Cugell, 1985; Walraven, Enroth-Cugell, Hood, et al., 1989). It is also rather more compression than commonly reported for retinal-ganglion and LGN cells, although not extraordinarily more than that reported for some retinal and LGN M cells (e.g., Derrington & Lennie 1984; Sclar, Maunsell & Lennie, 1990; Shapley & Perry, 1986; Spekreijse, van Norren & van den Berg, 1971).

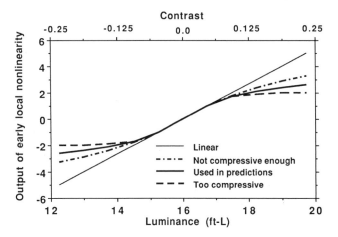

Fig. 18.10
Early-local nonliearity used in predictions of figure 18.9

Normalization Across Channels—Another Possibility

Perhaps a better candidate for the intensity-dependent nonlinearity displayed in our texture segregation results lies in some known properties of cortical cells. Experiments on cortical cells produce results often described as involving cross-orientation or cross-frequency inhibition (e.g., Bonds, 1989; De Valois & Tootell, 1983; Morrone, Burr & Maffei, 1982). Further, the relationship between contrast and cortical cells' responses is known to be very compressive; some cortical cells do show compression at 10 or 20 percent contrast (e.g., Albrecht & Hamilton, 1982; Ohzawa, Sclar & Freeman, 1982; Sclar, Lennie & DePriest, 1989; Sclar, Maunsell & Lennie, 1990). As has been recently pointed out (see chapter 9; Heeger & Adelson, 1989; Robson, 1988a,b), both the intracortical inhibition and the response compression may result from

---

1. The early-local-nonlinearity model of equation has the following parameters: w_s, w_c, k, and the values of the early-local nonlinearity at the five different incremental luminances used in the experiment. (The nonlinearity was assumed to be odd-symmetric around the background luminance.) The normalization model of equation 8 and 9 has the following parameters: w_c, w_c, w_0, σ, k', and k.

For each of the models, a crude grid search was done over the above parameters, varying each parameter by a factor of about 2 over a reasonable range. (For the normalization model, the value of k' was arbitrarily set at 1 in the calculations done so far.) For each chosen set of values of these parameters, the values of R_{seg} for the 66 stimuli in the experiment were calculated.

The observer's rating of perceived segregation is assumed to equal $f(R_{seg})$ where f is a monotonic function otherwise unspecified. In the fits shown here, however, we assumed that f was a member of a particular four-parameter family of functions. (This family is a slight generalization of the Weibull distribution function, the Quick psychometric function, and the asymptotic regression function. It was picked merely because it contained the right variety of shapes to fit for the task at hand.)

$$f(x) = a[b + 1 - 2^{-(c \cdot x)^d}] \qquad (7)$$

The Nelder-Meade algorithm (which is nicely described in *Numerical Recipes* by Press, Flannery, Teykolsky, and Vetterling, 1986) as instantiated in MAT-LAB (available from The MathWorks Inc., 21 Eliot St., South Natick, MA 01760) was used to find the four parameters for f producing the smallest mean-square error (over the 66 stimuli in the experiment) between $f(R_{seg})$ and the average rating of the observers.

The fits shown in figures 18.9 and 18.11 are the best ones found using this procedure, but many others were just as good, since there are strong interactions between these parameters. Trivially, making all the weights w larger by some factor or making the outputs of the early-local nonlinearity larger by some factor will be exactly compensated by making a smaller by that factor. Of particular note for the normalization model, it is generally only the ratio of w_0 to σ that matters rather than the values of either one. The predictions are not, overall, very sensitive to the value of k for either model.

the same process, a normalization process which keeps the total response from some set of neurons at or below a ceiling. It accomplishes this by doing something like dividing (normalizing) each individual neuron's response by the total response from the set (once thresholds have been exceeded) as is discussed in some detail in chapter 9. Normalization-type processes have also been used in visual models by, among others, Grossberg (1987), Grossberg and Mingolla (1985), Lubin, (1989), and Lubin and Nachmias (1990).

How could normalization act to produce the aspects of our results on texture segregation that suggest intensity-dependent nonlinearity? One first needs to assume that the set over which normalization occurs consists of neurons responsive to rather a broad range of spatial frequencies in the same region. The general idea is then that the greater amount of higher harmonics present in the same-sign-of-contrast patterns (relative to both one-element-type-only and opposite-sign-of-contrast patterns) produces larger responses to the same-sign-of-contrast patterns (than to other patterns) from certain channels, henceforth called *other* channels. These *other* channels can be either simple channels at higher harmonics or complex channels having their first-stage and third-stage filterings at higher harmonics. Notice these *other* channels are not capable of segregating the texture regions because they do not respond differentially overall to the two texture regions. The larger responses from the *other* channels to the same-sign-of-contrast patterns (than to one-element-type-only or opposite-sign-of-contrast patterns) would enter into the denominator of the normalization process, however. This larger denominator then leads to a smaller postnormalization response to the same-sign-of-contrast patterns (than to the other patterns) from all channels over which normalization occurs, in particular, from the channels that do lead to segregation of the texture regions (the simple channels at the fundamental and high-low complex channels).

The simplistic approximating approach of equations 4 to 6 can be extended to model normalization instead of early local nonlinearity. To do this we need an expression for R_0, the responses of the *other* channels. Since these channels respond to the higher harmonics (and thus roughly in proportion to the edge contrast of the individual elements), the total response of all such channels in any not-too-small region of the pattern can be approximated

by the following expression (and the approximation is very good; Graham, Beck, and Sutter, in preparation):

$$R_0 = w_0 \cdot \{ ||\Delta L_1|^{k'} + |\Delta L_2||^{k'} \}^{1/k'}. \tag{8}$$

In words, R_0 is proportional to a power-sum of the absolute values of the incremental luminances at the edges of the two types of individual elements, where the constant of proportionality is called w_0 and the exponent k' is from the spatial-pooling asssumption of equation 1. It might be useful to think through what a plot of R_0 vs. contrast-ratio angle looks like for a constant-difference series of patterns: It is flat for angles between -45 and $+45$ and then increases precipitously as the angle gets smaller than -45 or larger than $+45$.

To finish the prediction of perceived segregation one puts the response of these *other* channels into a denominator that normalizes the responses of all the channels but does not put it into the numerator (representing the fact that the *other* channels do not respond differentially in the two texture regions):

$$R_{seg} = \frac{\{ R_S^{k'} + R_C^{k'} \}^{1/k'}}{\{ \sigma + R_S^{k'} + R_C^{k'} + R_0^{k'} \}^{1/k'}}. \tag{9}$$

The parameter σ is necessary to keep the equation from blowing up at zero. When σ is so large that it dominates the rest of the denominator, this equation is equivalent to equation 6 above (except that the weights have been divided by σ).

As an aside, notice that one might just take equation 9 to be a formulation of some kind of "masking" of the responses at the fundamental frequency by responses to the higher harmonics. It is not clear that this last sentence has much content but it does suggest that one might profitably search for analogies between these psychophysical results and others commonly called "masking."

Figure 18.11 shows some predictions from equation 9 where the top panel shows the R_{seg} values themselves and the bottom panel shows R_{seg} transformed by a monotonic transformation to produce a better fit of R_{seg} to the data of figure 18.7. These predictions fit the data of figure 18.7 very well, almost exactly as well as those of figure 18.9 from the early local nonlinearity. (The r^2 between $f(R_{seg})$ and the average observer rating across all 66 stimuli was 0.9874.) Again the parameter values are given in the figure inset but should not be overinterpreted. See note 1 for further details.

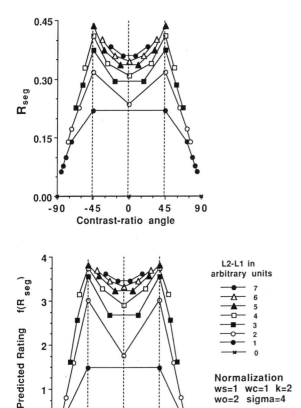

Fig. 18.11
Predictions for on-off experiment from a model incoporating complex channels and normalization (perhaps a result of intracortical inhibition).

To decide between early local nonlinearity and normalization on the basis of their predictions' fits to this data would be foolish. To decide between them totally on the basis of properties of their presumed physiological substrates (that the early local nonlinearity may not be plausible for the retina or the LGN) is at least premature. However, the processes differ in so many other properties (in particular, their spatial properties), not tested by this data, that further psychophysical experiments should be able to decide between them. The relationship of either of these processes in conjunction with complex channels to other nonlinear relationships that have been or are being suggested by others (e.g., the opponency in Bergen and Landy's model in this volume, the spatial inhibition in Malik and Perona 1989a,b, the thresholding in Victor and Conte 1989b) needs also to be made clearer conceptually

and/or experimentally. Certain other experimental results (e.g., Victor & Conte 1987, 1989a,b) suggest that even more complicated nonlinearities may be necessary to explain texture discrimination and perhaps also texture segregation.

Perceived Lightness

Whatever the process underlying the intensity-dependent saturating nonlinearity in the region segregation judgments, the same kind of saturation may not appear in judgments of the perceived lightness of individual elements in the pattern. For the relationship between region segregation judgments and perceived lightness judgments is not simple for element-arrangement texture patterns such as those in figure 18.1 and 18.4 (Beck, Graham & Sutter, 1991; Beck, Sutter & Ivry, 1987).

Summary

Although much of what determines whether different regions in the visual field segregate immediately is accounted for by linear spatial-frequency channels models, there is clear nonlinear behavior. The nonlinear behavior exhibited in our experiments can probably all be accounted for by two different nonlinearities of types we know to exist at relatively low levels in the visual pathways: (1) A rectification-type (spatial) nonlinearity quite like that used to describe complex cortical cell behavior; (2) a very dramatic compressive nonlinearity, occurring at contrasts far less than 25 percent, which can be quantitatively predicted either by an early local nonlinearity occurring before the channels or by normalization among the channels (perhaps intracortical inhibition). In any case, ignoring this dramatic compressive nonlinearity in future attempts to explain region (texture) segregation would seem unwise.

Thus, as we and others are currently showing, models involving well-known low-level visual processes can explain a great deal about perceived region (texture) segregation and at a quantitative level. This is not to deny that still higher-level processes—perhaps more like that grouping processes of the Gestalt psychologists and even perhaps acting at a more categorical level—play a role in region segregation but only to suggest that such processes should not be invoked until they are needed. (For further discussion down this line, see Bergen, 1991.) Perhaps, after all, such higher-level processes may *not* play a substantial role in region segregation if region segregation is a quick and easy computation done early in visual processing in order to ease the overload on higher processes by delimiting regions beyond which a given computation need not be done.

References

Adelson, E. H. & Bergen. J. R. (1985). Spatiotemporal energy models for the perception of motion. *Journal of the Optical Society of America A, 2,* 284–299.

Albrecht, D. G. & Hamilton, D. B. (1982). Striate cortex of monkey and cat: Contrast response function. *Journal of Neurophysiology, 48,* 217–237.

Beck, J., Prazdny, K. & Rosenfeld, A. (1983). A theory of textural segmentation. In J. Beck, B. Hope & A. Rosenfeld (Eds.), *Human and Machine Vision* (pp. 1–38). New York: Academic.

Beck, J., Graham, N. & Sutter, A. (1991). Perceived lightness and perceived segregation. *Perception and Psychophysics 49,* 257–269.

Beck, J., Sutter, A. & Ivry, R. (1987). Spatial frequency channels and perceptual grouping in texture segregation. *Computer Vision, Graphics, and Image Processing, 37,* 299–325.

Bergen, J. R. (1988). Visual texture segmentation based on oriented energy pyramids. Presented at Optical Society of America Annual Meeting, 30 Oct.-4 Nov. 1988. *Technical Digest Series, 11,* 162.

Bergen, J. R. (1991). Theories of visual texture perception. In D. Regan, (Ed.), *Vision and Visual Dysfunction, Vol. 10B: Spatial Vision* (pp. 114–134). New York: Macmillan.

Bergen, J. R. & Adelson, E. H. (1986). Visual texture segmentation based on energy measures. *Journal of the Optical Society of America A, 3,* 98.

Bergen, J. R. & Adelson, E. H. (1988). Early vision and texture perception. *Nature, 333,* 363–364.

Bonds, A. B. (1989). Role of inhibition in the specification of orientation selectivity of cells in the cat striate cortex. *Visual Neuroscience, 2,* 41–55.

Bovik, A. C., Clark, M. & Geisler, W. S. (1987). Computational texture analysis using localized spatial filtering. *Proceedings of Workshop on Computer Vision.,* Miami Beach, FL, Nov. 30–Dec. 2, 1987 (pp. 201–206). The IEEE Computer Society Press.

Caelli, T. M. (1982). On discriminating visual textures and images. *Perception and Psychophysics, 31,* 149–159.

Caelli, T. M. (1985). Three processing characteristics of visual texture segregation. *Spatial Vision, 1,* 19–30.

Caelli, T. M. (1986). Three processing characteristics of texture discrimination. *Vision Interface, '86,* Proceedings, 343–348.

Caelli, T. M. (1988). An adaptive computational model for texture segmentation. *IEEE Transactions on Systems, Man, and Cybernetics, 18,* 1

Chubb, C. & Sperling, G. (1988). Processing stages in non-Fourier motion perception. *Supplement to Investigative Ophthalmology and Visual Science, 29,* 266.

Clark, M., Bovik, A. C. & Geisler, W. S. (1987). Texture segmentation using a class of narrowband filters. *Proceedings of the IEEE International Conference on Acoustics, Speech, and Signal Processing.*

Coggins, J. M. & Jain, A. K. (1985) A spatial filtering approach to texture analysis. *Pattern Recognition Letters 3,* 195–203.

Daugman, J. G. (1987). Image analysis and compact coding by oriented 2D Gabor primitives. *SPIE Proceedings, 758,* 19–30.

Daugman, J. G. (1988). Complete discrete 2-D Gabor transforms by neural networks for image analysis and compression. *IEEE Transactions on Acoustics, Speech, and Signal Processing, 36,* 1169–1179.

Derrington, A. M. & Lennie, P. (1984) Spatial and temporal constant sensitivities of neurones in lateral geniculate nucleus of macaque. *Journal of Physiology, 357,* 219–240.

De Valois, K. K. & Tootell, R. B. (1983). Spatial-frequency-specific inhibition in cat striate cortex cells. *Journal of Physiology, 336,* 339–376.

Field, D. J. (1987). Relations between the statistics of natural images and the response properties of cortical cells. *Journal of the Optical Society of America A, 4,* 2379–2394.

Fogel, I. & Sagi, D. (1989) Gabor filters as texture discriminators. *Biological Cybernetics, 61,* 103–113.

Graham, N. (1985). Detection and identification of near-threshold visual patterns. *Journal of the Optical Society of America A, 2,* 1468–1482.

Graham, N. (1989a). Low-level visual processes and texture segregation. *Physica Scripta. 39,* 147–152.

Graham, N. (1989b). *Visual pattern analyzers.* New York: Oxford University Press.

Graham N., Beck, J. & Sutter, A. K. (1989). Two nonlinearities in texture segregation. *Supplement to Investigative Ophthalmology and Visual Science, 30,* 161.

Graham, N., Beck, J. & Sutter, A. K. (in preparation). Effects of sign and amount of contrast on perceived segregation of element-arrangement textures: Evidence for two nonlinear processes.

Grossberg, S. (1987). Cortical dynamics of three-dimensional form, color, and brightness perception: Monocular theory. *Perception and Psychophysics, 41,* 87–116.

Grossberg, S. & Mingolla, E. (1985). Neural dynamics of perceptual grouping: Textures, boundaries, and emergent features. *Perception and Psychophysics, 38,* 141–171.

Heeger, D. J. & Adelson, E. H. (1989). Mechanisms for extracting local orientation. *Supplement to Investigative Ophthalmology and Visual Science, 30,* 110.

Hochstein, S. & Spitzer, H. (1985). One, few, infinity: Linear and nonlinear processing in the visual cortex. In D. Rose and V. G. Dobson (Eds.), *Models of the Visual Cortex* (pp. 341–350). New York: Wiley.

Hood, D. C. & Finkelstein, M. A. (1986). Sensitivity to light. In K. R. Boff, L. Kaufman, & J. P. Thomas (Eds.), *Handbook of perception and performance. Vol. I. sensory processes and perception.* New York: Wiley, Chapter 5.

Klein, S. A. & Tyler, C. W. (1986). Phase discrimination of compound gratings: Generalized autocorrelation analysis. *Journal of the Optical Society of America A, 3,* 868–879.

Landy, M. S. & Bergen, J. R. (1988). Texture segregation by multiresolution energy or by structure gradient? Presented at the Annual Meeting of the Optical Society of America, 30 Oct.–4 Nov. *Technical Digest Series, 11,* 162.

Landy, M. S. & Bergen, J. R. (1989). Texture segregation for filtered noise patterns. *Supplement to Investigative Ophthalmology and Visual Science, 30,* 160.

Lubin, J. (1989). Discrimination contours in an opponent motion stimulus space. *Supplement to Investigative Ophthalmology and Visual Science, 30,* 426.

Lubin, J. & Nachmias, J. (1990). Discrimination contours in an F/3F stimulus space. *Supplement to Investigative Ophthalmology and Visual Science, 31,* 409.

Malik, J. & Perona, P. (1989a). *A computational model of texture perception.* (Report No. UCB/CSD 89/491). Computer Science Division (EECS), University of California, Berkeley, California.

Malik, J. & Perona, P. (1989b). Computational model of human texture perception. *Supplement to Investigative Ophthalmology and Visual Science, 30,* 161.

Morrone, M. C., Burr, D. C. & Maffei, L. (1982) Functional implications of cross-orientation inhibition of cortical visual cells. I. Neurophysiological evidence. *Proceedings of the Royal Society B, 216,* 335–354.

Nothdurft, H. C. (1985a). Orientation sensitivity and texture segmentation in patterns with different line orientation. *Vision Research, 25,* 551–560.

Nothdurft, H. C. (1985b). Sensitivity for structure gradient in texture discrimination tasks. *Vision Research, 25,* 1957–1968.

Ohzawa, I., Sclar, G. & Freeman, R. D. (1982). Contrast gain control in the cat visual cortex. *Nature, 298,* 266–268.

Peli, E. (1987). Seeing the forest for the trees: The role of nonlinearity. *Supplement to Investigative Ophthalmology and Visual Science, 28,* 365.

Press, W. H., Flannery, B. P., Teukolsky, S. A. & Vetterling, W. T. (1986). *Numerical recipes.* Cambridge: Cambridge University Press.

Robson, J. G. (1980). Neural images: The physiological basis of spatial vision. In C. S. Harris (Ed.), *Visual coding and adaptability* (pp. 177–214). Hillsdale, N.J.: Erlbaum.

Robson, J. G. (1988a). Linear and non-linear operations in the visual system. *Supplement to Investigative Ophthalmology and Visual Science, 29,* 117.

Robson, J. G. (1988b). Linear and non-linear behavior of neurones in the visual cortex of the cat. Presented at *New Insights on Visual Cortex,* the Sixteenth Symposium of the Center for Visual Science, University of Rochester, Rochester, New York, June, 1988. Abstract p. 5.

Rubenstein, R. S. & Sagi, D. (1989). *Spatial variability as a limiting factor in texture discrimination tasks: Implications for performance asymetries.* (Technical Report CS89-12). The Weizmann Institute of Science, Department of Applied Mathematics and Computer Science, Rehovot, Israel.

Sagi, D. (1989). Hierarchy of spatial filtering in early vision. *Supplement to Investigative Ophthalmology and Visual Science, 30,* 161.

Sclar, G., Lennie, P. & DePriest, D. D. (1989). Contrast adaptation in striate cortex of macaque. *Vision Research, 29,* 747–755.

Sclar, G., Maunsell, J. H. R. & Lennie, P. (1990). Coding of image contrast in central visual pathways of the macaque monkey. *Vision Research, 30,* 1–10.

Shapley, R. & Enroth-Cugell, C. (1985). Visual adaptation and retinal gain controls. In N. N. Osborne and G. J. Chader (Eds.), *Progress in retinal research, Vol. 3* (pp. 263–343). Oxford: Pergamon Press.

Shapley, R. & Perry, V. H. (1986). Cat and monkey retinal ganglion cells and their visual functional roles. *Trends in Neurosciences,* May, 229–235.

Spekreijse, H., van Norren, D. & van den Berg, T. J. T. P. (1971). Flicker responses in monkey lateral geniculate nucleus and human perception of flicker. *Proceedings of the National Academy of Science, USA, 68,* 2802–2805.

Sperling, G. (1989). Three stages and two systems of visual processing. *Spatial Vision, 4,* 183–207.

Sperling, G. & Chubb, C. (1989). Apparent motion derived from spatial texture. *Supplement to Investigative Ophthalmology and Visual Science, 30,* 161.

Sutter, A. (1987). The interaction of size and contrast in perceived texture segregation: A spatial frequency analysis. Doctoral Dissertation, University of Oregon, Eugene.

Sutter, A., Beck, J. & Graham, N. (1989). Contrast and spatial variables in texture segregation: Testing a simple spatial-frequency channels model. *Perception and Psychophysics, 46,* 312–332.

Turner, M. R. (1986). Texture discrimination by Gabor functions. *Biological Cybernetics, 55,* 71–82.

Victor, J. D. (1988). Models for preattentive texture discrimination: Fourier analysis and local feature processing in a unified framework. *Spatial Vision, 3*, 263–280.

Victor, J. D. & Conte, M. (1987) Local and long-range interactions in pattern processing. *Supplement to Investigative Ophthalmology and Visual Science, 28*, 362.

Victor, J. D. & Conte, M. (1989a) Cortical interactions in texture processing: Scale and dynamics. *Visual Neuroscience, 2*, 297–313.

Victor, J. D. & Conte, M. (1989b) What kinds of high-order correlation structure are readily visible? *Supplement to Investigative Ophthalmology and Visual Science, 30, 3*, 254.

Walraven, J., Enroth-Cugell, C., Hood, D. C., MacLeod, D. I. A. & Schnapf, J. (1989). Control of visual sensitivity. In L. Spillman and J. Werner (Eds.), *Physiological foundations of perception*. New York: Springer-Verlag.

Watson, A. B. (1983). Detection and recognition of simple spatial forms. In O. J. Braddick and A. C. Sleigh, (Eds.), *Physiological and biological preprocessing of images* (pp. 110–114). New York: Springer-Verlag.

Yellott, J. & Iverson, G. (1990). Triple correlation and texture discrimination. *Supplement to Investigative Ophthalmology and Visual Science, 31*, 561.

19

Orthogonal Distribution Analysis: A New Approach to the Study of Texture Perception

Charles Chubb and
Michael S. Landy

It has been recognized for a long time that the visual system is capable of using textural cues to segment the visual field. A region of one sort of texture will often appear distinct from a surrounding background texture. Chapters 17 by Bergen and Landy and 18 by Graham report results of experiments and modeling in this area, and a general review may be found in Bergen (1991). In this chapter we describe a new psychophysical measurement technique called *orthogonal distribution analysis* that is useful for the analysis of models of texture perception.

IID Textures

We concentrate here on a specific class of textured images that we call *IID* textures ("IID" stands for "independent, identically distributed"). Any IID texture can be produced in the following way:

1. Get a large urn.

2. Fill the urn with balls painted with various graylevels, keeping track of the proportion of balls painted each graylevel.

3. For each pixel in the texture, mix up the balls in the urn, and choose one at random. Paint the pixel the graylevel of the ball, and return the ball to the urn.

Obviously, the probability that a given pixel in this texture will be painted a particular graylevel is equal to the proportion of balls in the urn painted that graylevel, and if you know these probabilities for all graylevels, then you know all there is to know about the texture. That is, any IID texture is completely characterized by the probability distribution on graylevels that is used to paint the pixels of the texture. We call this distribution the *pixel distribution* of the texture.

If we consider a large patch of IID texture, it should be clear that the proportion of pixels in the patch that are painted a given graylevel is going to be approximately equal to the probability of that graylevel under the pixel distribution of the texture. Thus, if we generate a histogram of the graylevels occurring in this large patch, this histogram should closely resemble the pixel distribution.

In orthogonal distribution analysis, we manipulate pixel distributions in order to obtain thresholds for discriminating between IID textures of various sorts. As we shall show, the thresholds we obtain are informative about the visual processes underlying texture perception.

Before we describe the method itself, let us look at a variety of IID textures. Figure 19.1A shows a patch of IID texture whose pixel distribution is *uniform* on a set of 16 graylevels. That is, each pixel in this texture is assigned one of the graylevels 0, 1, ..., 15 with equal probability. If we are using an urn to produce this texture, we simply load the urn with 16 balls, with each ball painted one of the graylevels 0, ..., 15, and no two balls the same. Part B shows the graylevel histogram of this patch of texture. As expected, since the pixel distribution of the texture is uniform, the histogram is approximately flat across the 16 graylevels.

Figure 19.1C shows a patch of IID texture whose pixel distribution is *binomial*. Specifically, to paint any pixel of this texture, we flip a coin 15 times, and paint the pixel with that graylevel equal to the number of times the coin comes up heads. (Alternatively, we can use an urn filled with the appropriate distribution of balls to reflect the same probabilities.) Part D shows the graylevel histogram of this patch of texture.

Note first that the patch of binomial texture in Figure 19.1C has roughly the same overall lightness as the patch of uniformly distributed IID texture in part A. This is to be expected. The two texture patches have approximately the same average graylevel (and thus they reflect the same average amount of light). This is because the pixel distributions of the two textures have the same *mean*. In other words, the sum of all graylevels weighted by their respective probabilities is the same for each of these two textures (it is equal to 7.5).

The patch of uniformly distributed texture (figure 19.1A) has a higher apparent contrast than the patch of binomially distributed IID texture (part C). This difference in apparent contrast results from the fact that the uniformly distributed texture gives higher probabilities to the more extreme graylevels (i.e., has higher variance) than does the binomially distributed texture, which heaps most of its probability on graylevels near its mean.

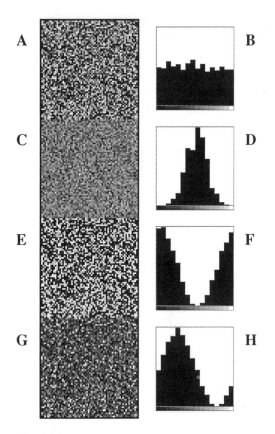

Fig. 19.1
IID textures for various pixel value distributions: (A) uniform distribution, (C) binomial distribution, (E) cosinusoidally modulated distribution, and (G) sinusoidally modulated distribution. Panels (B), (D), (F), and (H) show greylevel histograms of the images in panels (A), (C), (E), and (G), respectively.

Figure 19.1E shows a patch of IID texture that has even higher apparent contrast than the uniformly distributed texture of part A. As the graylevel histogram of this texture patch indicates (part F), the pixel distribution of this texture assigns the highest probabilities to the most extreme graylevels. In fact, these probabilities are modulated by a sinusoidal curve that runs through one full period as it covers the 16 graylevels. The phase of this sinusoid is chosen to yield an IID texture whose mean is equal to the means of the uniformly and binomially distributed textures (parts A and C).

By shifting the phase of the modulating sinusoid 1/4 cycle to the right, we obtain the IID texture shown in figure 19.1G. When we consider the histogram of this texture (part H), we note that the lower graylevels are more frequent than the higher graylevels. As a result, the mean graylevel of this texture is lower than the mean graylevels of the textures shown in parts A, C, and E.

A Simple Segmentation Model for IID Textures

We immediately see the boundaries between the four texture patches of figure 19.1. This suggests that the visual system uses both textural lightness and apparent textural contrast to segment the visual field.

But what exactly does it mean to say that the visual system uses a given property to segment the visual field? In essence, it means that the visual system constructs perceptual boundaries between regions that are internally homogeneous with respect to that property, but that differ significantly from each other with respect to that property.

It stands to reason that in order to use a property to segment the visual field, the visual system must first measure that property at each point in the visual field. Of course, after this initial computation there will doubtless be a great deal of sophisticated processing needed to actually complete the refined, sharp-bordered segmentation (see, e.g., Caelli, 1985).

When the visual system measures a property at each point in the visual field, it takes the input image (for us, this will always be a combination of IID textures) and produces a new output image. However, this output image is not captured on film; nor is it stored in the memory of a computer; rather, we presume, it is registered in an array of neurons somewhere in the visual pathway, an array of neurons corresponding to locations in the visual field, where the intensity of this hypothetical *neural image* (Robson, 1980) at a point in space is coded by the firing rate of the neuron corresponding to that point. Whereas the input image has a specific graylevel at each location in the visual field, the output image has a specific value of the given property at each location. This value is the result of a particular computation applied to the constellation of graylevels surrounding that point in the input image. In fact, this computation defines the property being measured.

In this context, the simplest possible property is luminance itself. For this property, segmentation could be performed on the input image, unmodified by any local computation. A more realistic model given what we know about light adaptation, is that an output image is generated, where each point is the *local stimulus contrast* of the input image (corresponding to apparent lightness). This value is obtained by

1. Computing the average of the input image luminance around that point

2. Subtracting this local average luminance from the luminace at that point

3. Dividing the result by the local average luminance

This computation is more in line with the notion of an early light adaptation mechanism.

One way the visual system might measure apparent contrast is to compute the absolute value of this (signed) local stimulus contrast at each point in the visual field.

Our observations about the textures in figure 19.1 thus suggest a simple model to explain segregation between different IID textures: The visual system processes the input image to produce two neural output images, (1) a lightness image, where lightness is actually local stimulus contrast, and (2) an apparent contrast image, where apparent contrast is actually the absolute value of (signed) stimulus contrast. Each neural image is subjected to a segmentation computation whose purpose is to construct perceptual boundaries between internally homogeneous regions that differ from each other sufficiently in average value.

This model may still be more complicated than we need. Would it be possible to handle all instances of IID texture segregation by segmenting only a *single* neural image? Obviously the lightness image is not sufficient by itself, since we can produce IID textures with the same lightness that segregate because they differ in apparent contrast. Likewise, the apparent contrast image is insufficient because we can produce IID textures with the same apparent contrast that segregate due to a difference in lightness. However, maybe we can produce a neural image that merges information from both the lightness image and the apparent contrast image. For instance, suppose we simply add the lightness and apparent contrast images. Is it possible that segmentation of this single image (or some similar image) predicts all instances of IID texture segregation? This seems unlikely because if it were true, then we would be able to cancel apparent contrast-driven segregation between two IID textures by adjusting the average lightness of one of the textures.

In spite of its implausibility, however, let us assume for the moment that the following very simple model holds:

Simple Model: There exists a single (unknown) function f that is applied by the visual system to the input image, point by point over the visual field, to produce a single neural output image. Segregation of IID textures results from segmentation of this single neural image.

Suppose we had such a system with an unknown *f*. How could we estimate *f* psychophysically? Consider the textures shown in figure 19.2. In each panel, the left half of the texture image is uniformly distributed. The pixel distribution of each of the textures on the right is modulated by a cosine function that cycles through one full period as it assigns probabilities to the graylevels 0, 1, ..., 15. However, the *amplitude* of the modulating cosine function is different for each of the right hand textures. Now let us ask a subject to try to detect a boundary between the uniformly distributed texture on the left and each of the various sinusoidally distributed textures on the right in order to determine the threshold amplitude (of pixel distribution modulation) for which the subject can just barely perform the task. (For instance, we might define this threshold amplitude to be the pixel distribution amplitude for which the subject can perform the border detection task successfully on 75 percent of the trials.)

Suppose this threshold amplitude turns out to be α. The pixel distribution of the corresponding IID texture is defined as follows for any graylevel *v*:

$$Probability[\,pixel\ painted\ v\,] = \frac{1 + \alpha \cos(2\pi v/16)}{16}. \tag{1}$$

The pixel distribution of the uniformly distributed texture is

$$Probability[\,pixel\ painted\ v\,] = \frac{1}{16}. \tag{2}$$

Our simple model of IID texture segregation implies that any two IID textures will segregate only if the average value of the unknown function *f* applied to one texture is

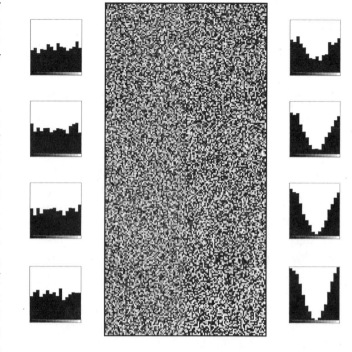

Fig. 19.2
Orthogonal distribution analysis. Each panel consists of two IID textures. In the left half of each panel, the pixel values are distributed uniformly. In the right half, the distributon is modulated cosinusoidally, with increasing modulation amplitude in each panel. The analysis proceeds by finding the distribution modulation amplitude for which the two textures are at threshold in a texture segregation task.

sufficiently different from the average value of *f* applied to the other texture. This condition can be expressed by saying that the two IID textures will segregate only if the following inequality holds, where $proportion_1(v)$ is the proportion of pixels in the first texture that have graylevel *v*, and $proportion_2(v)$ is the proportion of pixels in the second texture that have graylevel *v*:[1]

$$\left| \sum_{\substack{graylevel\\v=0}}^{15} f(v)\,proportion_1(v) - \sum_{\substack{graylevel\\v=0}}^{15} f(v)\,proportion_2(v) \right|$$

---

1. The model expressed in equation 4 is a simplification adopted in order to clarify the basic strategy behind orthogonal distribution analysis. An ideal discriminator which views the two textures as modified by the unknown function *f* will be able to segregate them if the difference between them is large relative to their variabilities, that is, the difference must be *statistically significant*. Thus, T_A and T_B will segregate if

$$\frac{expectation[\,f(a\ pixel\ in\ T_A) - f(a\ pixel\ in\ T_B)\,]}{standard\ deviation[\,f(a\ pixel\ in\ T_A) - f(a\ pixel\ in\ T_B)\,]} \geq threshold. \tag{3}$$

Surprisingly, this statistical viewpoint makes no essential difference to the arguments that follow. In particular, suppose we determine the threshold modulation α required to segregate a texture modulated by the function $\alpha\phi$ from a texture modulated by $-\alpha\phi$. It can be shown that under these conditions, assuming the model of equation 3, α is inversely proportional to $|\sum_{v=0}^{15} f(v)\phi(v)|$ as in equation 6. Additional ramifications of this viewpoint will be discussed in a subsequent paper.

$\geq$ *threshold.* $\qquad$ (4)

Thus, for IID textures that are just barely discriminable in a segregation task, we have

$$\left| \sum_{\substack{graylevel \\ v=0}}^{15} f(v)\,(proportion_1(v) - proportion_2(v)) \right|$$

$$= threshold. \qquad (5)$$

For sufficiently large patches of IID texture, $proportion_1(v)$ and $proportion_2(v)$ approximate the probabilities assigned to graylevel v in the pixel distributions of the two IID textures. Thus, for uniformly distributed texture (figure 19.2A), with pixel distribution given by equation 2, and the sinusoidally distributed texture with pixel distribution given by equation 1, we obtain

$$\left| \sum_{\substack{graylevel \\ v=0}}^{15} f(v)\cos(2\pi v/16) \right| = \frac{16\ threshold}{\alpha}. \qquad (6)$$

If you are familiar with the concept of the discrete Fourier series representation of a function (Bracewell, 1978), you will recognize the left side of equation 6. It is the absolute value of one of the Fourier series coefficients of our unknown function f. Specifically, when f is expressed as a weighted sum of sinusoids in its Fourier series representation, the left side of equation 6 is the absolute value of the weight in that sum given to the cosine phase component of frequency 1 cycle per 16 graylevels. Equation 6 shows that *the absolute value of this Fourier coefficient is inversely proportional to the threshold amplitude by which we need to modulate our cosinusoidal pixel distribution in order to just discriminate the resulting IID texture from uniformly distributed IID texture.* We can repeat the border detection experiment with sinusoids of different frequencies and different phases in order to obtain the absolute values of the entire set of Fourier series coefficients of f.[2]

Thus we can obtain the absolute values of all of the Fourier series coefficients of f. If we can determine the signs of these coefficients relative to one another, then we have determined the actual waveform of f. There is a

simple psychophysical method we can use to determine the signs of all of the different Fourier series coefficients, relative to each other. To see how this works, suppose that α is, as above, the amplitude needed in the pixel distribution of equation 1 in order for the corresponding IID texture to be threshold discriminable from uniformly distributed IID texture. Suppose that, in similar fashion, we find the amplitude β so that the IID texture with pixel distribution

$$Probability[pixel\ painted\ v] = \frac{1 + \beta\cos(2\pi\omega v/16)}{16} \qquad (7)$$

is also threshold discriminable from uniformly distributed texture. (The pixel distribution of equation 7 oscillates up and down through ω full cycles as it modulates probabilities over the 16 graylevels.)

Consider what happens when we try to discriminate the IID texture with the pixel distribution of equation 1 from the IID texture with the pixel distribution of equation 7. If our simple model holds, then the degree to which we can discriminate these two textures depends on the magnitude of the difference between the average of f applied to one texture and the average of f applied to the other: That is, for spatial averages taken over large enough regions, the discriminability of these two textures depends upon the magnitude of

$$\left| \sum_{\substack{graylevel \\ v=0}}^{15} f(v)\frac{1 + \alpha\cos(2\pi v/16)}{16} \right.$$

$$\left. - \sum_{\substack{graylevel \\ v=0}}^{15} f(v)\frac{1 + \beta\cos(2\pi\omega v/16)}{16} \right|, \qquad (8)$$

which is equal to

$$\left| \sum_{\substack{graylevel \\ v=0}}^{15} f(v)\frac{\alpha\cos(2\pi v/16)}{16} \right.$$

$$\left. - \sum_{\substack{graylevel \\ v=0}}^{15} f(v)\frac{\beta\cos(2\pi\omega v/16)}{16} \right|. \qquad (9)$$

However, from equation 6 we see that

---

2. Actually, it is impossible to measure the zero frequency (constant, or DC) term. In equation 1, if we substitute a constant function for $\alpha\cos(2\pi v/16)$, unless that constant is 0, the result is no longer a probability function (it does not sum to one). However, the zero frequency term of the function f has no effect on how well f discriminates pairs of textures. A system which used $f + C$ (where C is a constant) would make precisely the same discriminations as a system using f, because the constant C would drop out of equation 4.

$$\left| \sum_{\substack{graylevel \\ v=0}}^{15} f(v) \frac{\alpha \cos(2\pi v/16)}{16} \right.$$

$$= \left. \sum_{\substack{graylevel \\ v=0}}^{15} f(v) \frac{\beta \cos(2\pi\omega v/16)}{16} \right| = threshold. \quad (10)$$

This means that either

$$\left| \sum_{\substack{graylevel \\ v=0}}^{15} f(v) \frac{\alpha \cos(2\pi v/16)}{16} \right.$$

$$\left. - \sum_{\substack{graylevel \\ v=0}}^{15} f(v) \frac{\beta \cos(2\pi\omega v/16)}{16} \right| = 0, \quad (11)$$

or

$$\left| \sum_{\substack{graylevel \\ v=0}}^{15} f(v) \frac{\alpha \cos(2\pi v/16)}{16} \right.$$

$$\left. - \sum_{\substack{graylevel \\ v=0}}^{15} f(v) \frac{\beta \cos(2\pi\omega v/16)}{16} \right| = 2\, threshold. \quad (12)$$

If equation 11 turns out to be true, then the signs of the two Fourier series coefficients, $(\sum_v f(v) \cos(2\pi v/16)$ and $\sum_v f(v) \cos(2\pi\omega v/16))$ are the same, and we will be completely unable to discriminate the two textures. Otherwise equation 12 must hold, in which case the two Fourier series coefficients are of opposite sign, and the two textures are readily discriminable.

This means that we can determine the relative signs of the different Fourier coefficients of f by testing the discriminability of each of our threshold textures (that is, of the sinusoidally distributed IID textures found to be threshold discriminable from uniformly distributed IID texture) from an arbitrary threshold texture chosen as a standard.

Once we have sorted out the relative signs and magnitudes of the Fourier components of f, we may also test the simple model we have been assuming all along. Suppose we have determined that the IID textures with pixel distributions defined by equations 1 and 7 are, in fact, indiscriminable. In this case, our simple model implies that equation 11 holds. Next, we multiply both sides of equation 11 by the largest number we can, under the constraint that the amplitudes of the sinusoids on both sides of the resultant equality be no greater than 1 (if $\alpha < \beta$, this number is $1/\beta$; otherwise this number is $1/\alpha$). To make things concrete, suppose that $\alpha < \beta$. Then, multiplying both sides of equation 11 by $1/\beta$, we obtain

$$\sum_{\substack{graylevel \\ v=0}}^{15} f(v) \frac{(\alpha/\beta) \cos(2\pi v/16)}{16}$$

$$= \sum_{\substack{graylevel \\ v=0}}^{15} f(v) \frac{\cos(2\pi\omega v/16)}{16}, \quad (13)$$

from which we derive

$$\sum_{\substack{graylevel \\ v=0}}^{15} f(v) \frac{1 + (\alpha/\beta) \cos(2\pi v/16)}{16}$$

$$= \sum_{\substack{graylevel \\ v=0}}^{15} f(v) \frac{1 + \cos(2\pi\omega v/16)}{16}. \quad (14)$$

But if equation 14 is true, then the IID textures with pixel distributions

$$Probability[\,pixel\ painted\ v\,] = \frac{1 + (\alpha/\beta) \cos(2\pi v/16)}{16} \quad (15)$$

and

$$Probability[\,pixel\ painted\ v\,] = \frac{1 + \cos(2\pi\omega v/16)}{16} \quad (16)$$

are indiscriminable. Thus, we have amplified the pixel distribution modulation of each of these IID textures *above* the level required for threshold discrimination of the texture from uniformly distributed texture (assuming β was strictly less than one). Nonetheless, the simple model requires that these two new textures be indiscriminable from each other in the texture segregation task. We thus obtain a strong test of the simple model by verifying, for each pair of threshold-modulated, sinusoidally distributed textures satisfying equation 11, that the two textures remain indiscriminable even after maximal amplification of their individual pixel distributions by the same factor.

The psychophysical method we have described allows us to determine the waveform of the unknown function f of the *simple model*. This is done by comparing textures whose pixel distributions are modulated by a set of functions, which in our discussion so far has been the set of sine waves. By equation 6, this analysis allows us to determine the Fourier (sine wave) decomposition of f term by term. In addition, we have shown how the method can be used to *test* the simple model it presumes. The only essential property of the sine waves is that they are *mutually orthogonal*. Any other mutually orthogonal set of functions can be used as well, hence the name *orthogonal distribution analysis*. Below, we will in fact introduce a different set of functions we have used that allow us to investigate aspects of texture segregability other than lightness and apparent contrast.

The Back Pocket Model of Texture Segregation

In this section we briefly describe a general model that texture perception researchers routinely "pull out from their back pocket" to make sense of new instances of preattentive texture segregation. This *back pocket model* is a simple general model that appears to be adequate to account for most instances of preattentive texture segregation.

In order to describe the class of back pocket models, we need to begin with the concept of a *linear neuron*. A neuron is called *linear* if its response is a weighted sum of the luminances at different locations in the visual field. Those points in the visual field whose luminances receive nonzero weights make up the neuron's *receptive field*. Two linear neurons are said to have the same receptive field *profile* if they apply the same array of weights to different regions of the visual field. An array of linear neurons applied to a given image yields a neural image whose value at a given location is equal to the output of the neuron in the array whose receptive field is centered at that location. If every neuron in such an array has the same receptive field profile, then we shall call the array of neurons a *linear spatial filter*.

Most models of texture segregation suppose that the visual system is equipped with a variety of such linear spatial filters, each with a different receptive field profile. The key to the back pocket model of texture segregation lies in the fact that a linear spatial filter with a given profile will respond differently to different textures; that is, *the histogram of values in the neural image resulting from the application of the filter will vary systematically across different classes of textures*. Thus different filters can signal different types of textures by the differences in their response histograms.

These models are typically employed to explain segregation of textures which vary in spatial structure. For example, a linear spatial filter with a receptive field profile that is oriented vertically might be used to emphasize texture regions with a large amount of vertically oriented structure. Figure 19.3B shows a vertically oriented receptive field profile. When applied to the texture pair in part A, the resulting output image is part C. Note that the two texture regions produce the same average output value, but the vertically oriented texture results in a greater number of extreme output values (both positive and negative). In other words, in that region the output image has higher contrast.

These images have very different histograms, but have the same average value over space. Thus a segmentation process that draws boundaries between image regions differing only in *average value* can miss *histogram* differences between regions. However, whenever two images differ significantly in their histograms, then we can find some function to apply to both of them, point by point across the visual field, so that the average values over space of the two resultant images are very different. For the IID textures shown in figure 19.1, parts A, C, and E, as well as the filtered image of figure 19.3C, taking the absolute value of the pixel values does the job (figure 19.3D).

We can now simply state the back pocket model of texture segregation. This model proposes that the visual system

1. Applies a variety of linear filters to the retinal input, to produce a set of neural images, one for each filter

2. Further transforms each neural image by taking some nonlinear function (e.g., the square or the absolute value) of the neural image value at each location in the visual field

3. Passes the entire set of spatial output functions resulting from step 2 to a segmentation system whose purpose is to partition the visual field into regions within which these output functions are all relatively constant in value, and between which (at least some of) these output functions diverge in value

Most texture perception researchers feel that the three steps of this model are *necessary* to explain texture segregation (see references in chapter 18). However, there is empirical evidence indicating that these three steps are probably not *sufficient* to account for texture segregation (see, for instance, chapters 17 by Bergen and Landy and 18 by Graham).

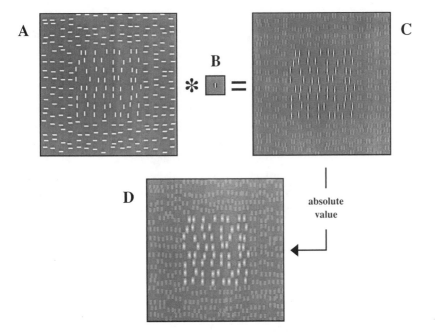

Fig. 19.3
The back pocket model of texture segregation. (A) A texture pair. (B) A vertically tuned linear receptive field. (C) The texture in (A) filtered by an array of linear neurons with the receptive field profile shown in (B). (D) The absolute value of the neural image shown in (C).

IID Textures and The Back Pocket Model

Figure 19.4 shows the result of applying a linear filter (with the garden variety, oriented receptive field profile of part B), to the IID texture of part A. The neural image that results is shown in part C. The important point to note about this texture is that its graylevel histogram has a Gaussian waveform. This is not surprising. Each pixel value in part C is a weighted sum of a moderately large number of pixels in part A, and these are jointly independent, identically distributed random variables. In this case, the central limit theorem (e.g., Feller, 1968) tells us that the output value will be approximately normally distributed. We emphasize that the normality of the output image pixel distribution depends neither on the pixel distribution of the input IID texture, nor on the particular form of the receptive field profile characterizing the filter. As long as the receptive field profile sums at least a

moderate number of input image values, the pixel distribution of the output image will be normal.

A normal distribution is completely characterized by its mean and variance. This implies some interesting things about the way in which the back pocket model deals with IID textures. Specifically, for any pair of IID textures whose pixel distributions have the same mean and variance, if we apply a linear filter with a moderately large receptive field profile to both textures, then we *obliterate any difference there may have been between the two textures prior to the application of the filter*. (Formally, the pixels in each of the two output images will be jointly normal, and the two images will have identical means and covariance matrices.)

Obviously, it is possible to produce IID textures with different pixel distributions which nonetheless have the same mean and variance. Examples of such texture pairs are shown in figures 19.5 and 19.6. The textures of figures 19.5A and 19.6A have pixel distributions modulated by polynomials obtained by performing Gram-Schmidt orthogonalization on the sequence of polynomials $l_i(v) = v^i$, taken over the discrete set $v = 0, 1, \ldots, 15$ of graylevels. This process results in a sequence L_i, $i = 0, 1, \ldots, 15$, of *orthogonal polynomials*.[3] This means that, for any i,

---

3. These are closely related to the set of Legendre polynomials (Hochstrasser, 1964).

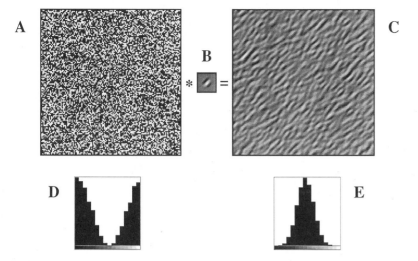

Fig. 19.4
IID textures and linear spatial filters. (A) An IID texture with a cosinusoidal pixel distribution. (B) A linear receptive field. (C) The result of filtering (A) with an array of linear neurons with the receptive field shown in (B). (D) The graylevel histogram of the patch of texture in (A). (E) The graylevel histogram of the texture patch in (C). Note that the distribution of pixel values is now approximately normal.

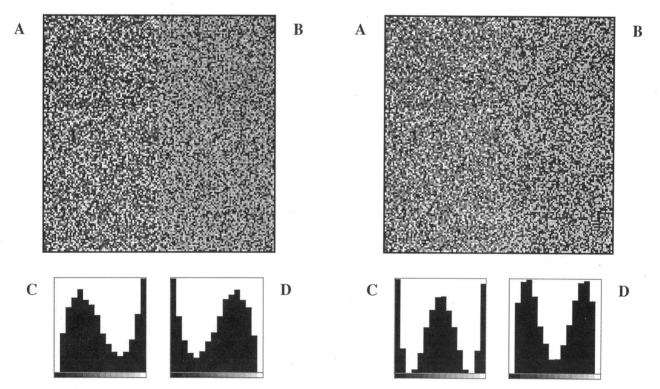

Fig. 19.5
(A) An IID texture using polynomial L_3. (B) An IID texture using polynomial $-L_3$. (C) the histogram of the texture patch of (A). (D) the histogram of the texture patch of (B).

Fig. 19.6
(A) An IID texture using polynomial L_4. (B) An IID texture using polynomial $-L_4$. (C) the histogram of the texture patch of (A). (D) the histogram of the texture patch of (B).

$j = 0, 1, \ldots, 15$, with $i \neq j$,

$$\sum_{\substack{graylevel \\ v=0}}^{15} L_i(v)L_j(v) = 0. \tag{17}$$

Consider the family of IID textures with pixel distributions

$$Probability[pixel\ painted\ v] = \frac{1 + \alpha L_i(v)}{16}$$

$$i = 3, 4, \ldots, 15 \tag{18}$$

(where α is some amplitude). The mean and variance of these distributions are equal to the mean and variance of the uniform pixel distribution of equation 2 (since L_3, L_4, etc., are orthogonal to L_1, which characterizes the mean, and to L_2, which along with L_1 characterizes the variance).

The pixel distribution of the IID texture in figure 19.5A is modulated by L_3, whereas that of the IID texture in figure 19.5B is modulated by the negative of this function, $-L_3$. Similarly, the pixel distributions of the IID textures in figure 19.6A and B are modulated by L_4 and $-L_4$, respectively. Although the differences between these texture pairs are small, nevertheless they can be segregated. The important fact to bear in mind is that all differences between IID textures whose pixel distributions have equal mean and variance (e.g., figures 19.5A, B and 19.6A, B) are effectively obliterated by applying any linear filter with a receptive field profile that sums the values of even a moderate number of input image pixels. This means that in order to discriminate between pairs of such textures, *the visual system must be using arrays of neurons whose responses depend on very few input values* (i.e., must be using an early, pointwise nonlinearity).

This brings us back to our original simple model. Since the textures in figures 19.5 and 19.6 do segregate, then the visual system can not consist solely of linear spatial filters with moderate-sized receptive fields (relative to the pixel sampling in the figures), but must include at least one array similar to that posited in the simple model, which applies the function f directly to the input image. Of course, if the neural output image of such a pointwise operator is to be of use in segmenting the visual field, then the function applied to each input value by the pointwise operator must be *nonlinear*. Moreover, if this nonlinear function used by our visual system is to be of any use in discriminating between IID textures whose

pixel distributions have the same mean and variance, then it must be something other than a second order polynomial.

We mentioned above that orthogonal distribution analysis may be used with sets of functions other than sine waves, as long as those functions are mutually orthogonal. The polynomials L_i are just such a set of functions. In addition, the polynomials L_i (for $i > 2$) result in textures which would be indiscriminable if the visual system were using only the neural images constructed using moderate-sized receptive fields. If there were only one pointwise operator available to the observer, then we could determine its properties by using orthogonal distribution analysis with textures using pixel distributions as in equation 18 to measure the higher order (i.e., > 2) polynomial components of the function used by that operator. If the "single pointwise operator" model does not hold, then the tests provided by the analysis should allow us to reject it. There is a distinct perceptual difference between the IID texture patches of Figure 19.5A and B, and between the patches in figure 19.6A and B. If this difference has the same characteristics as other textural differences (i.e., can define two-dimensional form in a brief flash), this suggests that there is such a pointwise operator, and orthogonal distribution analysis provides a means of studying that operator, bypassing other channels of the back pocket model.

Conclusions

We have defined a new method called *orthogonal distribution analysis* for psychophysically estimating some of the parameters of a generic model of texture segregation. The method can also be used to test the validity of that model. We are currently devising experiments which use this orthogonal distribution analysis with IID noise.

Acknowledgments

The research reported here was supported in part by AFOSR Visual Information Processing Program grant 88-0140, in part by a 1989 Henry Rutgers Research Fellowship to Dr. Chubb from Rutgers University, and by NIH grant EY08266. We thank Anne Sutter and John Econopouly for their helpful comments.

References

Bergen, J. R. (1991). Theories of visual texture perception. In D. Regan, (Ed.), *Vision and visual dysfunction, Vol. 10B* (pp. 114–134). New York: Macmillan.

Bracewell, R. N. (1978). *The Fourier transform and its applications.* New York: McGraw-Hill.

Caelli, T. M. (1985). Three processing characteristics of visual texture segmentation. *Spatial Vision, 1,* 19–30.

Feller, W. (1968). *An introduction to probability theory and its applications.* New York: Wiley.

Hochstrasser, U. W. (1964). Orthogonal polynomials. In M. Abramowitz & I. E. Stegun (Eds.), *Handbook of mathematical functions* (Ch. 22), Washington, DC: National Bureau of Standards, U.S. Government Printing Office.

Robson, J. G. (1980). Neural images: The physiological basis of spatial vision. In C. Harris, (Ed.), *Visual coding and adaptability* (pp. 177–214). Hillsdale, NJ: Erlbaum.

Part VII

3D Shape

The visual world is a three-dimensional place, and the retinal image is two-dimensional. Many cues exist to allow human observers to overcome this difficulty and deduce the structure of three-dimensional space and objects. These include relative motion, motion parallax, binocular disparity, occlusion, texture perspective, and many others. Marr (1982) suggested that these cues can be computed by independent "shape from X" modules, each of which calculates a depth map based on the information available from cue "X." Each of these partial depth maps are then combined into a single depth map, the "2-1/2D sketch." This representation then is used as the input to modules that look for three-dimensional objects.

This approach has had a major influence on studies of both computer and human vision. In computer vision, dozens of algorithms have been proposed for computing depth from various isolated cues. At the same time, it has also been suggested that multiple cues might be processed simultaneously to some advantage (Aloimonos & Shulman, 1989). The problem of combining these multiple depth maps into a single map is essentially a problem of statistical estimation (Maloney & Landy, 1989), and has only recent been examined psychophysically.

The chapter by Bülthoff reviews a number of studies he has carried out which measure the depth representation resulting from multiple depth cues. In addition, he examines the way in which multiple depth cues interact to produce a unified depth percept. Frisby reviews a number of computational issues in computing depth from stereo and describes recent machine vision algorithms for stereo vision. Parker, Johnston, Mansfield, and Yang review several psychophysical experiments on binocular stereopsis and consider the way in which stereoscopic cues combine to yield information about the shape of three-dimensional surfaces. Each of these chapters reflects the new awareness—derived from Marr's work—that the integration of multiple cues to depth is a critical part of the complex mechanism that gives us our impression of the full richness of the three-dimensional structure of the world.

References

Aloimonos, J. & Shulman, D. (1989). *Integration of visual modules.* New York: Academic Press.

Maloney, L. T. & Landy, M. S. (1989). A statistical framework for robust fusion of depth information. In W. A. Pearlman (Ed.), *Visual Communications and Image Processing IV, Proceedings of the SPIE, 1199,* 1154–1163.

Marr, D. (1982). *Vision.* San Francisco: W. H. Freeman.

20

Shape from X: Psychophysics and Computation

Heinrich H. Bülthoff

The Many Routes to Shape

The human visual system derives a variety of information about the three-dimensional (3D) structure of the environment from different cues. This is illustrated in figure 20.1, where computer simulations of surface properties of a simple geometric form under different lighting conditions can lead to quite different 3D impressions. If an ellipsoid of rotation with Lambertian reflectance properties (like a table tennis ball) is simulated to be illuminated only by ambient light (equal amount of light from all directions), no inference of the 3D shape of the object can be made. The addition of a single point light source in the far distance (i.e., parallel illumination) allows our visual system to interpret the shading variations as a three-dimensional form; in other words, it computes shape from shading. The 3D impression of the ellipsoid becomes stronger when a highlight is added to the image by using a different shading model (Phong, 1975) for the computer graphic simulation. We get the strongest impression of the 3D shape of the object in the lower right of figure 20.1, where an additional source of information is available through simulation of surface texture. Note that not only the form of the object but also the perceived orientation of the object changes with the number of simulated depth cues. By observing figure 20.1 we can ask ourselves, what are the correct form and orientation of the object? Can we infer the correct 3D shape from 2D images? What are the best cues for shape? Which are better for orientation? We hope to answer some of these questions in the next few sections.

The outline of this chapter is as follows. First we motivate the need for cue integration in human and machine vision. In the next section we describe different representations of depth and how they can be assessed in psychophysical experiments. We discuss in detail two different techniques to measure shape-from-X, local and global shape probes, and how they are used to measure

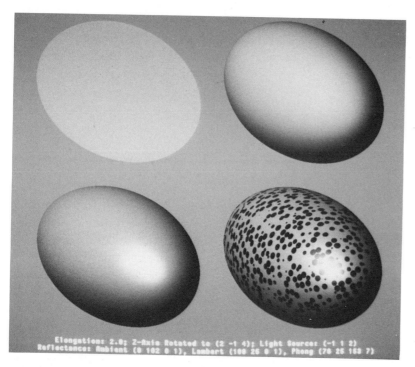

Fig. 20.1
Shape from X. The shape of the four objects looks quite different because the visual system derives different shape information from different shape cues. All four images were generated for the same 3D shape (ellipsoid of rotation) but with different simulated surface properties and under different lighting conditions.

shape from stereo, shading, and texture. In the following section we discuss an important and often neglected aspect of stereo vision: intensity-based stereo or shape from disparate shading. Bülthoff and Mallot (1988) showed that the human visual system can perceive depth in disparate images which have no discontinuities (zero crossings in the Laplacian of filtered images). This is a surprising finding because many theories in human and machine stereo vision are based on matching discontinuities in image intensities. An intensity-based stereo mechanism can be very useful for "direct" surface interpolation of surfaces with large smooth regions and should integrate with more robust measurements of edge-based stereo. In the section entitled Shape from Highlights we demonstrate an additional source of shape information that has been regarded previously as more of a nuisance than a useful cue to shape. Blake and Bülthoff (1990) showed that the human visual system can make use of the relative disparity of highlights in glossy images. For

most machine vision algorithms these highlights are most undesirable because the disparity (or motion) of the highlight is different from the underlying structure and therefore can lead to false depth (or motion) measurements. The human visual system, on the other hand, can use this information in situations where only ambiguous information about surface shape is available, for example, in order to disambiguate the convex-concave ambiguity of shape-from-shading. This is a perfect example of the "disambiguation" type of cue integration. Other types of cue integration are discussed in Integration of Depth Modules. In the final section, a theoretical framework for cue integration is discussed briefly. A more detailed description of this framework can be found in Bülthoff and Yuille (1990).

The Need for Integration

The shape and depth cues simulated in figure 20.1 (and others) have been formalized in terms of computational theory and have been implemented as single modules in machine vision systems. Related studies from psychophysics and computational vision exist mainly for stereo (Julesz, 1971; Marr & Poggio, 1976, 1979; Mayhew & Frisby, 1981; Prazdny, 1985) and shading (Blake, Zisser-

306   3D Shape

man & Knowles, 1985; Ikeuchi & Horn, 1981; Mingolla & Todd, 1986; Pentland, 1984). There are also a number of studies on depth from texture (Aliomonos & Swain, 1985; Bajcsy & Lieberman, 1976; Cutting & Millard, 1984; Kender, 1979; Pentland, 1986; Witkin, 1981), line drawings (Barrow & Tenenbaum, 1981), surface contours (Stevens, 1981; Stevens & Brookes, 1987) and structure-from-motion (Koenderink, 1986; Longuet-Higgins & Prazdny, 1981; Landy, 1987; Ullman, 1979,1984), accommodation (Pentland, 1985), and occlusion (Haynes and Jain, 1987). Most implementations are quite successful for synthetic images but less reliable for natural images. On the contrary, the human visual system more easily extracts depth from the multiple 3D cues available in natural images compared to the isolated cues found in synthetic images (e.g., random dot stereograms). In order to study how the human visual system can integrate the information from multiple cues so successfully, we developed methods for quantitative measurement of perceived depth and shape with stimuli that are closer to natural images than those used in most psychophysical experiments. Using computer graphic techniques, we have precise control over the different shape and depth cues and we can use them in supportive or contradictory combinations to study the interaction between them and get a better idea how different cues are integrated into a stable representation of the 3D world. But before we discuss this, we will examine the question of what kinds of representations can be used by our visual system.

How to Represent the Third Dimension?

Raw data, such as a range map from depth and shape cues, can be thought of as a trivial, or *zero-order representation* of the spatial structure of a scene. *Higher-order descriptors* can be derived from image data that make interesting spatial properties of the viewed scene explicit. The question of what constitutes a useful 3D descriptor can be answered in the light of the action that it should subserve. For example, a *pointwise depth map* can be useful for precise manipulation of objects while *surface curvature* (without exact range data) might be useful for the recognition of complex 3D shapes such as faces.

Which cues are relevant to one particular 3D descriptor? Occlusion contributes more readily to depth ordering than to surface curvature. Shading contributes more qualitatively to curvature than quantitatively to a depth map,

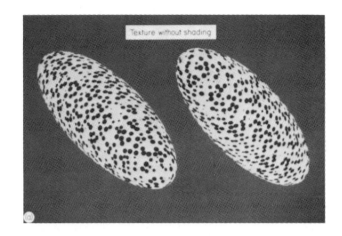

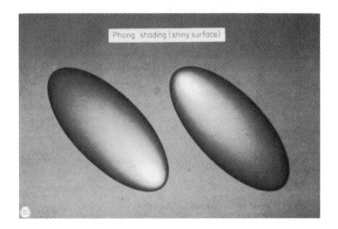

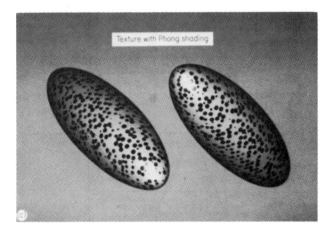

Fig. 20.2
3D descriptors. Different depth cues provide information about different 3D descriptors (e.g., range, shape, orientation). Try to estimate the angle between the long axes of the ellipsoids (for the correct answer, see text). (After Bülthoff & Mallot, 1990.)

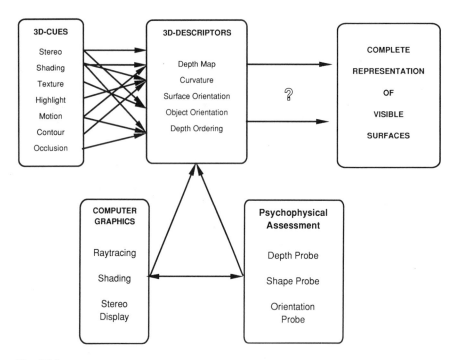

Fig. 20.3

Shape representation. 3D structure perceived from 2D image can be represented at different levels of abstraction. The depth cues themselves constitute multiple *zero-order* representations. Higher-order representations, i.e., *3D descriptors*, can be derived from interaction and integration of several of these zero-order representations. Different psychophysical experiments (much as computer vision tasks) involve various combinations of 3D descriptors. It is not clear whether a unique 3D representation exists that serves as a common data basis for all types of behavior dealing with the spatial structure of the environment. (Redrawn from Bülthoff & Mallot, 1990.)

and texture more to object orientation than to object form. This is illustrated in figure 20.2, where three pairs of ellipsoids are shown whose long axes of elongation are orthogonal to each other. The orthogonal orientation is best seen in part C, where texture and specular shading provide sufficient 3D information. If texture is used without shading (part A), the orientation of the objects can usually be perceived correctly, while the objects themselves appear flat. On the contrary, if shading is the only cue (part B), the objects appear nicely curved but it is difficult to see them orthogonal to each other.

How to Assess Properties of Multiple Representations?

Since the perception of three-dimensional scenes relies on so many different depth cues, which can lead to various descriptions of that scene in terms of distance, surface orientation, surface curvature and shape, we measured some of these 3D descriptors (depth map, curvature, and object orientation) for different depth cues (stereo, shading, highlight, texture, see figure 20.3).

The relation of shading (with and without highlights), stereo, and texture in the 3D perception of smooth and polyhedral surfaces was studied with computer graphic psychophysics (see appendix A). For polyhedral and textured objects, stereo disparities were associated with localized features, that is, the intensity changes at the facet or texel boundaries, while for the smooth surfaces only shading disparities occurred. For most of our experiments we used ellipsoids of revolution (viewed end-on) for the following reasons:

• As is shown later (Images Without Zero-Crossings), images of Lambertian shaded smooth ellipsoids with moderate eccentricities do not contain Laplacian zero-crossings when illuminated centrally with parallel light. This allows us to study intensity-based stereo mechanisms.

• The surfaces are closed and are naturally outlined by a planar occluding contour. This contour was placed in the zero disparity plane and did not allow the subjects to derive depth from binocular disparities.

• Convex objects such as ellipsoids do not cast shadows

or generate reflections on their own surface. Therefore, shading (attached shadows) could be studied without interference from cast shadows.

- End-on views of ellipsoids can be thought of as a model example of depth interpolation of a surface patch between sparse edge data.

Local and Global Depth Probes

Depending on the type of representation we wanted to measure quantitatively, we used two different types of probes (see appendix B). The depth probe can measure locally perceived depth, but has some disadvantages with depth cues which are better viewed monocularly (e.g., shading and texture). The global shape probe is more appropriate for the latter case but cannot be used to derive a precise depth map for all points in the image:

- *Local depth.* We mapped perceived depth with a small probe or cursor that was interactively adjusted to match the depth of the perceived surface (further details in appendix B). The depth of this probe was defined by edge-based stereo disparity and all other cue combinations were compared to the percept generated by edge-based stereo. All images were viewed binocularly with the depth cursor superimposed and hence had a zero disparity cue in them. Each adjustment of the probe gives a graded measurement of distance, or local depth, that is, this experiment corresponds to the 3D descriptor *depth map* in the scheme of figure 20.3. Note that the binocularly viewed local probe can interfere with monocular cues like shading and texture. Therefore, a more global shape probe was used to extend the range of possible shape measurements.

- *Global shape.* The global shapes of two objects with different combinations of depth cues were compared directly (further details in appendix B). Since all images showed end-on views of ellipsoids with different elongation, this measurement corresponds to *curvature* or *form* as a 3D descriptor.

- *Global orientation.* Object orientation can be measured in a matching task where long ellipsoids of different orientation are compared. While surface orientation is apparently hard to determine for human observers (Min-

golla & Todd, 1986; Todd & Mingolla, 1983), the orientation of entire objects (e.g., orientation of *generalized cylinders*) can be measured easily in a matching task.

Shape From Stereo and Shading (Local Measurements)[1]

In the first series of experiments, 165 measurements were performed, each consisting of 45 adjustments of the depth probe to the perceived surface. Results were consistent in all three subjects and were pooled, since the differences were noticeable only in the standard deviation. The 16 plots of figure 20.4 show the averaged results of all subjects for the four types of experiments and four different elongations of Lambertian shaded ellipsoids.

The perceived elongation in the images with consistent cue combinations depends on the amount of information available. In figure 20.5 a measure of perceived elongation is derived from the depth map shown in figure 20.4 by a principle component analysis (see appendix C) and plotted as a function of displayed elongation. As can be seen from figure 20.5, the perceived elongation is almost correct when shading, intensity-based and edge-based disparity information are available (D^+E^+). This is not too surprising because this condition involves basically a disparity-to-disparity match (the probe is a disparity cued probe). This disparity match should work perfectly as long as the probe is not too distant from the grid intersections (edges) of the polygonal ellipsoid. In the case of smooth-shaded disparate images (D^+E^-), the edges are missing and depth perception is reduced. When shading is the only cue (D^-E^-), perceived elongation is much smaller and almost independent of the displayed elongation. Phong shading (highlights) instead of Lambertian shading did not change perceived depth significantly (dashed lines). A much stronger influence on the type of shading can be measured with the shape probe (see below).

In experiment D^-E^+, two identical images (zero disparity) of polyhedral ellipsoids (edges) were shown. Although shading alone provided some depth information as shown in experiment D^-E^-, the fact that edges occurred at zero disparity was decisive. The perceived depth did not vary with the elongation suggested by the shad-

---

1. In collaboration with Hanspeter Mallot, Ruhr Universität Bochum.

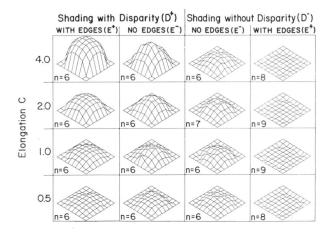

Fig. 20.4
Perceived surfaces. Each plot shows the average of six to nine sessions from three subjects. Perceived depth decreases with the following sequence of cue-combinations: disparity, edges, and shading ($D^+ E^+$); disparity and shading but no edges ($D^+ E^-$); shading only ($D^- E^-$); contradictory disparity and shading ($D^- E^+$). The elongation of the displayed objects is denoted by c (depth not drawn to scale). (Redrawn from Bülthoff & Mallot, 1988.)

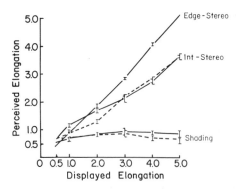

Fig. 20.5
Perceived elongation. Depth perception decreases with fewer cues available. The significant separation between the middle and lower curves (smooth shading with and without disparity) illustrates the influence of disparity information even in the absence of edges. Solid lines: Lambertian shading; dashed lines: Phong shading. (Redrawn from Bülthoff & Mallot, 1988.)

ing (and perspective) information and took slightly negative values which, however, were not significantly different from zero. This veto type of relationship between stereo and shading is probably due to the depth probe technique, which enforces disparity-to-disparity matching. A different type of integration between stereo and shading or texture (see, for example, Buckley, Frisby &

Mayhew, 1989) might go unnoticed with this technique and therefore a more global shape probe was used in other experiments.

Depth can still be perceived when no disparate edges are present. This is not surprising, since shading information was still available. A comparison of the results (figure 20.5) for smooth-shaded images with and without disparity information, however, establishes a significant contribution of shading disparities (intensity-based stereo). The curves for $D^+ E^-$ and $D^- E^-$ are significantly separated for all elongations except 0.5.

Shape from Shading and Texture (Global Measurements)

As discussed earlier, global shape cues like shape from shading and texture cannot be assessed with the local depth probe without interference with the shape-from-stereo module. Therefore we measured all cues, which are better viewed monocularly to eliminate zero disparity cues, with our global shape comparison technique (appendix B). All of our images with single monocular cues lead to large errors in perceived shape. With *shading* and *texture* curvature is underestimated (figure 20.6A, B), with a highlight it is overestimated (figure 20.6C). Note, that the reference ("given elongation") was displayed in stereo and that the elongation of the shaded or textured ellipsoid was chosen by the subject ("chosen elongation"). Underestimation of elongation corresponds therefore to chosen values above the dashed line and overestimation to values below the line.

Shape from Shading

One remarkable result of the comparison technique is that the shape-from-shading performance is much better with this technique than with the local depth probe technique. The adjusted shading scales with the displayed elongation of the stereoscopically displayed reference ellipsoid and does not level off as in the case of the depth probe measurements. There is still a strong underestimation of the elongation of the shaded ellipsoid for a given stereoscopically displayed reference ellipsoid, but in conjunction with a texture cue (figure 20.6D) the slope of the shape-from-texture-and-shading curve is close to 1.0 (veridical).

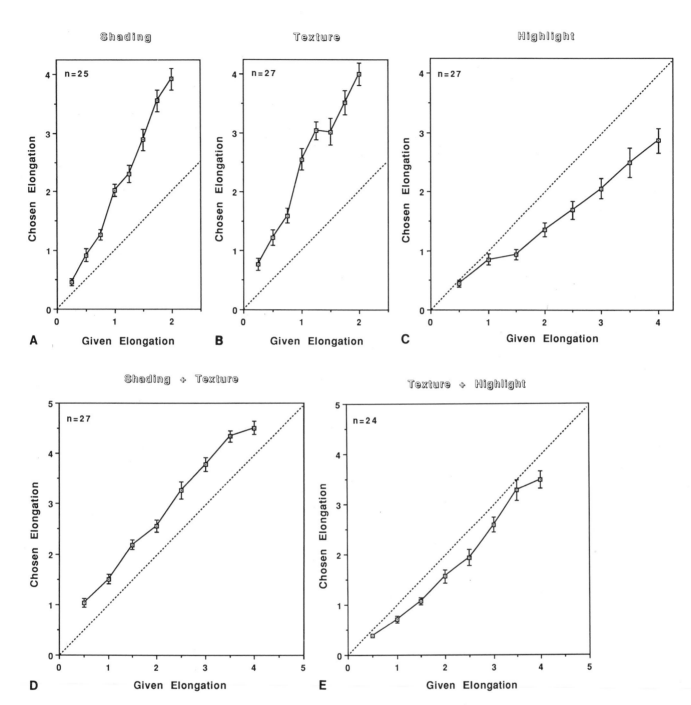

Fig. 20.6
Global shape. (A, B) Shape-from-shading and shape-from-texture lead to an underestimation of shape (slope > 1). (C) If a highlight is added to the shading (Phong shading model) the shape is overestimated in the adjustment task. (D) If shading and texture are presented simultaneously the shape is adjusted almost correctly (slope = 1) with a bias to adjust a larger elongation than necessary. (E) If a highlight is added the slope stays the same but the bias changes towards an overestimation of shape. (Redrawn from Bülthoff & Mallot, 1990.)

Shape from Texture

The performance of shape-from-texture and shape-from-shading is very similar. Both curves have almost the same offset and slope. This is not so surprising because the computational problem of shape-from-texture and shape-from-shading is very similar (Aliomonos & Swain, 1985). This similarity in the computational structure could be the reason for the strong cooperativity and almost veridical perception if both cues are present (figure 20.6D).

Shape from Highlights

A highlight on the shaded surface also seems to have a much larger influence with this technique and leads to an overestimation of curvature (figure 20.6C). This overestimation can be seen also if both texture and highlights are used (figure 20.6E). Again, in this case the cooperativity between modules shows up in the much more veridical perception of shape than with single modules. But compared to texture with shading (figure 20.6D), the texture and highlight curve (figure 20.6E) signals an overestimation of shape.

Shape from Disparate Shading (Intensity-Based Stereo)

As mentioned earlier, a very surprising finding is the strength of depth perception (70 percent) obtained from disparate shading under various illuminant conditions and reflectance functions. In computational theory, most studies have focused on edge-based stereo algorithms (for review, see Poggio & Poggio, 1984). This is due to the overall superiority of edge-based stereo, which is confirmed by the finding that edge-based stereo gives a better depth estimate than disparate shading (Blake et al., 1985). However, in the absence of edges and for surface interpolation, graylevel disparities appear to be more important than is usually appreciated.

Images Without Zero-crossings

One of the most important constraints in early vision for recovering surface properties is that the physical processes underlying image formation are typically smooth. The smoothness property is captured well by standard regularization (Poggio, Torre & Koch, 1985) and exploited in its algorithms. On the other hand, *changes of image intensity* often convey information about physical edges in the scene. The locations of sharp changes in image intensity very often correspond to depth discontinuities in the scene. Many stereo algorithms use dominant changes in image intensity as features to compute disparity between corresponding image points. In order to localize these sharp changes in image intensity, zero-crossings in Laplacian-filtered images are commonly used (Marr & Hildreth, 1980).

The disadvantage of these feature-based stereo algorithms is that only sparse depth data (at image features) can be computed. This forces an additional stage in which sophisticated algorithms (Blake & Zisserman, 1987; Grimson, 1982) interpolate the surface between data points. In order to test for the ability of human stereo vision to get denser depth data by using features other than edges, or even a completely featureless mechanism, we computed images without sharp changes in image intensity. We show that for an orthographically projected image of a sphere with Lambertian reflection function and parallel illumination, zero-crossings in the Laplacian are missing. Consider a hemisphere given in cylindrical coordinates by the parametric equation

$$z = \sqrt{1 - r^2}. \tag{1}$$

In the special case of a sphere, the surface normal simply equals the radius, that is,

$$\mathbf{n} = (r \cos \varphi, r \sin \varphi, \sqrt{1 - r^2}). \tag{2}$$

For the illuminant direction $\mathbf{l} = (0, 0, 1)$ and the Lambertian reflectance function, we obtain the luminance profile

$$I(r) = I_0(\mathbf{l} \cdot \mathbf{n}) = I_0\sqrt{1 - r^2}, \tag{3}$$

where I_0 is a suitable constant, i.e., the image luminance is again a hemisphere. For the Laplacian of I, we obtain

$$\nabla^2 I(r) = I''(r) - \frac{1}{r}I'(r) = -I_0\frac{r^2}{(1 - r^2)^{3/2}}. \tag{4}$$

This is a nonpositive function of r, with $\nabla^2 I(0) = 0$; i.e., the Laplacian of I has no zero-crossings.

Unfortunately, this result does not hold for ellipsoids with $c \neq 1$. A similar computation for an ellipsoid with elongation c yields

$$I_c(r) = I_0\frac{\sqrt{1 - r^2}}{\sqrt{1 - (1 - c^2)r^2}}, \tag{5}$$

which reduces to equation 3 for $c = 1$. The luminance-profiles for elongations $c \geqslant 2$ are no longer convex. That is to say that the second derivatives of these profiles in fact have zero-crossings, and a similar result holds for the Laplacians. However, when filtering with the Laplacian of a Gaussian or with the difference of two Gaussians (DOG) is considered, it turns out that these zero-crossings are insignificant for the elongations used here. Pixel-based convolutions failed to show the "edges" unequivocally, and even a Gaussian integration algorithm run on the complete function rather than on the sampled array produced no zero-crossings beyond the single-precision truncation error. We therefore conclude that the slight zero-crossings in the unfiltered Laplacian of our luminance profiles do not correspond to significant edges. For oblique illumination we found numerically that the self shadow boundary corresponds to a level rather than a zero-crossing in the DOG-filtered image.

Independently of our own work, images of ellipsoids may be useful in the study of the psychophysical relevance of Laplacian zero-crossings.

Local or Global Mechanisms?

Are there features other than zero-crossings that can account for the shape-from-disparate-shading performance found in our experiments? Possible candidates include the intensity peak as proposed by Mayhew and Frisby (1981) and level-crossings in the DOG-filtered image which, according to Hildreth (1983), might account for Mayhew and Frisby's data as well.

In order to distinguish between a localized (feature-based) and a distributed mechanism for shape-from-disparate-shading we tested the effect of a small disparate token displayed in front of a nondisparate background with the depth probe (figure 20.7). Our data show that for large elongations, a single stereo feature (ring) is not sufficient to produce the same percept as full disparate shading (compare part A of figure 20.7 with parts B to D). For small elongations (0.5 to 2.0; not shown in figure 20.7) the differences were not pronounced. We therefore conjecture that disparate shading does not rely on feature matching and thus can be used for surface interpolation when edges are sparse. This view is well in line with the

finding that edge information, whenever present, over-rides shape-from-disparate-shading (figure 20.8).

Note, however, that we do not propose the naive idea of pointwise intensity matching as a mechanism for shape-from-disparate-shading because of its sensitivity to noise in both the data and in neural processing. Even in the absence of image noise, intensity-based algorithms (e.g., Gennert, 1987) can lead to severe matching errors when run on our stimuli (see Psychophysical Support for the Bayesian Framework). A window-based correlation mechanism like the one used for optical flow computation (Bülthoff, Little & Poggio, 1989) might be more appropriate for shape-from-disparate-shading. This type of algorithm has been successfully used for stereo (D. Weinshall, personal communication). For a comparison see also the SWITCHER algorithm described in chapter 21. In the next section we will look at one additional cue (highlights) that is used by the visual system in cases where shape-from-shading or shape-from-texture does not provide unambiguous shape information.

Shape from Highlights[2]

Many images of artificial and natural scenes contain "highlights" generated by mirrorlike reflections from glossy surfaces. Computational models of visual processes have tended to regard these highlights as *obscuring* underlying scene structure. Mathematical modeling shows that, on the contrary, highlights are rich in local geometric information. This section will demonstrate that the brain can apply that information. Stereoscopically viewed highlights or "specularities" can serve as cues for 3D local surface geometry. The human visual system seems to employ a physical model of the interaction of light with curved surfaces—a model firmly based on ray optics and differential geometry. We develop such a model in the next section.

The Computational Model

The basic principle of the "specular stereo" model is quite simple (figure 20.9). According to ray optics, the image of a light source—a specularity—appears behind a glossy, convex surface and (generally) in front of a concave one,

---

2. In collaboration with Andrew Blake, Oxford University.

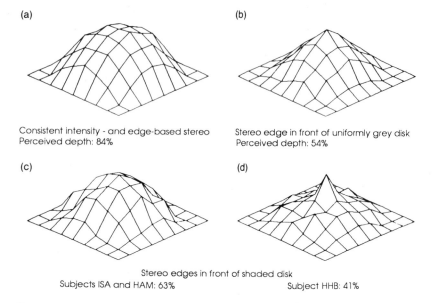

(a)

Consistent intensity - and edge-based stereo
Perceived depth: 84%

(b)

Stereo edge in front of uniformly grey disk
Perceived depth: 54%

(c)

(d)

Stereo edges in front of shaded disk

Subjects ISA and HAM: 63%   Subject HHB: 41%

Fig. 20.7

Surface interpolation. (a) Shape-from-disparate-shading plus disparate edge information leads to an almost correct percept ($n = 6$). (b) A single edge token in front of a uniformly gray disk yields a cone-like subjective surface ($n = 6$). (c, d) Shape-from-shading plus disparate edge information leads to an ambiguous perception ($n = 3 + 3$). Some subjects fused the edge-token and the surround into one coherent surface (c) while others saw the edge-token floating in front of a rather flat surface (d). Only data for elongation 4.0 are shown. (Redrawn from Bülthoff & Mallot, 1988.)

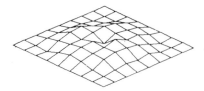

Shape-from-shading and zero-disparity edge
Perceived depth: 16%

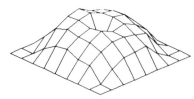

Intensity-based stereo and zero-disparity edge
Perceived depth: 66%

Fig. 20.8

Veto. (A) A zero-disparity edge token vetoes shape-from-shading ($n = 7$) and (B) shape-from-disparate-shading ($n = 6$). Only data for elongation 4.0 are shown. (Redrawn from Bülthoff & Mallot, 1988.)

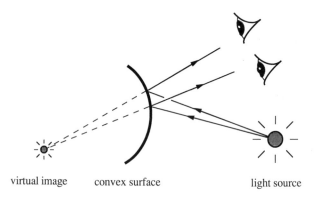

virtual image   convex surface   light source

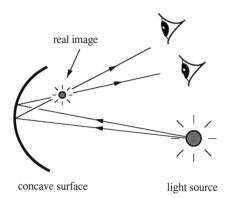

real image

concave surface   light source

Fig. 20.9

Specular stereo—the basic principle. Specularities appear behind a convex mirror but in front of a concave one. (Redrawn from Blake & Bülthoff, 1990.)

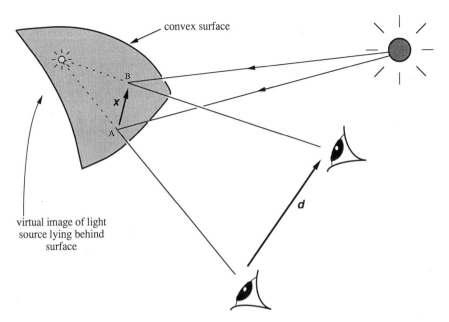

Fig. 20.10

Geometry of specular stereo. Ray optics establishes direct relationship between surface shape and measured disparity. Stereoscopic relative disparity δ is a projection of the displacement vector $\mathbf{x}$ of the specularity on the reflecting surface. Displacement $\mathbf{x}$, in turn, is related linearly to baseline vector $\mathbf{d}$, the coefficients of the relation being a function solely of surface geometry. If the visual system knows the physics of specular reflection and the light source position, then the relative disparity of a specularity would be consistent only with certain values of local surface curvature.

provided both viewer and source are sufficiently distant from the surface. But this simple idea must be expanded. How, for example, does a specularity appear in a surface that is hyperbolic? Whether it appears behind or in front depends on the orientation of the surface. Even on an elliptic surface, the apparent depth of the image varies if the surface is rotated about the line of sight.

In fact we are forced to hesitate at the notion of apparent "depth." What we actually observe is determined by *horizontal and vertical relative disparities*. Stereoscopic disparity is a vector quantity, conventionally taken (Mayhew & Longuet-Higgins, 1982) to have a horizontal and a vertical component equal to the differences in x, y coordinates of corresponding image points in left and right planar projections. Horizontal disparity is the component of the disparity vector parallel to the stereoscopic baseline ($\mathbf{d}$ in figure 20.10) and vertical disparity is the orthogonal component. *Relative* disparity of a specularity is (roughly) the difference between its disparity and that of

a nearby point on the surface. Surface features (scratches, for example) obey the "epipolar" constraint (Arnold & Binford, 1980; Mayhew & Frisby, 1981). Once the epipolar lines are known—a nontrivial problem of camera calibration in computer vision (see chapter 21)—vertical disparity of one surface point relative to another is zero. Specularities, however, are not surface features (that is, they are not stuck to a surface) so they do not obey the epipolar constraint. They frequently have nonzero vertical relative disparities. Both horizontal and vertical relative disparities of a specularity vary as the surface is rotated about the line of sight. Now, the actual depth of a *surface* feature is approximately proportional to horizontal disparity, but perceived depth could be affected by the introduction of vertical disparity (Koenderink & van Doorn, 1976). Only in cases where vertical disparity is negligible (e.g., on a spherical surface with slant less than about 30°) can we confidently talk about the depth of a specularity.

Ray optics establishes a direct relationship between surface shape and measured disparity (Blake, 1985; Blake & Brelstaff, 1988; Zisserman, Giblin & Blake, 1989). To a good approximation, the relative disparity vector δ depends linearly on the stereo baseline $\mathbf{d}$, and the coefficients of the linear relation are solely a function of surface geometry (figure 20.10). Suppose this model were fully utilized by the visual system, and light source position were known, then the relative disparity of a specularity would be consistent only with certain values of local surface curvature. Even if nothing is known about source position, relative disparity still constrains curvature: No convex surface can generate a negative horizontal relative disparity; a concave surface hardly ever generates a positive one. The experiments described in this section aim to test whether the human visual system exploits such constraints.

The idea that human vision employs physical constraints is, of course, not new—it has been argued vigorously by Marr (1982) and is exemplified by surface continuity and epipolar constraints in theories of stereo vision (Julesz, 1971; Marr & Poggio, 1979; Mayhew & Frisby, 1981). Continuity constraints also underly certain theories of motion perception (Bülthoff et al., 1989; Hildreth, 1984; Yuille & Grzywacz, 1988) that also have some psychophysical support. While continuity is a mathematically precise notion, its application to the physical world is intrinsically imprecise—it is scale dependent. However, the epipolar constraint *is* precise, and expressible in terms of the equations of projective geometry. But it is "internal"—a consequence of the physics of the eye itself rather than of the external world. In the case of the analysis of specularities, however, it seems that the visual system may have summarized an algebraic theory that describes the physics of surfaces in the world. The theory is both "external" and precise. The next two sections describe two experiments aimed to test whether the human visual system exploits such constraints.

Surface Quality from Highlights

An adjustment task was devised in which the subject interactively changes both horizontal and vertical disparities of a highlight. Images of glossy, textured, curved surfaces are generated with a computer graphics workstation (Symbolics, Inc.) and displayed on a high-resolution color monitor with a stereo viewing system (see appendix A). The texture is of sufficient density to furnish strong cues for curvature from edge-based stereo. Simulation of surface gloss causes a specularity to appear superimposed on the texture, as in figure 20.11A. As discussed earlier, edge-based stereo cues can override cues such as monocular or disparate shading. We might therefore expect also that specularity cues should be overridden; that is precisely what happens. When the specular relative disparities are veridical the whole surface appears glossy as in

figure 20.11A and not just in the vicinity of the specularity (Beck, 1972). However, when horizontal relative disparity is nonveridical the surface ceases to look glossy. For example, if the specularity is in front of the surface with large convergent (−) relative disparity, surface quality is reported to be matte and opaque, with a puff of cloud in front of the surface (figure 20.11B). The cloud patch is not perceived as a specularity and therefore there is no reason for the surface to look glossy. For excessively divergent (+) relative disparity, subjects usually report that the surface looks transparent, with a source of light behind it (like a frosted glass light bulb). Again, an incorrect position (relative disparity) of the specularity discounts the bright patch as a specularity and the visual system finds a different interpretation for the way in which the patch was generated. The interpretation of surface property changes from opaque to transparent. When the relative disparity is zero the simulated specularity looks like a powdery patch on the surface and the surface does not look glossy. Note, however, that in nonstereo images (like any photograph) surfaces can look glossy even with zero relative disparity. In this case a cue conflict does not really exist because all surfaces are flat and relative disparity does not have any meaning in these images.

In an informal two-alternative, forced-choice (2AFC) experiment, 11 out of 12 naive observers who were asked which of two presented surfaces was the "polished" surface chose the surface shown in figure 20.11A, in agreement with the prediction of the model.

In an adjustment task naive subjects were asked to achieve the most realistic looking glossy surface. They repeatedly pressed buttons which (unknown to the naive subjects) caused the relative disparity of a specularity to vary. They were simply told that pressing the two buttons would make the surface appear more or less shiny. Either vertical disparity was held constant (at the value determined by the ray-optic model) while horizontal disparity was varied or vice versa. Steps in specular disparity for each button press were sufficiently small (2 pixels or about 1.5 min arc) that most of the subjects did not perceive the specularity to be moving in depth. Four test surfaces were used in the adjustment task—a convex sphere, two convex ellipsoids and one concave ellipsoid.

Results for the convex sphere (figure 20.11C) show that, on average, subjects' adjusted values were not significantly different from veridical for horizontal

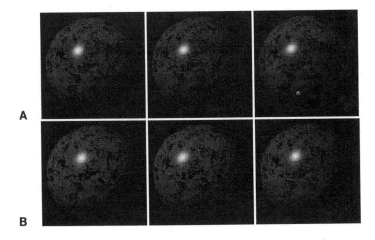

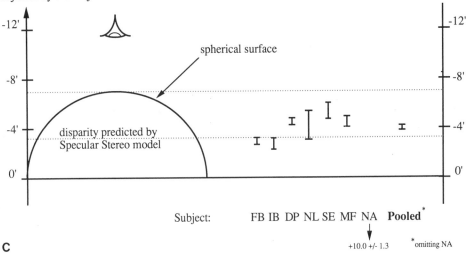

C

Fig. 20.11

Surface property. The perception of surface properties can change by moving a specular highlight relative to the surface. The surface of the sphere (A) (stereo view) looks metallic because the highlight is in the correct position behind the surface. If the highlight is in front of the surface (B) the surface looks more dull and not metallic (mirrorlike) at all. The human visual system seems to exploit the laws of reflection in the 3D interpretation of 2D images. In the psychophysical adjustment task most subjects put the specular highlight slightly (not significantly) displaced from the correct position for the sphere (C).

$(P < 0.001, F = 2)$. Note that the *sign* of the horizontal relative disparity after adjustment is always correct. This corresponds to robust discrimination between convex and concave surfaces as mentioned earlier. It is difficult to get significant vertical disparity effects for this surface because the veridical vertical disparity is close to zero (0.5 min arc). Four naive subjects adjusted the circumpolar disparity close to zero, but it is conceivable that there is some regression toward zero. Therefore, we tested a situation in which the correct vertical disparity of a specularity was quite different from zero. This is the case for the oblique-oriented ellipsoid. Five naive subjects and the two authors made adjustments whose signs were as predicted by the model. The visual system apparently has some dedicated competence for analysis of specularities and apparently "knows" enough about the physics of specularity to predict the sign of the vertical disparity correctly. Similar results are obtained for the two convex ellipsoids; the average adjusted disparities are close to veridical. Poorer agreement is obtained in the case of the concave ellipsoid, and the sign of the relative horizontal disparity after adjustment is inconsistent. Subjects reported that, for this surface, the adjustment task was relatively difficult to perform.

The conclusion of this experiment is that the human visual system models the physics of specular reflection well enough to predict relative disparity effects. Agreement with predictions is good qualitatively (sign is preserved), and there even is a degree of quantitative agreement. In particular, in the case of a convex sphere for which we can associate horizontal disparity with depth, the visual system "expects"—correctly—that a specularity lies behind not on the surface.

Surface Curvature from Highlights

The second experiment is complementary to the first. Can the visual system accommodate to variations in specular relative disparities by changing its hypothesis about surface curvature, rather than its hypothesis of glossiness?

We devised the stimulus of figure 20.12A—a stereo, textured variant of an ambiguous (reversible) shaded surface. The texture elements all have zero disparity, consistent with a frontoparallel surface. Nonetheless, monocular shading/texture cues are not entirely overridden, so that subjects can usually see both convex and concave (like a dog bowl) interpretations. A superimposed specularity (figure 20.12B), with either convergent or diver-

gent relative disparity ($\pm 5'$) biases the interpretation. As the physics predicts, convergent relative disparity biases subjects' interpretation toward concave and divergent toward convex (figure 20.12C). The effect develops gradually with repeated exposures. Naive subjects made a forced choice (2AFC) between a convex or a concave interpretation. Time sequences (figure 20.12C) show that while initially subjects may be locked into one or the other interpretation, after around 20 exposures they reliably pick the interpretation that is consistent with the sign of horizontal relative disparity. Note that the change in position of the specularity is contrary to that of the surface—when the specularity is furthest away (divergent horizontal disparity) the center of the surface is nearest to the viewer (convex) and vice versa. Any explanation in terms of a pulling effect exerted by the specularity on the surface is thereby excluded.

How Important are Specularities?

It could be argued that specularity is a marginal visual phenomenon since specularities are relatively sparse in images compared with texture edges and other features. Moreover, it is associated more with artifacts, relatively recent on an evolutionary timescale, than with "natural" objects. Is it really likely, as we claim, that we have developed mechanisms to analyze specularities? In reply, it is worth noting first that specularities do commonly occur on (hairless) faces and that facial recognition is, presumably, important for survival. More significant though, it is not necessary to claim that the ability to deal with specular motion and stereo developed via evolution. The processing of specularities, therefore, could simply be an extended usage of the parallax mechanism, *learned* in a modern environment filled with specular artifacts.

Cognitive vs. Early Vision

Naive observers, asked where a specularity appears to be in relation to the surface that generated it, usually reply that it appears to lie *on* the surface. What we tried to show with the first experiment is that the early visual system "knows" better, choosing configurations that are broadly consistent with the physics of specular reflection. The second experiment demonstrates that the early visual system can use the information about the 3D position of the specularity to make some inference about the curvature of the underlying surface. One reason that the more

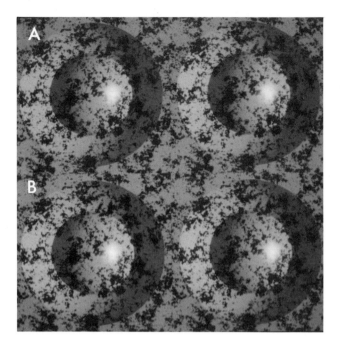

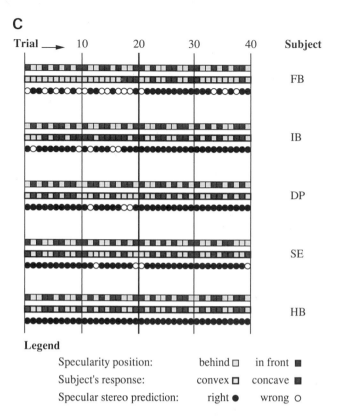

Fig. 20.12

Surface curvature. The perception of surface curvature can change with the position of a specular highlight. In order to demonstrate that the human visual system knows the physics of light reflection we used an image of a surface whose three-dimensional interpretation can flip easily between two states (convex/concave). If a highlight is added to the image the 3D interpretation of the inner part of the surface is biased more towards convex. A stereo pair was made with zero disparity for the textured surface, and then a specularity superimposed either in front of (A) or behind (B) the textured surface (uncrossed view), flipping randomly between the two, with 5 or 10 sec exposures separated by a random-dot masking frame. Subjects made a two-alternative forced choice (2AFC) between convex and concave. After a short training period (20 exposures without feedback) they made more choices that conform to the predictions of the model (C). A control experiment with a white disk of about the size of the specularity that did not look like a highlight at all, did not show any consistent effect between subjects on the perceived curvature. It might be difficult to experience the curvature effect if the images are not displayed on a CRT monitor because of the limited contrast range in the print. In order to get the best effect it is essential that the highlight look like a real reflection of the light source. (Redrawn from Blake & Bülthoff, 1990.)

cognitive level ignores this position information might be that it is better to ignore the virtual images of light sources around us; otherwise, we would perceive them as obstacles and we would be very busy trying to avoid all those specularities around us.

Integration of Depth Modules

Before we get to the final section on a computational model of cue integration, we summarize the interactions of different depth cues (as derived from our depth probe experiments) in figure 20.13. In some experiments we presented conflicting information from stereo and shading cues. Whenever visible, edge-based disparities were decisive for the perceived depth (see figures 20.4, $D^- E^+$, 20.7, and 20.8). Edge-based stereo thus overrides both shape-from-shading and shape-from-disparate-shading in our experiments. It is possible, however, that this veto relationship occurs only in the locally derived depth map (disparity matching) because the global percept of the polyhedral ellipsoid in experiment $(D^- E^+)$ is not flat, but rather convex. Stevens and Brookes (1988) also reported that with conflicting monocular and stereo information

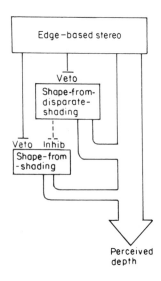

Fig. 20.13

Integration of depth cues. The size of the boxes and interaction channels reflects the contribution of the different depth cues to the overall perceived depth (accumulation). In contradictory cases, shape from both disparate and nondisparate shading is vetoed by edge-based stereo. An inhibitory influence of shape-from-disparate-shading on shape-from-shading is discussed in the text. (Redrawn from Bülthoff & Mallot, 1988.)

the 3D percept was dominated by the monocular information and not by stereo. Their task involved comparing the relative depth of two points on a planar surface that had contradictory monocular and stereo information and, in addition, surface orientation had to be estimated —which is a difficult task (see Todd & Mingolla, 1983). A conflicting cue combination of shape-from-shading and shape-from-disparate-shading was presented in the experiment with smooth-shaded nondisparate images ($D^- E^-$). In this case, shape-from-shading is not vetoed by the lack of shading disparities but leads to a reduced depth perception of about 25 percent. An inhibitory interaction between the two cues may account for this poor shape-from-shading performance and the ceiling effect in figure 20.5.

Another summary of our data that includes both depth probe and shape comparison techniques is shown in figure 20.14. This representation is based on the idea (sketched in figure 20.3) that the integration of different *3D cues* can lead to the perception of different *3D descriptors* (range,

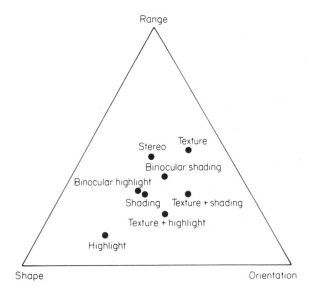

Fig. 20.14

Depth triangle. This representation of our depth probe and shape comparison data shows the relative importance of depth cues (stereo, shading, texture) for different 3D descriptors (range, shape, orientation); see also figure 20.3. Shading has a stronger influence on the perceived shape, while texture seems to be more important for orientation (compare with figure 20.2). Stereo is of equal importance for all 3D descriptors because the shape, orientation and distance to an object (range) can be easily derived from a complete depth map. (Redrawn from Bülthoff & Mallot, 1990.)

shape, orientation). The contribution of single monocular cues is different for the 3D descriptors. Object orientation is best recovered from texture cues (Bülthoff & Mallot, 1988) while surface curvature (shape) can be inferred more easily from shading. With binocular shading (Lambertian or Phong shading) range perception is rather strong (70 percent). It is even stronger for the perception of shape (100 percent). The addition of a highlight to a shaded surface has no effect in the range-matching task, while a strong effect was found in the shape comparison task. Highlights always led to an overestimation of shape, while dull surfaces (Lambertian shading) were judged too flat.

A Bayesian Framework for Cue Integration[3]

In this section a theoretical formulation for cue integration is introduced. This formulation is based on the Baye-

---

3. In collaboration with Alan Yuille, Harvard University, and Davi Geiger, MIT.

sian approach to vision, in particular in terms of coupled Markov random fields. This formalism is rich enough to contain most of the elements used in standard stereo theories with the additional advantage that it allows integration of cues from different matching primitives. These primitives can be weighted according to their robustness. For example, depth estimates obtained by matching intensity are unreliable, since small fluctuations in intensity (due to illumination or detector noise) might lead to large fluctuations in depth, hence they are less reliable than estimates from matching edges. The formalism can also be extended to incorporate information from other depth modules (e.g., shading and texture) and provides a model for sensor fusion (Clark & Yuille, 1990).

Unlike previous theories of stereo that first solved the correspondence problem and then constructed a surface by interpolation (Grimson, 1982), this framework proposes combining the two stages. The correspondence problem is solved to give the disparity field which best satisfies the a priori constraints.

The model involves the interaction of several processes and is introduced here in three stages at different levels of complexity.

At the first level, features (such as edges) are matched using a binary matching field V_{ia} determining which features correspond. In addition, smoothness is imposed on the disparity field $d(\mathbf{x})$, which represents the depth of the surface from the fixation plane. In this case the correspondence problem, determining the V_{ia}, is solved to give the smoothest possible disparity field. The theory is related to work by Yuille and Grzywacz (1988) on motion measurement and correspondence and, in particular, to work on long-range motion. It can be shown that the cooperative stereo algorithms of Dev (1975) and of Marr and Poggio (1976) are closely related to this theory (Bülthoff & Yuille, 1990; Yuille, Geiger & Bülthoff, 1989).

At the second level, line process fields $l(\mathbf{x})$ (which represents depth discontinuities) (Geman & Geman, 1984) are added to break the surfaces where the disparity gradient becomes too high. For a different approach making use of the disparity gradient constraint, see chapter 21.

The third level introduces additional terms corresponding to matching image intensities. Such terms are used in the theories of Gennert (1987) and Barnard (1986) which, however, do not have line process fields or matching fields. A psychophysical justification for intensity match-

ing is given in the section Shape from Disparate Shading. Thus the full theory is expressed in terms of energy functions relating the disparity field $d(\mathbf{x})$, the matching field V_{ia}, and the line process field $l(\mathbf{x})$.

By using standard techniques from statistical physics, particularly the mean field approximation, one can eliminate certain fields and obtain effective energies for the remaining fields (see Geiger & Girosi, 1989; Geiger & Yuille, 1989). As discussed in Yuille (1989), this can be interpreted as computing marginal probability distributions and allows us to show that several existing stereo theories are closely related to versions of the proposed framework. The three levels of this framework are presented in more detail in appendix D.

The Bayesian Formulation

Given an energy function model one can define a corresponding statistical theory. If the energy $E(d, V, C)$ depends on three fields: d (the disparity field), V the matching field, and C (the discontinuities), then (using the Gibbs distribution; see Parisi, 1988) the probability of a particular state of the system is defined by

$$P(d, V, C|g) = \frac{e^{-\beta E(d, V, C)}}{Z}, \tag{6}$$

where g is the data, β is the inverse of the temperature parameter, and Z is the partition function (a normalization constant).

Using the Gibbs distribution one can interpret the results in terms of Bayes' formula

$$P(d, V, C|g) = \frac{P(g|d, V, C)P(d, V, C)}{P(g)}, \tag{7}$$

where $P(g|d, V, C)$ is the probability of the data g given a scene d, V, C; $P(d, V, C)$ is the a priori probability of the scene; and $P(g)$ is the a priori probability of the data. Note that $P(g)$ appears in the above formula as a normalization constant, so its value can be determined if $P(g|d, V, C)$ and $P(d, V, C)$ are assumed known.

This implies that every state of the system has a finite probability of occurring. The more likely ones are those with low energy. This statistical approach is attractive because the β parameter gives us a measure of the uncertainty of the model (some refer to the temperature parameter $T = 1/\beta$). At zero temperature ($\beta \to \infty$) there is no uncertainty. In this case the only state of the system that has nonzero probability, hence probability 1, is the state that globally minimizes $E(d, V, C)$. In some nongeneric situations there could be more than one global minimum of $E(d, V, C)$.

Minimizing the energy function will correspond to finding the most probable state, independent of the value of β. The mean field solution,

$$\bar{d} = \sum_{d,V,C} dP(d, V, C | g), \tag{8}$$

is more general and reduces to the most probable solution as $T \to 0$. It corresponds to defining the solution to be the mean fields, the averages of the f and l fields over the probability distribution. This allows one to obtain different solutions depending on the uncertainty. A justification for using the mean field as a measure of the fields resides in the fact that it represents the minimum variance Bayes estimator (Gelb, 1974). More precisely, the variance of the field d is given by

$$Var(d : \bar{d}) = \sum_{d,V,C} (d - \bar{d})^2 P(d, V, C | g), \tag{9}$$

where $\bar{d}$ is the center of the variance and the $\sum_{d,V,C}$ represents the sum over all possible configurations of d, V, C. Minimizing $Var(d:\bar{d})$ with respect to all possible values of $\bar{d}$ we obtain

$$\frac{\partial}{\partial \bar{d}} Var(d : \bar{d}) = 0 \to \bar{d} = \sum_{d,V,C} dP(d, V, C). \tag{10}$$

This implies that the minimum variance estimator is given by the mean field value.

Statistical Mechanics and Mean Field Theory

One can estimate the most probable states of the probability distribution (equation 7) by, for example, using Monte Carlo techniques (Metropolis, Rosenbluth, Rosenbluth, Teller & Teller, 1953) and the simulated annealing (Kirkpatrick, Gelatt & Vecchi, 1983) approach. The drawback of these methods is the amount of computer time needed for the implementation.

There are, however, a number of other techniques from statistical physics that can be applied. They have recently been used to show (Geiger & Girosi, 1989; Geiger & Yuille, 1989) that a number of seemingly different approaches to image segmentation are closely related.

There are two main uses of these techniques: (1) we can eliminate (or average out) different fields from the energy function to obtain effective energies depending on only some of the fields (hence relating this framework to previous theories), and (2) one can obtain methods for finding deterministic solutions.

There is an additional important advantage in eliminating fields—one can impose constraints on the possible fields by only averaging over fields that satisfy these constraints. For example, Geiger and Yuille (1989) describe two possible energy function formulations of a winner-take-all network in which binary decision units determine the "winner" from a set of inputs. The constraint that there is only one winner can be expressed by (1) introducing a term in the energy function to penalize configurations with more than one winner, or (2) computing the mean fields by averaging only over configurations with a unique winner. The second method is definitely preferable in general because it enforces the constraint more strongly. Moreover, it leads to a very simple solution of the winner-take-all problem.

For the first level theory it is possible to eliminate the disparity field to obtain an effective energy $E_{eff}(V_{ij})$ depending only on the binary matching field V_{ij}, which is related to cooperative stereo theories (Dev, 1975; Marr & Poggio, 1976). Alternatively, one can eliminate the matching fields to obtain an effective energy $E_{eff}(d)$ depending only on the disparity. The second approach seems to be better since it incorporates the constraints on the set of possible matches implicitly rather than imposing them explicitly in the energy function (as the first method does).

One can also average out the line process fields or the matching fields or both for the second and third level theories. This leaves us again with a theory depending only on the disparity field.

Alternatively, one can use mean field theory methods to obtain deterministic algorithms for minimizing the first level theory $E_{eff}(V_{ij})$. These differ from the standard cooperative stereo algorithms and should be more effective (though not as effective as using $E_{eff}(d)$) since they can be interpreted as performing the cooperative algorithm at finite temperature, thereby smoothing local minima in the energy function.

Psychophysical Support for the Bayesian Framework

The experiments discussed earlier show that depth can be derived from images with disparate shading even in the absence of disparate edges. The perceived depth, however, was weaker for shading disparities (70 percent of the true depth). Putting in edges or features helped improve the accuracy of the depth perception. But in some cases these additional features appeared to decouple from the intensity and were perceived to lie above the depth surface generated from the intensity disparities.

These results are in general agreement with the Bayesian framework. The edges give good estimates of disparity and so little a priori smoothness is required and an accurate perception results. The disparity estimates from the intensity, however, are far less reliable (small fluctuations of intensity might yield large fluctuations in the disparity). Therefore, more a priori smoothness is required to obtain a stable result. This gives rise to a weaker perception of depth.

The use of the peak as a matching feature is vital (at least for the edgeless case) since it ensures that the image intensity is accurately matched (some stereo theories based purely on intensity give an incorrect match for these stimuli [M. Gennert, personal communication; see figure 20.15]). For these images, however, the peak is difficult to localize and depth estimates based on it are not very reliable. Thus the peak is not able to pull the rest of the surface to the true depth.

Pulling up did occur for the edgeless case if a feature (ring) was added at the peaks of the images (figure 20.16). This is consistent with our theory since, unlike the peaks, features are easily localized, and matching them would give a good depth estimate. Our present theory, however, is not consistent with a perception that sometimes occurred for this stimulus. In some cases the dots were perceived as lying above the surface rather than being part of it. This may be explained by the extension of our theory to transparent surfaces (Yuille, Yang & Geiger, 1990).

Additional support for this framework comes from the experiment of Bülthoff and Fahle (1989; see also Bülthoff, Fahle & Wegman, 1990) in which perceived depth for different matching primitives and disparity gradients was precisely measured. The results of these experiments suggest that several types of primitives are used for correspondence, but that some primitives are better than others. Perceived depth decreased as a function of the disparity gradient. This effect was strongest for horizontal lines, strong for pairs of dots or similar features, and weak for dissimilar features and nonhorizontal lines. An explana-

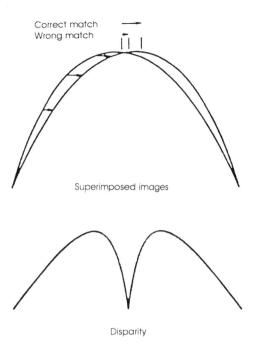

Fig. 20.15
False matching. The upper figure superimposes the left and right image and shows how the midpoints of the images (which have idential intensity) are incorrectly matched by some intensity-based stereo theories, giving rise to the disparity profile shown in the lower figure with a dip in the center.

tion in terms of the Bayesian framework assumes that these effects are due to the matching strategy and are based on the second level theory. The idea is that the smoothness term is required to give unique matching but that its importance, measured by λ, increases as the feature become more similar. If the features are sufficiently similar, then smoothness (or some other a priori assumption) must be used to obtain a unique match, leading to biases towards the frontoparallel plane. The greater the similarity between features, the more the need for smoothness and hence the stronger the bias toward the frontoparallel plane. The fall-off of perceived depth with increasing disparity gradient is modeled in detail by means of the second level theory in Yuille et al. (1989).

Final Remarks

In this chapter we discussed different modules for shape perception and their interaction. One can categorize these interactions in two broad classes. In one, the cues are *consonant* (noncontradictory). For example, consider view-

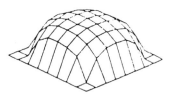

Dense edge-based and intensity-based stereo
Perceived depth: 100%

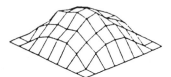

Intensity-based stereo
Perceived depth: 70%

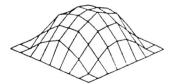

Consistent intensity - and edge-based stereo
Perceived depth: 84%

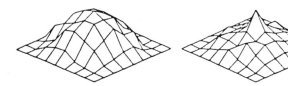

Stereo edges in front of shaded disk (without disparity)
Subjects ISA and HAM: 63%

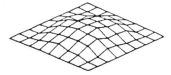

Shape from shading
Perceived depth: 23%

Fig. 20.16
Surface interpolation. The upper three figures show surface interpolation for: (1) dense edges and intensity-based stereo, (2) intensity-based stereo, and (3) sparse edges and consistent shading. The next two figures illustrate pulling: an edge token in front of intensity patterns with no relative disparity (no intensity-based stereo) pulls the surface up (*left*) but can sometimes cause a transparency percept (*right*) of the token lying in front of the intensity surface. The final figure shows the perceived depth without the edge token. (Redrawn from Bülthoff & Mallot, 1990.)

ing a golf ball with both eyes. There will be consistent depth information from stereo, shading, and texture cues. Viewing an image of the same golf ball in a photograph, however, puts the stereo cue into *conflict* with shading and texture.

Psychophysicists have attempted to deal with the first case by taking weighted linear combinations with some success (Bruno & Cutting, 1988; Dosher, Sperling & Wurst, 1986). Some experiments discussed in this chapter, however, do not seem consistent with such a model.

The case of conflicting cues seems to require significant nonlinearity and usually requires a different, and independent, mechanism. For example, this case is explicitly excluded in the statistical framework for fusion of depth information proposed by Maloney and Landy (1989).

Workers in computer vision have tended to use an alternative viewpoint. A recent book on sensor fusion (Clark & Yuille, 1990) proposed a distinction between *weak* methods in which modules compute depth independently and combine their results (perhaps by linear combination) and *strong* methods in which two modules interact during computation, usually in a very nonlinear way. They argue that strong methods are preferable since individual modules may be using conflicting assumptions. These theories also seem rich enough to encompass both the categories defined by psychophysicists.

These theories are expressed in a Bayesian framework that can be used both for describing the individual modules and for their integration. Although there are many other methods for dealing with individual modules, the Bayesian approach subsumes a number of these methods by isolating the key assumptions used by these theories.

Acknowledgments

The work in the first part of this chapter was done in close collaboration with Hanspeter Mallot, and parts of it were published in Bülthoff and Mallot (1988, 1990). The shape from highlights section is based on articles with Andrew Blake (Blake & Bülthoff, 1990, 1991; Bülthoff & Blake, 1989). The computational model for the integration of early vision models is based on a collaboration with Alan Yuille and Davi Geiger (Yuille, Geiger & Bülthoff, 1989). I thank all of them for many interesting discussions and a very enjoyable collaboration.

This chapter describes research done within the Center for Biological Information Processing (Whitaker College) at the Massachusetts Institute of Technology and in the Department of Cognitive and Linguistic Sciences, Brown University. Support for this work is provided by a grant from the Office of Naval Research, Cognitive and Neural Sciences Division and a NATO Collaborative Grant No. 0403/87.

Appendices

A.   Computer Graphic Psychophysics

Images of smooth- and flat-shaded (polyhedral) ellipsoids of revolution were generated by either ray-tracing techniques or with a solid modeling software package (S-Geometry, Symbolics Inc.; figure 20.17). The polyhedral objects were derived from quadrangular tessellations of the sphere along meridian and latitude circles. The objects were elongated along an axis in the equatorial plane of the tessellated sphere. Thus the two types of objects differed mainly in the absence or presence of edges. As compared to spheres, the objects were elongated by the factors 0.5, 1.0, 2.0, 3.0, 4.0, and 5.0. With an original radius of 6.7 cm, this corresponds to depth values between 3.3 and 33.3 cm. In the following, all semidiame-

ters (elongations) are given as multiples of 6.7 cm. In most experiments objects were viewed end-on, that is, the axis of rotational symmetry was orthogonal to the display screen. In an additional experiment, objects could be rotated around a diagonal axis in the display plane. As an example, the objects displayed in figure 20.2 are rotated around that axis by plus and minus $45°$, respectively.

For the computation of the smooth-shaded ellipsoids, a ray-tracing operation was performed (Bülthoff & Mallot, 1988). The illuminant was modeled as a point source at infinity (parallel illumination) centrally behind the observer. For some control experiments, oblique directions of illumination (upper left and lower right) were used. Surface shading was computed according to the Phong model (Phong, 1975), consisting of an ambient, a diffuse (Lambertian), and a specular component. For Lambertian shading, the ambient and specular components were zero, while for specular shading (highlight), a combination of 30 percent ambient, 10 percent diffuse, and 60 percent specular reflectance (specular exponent 7.0) was chosen. Since our objects were convex, no cast shadows or repeated reflections had to be considered.

B.   Experimental Procedure

We displayed either a pair of disparate images (stereo pair) or a nondisparate view of the object as seen from be-

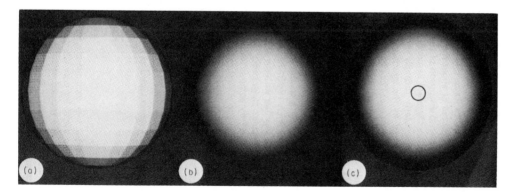

Fig. 20.17
Flat- and smooth-shaded surfaces. (a, b) Discontinuous and smooth intensity variations in images of polyhedra and ellipsoids provide cues for edge-based stereo, shape-from-disparate-shading, and shape-from-shading. (c) Smooth ellipsoids with sparse edge information have been used in experiments on the interaction of edge-based stereo and shape-from-shading. All images could be displayed as stereograms or as pairs of identical images. In image (c), the disparities of shading and the edge token (ring) could be varied independently. (Redrawn from Bülthoff & Mallot, 1988.)

tween the two eyes on a CRT Color Monitor (Mitsubishi UC-6912 High-Resolution Color-Display Monitor, Resolution (H × V) 1024 by 874 pixels; bandwidth ±3 dB between 50 Hz and 50 MHz, short persistence phosphor). The disparate images were interlaced (even lines for the left image and odd lines for the right image) with a frame rate of 30 Hz. This technique allows one to display the left and right view at about the same location on the monitor and therefore treats any geometric distortion of the monitor equally for both eyes. Errors in displayed disparities due to geometric distortions of the monitor are therefore avoided. Both disparate and nondisparate images were viewed binocularly through shutter glasses (Stereo-Optic Systems, Inc.) which were triggered by the interlace signal to present the appropriate images only to the left and right eye. The objects were shown in black and white with a true resolution of 254 graylevels using a 10-bit D/A-Converter. The background was uniformly colored in half-saturated blue. The screen was viewed in complete darkness.

Local Depth Probe Technique

Perceived depth was measured by adjusting a small, red, square (4 by 4 pixel) depth probe to match the perceived depth of the surface interactively (with the computer mouse). This probe was displayed in interlaced mode together with the disparate images. This is a computer graphics version of a binocular rangefinder developed by Gregory (1966) called "Gregory's Pandora's Box" by some investigators with the additional advantage that the accommodation cue is eliminated. Measurements were performed at 45 vertices of a Cartesian grid in the image plane in random order. The initial disparity of the depth probe was randomized for each measurement to avoid hysteresis effects. Subjects were asked to move the cursor back and forth in depth until it finally seemed to lie directly on top of the displayed test surface. After some training sessions, subjects felt comfortable with this procedure and achieved reproducible depth measurements. Subjects included the authors (corrected vision) and one naive observer, all with normal stereo vision as tested with natural and random dot stereograms.

Global Shape Comparison Technique

The global shape comparison technique was used mainly for those cues that required monocular viewing. It is also

useful for cues that are processed more globally and would be hindered by focussed attention on the local probe. Depending on the task, this technique was used in two different ways. To measure shape from shading and/ or texture with the global probe we displayed a stereoscopically viewed reference object in the same orientation as the probe. The task of the subject was to change the shading or the texture (or both together) in order to match the shape with the reference object. This could be done almost in real-time by fast recall from computer memory of precomputed images of different shapes and/ or orientations. The reference object did not contain any shading or texture cue beside the disparate rings on its surface to avoid any cross-comparison with the depth cues to be tested.

C. Data Evaluation

Depth Probe Technique

The depth probe technique leads to a depth map measured locally at 45 positions in the image plane. In order to derive a global measure of perceived depth we performed a principal component analysis on all data sets, treating each one as a point in 45-space. Variance of the perceived shapes was found mainly (94 percent) along the first principal axis, whose corresponding loading was very close to an ideal ellipsoid (or sphere). The second component accounted for only 1.4 percent of the total variance. We therefore chose the overall elongation, namely, the coefficient associated with the first principal component, as a measure of perceived depth for a given cue combination (see figure 20.5).

Global Shape Comparison Technique

The depth comparison data were averaged over different runs and over two to four subjects. The mean number of runs was about 180 and the average correlation between displayed and estimated shape was 0.83. In order to distinguish easily between over or underestimation of depth we give the mean slope for each depth cue. A slope of 1.0 is naturally the veridical perception and a slope > 1 is an underestimation of curvature (see figure 20.6).

D. A Bayesian Framework for Stereo

The First Level: Matching Field and Disparity Field

The basic idea is that there are a number of possible primitives that could be used for matching and that these all contribute to a disparity field $d(x)$. This disparity field exists even where there is no source of data. The primitives considered here are features such as edges in image brightness. Edges typically correspond to object boundaries, and other significant events in the image. Other primitives, such as peaks in the image brightness or texture features, can also be added. In the following, the theory is described for the one-dimensional case.

One can assume that the edges and other features have already been extracted from the image in a preprocessing stage. The matching elements in the left eye consist of features at positions x_{i_L}, for $i_L = 1, \ldots, N_l$. The right eye contains features at positions x_{a_R}, for $a_R = 1, \ldots, N_r$. A *matching field* is defined as a set of binary matching elements $V_{i_L a_R}$, such that $V_{i_L a_R} = 1$ if point i_L in the left eye corresponds to point a_R in the right eye, and $V_{i_L a_R} = 0$ otherwise. A *compatibility field* $A_{i_L a_R}$ is defined over the range $[0, 1]$. For example, it is 1 if i_L and a_R are compatible (i.e., features of the same type), 0 if they are incompatible (an edge cannot match a peak),

One can now define a cost function $E(d(x), V_{i_L a_R})$ of the disparity field and the matching elements. There are several methods to estimate the fields $d(x)$, $V_{i_L a_R}$ given the data. A standard estimator is to minimize $E(d(x), V_{i_L a_R})$ with respect to $d(x)$, $V_{i_L a_R}$.

$$E(d(x), V_{i_L a_R}) = \sum_{i_L, a_R} A_{i_L a_R} V_{i_L a_R} (d(x_{i_L}) - (x_{a_R} - x_{i_L}))^2$$

$$+ \lambda \left\{ \sum_{i_L} \left(\sum_{a_R} V_{i_L a_R} - 1 \right)^2 \right.$$

$$+ \sum_{a_R} \left(\sum_{i_L} V_{i_L a_R} - 1 \right)^2 \right\}$$

$$+ \gamma \int_M (Sd)^2 \, dx. \tag{11}$$

The first term gives a contribution to the disparity obtained from matching i_L to a_R. The fourth term imposes a smoothness constraint on the disparity field imposed by a smoothness operator S.

The second and third term encourage features to have a single match, they can be avoided by requiring that each column and row of the matrix $V_{i_L a_R}$ contains only one 1. Minimizing the energy function with respect to $d(\mathbf{x})$ and $V_{i_L a_R}$ will cause the matching that results in the smoothest disparity field. The coefficient γ determines the amount of a priori knowledge required. If all the features in the left eye have only one compatible feature in the right eye then little a priori knowledge is needed and γ may be small. If all the features are compatible then there is matching ambiguity which the a priori knowledge is needed to resolve, requiring a larger value of γ and hence more smoothing. This gives a possible explanation for the depth reduction effects discussed in Bülthoff, Fahle & Wegman (1990).

The theory can be extended to two dimensions in a straightforward way. The matching elements $V_{i_L a_R}$ must be constrained to only allow for matches that use the epipolar line constraint. The disparity field will have an additional smoothness constraint perpendicular to the epipolar line which will enforce figural continuity.

Finally, and perhaps most importantly, a form for the smoothness operator S has to be chosen. Marr (1982) proposed that, to make stereo correspondence unambiguous, the human visual system assumes that the world consists of smooth surfaces. This suggests that one should choose a smoothness operator that encourages the disparity to vary smoothly spatially. In practice the assumptions used in Marr's two theories of stereo are somewhat stronger. Marr and Poggio I (1976) encourages matches with constant disparity, thereby enforcing a bias to the frontoparallel plane. Marr and Poggio II (1979) uses a coarse to fine strategy to match nearby points, hence encouraging matches with minimal disparity and thereby giving a bias towards the fixation plane.

An alternative approach is to introduce discontinuity fields that break the smoothness constraint. For these theories the experiments described in Bülthoff et al. (1989, 1990) are consistent with S being a first order derivative operator. This is also roughly consistent with Marr and Poggio I (1976). A default choice is therefore $S = \partial/\partial x$.

The Second Level: Adding Discontinuity Fields

The first level theory is easy to analyze but makes the a priori assumption that the disparity field is smooth everywhere, which is false at object boundaries. There are several standard ways to allow smoothness constraints to break (Blake, 1983; Geman & Geman, 1984; Mumford &

Shah, 1985). Here, a discontinuity field $l(x)$ is introduced which is represented by a set of curves C.

Introducing the discontinuity fields C gives an energy function

$$E(d(x), V_{i_L a_R}, C) = \sum_{i_L, a_R} A_{i_L a_R} V_{i_L a_R}(d(x_{i_L}) - (x_{a_R} - x_{i_L}))^2$$

$$+ \lambda \left\{ \sum_{i_L} \left(\sum_{a_R} V_{i_L a_R} - 1 \right)^2 \right.$$

$$+ \sum_{a_R} \left(\sum_{i_L} V_{i_L a_R} - 1 \right)^2 \right\}$$

$$+ \gamma \int_{M-C} (Sd)^2 \, dx + M(C), \qquad (12)$$

where smoothness is not enforced across the curves C, and $M(C)$ is the cost for enforcing breaks.

The Third Level: Adding Intensity Terms

The final version of the theory couples intensity based and feature based stereo. The psychophysical results suggest that this is necessary. The energy function becomes

$$E(d(x), V_{i_L a_R}, C) = \sum_{i_L, a_R} A_{i_L a_R} V_{i_L a_R}(d(x_{i_L}) - (x_{a_R} - x_{i_L}))^2$$

$$+ \mu \int \left\{ L(x) - R(x + d(x)) \right\}^2 \, dx$$

$$+ \lambda \left\{ \sum_{i_L} \left(\sum_{a_R} V_{i_L a_R} - 1 \right)^2 \right.$$

$$+ \sum_{a_R} \left(\sum_{i_L} V_{i_L a_R} - 1 \right)^2 \right\}$$

$$+ \gamma \int_{M-C} (Sd)^2 \, dx + M(C). \qquad (13)$$

If certain terms are set to zero in equation 13, it reduces to previous theories of stereo. If the second and fourth terms are kept, without allowing discontinuities, it is similar to work by Gennert (1987) and Barnard (1986).

Thus the cost function (13) reduces to well-known stereo theories in certain limits. It also shows how it is possible to combine feature and brightness data in a natural manner. In addition it can be modified to include monocular cues (Clark & Yuille, 1990).

A similar theory for integrating different cues for motion perception was proposed by Yuille and Grzywacz (1988), although this theory did not involve discontinuity fields.

References

Aliomonos, J. & Swain, M. J. (1985). Shape from texture. IEEE Joint Conference on Artificial Intelligence, 926–931.

Arnold, R. D. & Binford, T. O. (1980). Geometric constraints in stereo vision. *Society of Photo-Optical Instrumentation and Engineering, 238*, 281–292.

Bajcsy, R. & Lieberman, L. (1976). Texture gradient as a depth cue. *Computer Vision, Graphics, and Image Processing, 5*, 52–67.

Barnard, S. (1986). *Proceeding of the Image Understanding Workshop*, Los Angeles.

Barrow, H. G. & Tenenbaum, J. M. (1981). Interpreting line drawings as three-dimensional surfaces. *Artificial Intelligence, 17*, 75–116.

Beck, J. (1972). *Surface color perception*. New York: Cornell University Press.

Blake, A. (1983). The least disturbance principle and weak constraints. *Pattern Recognition Letters, 1*, 393–399.

Blake, A. (1985). Specular stereo. *Proceedings of the 9th IJCAI Conference*, 973–976.

Blake, A. & Brelstaff, G. J. (1988). Geometry from specularities. In *Proceedings of the International Conference on Computer Vision* (pp. 394–403). Washington, DC: IEEE.

Blake, A. & Bülthoff, H. H. (1990). Does the brain know the physics of specular reflection? *Nature, 343*, 165–168.

Blake, A. & Bülthoff, H. H. (1991). Shape from specularities: Computation and psychophysics. *Philosophical Transactions of the Royal Society London B, 331*, 237–252.

Blake, A. & Zisserman, A. (1987). *Visual reconstruction*. Cambridge, MA: MIT Press.

Blake, A., Zisserman, A. & Knowles, G. (1985). Surface description from stereo and shading. *Image and Vision Computing, 3*, 183–191.

Bruno, N. & Cutting, J. E. (1988). Minimodularity and the perception of layout. *Journal of Experimental Psychology: General, 117*, 161–170.

Buckley, D., Frisby, J. P. & Mayhew, J. E. W. (1989). Integration of stereo and texture cues in the formation of discontinuities during three-dimensional surface interpolation. *Perception, 18*, 563–588.

Bülthoff, H. H. & Blake, A. (1989). Does the seeing brain know physics. *Investigative Ophthalmology and Visual Science, Suppl., 30*, 262.

Bülthoff, H. H. & Fahle, M. (1989). Disparity gradients and depth scaling. *MIT Artificial Intelligence Memo, 1175*.

Bülthoff, H. H., Fahle, M. & Wegman, M. (1990). Perceived depth scales with disparity gradient. *Perception*, in press.

Bülthoff, H. H., Little, J. J. & Poggio, T. (1989). A parallel algorithm for real-time computation of motion. *Nature, 337,* 549–553.

Bülthoff, H. H. & Mallot, H. A. (1988). Integration of depth modules: stereo and shading. *Journal of the Optical Society of America, 5,* 1749–1758.

Bülthoff, H. H. & Mallot, H. A. (1990). Integration of stereo, shading and texture. In A. Blake & T. Troscianko (Eds.), *AI and the eye.* New York: John Wiley and Sons.

Bülthoff, H. H. & Yuille, A. (1990). Models for seeing surfaces and shapes. *Comments in Theoretical Biology,* in press.

Clark, J. & Yuille, A. (1990). *Data fusion for sensory information processing.* Norwell, MA: Kluwer Academic Press.

Cutting, J. E. & Millard, R. T. (1984). Three gradients and the perception of flat and curved surfaces. *Journal of Experimental Psychology: General, 113,* 198–216.

Dev, P. (1975). Perception of depth surfaces in random-dot stereograms. *IEEE Transactions on Pattern Analysis and Machine Intelligence, PAMI-2,* 333–340.

Dosher, B. A., Sperling, G. & Wurst, S. (1986). Tradeoffs between stereopsis and proximity luminance covariance as determinants of perceived 3D structure. *Vision Research, 26,* 973–990.

Gelb, A. (1974). *Applied optimal estimation.* Cambridge, MA: MIT Press.

Geman, S. & Geman, D. (1984). Stochastic relaxation, Gibbs distributions and the Bayesian restoration of images. *IEEE Transactions on Pattern Analysis and Machine Intelligence, PAMI-6,* 721–741.

Geiger, D. & Girosi, F. (1989). Parallel and deterministic algorithms from MRFs: Integration and surface reconstruction. *MIT Artificial Intelligence Laboratory Memo, 1114.*

Geiger, D. & Yuille, A. (1989). *A common framework for image segmentation* (Harvard Robotics Laboratory Technical Report No. 89–7).

Gennert, M. A. (1987). A computational framework for understanding problems in stereo vision. *MIT Artifical Intelligence Laboratory Thesis.*

Gregory, R. L. (1966). *Eye and brain.* New York: McGraw-Hill.

Grimson, W. E. L. (1982). A computational theory of visual surface interpolation. *Philosophical Transactions of the Royal Society London B, 298,* 395–427.

Haynes, S. M. & Jain, R. (1987). A qualitative approach for recovering depth in dynamic scenes. *Proceedings of the of IEEE Workshop on Computer Vision,* Miami Beach, 66–71.

Hildreth, E. C. (1983). The detection of intensity changes by computer and biological vision systems. *Computer Vision, Graphics and Image Processing, 22,* 1–27.

Hildreth, E. C. (1984). Computations underlying the measurement of visual motion. *Artificial Intelligence Journal, 23,* 309–354.

Ikeuchi, K. & Horn, B. K. P. (1981). Numerical shape from shading and occluding boundaries. *Artificial Intelligence, 17,* 141–184.

Julesz, B. (1971). *Foundations of cyclopean perception.* London: The University of Chicago Press, Ltd.

Kender, J. R. (1979). Shape from texture: An aggregation transform that maps a class of textures into surface orientation. In *Proceedings, International Joint Conference on Artificial Intelligence,* Tokyo, Japan.

Kirkpatrick, S., Gelatt, C. D. Jr. and Vecchi, M. P. (1983). Optimization by simulated annealing. *Science, 220,* 671–680.

Koenderink, J. J. (1986). Optic flow. *Vision Research, 26,* 161–180.

Koenderink, J. J. & van Doorn, A. J. (1976). Geometry of binocular vision and a model for stereopsis. *Biological Cybernetics, 21,* 29–35.

Landy, M. S. (1987). Parallel model of the kinetic depth effect using local computations. *Journal of the Optical Society of America A, 4,* 864–877.

Longuet-Higgins, H. C. & Prazdny, K. (1981). The interpretation of a moving retinal image. *Proceedings of the Royal Society London B, 208,* 385–397.

Maloney, L. T. & Landy, M. S. (1989). A statistical framework for robust fusion of depth information. In W. A. Pearlman (Ed.), *Visual Communications and Image Processing IV. Proceedings of the SPIE, 1199,* 1154–1163.

Marr, D. (1982). *Vision.* San Francisco: Freeman.

Marr, D. & Hildreth, E. (1980). Theory of edge detection. *Proceedings of the Royal Society London B, 207,* 187–217.

Marr, D. & Poggio, T. (1976). Cooperative computation of stereo disparity. *Science, 194,* 283–287.

Marr, D. & Poggio, T. (1979). A computational theory of human stereo vision. *Proceedings of the Royal Society London B, 204,* 301–328.

Mayhew, J. E. W. & Frisby, J. P. (1981). Psychophysical and computational studies towards a theory of human stereopsis. *Artificial Intelligence, 17,* 349–386.

Mayhew, J. E. W. & Longuet-Higgins, H. C. (1982). A computational model of binocular depth perception. *Nature, 297,* 376–379.

Metropolis, N. Rosenbluth, A., Rosenbluth, M., Teller, A., and Teller, E. (1953). Equation of state calculations by fast computing machines. *Journal Physical Chemistry, 21,* 1087–1091.

Mingolla, E. & Todd, J. T. (1986). Perception of solid shape from shading. *Biological Cybernetics, 53,* 137–151.

Mumford, D. and Shah, J. (1985). Boundary detection by minimizing functionals, I, *Proceedings of the IEEE Conference on Computer Vision and Pattern Recognition,* San Francisco.

Parisi, G. (1988). *Statistical field theory.* Reading, MA: Addison-Wesley.

Pentland, A. P. (1984). Local shading analysis. *IEEE Transactions on Pattern Analysis and Machine Intelligence, PAMI-6,* 170–187.

Pentland, A. P. (1985). A new sense for depth of field. *IEEE Joint Conference on Artificial Intelligence,* 988–994.

Pentland, A. P. (1986). Shading into texture. *Artificial Intelligence, 29,* 147–170.

Phong, B. T. (1975). Illumination for computer generated pictures. *Communications of the ACM, 18,* 311–317.

Poggio, G. & Poggio, T. (1984). The analysis of stereopsis. *Annual Review of Neuroscience, 7,* 379–412.

Poggio, T., Torre, V. & Koch, C. (1985). Computational vision and regularization theory. *Nature, 317,* 314–319.

Prazdny, K. (1985). Detection of binocular disparities. *Biological Cybernetics, 52,* 93–99.

Stevens, K. A. (1981). The visual interpretation of surface contours. *Artificial Intelligence, 17,* 47–73.

Stevens, K. A. & Brookes, A. (1987). Probing depth in monocular images. *Biological Cybernetics, 56,* 355–366.

Stevens, K. A. & Brookes, A. (1988). Integrating stereopsis with monocular interpretations of planar surfaces. *Vision Research, 28,* 371–386.

Todd, J. T. & Mingolla, E. (1983). Perception of surface curvature and direction of illumination from patterns of shading. *Journal of Experimental Psychology: Human Perception and Performance, 9,* 583–595.

Ullman, S. (1979). *The interpretation of visual motion.* Cambridge, MA: MIT Press.

Ullman, S. (1984). Maximizing rigidity: The incremental recovery of 3-D structure from rigid and non-rigid motion. *Perception, 13,* 255–274.

Witkin, A. P. (1981). Recovering surface shape and orientation from texture. *Artificial Intelligence, 17,* 17–47.

Yuille, A. L. (1989). (Harvard Robotics Laboratory Technical Report 89–12).

Yuille, A. L., Geiger, D. & Bülthoff H. H. (1989). *Stereo integration, mean field theory and psychophysics* (Harvard Robotics Laboratory Technical Report 89–1).

Yuille, A. L. & Grzywacz, N. M. (1988). A computational theory for the perception of coherent visual motion. *Nature, 333,* 71–74.

Yuille, A. L., Tong Yang, & Geiger, D. (1990). *Robust statistics, transparency and correspondence* (Harvard Robotics Laboratory Technical Report 90-7).

Zisserman, A., Giblin, P. & Blake, A. (1989). The information available to a moving observer from specularities. *Image and Vision Computing, 7,* 38–42.

21

Computational Issues in Solving the Stereo Correspondence Problem

John P. Frisby and
Stephen B. Pollard

Due to their different positions, the two eyes receive slightly different images of the world. Differences between left and right images are termed *binocular disparities* (figure 21.1). The human visual system, as well as those of many other species, can detect and use these disparities to recover information about the three-dimensional (3D) structure of the scene being viewed. The *stereo correspondence problem* is, how can the two images be mapped into a single representation, called a *disparity map*, that makes explicit the disparities of all points common to both images?

A great deal of computer vision research has addressed this problem, because a disparity map is a useful first step towards building a representation of 3D scene structure. The goal of this chapter is to provide a tutorial overview of this work. Although references will be made to some biological studies that have helped shape computational models, the chapter will not be concerned with modeling biological stereo vision systems per se. The chapter is in three main parts: the first is a general review of the field, the second describes a particular stereo algorithm called PMF, and the third discusses practical problems in building an effective stereo algorithm, illustrating these with the evolution of PMF into PMF42. The chapter ends with a general discussion that includes issues arising for biological studies.

Background

A stimulus point can be positioned such that it has zero binocular disparity, that is, it projects to exactly corresponding retinal coordinates in the two eyes. The locus of all such points is termed the *point horopter*. For symmetric gaze on a fixation point nearer than infinity, this horopter comprises (1) a circle lying in a horizontal plane passing through the fixation point and the optical centres of the two eyes, together with (2) a single line passing through the fixation point and tilted away from the ob-

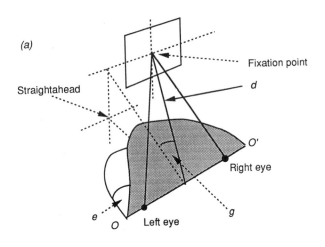

(a)

Fixation point

Straightahead

d

O'

Right eye

e

O

Left eye

g

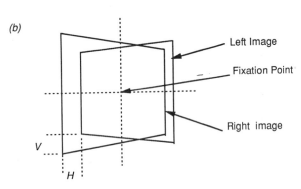

(b)

Left Image

Fixation Point

Right image

V

H

Fig. 21.1

Schematic illustration of geometry of stereo projections (as used by Porrill et al., 1987a). (A) The two eyes are shown fixating the center of a square located in the upper right quadrant of the visual field (in head coordinates). The angle of elevation *e* is the angle between (1) the plane defined by the line *OO'* running through the optical centers of the two eyes and the point labeled *straightahead*, and (2) the shaded plane containing *OO'* and the fixation point. The angle of gaze *g* lies in the latter plane. (B) The left and right images of the square. The differences between them can be described in terms of horizontal (*H*) and vertical (*V*) disparities, defined respectively as the difference in *x* and *y* image coordinates of matching points. It can be readily appreciated from the figure that the larger the observed square, the larger will be *H* and *V*; in other words, *H* and *V* will be scaled by retinal eccentricity. It is also true that *H* and *V* will vary with *g* and *e* and with the fixation distance *d* as all those factors help determine the relative sizes of the two images.

server. The tilt is due to the eyes being rotated slightly around their principal axes (Helmholtz, 1909/1962; Tyler & Scott, 1979, provide a good tutorial review of horopters). Any point not lying on the point horopter projects with either a vertical disparity, or with both a vertical and a horizontal disparity, between its left and right eye image coordinates (see figures 21.1 and 21.3). Horizontal disparities are termed crossed (or convergent) and uncrossed (or divergent) for points lying respectively in front of or behind the fixation point.

Tackling the stereo correspondence problem (building a disparity map) leads immediately to two questions. First, what image features should serve as points to be matched? Such features are often termed *matching primitives*. And second, how can true matches be distinguished from false ones? These questions are closely intertwined, as disambiguating matching algorithms suitable for one kind of primitive may not be suitable for another. Nevertheless, it will be convenient to deal with them in sequence.

Before doing so, it is worth emphasizing that a disparity map is simply another iconic (imagelike) representation that is of limited use for controlling visually guided behavior. This remains true even if the disparities attached to matched features are translated, using knowledge of the parameters of camera geometry such as intercamera separation, and so on, into a *depth map*, which represents the distances from the observing system, animal or robot, of the scene elements giving rise to the image points.

To be of most value for visual guidance, iconic disparity or depth maps need to be interpreted to yield useful descriptions of scene geometry, such as *"Depth discontinuity of size a in location x,y,z on the ground plane."* A representation of this form makes available *explicitly* information of the kind required for action, in this example scene structure useful for obstacle avoidance. Such information is only *implicit* in a disparity or depth map. (By explicit information is meant information delivered to subsequent processes in such a form that those processes need do no further work before being able to use the information represented.) The same general point is true if stereo vision is to be used for guiding grasp movements, although there the explicit 3D scene geometry required would of course be different. For example, if a robot is to pick something up, it needs visual information of a kind that can help it organize appropriate grasp movements, such as, "*Parallel plane faces bounding object M, with such and such size parameters.*"

A slogan that helps keep this sobering reality firmly in mind is *Perception is for action.* There is nothing new in this, of course (Helmholtz, 1909/1962), but trying to provide visual guidance for robotics is proving an admirably rigorous forcing domain for ensuring that it is taken seriously (Brady, 1982; Brooks, 1985). For the present topic, the point is that there is much more to stereo vision than solving the stereo correspondence problem. Indeed, it is now clear that it is possible to derive directly from stereo images some types of useful scene geometry without ever making explicit disparity or depth maps as intervening representations (Hoff & Ahuja, 1987; McLauchlan & Mayhew, 1989; McLauchlan, Mayhew & Frisby, 1990; Pollard, 1987).

Despite these cautionary remarks, this chapter will discuss in detail only the stereo correspondence problem. Aside from considerations of space, this is because most work has been done on it and because it forms a natural starting point for discussing other aspects of stereo processing. Work from both the biological and computational literatures will be intermingled but with emphasis given to the latter, and with no consideration given to modeling biological mechanisms *per se.* For a review of the psychophysical and neurophysiological literatures on stereopsis aimed at the same kind of readership as the present chapter, see Regan, Frisby, Poggio, Schor and Tyler (1990).

Matching Primitives

Image Point Intensities

Pixel values (cf. rod and cone activities) are generally not suitable as matching primitives for stereo because a given scene entity often produces pixels in the left and right images of different intensities. This fact is usually expressed by saying that *stereo projections do not preserve photometric invariance.* This is because scene surfaces are usually at slightly different angles to the principal optical axis of each camera (or eye), such that the same scene entity may reflect a different intensity into each one. This means that any attempt to match individual left and right pixels of identical intensity value is in general doomed to failure (Marr & Poggio, 1976).

Pixel intensity variation between images also arises from various sources of image noise. Moreover, the two cameras are most unlikely to be perfectly matched in their photometric sensitivities, which creates further problems of photometric variation—a simple fact, but one of great practical importance.

These considerations led Marr and Poggio (1976) to offer as a general rule: For matching primitives, choose features that stand in a close relation to scene entities, such as surface markings or object edges. This seems sensible advice not only because it helps avoid photometric variance problems but also because the ultimate goal is to deliver 3D information about scene structures.

Image Regions

Perhaps the simplest if rather indirect way to follow Marr and Poggio's general rule for choosing matching primitives is to try to match *regions* of pixels in the left and right images. This is the tack taken by stereo correspondence algorithms which rely on area cross-correlation. The usual sequence of steps is: (1) choose a window of pixels centered on a point in one image, (2) compute correlations with similarly sized windows in the other image whose center positions are shifted over some disparity range, and (3) use the highest correlation to select the best window match. These operations are performed (in principle in parallel, if so desired) for all image points of interest.

An example of this type of algorithm that has been developed to support a crude but useful ground plane obstacle detection capability is called SWITCHER (Zheng, Jones, Billings, Mayhew & Frisby, 1989). The key idea on which it is based is to use a statistical test to decide whether to switch (hence the algorithm's name) from one disparity plane to another in selecting "best correlating windows." Figure 21.2 illustrates how it works. It uses as inputs stereo image pairs that have been preprocessed (with high-pass filtering and gray scale equalization) to reduce photometric variance problems to manageable proportions. Note that SWITCHER's form of window correlation is based on subtraction (see Julesz, 1971, p. 123, for a discussion of why addition and multiplication would be inappropriate for stereo correlation).

The perennial problem with area correlation stereo algorithms is setting window size parameters. If the window is made very small, then poor disambiguation can

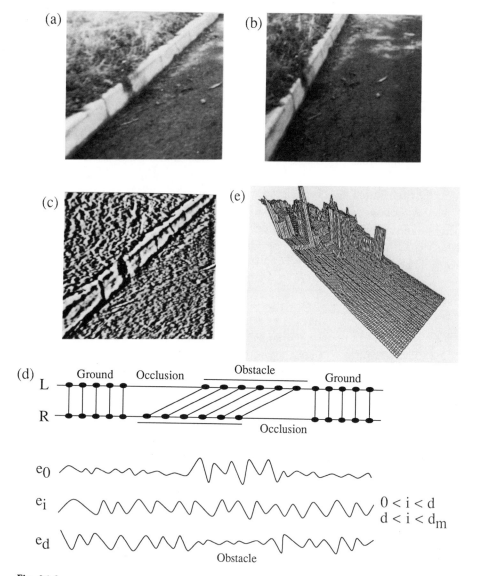

Fig. 21.2

The *SWITCHER* Stereo Algorithm (Zheng et al., 1989). (A) and (B) are the right and left halves of a stereo pair captured from video cameras mounted on a moving vehicle (here arranged for crossed-eye fusion). The task is to detect the disparity discontinuity created by the curb for the purposes of visual guidance of the vehicle. (C) The left stereo half following high-pass filtering and gray scale equalization (the latter being separate log transforms of intensities above and below the mean graylevel of the image). (D) The principle on which *SWITCHER* is based. L and R are two (notional) rasters comprising points lying in the ground plane, points associated with an obstacle, and points falling in occluded regions. The links between L and R show the correct disparities that must be found. The lines labeled e_0 to e_d show the results of subtracting L and R for various disparity shifts lying in the range 0 to the maximum disparity considered, d_m.

It can be seen that these show small excursions from zero (due to image noise, etc.) where the disparity shift is appropriate to the disparities contained in L and R but they are relatively large elsewhere. The *SWITCHER* algorithm works out variances in windows placed on the e lines. It then uses a statistical test (currently the F test) to decide whether a window at a different disparity shift from the one currently selected as correct has a significantly smaller variance. If it has, then *SWITCHER* shifts to that new disparity—hence its name. The test is applied sequentially in a left to right scan. The advantage in using a statistical test is that reasonable evidence has to emerge before a new disparity is selected. (E) A disparity map delivered by *SWITCHER* from the inputs shown in (A), from which it is a trivial matter to find the dicontinuity in the ground plane caused by the curb.

result due to insufficient image structure being used in computing correlations to overcome the problems of image noise, and so forth. If it is set to be large, then the window may too often straddle scene regions of greatly varying distances, again lowering the correlation score. Experiments on SWITCHER have shown that windows of 17 by 3 pixels (from images of 256 by 256 covering a viewing angle of about $27°$) are effective for the types of scene (and image noise levels) for which it has been used for the relatively simple business of ground plane obstacle detection. Nevertheless, perhaps some form of dynamic setting of window size driven by success in forming good matches might be preferable.

Human stereo vision may possess mechanisms that perform an analogous operation to intensity correlation. For example, Bülthoff and Mallot (1988) created stereo pairs depicting 3D ellipsoids whose gentle variations in left/right image shading produced a stereo depth effect that cannot, they argue convincingly, be explained in terms of any standard form of edge matching.

Edge Points

Edges extracted from images stand in a reasonably close relation to scene elements. Given the current state of the art in edge detection, this relationship is by no means a perfect one, but even so, image edges clearly satisfy the spirit of Marr and Poggio's general rule for choosing matching primitives. This is one reason, no doubt, why numerous edge-based stereo correspondence algorithms have now been described (see Barnard & Fischler, 1982, and Hoff & Ahuja, 1987, for reviews).

Working on the assumption that there exist human stereo mechanisms that use edge-based matching primitives, Mayhew and Frisby (1978a) asked whether such primitives were delivered by oriented or nonoriented channels. They created a series of demonstration stereograms whose textures were obtained by oriented filtering of random dots. These demonstrations indicated that an oriented stereo signal masked by similarly oriented noise was not released from masking when the orientation of the noise was rotated by $45°$, as would be expected on an oriented channels model. They concluded that edge points for human stereo matching were derived from nonoriented receptive fields, at any rate for the kind of dense complex random-dot textures used in their stereograms.

Mayhew and Frisby (1979a) reinforced this conclusion in a subsequent study which pointed out that oriented channels have grave difficulties *in principle* in dealing with surfaces made up of steep (high frequency) depth corrugations running in a direction orthogonal to oriented texture elements. This is because the extended receptive fields of oriented channels suitable for detecting the oriented texture would inevitably straddle several depth corrugations and hence blur together disparity information about different parts of the corrugated surface. Yet human vision copes well with such corrugations. This again indicates the use of nonoriented channels for human stereo matching.

Mayhew and Frisby's conclusions, however, have been challenged by Parker, Johnston, Mansfield, and Yang, who describe in their chapter of this book an experiment that used stimuli of the same general type as Mayhew and Frisby (1978a) but in a forced-choice paradigm involving many hundreds of trials. The two subjects in their experiment displayed orientationally tuned masking; that is, the effectiveness of the masking noise field was a function of the similarity between stereo and noise orientations. While noting general problems with the masking paradigm, Parker et al. conclude that the Mayhew and Frisby (1978a) result should no longer be taken as a firm indication of the contribution of nonoriented mechanisms to stereopsis.

In reply, we would note that the clear-cut character of the Mayhew and Frisby demonstrations for everyone to whom we have shown those stimuli is a fact that is not itself destroyed by the Parker et al. experiment. Moreover, the latter's forced-choice paradigm can be viewed as an extensive training exercise that culminates in showing once again how well the human visual system can seize upon slight cues and develop its use of them using impressive but as yet poorly understood mechanisms of perceptual learning. Indeed, Parker et al. themselves note that the ability of their observers to detect the stereo signal in the presence of masking noise improved as their experiment proceeded. We have here, then, demonstrations of no release of masking by rotation of noise orientation for untrained observers (Mayhew and Frisby) coupled with some release for highly trained psychophysical observers following extensive experience with the stimuli (Parker et al.)

Perhaps the deep underlying issue raised here, indeed one of the main themes of this book, is that psychophysical results need to be interpreted in the context of explicit computational models. The Mayhew and Frisby demonstration stimuli were used by them to rule out a version of the simple spatial frequency-tuned channels model of stereopsis considered by Mayhew and Frisby (1978b) in which the channels have oriented fields. Simulations of this model show that it copes easily (how could it fail?) with a stereo signal carried by an oriented texture upon which is superimposed rotated oriented noise because the noise is straightforwardly "cleaned off" by suitably oriented filtering. Hence, if this model is valid for human stereo vision dealing with the dense random noise textures in question, the stereo target in the Mayhew and Frisby demonstration stimuli ought to be perceived easily. In short, as far as the predictions of *that particular model* are concerned, release from masking should be observed without difficulty when the noise field is rotated well away from the orientation of the stereo signal. (Mayhew and Frisby further noted, as a practical point concerning their demonstrations, that this prediction is a reasonable one in general terms in that human stereopsis is remarkably resistant to noise of many types; see the many demonstrations to this effect in Julesz, 1971.)

The fact that the demonstration stimuli of Mayhew and Frisby do not show ready release from masking when the noise is rotated is therefore against the prediction of the particular model they were testing. This fact further suggests to us that the Parker et al. result is better interpreted as showing that, when pushed by extended training, human vision is able to make the best of a bad job. That is, human vision seems wonderfully able to recruit processes that are not normally used for a given task and press them into service to produce some kind of reasonable outcome, using mechanisms of perceptual learning to achieve results that are not characteristic of its hitherto normal means of operation. This is one reason why psychophysics is such a difficult business. In the present instance, with so many different "stereo tricks" at its disposal, each presumably having evolved for different purposes, the isolation of any one to the total exclusion of any other is problematic. This is particularly so if experimental paradigms are used that permit extensive training.

To sum up, our present view remains unchanged in the face of the Parker et al. experiment, namely that oriented processes do not seem to play an important part in the normal perception of stereopsis from complex random

textures, and that a simple form of oriented channels model is falsified for those circumstances. On the other hand, their experiment suggests oriented processes can be utilized following extensive experience, so that an oriented model may be a reasonable account of post-training performance.

"Corner" Points

Thacker and Mayhew (1989) have demonstrated a stereo algorithm that begins by finding highly distinctive "corner" points in each image, defining these as image features possessing a sharply peaked autocorrelation function (Harris & Stephens, 1988; cf. Barnard & Thompson, 1980, who used Moravec's, 1977, "busyness" operator to provide matching primitives for a stereo algorithm). Such "corner" points occur sufficiently sparsely in many natural images to permit matching of corresponding "corners" in the two images, using a simple correlation measure reflecting the similarity of the intensity levels comprising each such point. Thacker and Mayhew (1989) used the sparse set of matches thus provided as inputs to Trivedi's (1987) algorithm for camera calibration (the latter problem is discussed later).

It is worth noting here that Saye and Frisby (1975) found that random-dot stereograms to which have been added monocularly discriminable features such as highlighted corners and blobs produce shortened latencies for fusion. This led them to suggest that human vision may use such features to guide vergence eye movements necessary for fusing large disparities.

Higher-order Primitives

The random dot stereogram stands as a demonstration that stereo matching can be achieved without recourse to representations at the level of objects (chairs, faces, etc). This is because such entities are not discriminable in either half of a random-dot stereo pair prior to fusion. However, Ayache and Faverjon (1985; see also Vergnet, Pollard & Mayhew, 1989) have demonstrated the potential for using quite long image lines and curves as inputs to a stereo algorithm (see also Brint & Brady's 1989 report of stereo matching of image curves; Porrill & Pollard, 1990).

Before leaving the topic of matching primitives, it is worth noting that edge and corner points produce rather sparse disparity maps. It is possible to interpolate a dense disparity surface between the data points in such maps (e.g., Blake & Zisserman, 1987; Grimson, 1981; McLauchlan & Mayhew, 1989; McLauchlan et al., 1990). It seems that texture boundary cues help shape such interpolation processes in human vision (Buckley, Frisby & Mayhew, 1989). An alternative, or an addition, to interpolation might be some form of area intensity correlation to fill in the gaps (Baker, 1982; Bülthoff & Mallot, 1988).

Resolving Ambiguities

Highly distinctive matching primitives will sometimes be sufficient to establish correct matches (permitting what Julesz, 1971, termed "local stereopsis"). More generally, one or more algorithms will be necessary to resolve ambiguities in choosing which left and right primitives should be matched ("global stereopsis"; Julesz, 1971). These algorithms need to be founded on *constraints* discovered by a careful analysis of the stereo matching task (Marr, 1982; Marr & Poggio, 1976). Constraints are here defined as aspects of the viewed world and its projection into stereo images from which can be inferred *binocular matching rules* capable of eliminating false matches while preserving correct ones. The value of any given constraint needs to be tested in computational experiments, with its probable shortcomings at any rate as originally conceived, leading to an ever more refined analysis of the stereo matching task.

The main constraints that have been identified for stereo matching will be briefly described next (other reviews are provided by Barnard & Fischler, 1982; Marr, 1982; Mayhew, 1983; and Poggio & Poggio, 1984). This will be followed by a discussion of a particular stereo algorithm called PMF (*Pollard, Mayhew & Frisby, 1985a*) and its extended version PMF42, which is embedded in the TINATOOL computer stereo vision system (Porrill, Pollard, Pridmore, Bowen, Mayhew & Frisby, 1987). PMF42 exploits all the constraints listed below and has the additional merit for present tutorial review purposes of being founded on some psychophysical findings.

The Epipolar Constraint

Almost all stereo algorithms use the epipolar constraint. Figure 21.3 shows how the image locations of potential matches fall on geometrical constructs termed *epipolar lines* (see any photogrammetric textbook). The importance of this constraint is that it makes the stereo match-

ing problem a one-dimensional search. Without it, the stereo problem becomes formally identical to the two-dimensional motion correspondence problem. Figure 21.3 shows that epipolar lines in fact come in left-right pairs which together define the loci of image locations that can form potential matches. The ambiguities shown in that figure illustrate the classic false targets problem of global stereopsis to which Julesz's work drew attention (reviewed in Julesz, 1971).

Camera Calibration

If the epipolar geometry of stereo projections is to be exploited then it must be known *where* corresponding epipolar lines are to be found in the two images. Working out the location of epipolar lines for a given primitive requires a solution to the nontrivial problem of knowing the spatial relationships between the two cameras, as well as facts about focal length, optical centers, and so forth. This is the business of *camera calibration*, as it is termed in the computational literature. For a computer stereo camera rig it typically involves solving at least 12 free parameters! The usual approach for a fixed geometry rig is to infer most of them at start-up time from stereo images of an accurately measured test object (e.g., Tsai, 1986). Complications arise if the camera geometry is variable (i.e., capable of taking on different fixation directions, vergence angles, etc).

Thacker and Mayhew (1989) have developed a way of avoiding the need for a calibrated test object by using "corner" features (see above) as the inputs for Trivedi's (1987) camera calibration algorithm. The latter finds an optimal least-squares fit of the various camera parameters to the matched corner data. Dispensing with the need for a test object is obviously a more plausible approach to modeling biological systems. Another way of achieving that desirable outcome (Porrill, personal communication) is to refine camera calibration by exploiting the consistency discovered when deriving geometric edge descriptions from multiple views using the Gauss-Markov statistical combination techniques described in Porrill, Pollard, and Mayhew (1987b).

Camera Calibration from a Simplified Model of Vertical Disparities

Attention was drawn at the outset of this chapter to the fact that disparities have both vertical and horizontal com-

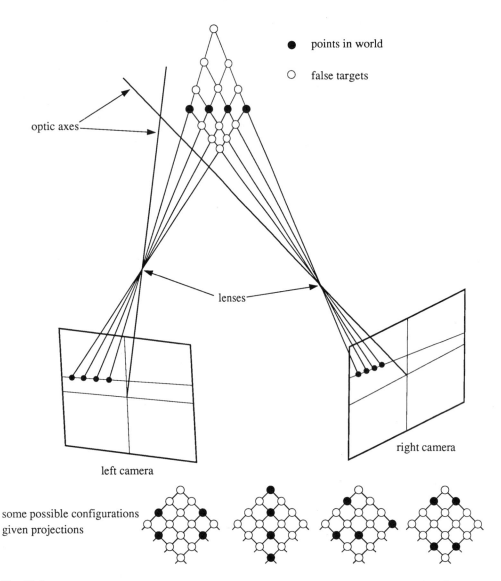

points in world
false targets

optic axes

lenses

left camera

right camera

some possible configurations
given projections

Fig. 21.3
Epipolar geometry and the stereo correspondence problem (courtesy
P. McLauchlan). The four points in the world (*solid circles*) happen to
lie in a single epipolar plane defined as a plane that includes a point
in the world and the optic centers of the left and right cameras. The
intersection of the epipolar plane with the image planes of the left
and right cameras results in a pair of epipolar lines. These lines have
the desirable property that they provide a restriction on allowable
matches between the two views based on geometry alone. This in
effect reduces the correspondence problem to a single dimension. The
possible ghost matches that exist in this case are shown in the upper
figure as open circles. A few of the 24 alternative matching scenarios
that enforce the uniqueness constraint (see text) are illustrated in the
lower figures: Each solid circle there illustrates a chosen match rather
than a correct one. The optic axes of the left and right hand cameras
need not necessarily meet at a common point of fixation for generic
stereo camera geometry, although it is helpful if the cameras are
facing roughly the same direction.

ponents (epipolar lines are generally tilted). Mayhew
(1982) derived some remarkably simple equations specifying to first order the vertical (V) and horizontal (H) disparities of any point as the sum of components due to: (1)
the retinal coordinates of the point, (2) the prevailing gaze
angle, and (3) depth of the point relative to the fixation
point (see figure 21.1). His equations hold to first order
using small angle approximations for trigonometric functions (see Longuet-Higgins, 1982a, b). These equations
were extended by Porrill to take account of the angle of
elevation of the eyes (Porrill, Mayhew & Frisby, 1987), in
which case they become:

$$V = V_{ecc} + V_g + V_e = \frac{xyI}{d} + \frac{gyI}{d} + \frac{exI}{2d}$$

$$H = H_{ecc} + H_g + H_e + H_z = \frac{x^2 I}{d} + \frac{gxI}{d} + \frac{eyI}{2d} + \frac{zI}{d^2},$$

where I is the interocular separation, d is the distance to the fixation point, z is the distance relative to the fixation point (all in centimeters), g is the angle of gaze, e is the angle of eye elevation, y is the vertical retinal coordinate, and x is the horizontal retinal coordinate (all in radians, as are V and H). The equations assume that $I \ll d$, which is a reasonable assumption for much of human vision.

What these equations say is that horizontal disparities arise when a point lies in front or behind the plane of the fixation point (hence the H_z term). Also, horizontal disparities have components due to angle of gaze (H_g), angle of eye elevation (H_e), and retinal eccentricity (H_{ecc}, determined by the retinal x coordinate of the point in question).

Vertical disparities are not determined by variations in the distance of scene elements: their equation has no term with z in it. Rather, they have just three components, V_g, V_e, and V_{ecc}, deriving from gaze angle, elevation angle, and eccentricity of retinal location, respectively. Vertical disparities arise for elements (lying off the horizontal meridian and for nonparallel camera geometry) that are nearer one eye than the other so that their vertical distances from the horizontal meridian project different sizes in the two eyes. Vertical disparities thus arise when a point is viewed with an off-center angle of gaze (asymmetric fixation); hence the the V_g term. In addition, like horizontal disparities, they also have a component due to retinal eccentricity but, unlike the equivalent H_{ecc} term, V_{ecc} has both x and y scaling factors.

The elegant Mayhew/Porrill equations for V and H constitute a theory of binocular depth perception showing that the absolute distances of all points in a scene can be recovered from visual information alone (see also Gillam & Lawergren, 1983; Petrov, 1980). Indeed, the equations are so simple that, at least in principle, V values for only three matched points (of differing x eccentricity and not falling too close to the horizontal meridian) are required for the solution of three simultaneous equations in V to recover the parameters d, g, and e. This is remarkable because it has been a commonplace belief that these parameters, which are essential for interpreting horizontal disparities, have to be obtained from extraretinal information about eye positions. Peek, Mayhew, and Frisby (1984)

have demonstrated a practical algorithm for exploiting Mayhew's equations.

Curiously, although Helmholtz (1909/1962) knew that information about absolute distance was contained in vertical disparities, he gave no details and his comments have been neglected, perhaps because it has been assumed—incorrectly for near distances—that vertical disparities are too small to be usable by the human visual system. In fact, a certain visual illusion called the induced effect, which is generated by vertical magnification of one image, is consistent with human vision using vertical disparities to recover d and g (Gillam & Lawergren, 1983; Mayhew & Longuet-Higgins, 1982; Petrov, 1980). That interpretation has been challenged by Westheimer (1984) because he found that human sensitivity to vertical magnification falls well below that for horizontal. This appears quite at odds with the requirement that vertical disparities be measured with great precision. Frisby (1984), however, points out in a general review of that study and others on the induced effect that Westheimer used a viewing distance of 3 m, which meant that the magnifications he studied would require impossibly large g values to generate them. The general conclusion reached by Frisby was that psychophysical predictions drawn from the so-called *d/g hypothesis* for exploiting vertical disparities have so far survived attempts to falsify them as long as the requirement is met that experimental conditions present vertical size differences between images which could arise in natural viewing.

An alternative account of the induced illusion and related effects suggests that it reflects an analysis of the disparity vector field in terms of differential invariants (Koenderink, 1986; Rogers & Koenderink, 1986). Porrill et al. (1987a) extended that theory to predict a new kind of induced effect but failed to find it. See also Blake and Bülthoff, 1990, for the use of vertical disparities in interpreting specularities.

Camera Calibration: Practical Difficulties

Whatever the mechanisms used by human vision for solving its version of the eye/camera calibration problem, the fact that we can adjust, given time, to perturbations imposed by various distorting lenses shows that these mechanisms are adaptive in character, suggesting that a process of continual recalibration is at work. Neural network models for eye movement control exhibiting this desirable property are now beginning to emerge (Anastasio & Robinson, 1989; Dean, Mayhew & Thacker, 1990).

The practical complexities in solving the stereo camera calibration problem are easy to overlook if attention is restricted to artificial images such as random-dot stereograms. For the latter, knowledge of which region to search in one image for the match of a primitive identified in the other is usually given directly from the method used to create the stimuli. For example, the search can be restricted to equivalent rasters in the two images if the disparity shifts used in the creation of the stereogram have been made along those rasters. But in a practical stereo vision system, biological or man-made, it will rarely be the case that matches lie on corresponding horizontal lines in the two images. Also, even given reasonably accurate knowledge of the camera geometry, errors in camera calibration and/or in image edge location may still make it desirable to search regions lying a little to either side of the predicted epipolar lines.

It conveys considerable computational convenience to use camera calibration parameters to transform images to parallel camera geometry so that searches can be made along rasters, thereby gaining all the benefits of simple rectangular array data structures as well as easier recovery of 3D structures such as planes, vertices and the like from matched points. If this so-called *stereo image rectification* process is conducted on edge primitives then aliasing problems are insignificant (Porrill et al., 1987c). However, if it is conducted on the graylevel images themselves then suitable antialiasing precautions must be taken.

Transforms into orthographic projections are not the only ones to convey convenient simplicities of implementation. Mallot, Schulze, and Storjohann (1988) have shown how inverse perspective projections that render the ground plane everywhere to have zero disparity permit simple image subtraction techniques for obstacle detection. They have implemented this idea, which was derived from a study of the topological projections found in biological vision systems (see also Epstein, 1984), in a visual guidance system for an autonomous warehouse vehicle.

If infinite resolution were available, the epipolar constraint would be sufficient in principle to solve the stereo correspondence problem: For generic views of generic point sets no two points would lie on the same epipolar line, and so every point would have a unique match. In practice, stereo does not deal with generic point sets and quantization error also forces many points into the same epipolar line. As a result, solving the stereo correspondence problem requires resolving matching ambiguities *along* epipolars, and this has to be achieved using one or more additional constraints derived from assumptions about the nature of the viewed world and its projections into stereo images. It is to these other constraints that we now turn.

Compatibility of Matching Primitives

It has often been suggested that the size of the ambiguity problem can be substantially reduced, if not altogether eliminated, by matching features of similar shape and contrast (e.g., Barlow, Blakemore & Pettigrew, 1967; Frisby & Roth, 1971; Mayhew & Frisby, 1980). This strategy has already been referred to above at some length in connection with choosing matching primitives such as "corner" points but note that even using those distinctive primitives is not enough in general for achieving disambiguation (Thacker & Mayhew, 1989).

Marr's (1982, p. 114) way of expressing this constraint, which he dubbed the *compatibility constraint*, is: Only match left and right features that could have arisen from the same scene entity. To implement this constraint requires careful attention to how scene features appear in stereo projections. This is necessary to determine bounds on the ranges of, for example, size (spatial frequency) and orientation differences allowed between left and right image features if they are to form potential matches. An example of one way of doing this will be given later in connection with the PMF stereo algorithm.

Marr gave as an example of using the compatibility constraint the binocular matching rule: *Black dots can match only black dots*. This was in the context of discussing problems posed by random dot stereograms, but it is tempting to extend the rule to: Match edge points of the same contrast sign. Yet computational experience in developing PMF has shown that a light-to-dark edge in one image not infrequently projects as a dark-to-light edge in the other image. An example where this happens is at occlusion edges for which the edge is seen against a light background from the vantage point of one eye but against a dark background in the other eye. This illustrates that stereo projections do *not* always preserve the sign of edge contrast, and the PMF42 version of PMF takes this into account (see later). Nevertheless, the failure of human stereo vision to cope with contrast reversed random-dot stereograms has been used to suggest that it implements invariably a "same-contrast" binocular matching rule (Julesz, 1971; Frisby, 1979, p. 153).

The image intensity area correlation algorithms referred to above can be viewed as relying to some degree on the compatibility constraint in that they try to find matches supported by highly similar local image structure in the two stereo projections.

The Ordering Constraint

If opaque surfaces can be assumed, then it is possible to exploit the fact that the order of primitives along an epipolar line in one image is preserved in the other image (Baker, 1982; Baker & Binford, 1981). This property can be seen in the same ordering of points along the left and right image epipolar lines shown in figure 21.3.

The Cohesivity Constraint

Marr and Poggio (1976) argued that it is reasonable to assume the visual world is made up of matter that is separated into objects whose surfaces are generally smooth compared with their overall distances from the viewer. In other words, the visual world is not usually made up only of clouds of dust particles or snowflakes. They termed this the *cohesivity constraint* and they used it to underpin their continuity binocular matching rule: *Prefer possible matches that could have arisen from smooth surfaces.* This rule is frequently referred to as imposing a smoothness constraint. (The notion of imposing smoothness is ubiquitous in early visual processing. Poggio, Torre and Koch, 1985, show how its use in stereo can be seen as just one instance of its more general use as a *regularizer* for solving what are mathematically known as *ill-posed* vision problems, because they are either under- or over-determined.)

The Uniqueness Constraint

Marr and Poggio (1976) also noted that *a scene entity cannot be in two places at the same time*, from which they derived the binocular matching rule: *Each matching primi-*

tive from each image may be assigned at most one disparity value.

The Figural Continuity Constraint

Mayhew and Frisby (1980, 1981) used Marr and Poggio's cohesivity constraint to justify a quite different matching rule: Because cohesive objects generate surface edges and surface markings that are spatially continuous, *prefer matches that preserve figural continuity.* That is, give preference to any point-for-point matches that are part of an edge whose other component points also have matches, such that the whole forms a figurally continuous structure of matched points. Mayhew and Frisby cited psychophysical evidence suggesting that human stereovision exploits this constaint and developed a correspondence algorithm, called STEREOEDGE, that relied on it.

The PMF Stereo Algorithm

The so-called *PMF* stereo algorithm of Pollard, Mayhew and Frisby (1985; see also Pollard 1987; Pollard, Porrill, Mayhew & Frisby, 1985b) is a *neighborhood support* algorithm. In this respect it is like many others, of which the best known is Marr and Poggio (1976; but see also Dev, 1975, the critique of Dev by Marr, 1982, and Sperling, 1970).

Matching Primitives Used in PMF

The disambiguating algorithm used by PMF requires only that matching primitives should be reasonably closely related to scene entities and that they should occur with reasonable density. For natural images, the primitives used in the early stages of PMF (higher-order primitives are used later) that satisfy these requirements are edge points of similar contrast sign delivered by a single scale, high-frequency Canny (1986) edge detector.[1] For the experiments using random-dot stereograms to develop PMF, the matching primitives were simply point locations defined when the stimuli were created. From results with the latter, it seems probable that PMF would work perfectly well with a variety of texture element primitives

---

1. The edge detector typically used for PMF has a sigma of 1 pixel and incorporates nonmaximal suppression and hysteresis (Canny, 1986). Subpixel edge location acuity of about ± 0.1 pixel is provided by quadratic interpolation of the peak of the convolution profile orthogonal to edge orientation, the latter being a parameter attached to each point.

(e.g., blobs, line endpoints, corners), as long as they occur with sufficient density.

Camera calibration is performed using an accurately measured checkered calibration tile. Being sparse, image locations of the corners of the checker squares are readily identified, by extrapolation from the edges of the squares. These are then fed into an implementation of Tsai's algorithm (see above). For subsequent processing convenience, camera calibration parameters are then used to "rectify" the Canny edge output to parallel camera geometry, thereby ensuring that the epipolar lines fall conveniently on horizontal rasters. Aliasing problems are avoided by rectifying the positions of the edge points, not the image intensity levels.

PMF's Gradient Limit Constraint

The key idea in PMF is that neighboring potential matches exchange support (mutual facilitation) *iff* their relative disparities are not too different. The latter is defined in terms of the disparity between potential matches not exceeding a *disparity gradient limit*. The butterfly shape in figure 21.4 illustrates the bounds on neighboring matches falling within and outside this limit.

Disparity gradient is defined in PMF as:

$$DG = \frac{\text{difference in disparities}}{\text{feature separation}}.$$

The denominator currently in use in PMF is the separation in the left image of the pair of features that participate in the pair of matches concerned. Originally, all operations were conducted in a cyclopean space, following Burt and Julesz's (1980b) definition of disparity gradient. The change to basing all operations on the left image (thereby creating a dominant "eye"?) is a computational convenience that has little bearing on the effectiveness of the algorithm. Note that DG is here defined one-dimensionally, as it is computed between pairs of potential matches.

In outline, the PMF support algorithm works as follows. The *matching strength* of each potential match is computed as the sum of the strengths of all potential matches in a local image neighborhood that satisfy a moderate DG limit (0.5 to 1.5; see later) with respect to it. Because the probability of a neighboring match falling within the DG limit by chance increases (almost linearly) with its distance away from the match under considera-

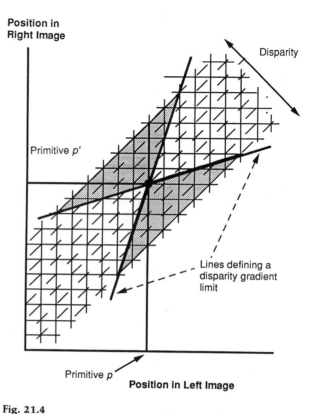

Fig. 21.4

The diaparity gradient limit used for defining neighborhood support. The two axes depict locations of primitives on a corresponding pair of left and right epipolar lines (cf. Marr & Poggio, 1976). The intersections of lines drawn perpendicularly from each primitive represent potential matches. Primitives with zero disparity fall on the principal diagonal; other disparity planes lie parallel to that diagonal. A potential match *pp′* formed from the primitives *p* and *p′* and lying in a nonzero disparity plane is shown as a solid circle. Extending from this point are two bold lines whose slope reflects a particular disparity gradient. The shaded areas on one side of these lines depict regions in which neighbors of *pp′* would have too steep a disparity gradient with *pp′* to be allowed to support that match in PMF.

tion (details in Pollard, 1985), the contribution of each match in the neighborhood is weighted inversely by its distance away. The uniqueness constraint is exploited at this stage by requiring that at most one match associated with a single primitive in one or other image makes a contribution to the matching strength.

Expressing this in more detail, consider the points in one image, the left say. Each point, for example point *p*, identified in that image can take part in a number of matches over some disparity range (figure 21.5). Experiments have shown no appreciable loss of disambiguating power if the latter parameter is set to be quite large, as

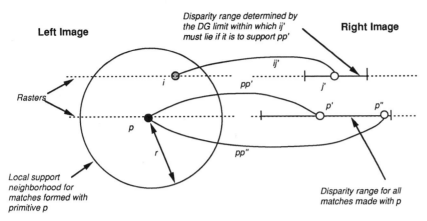

Left Image

Right Image

Disparity range determined by
the DG limit within which ij'
must lie if it is to support pp'

ij'

pp'

i

j'

p

p'

p"

pp'

r

pp"

Rasters

Local support
neighborhood for
matches formed with
primitive p

Disparity range for all
matches made with p

Fig. 21.5

Neighborhood Support in PMF. The circles p, p', p'', i, and j' represent
edge point primitives (the edge strings of which they form a part are
not shown). Matching is initiated from left image primitives, and two
potential matches for p are illustrated with the lines labeled pp' and
pp''. Support for each of these matches is sought from the potential
matches of other left image primitives lying within the neighborhood
support circle (of radius r not drawn to scale) shown around p. Just
one supporting match, ij', is illustrated for the match pp'. Note that ij'
lies within the disparity gradient limit with respect to pp'. See text
for details.

judged by the standard of Panum's fusional area in human
vision: Currently the disparity range used in PMF is 20°!
This goes a long way to compensate for the use of fixed
camera rig geometry (i.e., PMF, at present, has only been
used without the benefits conveyed by vergence eye
movements in human vision).

A support neighborhood of radius r pixels is defined in
the left image (figure 21.5). Only those matches associated with points that lie within this neighborhood are
allowed to contribute support to each of the possible
matches for p, and only then if the disparity gradient
between them and p is less than a moderate predetermined limit. Furthermore, in accordance with the uniqueness constraint only a single match for each primitive in
the neighborhood is allowed to convey support.

The matching strength can be expressed more formally
as

$$MS_{pp'} = \sum_{i \in N(p)} \left(\max \text{ all } j' \frac{C_{ij'} \times DG(M_{pp'}, M_{ij'})}{S(p, i)} \right),$$

where $N(p)$ is the set of points in the neighborhood of p.
DG $(M_{pp'}, M_{ij'})$ is a function of the disparity gradient that
exists between match $M_{pp'}$ and $M_{ij'}$: It has value one if
the gradient is less than the chosen limit, zero otherwise.

$S(p, i)$ is the magnitude of the separation between points
p and i. $C_{ij'}$ reflects the goodness of the match between
primitives i and j'; it is defined as the contrast strength of
the weaker of the two constituent edges participating in
the match and its role is to give most weight to the most
reliable data (the stronger the contrast, the less likely the
edge is noise). In those situations where there is more
than one match for a single primitive satisfying the gradient limit, only the strongest contributes to the matching
strength.

Rationale Underlying The Gradient Limit Constraint

The idea of using a disparity gradient limit was prompted
by psychophysical studies (Burt & Julesz, 1980a,b; see
also Tyler, 1973a,b) which showed that if two disparate
dots are brought closer and closer together while their
disparity is maintained, there comes a point at which
binocular fusion breaks down into diplopia. The breakdown occurs for a disparity gradient between the pair of
dots of about 1.0. Although it is well known that humans
can perceive depth differences between stimuli whose
disparity differences are so large that they are diplopic
(Ogle, 1950), this observation of fusional breakdown
nevertheless led Pollard to have the idea of imposing a
DG limit as a way of solving the stereo correspondence
problem. (Prazdny, 1985, independently made different use
of disparity gradients in a stereo algorithm; see below.)

Steeply slanted surfaces give rise to steeper disparity
gradients than gently slanting ones at the same distance.
Note that disparity gradient is scaled by I/d where I is
interocular separation, d is distance to the fixation point,
and s is the slant angle (that between the frontoparallel
plane and the tangent to the surface), the equation being:

$$DG = \frac{I \tan s}{d}.$$

If $I \ll d$, as is customary for human stereo vision, then even quite large slant angles project modest disparity gradients. Pollard (1985; see also Arnold & Binford. 1980; Kass, 1984) computed the probability density function based on the assumption that scene surface orientations are uniformly distributed over the Gaussian sphere. It turns out that less than 10 percent of the surfaces in such a world viewed from 26 cm will present with a disparity gradient in excess of 0.5. But crucially for the rationale of using a disparity gradient limit to determine whether matches should be allowed to exchange support, Pollard also demonstrated that false matches typically generated disparity gradients larger than 0.5 to 1.0. In general, the lower the disparity gradient limit allowed, the greater the probability of excluding false matches.

To get a feel for disparity gradient, it is helpful to consider what happens when an opaque planar patch is made to slant more and more steeply by rotating it about a vertical axis. There comes a point at which one eye loses all sight of the texture on the surface because it is looking exactly along the surface. At that surface slant, for which the other eye can still see some texture because it is looking at the surface from a vantage point that is a little more square on, the disparity gradient in cyclopean disparity space happens to be 2.0—which is therefore the theoretical limit for disparity gradients between texture elements on opaque surfaces rotated around vertical. The theoretical limit for surfaces rotated around horizontal is infinity.

The particular value chosen for the DG limit in PMF is not crucial, although values near the 2.0 limit provide little disambiguating power—false matches then often receive as much support as correct ones (Pollard et al., 1985b). It is interesting to note that the disparity gradient limit for fusion in human stereo vision was found by Burt and Julesz to be about 1.0 (isotropically over all the orientations they tested but note the anisotropy in Bülthoff and Fahle, 1989). Hence a value of 1.0 was used successfully in early versions of PMF for many types of scenes. This is an unusually clear case of a psychophysical result leading to a quite detailed design feature of a computer vision algorithm. In PMF42, different DG values are used at different stages. For the equivalent (and still initial) phase to that described here, the DG limit is set to 0.5,

which is quite a severe and strongly disambiguating value, by way of selecting strong "seed point" matches (see later).

It is important to emphasize that PMF is interested only in the quantity of within-disparity-gradient-limit *support* that exists for a particular match. Hence the extent to which the disparity gradient limit is offended in the neighborhood of a candidate match does not directly affect the selection procedure of PMF. This design feature is perfectly in line with the justification given above for seeking within-DG-limit support as the disparity gradient limit need not necessarily be satisfied everywhere. Indeed, a large step in a scene will create large disparity gradients across it but not along it; within-DG-limit support exchanged between neighboring matches lying on either side of the edge can thereby lead to their selection. This avoids the problems that would arise if correct matches had to pay a cost by having neighbors from across the step whose disparity gradients were large. The same line of reasoning explains why the support-only basis for PMF leads to it being able to deal successfully with points arising from overlapping transparent surfaces (Pollard & Frisby, 1990; Pollard et al., 1985).

We have also thought it sensible not to weight contributions by the actual magnitude of their disparity gradients, but instead to treat all within-DG-limit contributions homogeneously. This makes sense for the stereo correspondence problem, as there seems to be no reason to penalize any pertubations that lie within the range expected in stereo projections of the scenes of interest. However, many other functions using disparity gradients could be employed. In one interesting example suggested by Prazdny (1985), the strength of the support that flows between a pair of matches is scaled in a Gaussian fashion with respect to the size of the disparity gradient between them.

A further point to notice in this implementation of PMF is that within-DG-limit support is sought independently from all possible matches in the neighborhood of the match under consideration. This means that it is possible that two or more matches that give within-disparity-gradient-limit support might not themselves share a within-DG-limit disparity gradient. This design feature has been dictated by considerations of computational efficiency but Pollard et al. (1985b) found little benefit in practice from insisting on within-neighborhood support consistency.

Selection of Strongest Matches

Once the matching strengths have been computed, correct matches are selected using a form of winner-take-all discrete relaxation (Ballard & Brown, 1982). At the first iteration, any potential matches which have the highest matching score for *both* the left and the right image primitives that gave rise to them are immediately chosen as "correct." Other potential matches deriving from these primitives are eliminated from further consideration, a procedure justified by the uniqueness constraint. This allows in the next iteration further potential matches that were neither accepted nor eliminated in the previous one to be selected as correct because they now have the highest matching strengths for both constituent primitives. Usually only four or five iterations are needed to propagate the uniqueness constraint in this way to a satisfactory endpoint. In fact, the overwhelming majority of correct matches are selected on the first iteration, so PMF is hardly an iterative algorithm at all, if by this term is meant an algorithm relying on hundreds or thousands of iterations (as does Marr and Poggio's, 1976, stereo algorithm).

PMF as a Parallel Algorithm

Although the use of a disparity gradient limit in PMF was stimulated by observations of the human visual system, various details of its design were shaped by more practical constraints introduced by the need to achieve reasonable efficiency and robustness on near-state-of-the-art computer machinery. The speed criterion is met by the intrinsically parallel nature of the structure chosen for PMF: Each matching strength could, on appropriate computer architecture, be computed independently. Recent work in our laboratory using a 24-transputer device (specially designed in-house for stereo vision processing) has shown that PMF can be run in about a second on 512 by 512 images of quite densely textured scenes (Rygol & Brown, 1990). Moreover, extensive examination of PMF's performance on various artificial and natural stereo images shows it to be robust. These twin factors of speed and robustness suggest that PMF might prove valuable for industrial application in the short to medium term.

Constraints Imposed by Using a Disparity Gradient Limit

Imposing a disparity gradient limit for disambiguation can be viewed as a technique for implementing several of the constraints listed above.

First and foremost, it amounts to enforcing a form of scene-to-image and left-image-to-right-image continuity that can be described as imposing a bound on the allowable degree of *scene surface jaggedness* (Pollard et al., 1985a). In so doing, using the disparity gradient concept breaks away from the restrictive notion of surface smoothness implemented by Marr and Poggio (1976). Essentially they imposed a disparity gradient limit of zero, by allowing only matches with the same disparity to exchange support. That is, facilitation was exchanged only between potential matches lying on the diagonally oriented lines in figure 21.4. Restricting facilitation in that way amounts to insisting that surfaces should be locally flat and viewed square on if their elements are to be allowed to exchange support.

Yet it is evident from simple inspection of tufts of hair, bunches of flowers, and the like, that human stereo vision can cope magnificently with scenes that are full of a wide variety of slants and depth discontinuities, scenes comprising just about anything but (even locally) frontoparallel planar patches! Using a disparity gradient limit of around 1.0 is much less restrictive; for example, 1.0 is the maximum disparity gradient that can be generated between features on a planar patch viewed at a distance of 65 cm with an interocular separation of 6.5 cm and with a slant of 84°. Figure 21.6 shows a stereo pair that satisfy a DG limit of 1.0: The 3D structure it portrays is far from even locally "smooth."

The technical mathematical term for defining surface continuity with reference to a gradient limit is *Lipschitz* continuity. Pollard et al. (1985b) discuss formally the mathematical basis for using this notion of continuity in stereo algorithms (see also Trivedi & Lloyd, 1986).

To sum up this section on the disparity gradient and the continuity constraint, it seems best to view the use of a disparity gradient limit as a way of "parameterizing" the binocular matching rule of seeking matches that preserve surface smoothness. If the DG is set close to zero, then the disambiguating power is great but the range of surfaces that can be dealt with is correspondingly small;

(a)

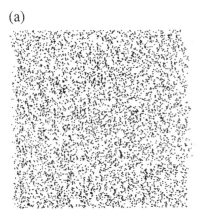 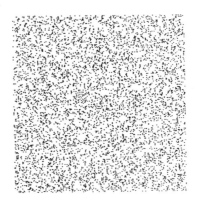

(b)

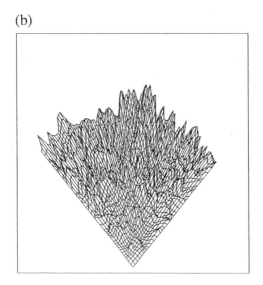

Fig. 21.6

A random-dot stereogram demonstrating the capacity of PMF to deal with jagged surfaces. (A) A sterogram (256 units square) in which disparities have been randomly selected over a range of 5 units except that everywhere they satisfy a disparity gradient limit of 0.5. (B) The depth profile recovered by the PMF stereo algorithm. Over 95 percent of matches are correctly located. Note that this profile is far from smooth (see text).

mutatis mutandis if the DG limit is increased towards the theoretical limit of 2.0.

Second, the disparity gradient limit also provides a principled way of determining bounds for implementing the *compatibility constraint*. For example, a disparity gradient of 1.0 permits the derivation of allowable orientation differences between left and right edge primitives (details in Pollard, 1985). Equally, the DG limit could in principle be used to produce spatial frequency bounds on left and right primitives but PMF does not exploit this, so far being used in connection with a single high spatial frequency edge detector.

Third, it has often been noted that order reversals correspond to disparity gradients of 2.0 or greater. Hence the 1.0 limit used in PMF automatically imposes a conservative version of the *ordering constraint*. However, it would be wrong to see PMF's use of the disparity gradient limit as doing no more than implementing a version of the ordering constraint, for two reasons. First, a DG limit of 2.0 provides far too little disambiguating power for PMF's support scheme to work (Pollard et al., 1985b), so some rationale over and above the ordering constraint must be given for choosing a DG limit well within 2.0. And second, PMF imposes its limit isotropically, whereas the ordering constraint is justified only along epipolars.

Fourth, the *uniqueness constraint* is also implied by a

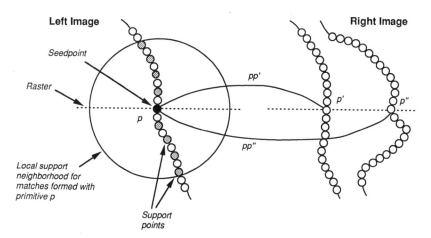

Left Image

Seedpoint

Raster

p

pp'

pp"

Local support
neighborhood for
matches formed with
primitive *p*

Support
points

Right Image

p'

p"

Fig. 21.7
Selection of seed point matches in PMF42. The circles represent edge
point primitives comprising edge strings. Matching is initiated from
left image strings and at first only every *n*th point comprising a left
hand string is considered for matching (currently *n* = 4). Such points
are termed seed points. Two potential matches for the seed point
primitive *p* are shown, *pp'* and *pp"*. Support for each of these matches
is sought within the neighborhood support circle shown around *p*
(radius not drawn to scale), with every *m*th primitive along the string
evaluated for the support it offers (the shaded circles illustrate
m = 2). See text for details.

disparity gradient of less than 2.0. This is because if a
single point from one image is allowed to match with a
pair of points from the other (cf. the usual, but not the
only, interpretation of Panum's limiting case; Krol, 1982),
then the disparity gradient between the two matches so
obtained would be 2.0. This comment should not, however, obscure the fact that the uniqueness constraint is
also imposed during the winner-take-all selection phase of
PMF. Also, it is worth noting that Pollard and Frisby
(1990) show that PMF's use of the uniqueness constraint
is entirely compatible with the psychophysical observation of multiple depth planes from random-dot versions
of the double nail illusion, despite claims to the contrary
by Weinshall (1989).

From PMF to PMF42

The main difference in philosophy between PMF and
PMF42 is that the latter adds to the former's relatively
local operations various selection strategies that exploit
more global constraints. These are: (1) figural continuity
along strings of edge points, and (2) greater use of the
ordering constraint along epipolars. These will be ex-

plained and at the same time various other features of
PMF not so far covered will be addressed.

In addition, some of PMF42's detailed features that
relate to speeded-up processing will be outlined. The ones
chosen for mention illustrate general implementation strategies that might have a bearing on the understanding of
any stereo algorithm, including those embedded in biological vision systems.

PMF42—Stage 1: Selection of a Sparse Set of Seed Point Matches

A control strategy used in PMF42 aimed at speeded-up
yet reliable matching is to begin by seeking a set of
strong *seed point matches*, which can be used to guide
selection of subsequent matches. This is done by trying to
match at first only a subset of all the edge points available. So, only every nth point on an edge string is considered; currently *n* = 4. For the same reason, only every
mth point along a string can give support; currently *m* =
2. Figure 21.7 illustrates these concepts.

The local neighborhood support scheme already described for PMF is run with the DG limit set to 0.5 for this
limited set of potential matches. The 0.5 value provides
better disambiguating power than 1.0 (Pollard, 1985). The
size of the support neighborhood is set to be a function
of the image size; currently, a default radius of 20 pixels
for 256 by 256 images, a radius 40 pixels for 512 by 512
images, and so on, has been found satisfactory. The underlying concern here is to ensure that the support neighborhood is large enough to cover a sufficient amount of
scene structure to provide good disambiguation while not
being so large that processing time is spent needlessly
trying to use unrelated scene events. It is doubtful whether

it is possible to find a way of setting the size of neighborhood support parameter in a principled way that would suit many types of images. In lieu of that, it might be preferable to set it dynamically according to what is being found, but as support is scaled by distance between matches, in practice little benefit is gained by enlarging the support window greatly (unless the primitives are very sparse).

The output at this stage is a list of potential matches for every nth point in the left image, with the list ordered by *strength*. The latter measure reflects both the degree of support each match has received and the contrast strength of the weakest edge point, as in PMF.

The next step is to select a match for each *seed point* from its list of potential matches. The goal is to choose seed point matches that are sufficiently strong to form a reliable basis for eliminating other potential matches. (Brady, 1987, has discussed the merits of seed points in other contexts). These points (which are not treated as absolutes; they can be, and not infrequently are, killed off later) are chosen using the following winner-take-all selection rule:

From the list of potential matches for a given left image edge point, choose as a seed point match the strongest match *unless* there exists in the neighborhood of this match a stronger match that exceeds $DG = 1.5$ with respect to the match under consideration. If a selection is made, eliminate from further consideration at this stage (they may get resuscitated later) (1) all other matches for the given left image edge primitive, and (2) those that violate the gradient limit with respect to the selected match.

The idea behind the *unless* proviso is that a stronger match in the neighborhood that is offending a quite steep disparity gradient limit is evidence that the match under consideration might well be false. It should not therefore be selected as a seed point on which to base other selections.

The selection rule is applied iteratively. If a stronger match exists, then no selection is made on that iteration. If the stronger match gets killed off (by not getting selected as a seed point itself), then any selection held over may be allowed to proceed on the next iteration.

The above selection procedure implements the uniqueness constraint by allowing only one match per primitive but it does so only with respect to the left image points. Uniqueness is not imposed with respect to right image

points as well (as happened in PMF) *except* later on via a greater use of the ordering constraint.

The selection of a sparse set of seed points likely to form a reliable basis for subsequent processing is akin, albeit not identical, to the *coarse-to-fine processing* strategy used widely in computer vision systems. This strategy was used for stereo matching by Marr and Poggio's second stereo algorithm (Marr & Poggio, 1979; see also Grimson's, 1981, 1983, implementations of this algorithm). The key idea in that algorithm is that at a coarse image resolution (low spatial frequencies) there is little or no ambiguity problem (for an edge-based algorithm) because there are so very few "edges" to contend with. This enables a rough solution to be attained to the stereo matching problem in a given region without need of computationally expensive neighborhood facilitation/inhibition interactions (i.e., little or no need of cooperative processes of the kind embedded in PMF). The approximate coarse solution can then be used to guide the search for matches at a finer resolution (higher spatial frequencies) and so on, in a coarse-to-fine sequence to the finest resolution required.

Prazdny (1987) has noted that Marr and Poggio's coarse-to-fine strategy relies on an *assumption of spectral continuity*. Thus it fails if different spatial frequencies carry different depth information, as when objects generating low frequencies are seen through semitransparent lacy surfaces generating mainly high frequencies. Here the outputs of a low spatial frequency channel would give incorrect information about where to seek matches for the lacework.

It is also of interest to note that Marr and Poggio's (1979) algorithm, which relied on vergence movements driven by coarser channels to bring finer resolution channels into their more limited disparity processing range, has been falsified as a general model of human stereopsis by experiments showing that matches can be resolved over a greater spatial extent than that predicted by the Marr/Poggio theory (Mayhew & Frisby, 1979b). In short, it seems that human stereopsis really is cooperative, in the sense that it uses neighborhood relations between primitives to solve the stereo ambiguity problem, as Julesz (1971, 1986) has always claimed. On the other hand, the link between spatial frequency and disparity range used by Marr and Poggio does seem to apply at the coarse end of the spatial frequency spectrum (Schor & Wood, 1985). But the very large disparities investigated in that study for low spatial frequencies were much too big to arise naturally from scene depth variations in human vision, so the observed coupling may have more to do with maintaining eye alignment than with solving the stereo correspondence problem addressed by Marr and Poggio.

In any event, the coarse-to-fine strategy built into PMF42 is of a quite different kind. It achieves an initial sparseness not by using a coarse image scale but by starting its operations from just a sample of potential matches at a single scale, and then from this sample selecting only those that are relatively strong in terms of degree of local support and contrast.

PMF42—Stage 2: Match Strings as a Whole

The figural continuity constraint is exploited by counting the seed points along each string of edge points, finding out which other string most seeds want to match, and selecting the choice that is most often made. This operation marks a shift from the fairly local operations embedded in the neighborhood support stage to much more global operations that can in principle span quite large regions of the image (indeed, the whole image if an edge happens to traverse right across it). Seed points that choose to go to the wrong edge string get killed off at this stage (figure 21.8).

This stage copes with mild "wallpaper illusion" prob-

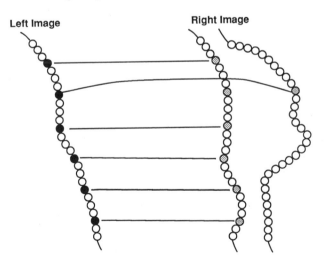

Fig. 21.8
Exploiting the figural continuity constraint by matching strings of edge points as a whole in PMF42. Lines connecting left and right image strings depict matches between initial seed points. The second line from the top shows a match whose right image primitive lies within a different edge string from those of all other matches. This fact is discovered and the discrepant match killed off.

lems caused by similar but not identical edge strings. Of course, there is no way to solve the ambiguity problem posed by repeating identical surface texture elements (the *real* wallpaper illusion problem) unless some disambiguating information can be propagated from the edges of the "wallpaper."

PMF42—Stage 3: Finding Matches In Between Seed Points

This is also done by a species of figural grouping. The procedure employed simply extrapolates from seed points along edge strings except that it can jump over gaps caused by unmatchable edge points. The latter typically arise when left and right image edge points fall outside the allowable orientation limit required for matching (justified by the compatibility constraint and guided by the disparity gradient limit, as in PMF). This tends to happen when the edge string meanders due to local image noise, or closely neighboring edges cause interference in the locations of Canny edge point locations. When small gaps of this kind are crossed, left image edge points lacking a match due to the gap in the right image do not have a disparity value attached to them.

PMF42—Stage 4: Applying the Ordering Constraint Explicitly

It sometimes happens, particularly in image regions with few edges, that whole strings of edges points are incorrectly matched using the figural continuity procedures of stage 3. A check is imposed to discover and remedy such problems using the ordering constraint explicitly and qualitatively. For example, suppose there exist strings A, B, C, D in the left image, each with a strength that is the sum of the strengths of the matches along them (not just length of string). If the matches for these strings in the right image violate the ordering constraint (figure 21.9), then the rule is to kill the weakest strings that result in the ordering constraint being satisfied. The primitives thereby released from matching are considered (along with others also remaining unmatched) in subsequent stages.

PMF42—Stage 5: Imposing an Allowable Disparity Range for Unmatched Points

Some of the remaining ambiguities can be resolved using the ordering constraint to reset the allowable disparity

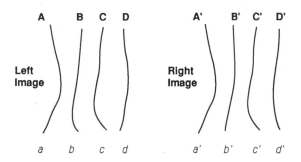

Fig. 21.9
Imposing the ordering constraint explicitly in PMF42. Suppose strings of points existed in the two images as shown, each with associated strengths a, b, ..., c', d'. Suppose also that the correct matches were AA', BB', CC', and DD'. If matches AA', BD', CC', and DB' were initially chosen by PMF42, then the violation of the ordering constraint by matches BD' and DB' would be noted. The weakest strings whose elimination from matching would remove the violation are then discovered and their primitives freed for reconsideration by later stages of matching.

range. That is, matched strings are used to set disparity bounds within which matches must be found for intervening *un*matched points if the ordering constraint is not to be violated. This allows a principled basis on which to eliminate some false matches. Note that this procedure has the advantage of avoiding a fixed disparity range for the whole image.

PMF42—Stage 6: Allow Matches of Opposite Contrast

If all else fails, PMF42 allows matches between left and right edge points of reversed contrast. These can and do occur, typically created by occlusion relationships, as described earlier.

PMF42—Stage 7: Horizontal Edges

As always, horizontal edges present a special problem due to the intractable nature of the matching problem that they pose, namely, there are an infinite number of possible solutions to matching the points comprising horizontal edges. (Think of looking at a dark clothes line against a clear sky: It is reasonable to presume that it is stretched tightly between its supports but the images are also consistent with it being a rigid wire bent to and fro in depth between those supports). PMF42 copes with each horizontal edge point in the left image by positing a range of possible disparity values determined by the size of the horizontal string in the other image which could be

matched with the point in question. This makes no assumptions about the depth variations along horizontal edges.

Performance Examples of PMF42

Figures 21.10 and 21.11 show examples of the output achieved by PMF42.

Discussion

Overview on Constraints

Marr (1982) stated what he called the *fundamental assumption of stereopsis*: "If a correspondence is established between physically meaningful primitives extracted from the left and right images of a scene that contains a sufficient amount of detail, and if the correspondence satisfies the three matching constraints [of compatibility, uniqueness, and continuity] then that correspondence is physically correct (p. 115)."

Marr goes on to point out that this assumption takes the debate away from simply identifying necessary consequences of the way the viewed world projects into stereo images and toward the statement that these consequences are actually *sufficient* to determine unique correspondences. He remarks that "to isolate this fundamental assumption and to establish that it is valid is precisely what I mean by the computational theory of a process (p. 115)." What this amounts to is developing the assumption in more precise terms and then proving that the constraints do indeed force unique correspondences. Marr noted that phrases such as "scene contains a sufficient amount of detail" and "physically meaningful primitives" are stated too imprecisely for mathematical demonstrations.

The theorems provided in Pollard et al. (1985b) proving that use of the disparity gradient imposes a form of scene-to-view and view-to-view continuity during stereo matching seem to satisfy Marr's requirement for a computational theory of the stereo matching process. Moreover, in developing our stereo algorithm from PMF through its various stages to the current version PMF42, we have at all stages been at pains to guide its design by the constraints discussed above.

In so doing, however, it has to be said that the business of implementing constraints in PMF42 has not infrequ-

(a)

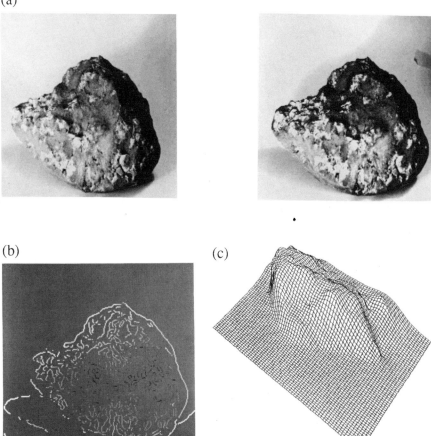

(b)

(c)

Fig. 21.10
Performance of PMF42 on a rock stereogram. (A) Graylevel stereo images arranged for cross-eyed fusion. (B) Matched Canny edge points from the left image coded for relative depths with far = light and near = dark. (C) Smooth depth profile obtained from matches in *b* with the viewpoint from the top left hand side with respect to the other images.

ently taken on the uncomfortable character of a hack, as the difficulties experienced in dealing with natural images lead to an ever greater list of programming refinements. Each one depends in general terms on an heuristic derived from one or other constraint, but the relevance of, for example, the mathematical theorems in Pollard et al. (1985b) are of rather little help when developing a practical and effective stereo algorithm. This experience has led some to regard a great deal of the mathematics in the computer vision literature as "mathematical hair," the implication being that it can be trimmed off without serious loss.

The point being made here is, however, *not* that the theorems of Pollard et al. (1985b) are irrelevant: far from it. They provide the justification for proceeding with a disparity gradient limit at all. But there is an awful lot of hard work involved in moving from that secure mathematical basis to an efficient and reliable stereo system. Much of this effort is at what Marr (1982) calls the *algorithm level*, and its importance should not be underestimated.

Yet it is a moot point whether the numerous refinements incorporated into PMF42 during its development constitute a good example of the kind of work that Marr believed appropriate at the algorithm level, despite each added "bell and whistle" being principled by virtue of being carefully underpinned by constraints. Andrew Parker (personal communication) wonders whether the numerous features incorporated into PMF42 for dealing with the wide variety of different problems thrown up by natural stereo images could be the result of a poor specification of the stereo computation in the first place. Only

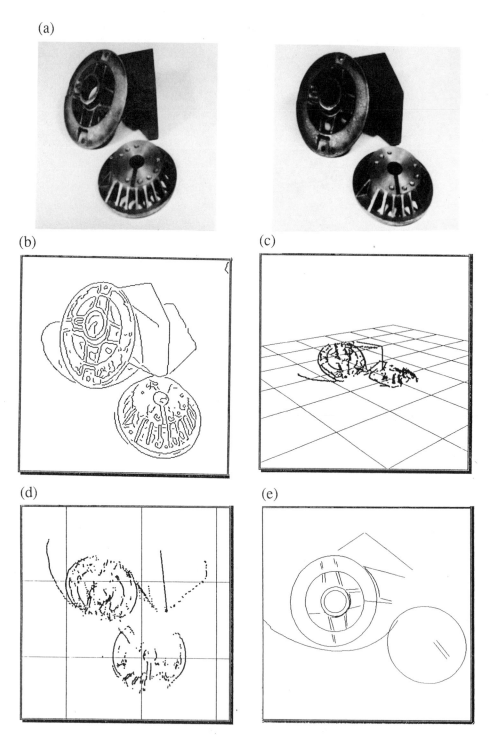

(a)

(b)

(c)

(d)

(e)

Fig. 21.11

Performance of PMF42 on a cluttered scene of industrial objects.
(A) Graylevel stereo images arranged for cross-eyed fusion. (B)
Canny edges for the left image. (C) Perspective view of depth data
recovered by PMF using same program parameters as for the rock in
figure 21.10. (D) Plan view of depth data. (E) Some of the final 3D
descriptions fitted to the depth data as recovered by the TINA
system (Porrill et al., 1987c).

time will tell whether a new specification of the stereo correspondence problem will be found that will lead to a less complex algorithm able to cope straightforwardly with a wide range of natural images. Meanwhile, the multiple modules and stages of PMF42 are typical of state-of-the-art effective computer vision systems. They reflect in part the requirement for reasonable efficiency given the nature of currently available and affordable hardware.

Interpreting Matches to Recover Useful Descriptions of Scene Geometry

The point was made at the outset of this chapter that providing correct stereo matches is not in itself always enough for guiding action. Generally, those matches will need to be interpreted in some way to provide descriptions of 3D scene structures useful for guiding the particular behavior required.

Perhaps the simplest approach in the computational literature to acquiring useful scene geometry from a range map is to *group up connected edge points into strings* (cf. *Gestalt* grouping) and then fit straight lines, circular arcs, and so on to those groupings. This approach has been taken by Porrill et al. (1987c), who used the resulting 3D geometrical entities for model matching. Those entities can also be used as the input for further stages of processing whose goal is to make explicit scene surface topology (i.e., labeling regions and their neighborhood relationships).

An alternative approach is to begin by *reconstructing surfaces by interpolation* between the sparse edge matches and then obtain descriptions of the properties (e.g., planar, quadratic) of surface regions so discovered (Grimson, 1981; see Blake & Zisserman, 1987, for a recent review; McLauchlan et al., 1990). Interpolation over stereo matches can be guided by other depth cues (see later).

A quite different approach to interpreting matched disparity data is to treat them as a vector field and to find the deformation term of its partial derivatives, which gives information about surface structure directly (Koenderink & van Doorn, 1976; Koenderink, 1986 gives a tutorial review). Space forbids an explanation of the technical details, but the reader should be aware that this approach, is being used to guide some current psychophysical studies of human stereo vision (e.g., Rogers & Koenderink,

1986) and has been used to explain the induced effect (see earlier).

Finally, it is worth mentioning approaches that attempt to obtain surface descriptions at the same time as solving the stereo correspondence problem. Pollard (1987) reports a version of the PMF algorithm in which potential matches "vote" for best-fit planar patches, an approach which he notes can be regarded as an implementation of some of the ideas of Koenderink and van Doorn just referred to. Hoff and Ahuja (1987) describe an algorithm that integrates processes of feature matching, contour detection, and smooth surface interpolation using a coarse-to-fine strategy (see also Kass, Witkin & Terzopoulos, 1987). McLauchlan and Mayhew (1989) and McLauchlan et al. (1990) have developed fast Hough transform techniques for integrating 3D surface reconstruction into the stereo matching process, including the detection of surface discontinuities.

Issues for Studies of Biological Binocular Vision Arising from Computational investigations

Regan et al. (1990) discuss the following under this heading.

Many Different Types of Stereo Matching

There seems no reason to believe in "The One True Stereo Algorithm" capable of dealing efficiently with all types of scenes and situations.

Evolving Spatial Structures Over Time

Many algorithms have now been described for solving the stereo correspondence problem for a wide range of natural and artificial images. Typically, however, the image data come from a single "stereo snapshot" (motion algorithms are rarely any better—their "temporal snapshot" is usually just two or three frames long). This neglects the fact that most scenes remain largely unchanged from moment to moment, offering huge potential for speeded-up stereo processing in that there should be no need to solve the stereo correspondence problem ab initio for all parts of the field of view at frame rate, even given a change of viewpoint. This opens up opportunities for predictive feedforward stereo tracking (Pollard, Porrill & Mayhew, 1989).

Are there human stereo mechanisms that integrate matching and surface fitting?

Cue integration

The question of how to integrate disparity information with that from other cues has often been considered from a computational perspective (e.g. Aloimonos & Shulman, 1989; Kass et al., 1987; Marr, 1982). That question has a much longer history of psychophysical studies, some recent stereo/motion examples being the work of Regan (1985), Rogers and Graham (1982), and Rogers and Collett (1989). Buckley et al. (1989; see also Collett, 1985) provide a series of demonstration stereograms suggesting that human vision uses texture boundaries to guide its processes of surface interpolation over sparse stereo cues. Bülthoff's chapter in this book also discusses many studies of how stereo is integrated with other cues.

The Role of Vertical Disparities for "Camera Calibration" in Human Vision

The issue here is whether Mayhew's (1982) equations for obtaining from vertical disparities the viewing parameters of distance to the fixation point d and gaze angle g are implemented in the human visual system (see earlier comments).

Implications for Neurophysiology

Poggio and Poggio (1984) raise many questions on how neurophysiological studies of binocular vision might be profitably guided by computational considerations. One important question is, what exactly is the nature of the computation being performed by cells found to be selectively responsive to disparity? One possibility that might repay investigation is to explore the extent to which the sensitivity of those cells is explicable in terms of the disparity gradient concept. Pollard et al. (1985a) point out that their PMF stereo algorithm can be interpreted as effecting a correlation between images in which the figural distortions that characterise the differences between left and right stereo projections are not allowed to lower the correlation score. Do disparity-selective cells perform their correlation on a similar basis?

Acknowledgments

Our thanks to David Buckley who helped to clarify the paper considerably. We are also grateful for innumerable discussions with John Mayhew, John Porrill, and Neil Thacker, and the useful comments of our referees, Heinrich Bülthoff and Andrew Parker.

References

Aloimonos, J. & Shulman, D. (1989). *Integration of visual modules: An extension of the Marr paradigm.* San Diego, CA.: Academic Press.

Anastasio, T. J. & Robinson, D. A. (1989). Distributed representation of vestibulo-oculomotor signals by brain-stem neurons. *Biological Cybernetics, 61,* 79—88.

Arnold, R. D. & Binford, T. O. (1980). Geometric constraints in stereo vision. *Society of Photo-Optical Instrumentation and Engineering, 238,* 281—292.

Ayache, N. & Faverjon, B. (1985). A fast stereo vision matcher based on prediction and recursive verification of hypotheses. *Proceedings of the Third Workshop on Computer Vision: Representation and Control* (pp. 13—16). Bellaire, U.S.A.

Baker, H. H. (1982). *Depth from edge and intensity based stereo.* PhD thesis, University of Illinois.

Baker, H. H. & Binford, T. O. (1981). Depth from edge and intensity based stereo. In *Proceedings of 7th International Joint Conference on Artificial Intelligence* (pp. 631—636). Los Altos, CA: William Kaufman.

Ballard D. H. & Brown, C. M. (1982). *Computer vision.* New Jersey: Prentice-Hall.

Barlow, H., Blakemore, C. & Pettigrew, J. D. (1967). The neural mechanism of binocular depth discrimination. *Journal of Physiology, 193,* 327—342.

Barnard, S. T. & Fischler, M. A. (1982). Computational stereo. *Computing Surveys, 14,* 553—572.

Barnard, S. T. & Thompson, W. B. (1980). Disparity analysis of images. *IEEE Transactions on Pattern Analysis and Machine Intelligence, PAMI-2,* 333—340.

Blake, A. & Bülthoff, H. H. (1990). Does the brain know the physics of specular reflection? *Nature, 343,* 165—168.

Blake, A. & Zisserman, A. (1987). *Visual reconstruction.* Cambridge, MA: MIT Press.

Brady, M. (1982). Computational approaches to image understanding. *Computing Surveys, 14,* 3—71.

Brady, M. (1987). Seeds of perception. *Proceedings of the Third Alvey Vision Conference* (pp. 259—266). Cambridge, U.K.

Brint, A. T. & Brady, M. (1989). Stereo matching of curves. *Proceedings of the Fifth Alvey Vision Conference* (pp. 187–192). Reading, U.K.

Brooks, R. A. (1985). A robust layered control system for a mobile robot. *IEEE Journal of Robotics and Automation, RA-2,* 14–23.

Buckley, D., Frisby, J. P. & Mayhew, J. E. W. (1989). Integration of stereo and texture cues in the formation of discontinuities during three-dimensional surface interpolation. *Perception, 18,* 563–588.

Bülthoff, H. H. & Fahle, M. (1989). Disparity gradients and depth scaling. *MIT Artificial Intelligence Memo, 1175.*

Bülthoff, H. H. & Mallot, H. A. (1988). Integration of depth modules: Stereo and shading. *Journal of the Optical Society of America A, 5,* 1749–1758.

Burt, P. & Julesz, B. (1980a). A disparity gradient limit for binocular fusion. *Science, 208,* 615–617.

Burt, P. & Julesz, B. (1980b). Modifications of the classical notion of Panum's fusional area. *Perception, 9,* 671–682.

Canny, J. (1986). A computational approach to edge detection. *Transactions on Pattern Analysis and Machine Intelligence, PAMI-8,* 679–698.

Collett, T. S. (1985). Extrapolating and interpolating surfaces in depth. *Proceedings of the Royal Society of London B, 244,* 43–56.

Dean, P., Mayhew, J. E. W. & Thacker, N. (1990) Saccade control in a simulated eye-head system: neural net architectures for efficient learning of inverse kinematics. *AI Vision Research Unit Memo 47,* University of Sheffield, U.K.

Dev, P. (1975). Perception of depth surfaces in random-dot stereograms: A neural model. *International Journal of Man-Machine Studies, 7,* 511–528.

Epstein, L. I. (1984). An attempt to explain the differences between the upper and lower halves of the striate cortical map of the cat's field of view. *Biological Cybernetics, 49,* 175–177.

Frisby, J. P. (1979). *Seeing: Illusion, brain and mind.* Oxford: Oxford University Press.

Frisby, J. P. (1984). An old illusion and a new theory of stereoscopic depth perception. *Nature, 307,* 592–593.

Frisby, J. P. & Roth, B. (1971). Orientation of stimuli and binocular disparity coding. *Quarterly Journal of Experimental Psychology, 23,* 367–372.

Gillam, B. & Lawergren, B. (1983). The induced effect, vertical disparity, and stereoscopic theory. *Perception & Psychophysics, 34,* 121–130.

Grimson, W. E. L. (1981). *From images to surfaces: A computational study of the human early visual system.* Cambridge, MA: MIT Press.

Grimson, W. E. L. (1983). An implementation of a computational theory of visual surface interpolation. *Computer Vision, Graphics and Image Processing, 22,* 39–69.

Harris, C. & Stephens, M. (1988). A combined and corner and edge detector. *Proceedings of the Fourth Alvey Vision Conference* (pp. 147–152). Manchester, U.K.

Helmholtz, H. von (1909/1962). *Physiological Optics Volume 3.* New York: Dover, 1962; English translation by J. P. C. Southall for the *Optical Society of America* (1924) from the 3rd German edition of *Handbuch der physiologischen Optik* (Hamburg: Voss, 1969).

Hoff, W. & Ahuja, N. (1987). Extracting surfaces from stereo images: An integrated approach. *Proceedings of First International Conference on Computer Vision* (pp. 284–294). London: IEEE Computer Society Press.

Julesz, B. (1971). *Foundations of cyclopean perception.* Chicago: University of Chicago.

Julesz, B. (1986). Stereoscopic vision. *Vision Research, 26,* 1601–1612.

Kass, M. H., (1984). Computing stereo correspondence. MSc Thesis, Department of Electrical Engineering and Computer Science. Cambridge, MA: MIT Press.

Kass, M., Witkin, A. & Terzopoulos, D. (1987). Snakes: Active contour models. In *Proceedings of First International Conference on Computer Vision* (pp. 259–268). London: IEEE Computer Society Press.

Koenderink, J. J. (1986). Optic flow. *Vision Research, 26,* 161–180.

Koenderink, J. J. & van Doorn, A. J. (1976). Geometry of binocular vision and a model for stereopsis. *Biological Cybernetics, 21,* 29–35.

Krol, J. D. (1982). *Perceptual ghosts in stereopsis.* PhD thesis, University of Amsterdam.

Longuet-Higgins, H. C. (1982a). The role of the vertical dimension in stereoscopic vision. *Perception, 11,* 377–386.

Longuet-Higgins, H. C. (1982b). Appendix to paper by John Mayhew entitled: The interpretation of stereo information: The computation of stereo orientation and depth. *Perception, 11,* 405–407.

Mallot, H. A., Schulze, E. & Storjohann, K. (1988). Neural network strategies for robot navigation. In G. Dreyfus & L. Personnaz (Eds.), *Proceedings of Euro'88,* Paris.

Marr, D. (1982). *Vision.* San Francisco: Freeman.

Marr, D. & Poggio, T. (1976). A cooperative computation of stereo disparity. *Science, 194,* 283–287.

Marr, D. & Poggio, T. (1979). A theory of human stereopsis. *Proceedings of the Royal Society of London B, 204,* 301–328.

Mayhew, J. E. W. (1982). The interpretation of stereo information: The computation of stereo orientation and depth. *Perception, 11,* 387–403.

Mayhew, J. E. W. (1983). Stereopsis. In O. J. Braddick & A. C. Sleigh (Eds.), *Physiological and biological processing of images* (pp. 204–216). Berlin: Springer-Verlag.

Mayhew, J. E. W. & Frisby, J. P. (1978a). Stereopsis masking is not orientationally tuned. *Perception, 7,* 431–436.

Mayhew, J. E. W. & Frisby, J. P. (1978b). Contrast summation effects and stereopsis. *Perception, 7*, 537–550.

Mayhew, J. E. W. & Frisby, J. P. (1979a). Surfaces with steep variations in depth pose difficulties for orientationally tuned disparity filters. *Perception, 8*, 691–698.

Mayhew, J. E. W. & Frisby, J. P. (1979b). Convergent disparity discriminations in narrow-band-filtered random-dot stereograms. *Vision Research, 19*, 63–71.

Mayhew, J. E. W. & Frisby, J. P. (1980). Psychophysical and computational studies towards a theory of human stereopsis. *Artificial Intelligence, 17*, 349–385.

Mayhew, J. E. W. & Frisby, J. P. (1981). Computation of binocular edges. *Perception, 9*, 69–86.

Mayhew, J. E. W. & Longuet-Higgins, H. C. (1982). A computational model of binocular depth perception. *Nature, 297*, 376–379.

McLauchlan, P. & Mayhew, J. E. W. (1989). Needles: A stereo algorithm for texture. *Proceedings of Conference on Image Understanding and Machine Vision* (pp. 88–91). Cape Cod, MA.

McLauchlan, P., Mayhew, J. E. W. & Frisby, J. P. (1990). Stereoscopic recovery and description of smooth textured surfaces. *Proceedings of First British Machine Vision Conference* (pp. 199–204). Oxford, U.K.

Moravec, H. P. (1977). Towards automatic visual obstacle avoidance. *Proceedings of 5th Joint International Conference on Artificial Intelligence* (p. 584). Cambridge, MA.

Ogle, K. N. (1950). *Researches in binocular vision*. Philadelphia: Saunders.

Peek, S. A., Mayhew, J. E. W. & Frisby, J. P. (1984). Obtaining viewing distance and angle of gaze from vertical disparity using a Hough-type accumulator. *Image & Vision Computing, 2*, 180–190.

Petrov, A. P. (1980). A geometrical explanation of the induced size effect. *Vision Research, 20*, 409–413.

Poggio, G. F. & Poggio, T. (1984). The analysis of stereopsis. *Annual Review of Neuroscience, 7*, 379–412.

Poggio, T., Torre, V. & Koch, C. (1985). Computational vision and regularisation theory. *Nature, 317*, 314–319.

Pollard, S. B. (1985). *Identifying correspondences in binocular stereo*. PhD thesis, University of Sheffield.

Pollard, S. B. (1987). The PMF stereo algorithm: theory and implementation. *British Computer Society Parallel Architectures and Computer Vision Workshop*. Oxford: Oxford University Press.

Pollard, S. B. & Frisby, J. P. (1990). Transparency and the Uniqueness Constraint in Human and Computer Stereo Vision. *Nature, 347*, 553–556.

Pollard, S. B., Mayhew, J. E. W. & Frisby, J. P. (1985a). PMF: A stereo correspondence algorithm using a disparity gradient limit. *Perception, 14*, 449–470.

Pollard, S. B., Porrill, J. & Mayhew, J. E. W. (1989). Predictive feedforward stereo processing. *Proceedings of the Fifth Alvey Vision Conference* (pp. 97–102). Reading, U.K.

Pollard, S. B., Porrill, J., Mayhew, J. E. W. & Frisby, J. P. (1985b). Disparity gradient, Lipschitz continuity and computing stereo correspondences. In *Proceedings of the Third International Symposium of Robotics Research* (pp. 19–26), Gouvieux, France. Cambridge, MA: MIT Press.

Porrill, J., Mayhew, J. E. W. & Frisby, J. P. (1987a). Cyclotorsion, conformal invariance, and induced effects in stereoscopic vision. In *Frontiers of Visual Science: Proceedings of the 1985 Symposium* (pp. 90–108). Washington, DC: National Academy Press

Porrill, J. & Pollard, S. B. (1990). Curve matching and stereo calibration. *Proceedings of First British Machine Vision Conference* (pp. 37–42). Oxford, U.K.

Porrill, J., Pollard, S. B. & Mayhew, J. E. W. (1987b). Optimal combination of multiple sensors including stereo vision. *Image and Vision Computing, 5*, 174–180.

Porrill, J., Pollard, S. B., Pridmore, T. P., Bowen, J. B., Mayhew, J. E. W. & Frisby, J. P. (1987c). TINA: The Sheffield Vision System. *Proceedings of the Ninth International Joint Conference on Artificial Intelligence* (pp. 1138–1144). Milan.

Prazdny, K. (1985). Detection of binocular disparities. *Biological Cybernetics, 52*, 93–99.

Prazdny, K. (1987). On the coarse-to-fine strategy in stereomatching. *Bulletin of the Psychonomic Society, 25*, 92–94.

Regan, D. (1985). Visual processing of four kinds of relative motion. *Vision Research, 26*, 127–145.

Regan, D., Frisby, J. P., Poggio, G., Schor, C. M. & Tyler, C. (1990). Binocular vision. In L. Spillman & J. Werner (Eds.), *Visual perception: The neurophysiological foundations* (pp. 317–347). San Diego, CA: Academic Press.

Rogers, B. J. & Collett, T. S. (1989). The appearance of surfaces specified by motion parallax and binocular disparity. *The Quarterly Journal of Experimental Psychology, 41*, 697–717.

Rogers, B. J. & Graham, M. (1982). Similarities between motion parallax and stereopsis in human depth perception. *Vision Research, 22*, 261–270.

Rogers, J. & Koenderink, J. (1986). Monocular aniseikonia: A motion parallax analogue of the disparity-induced effect. *Nature, 322*, 62–63.

Rygol, M. & Brown, C. R. (1990). MARVIN: A transputer-based system for computer stereo vision. In J. E. W. Mayhew & J. P. Frisby (Eds.), *3D model recognition from stereoscopic cues* (in press). Cambridge, MA: MIT Press.

Saye, A. & Frisby, J. P. (1975). The role of monocularly conspicuous features in facilitating stereopsis from random-dot stereograms. *Perception, 4*, 159–171.

Schor, C. M. & Wood, I. (1985). Disparity range for local stereopsis as a function of luminance spatial frequency. *Vision Research, 23,* 1649–1654.

Sperling, G. (1970). Binocular vision: A physical and neural theory. *American Journal of Psychology, 83,* 461–534.

Thacker, N. & Mayhew, J. E. W. (1989). Stereo camera calibration from arbitrary images (*AI Vision Research Unit Memo 41*). University of Sheffield, Sheffield, U.K.

Trivedi, H. P. (1987). Estimation of stereo and motion parameters using a variational principle. *Image & Vision Computing, 5,* 181–183.

Trivedi, H. P. & Lloyd, S. A. (1986). The role of disparity gradient in stereo vision. *Perception, 14,* 685–690.

Tsai, R. Y. (1986). An efficient and accurate camera calibration technique for 3D machine vision. *Proceedings IEEE Computer Vision and Pattern Recognition, 86* (pp. 364–374).

Tyler, C. W. (1973a). Stereoscopic vision: Cortical limitations and a disparity scaling effect. *Science, 181,* 276–278.

Tyler, C. W. (1973b). Depth perception in disparity gratings. *Nature, 251,* 140–142.

Tyler, C. W. & Scott, A. B. (1979). Binocular vision. In R. Records (Ed). *Physiology of the human eye and visual systems* (pp. 643–671). Hagerstown, Md.: Harper & Row.

Vergnet, R. L., Pollard, S. B. & Mayhew, J. E. W. (1989). Stereo-matching of line segments based upon a 3-dimensional heuristic with potential for parallel implementation. *Proceedings of the Fifth Alvey Vision Conference* (pp. 181–186). Reading, U.K.

Weinshall, D. (1989). Perception of multiple transparent depth planes in stereo vision. *Nature, 341,* 737–739.

Westheimer, G. (1984). Sensitivity for vertical retinal image differences. *Nature, 307,* 632–633.

Zheng, Y., Jones, D. G., Billings, S. A., Mayhew, J. E. W. & Frisby, J. P. (1989). SWITCHER: a stereo algorithm for ground plane obstacle detection. *Proceedings of the Fifth Alvey Vision Conference* (pp. 91–96). Reading, U.K.

22

Stereo, Surfaces, and Shape

Andrew J. Parker,
Elizabeth B. Johnston,
J. Stephen Mansfield,
and Yuede Yang

One of the striking accomplishments of computational vision has been the study of natural images. The physics and mathematics (particularly geometry) of image formation are much better understood than 10 to 15 years ago. The improved understanding has assisted the development and analysis of mechanisms for extracting useful information from images. Figure 22.1 illustrates a common assumption of the role that might be played by stereoscopic depth in providing information about the three-dimensional (3D) shape of objects. The scheme is part of a wider view of early visual processing put forward by the MIT school of computational vision in the early 1980s (Horn, 1986; Marr, 1982). Several machine vision systems have been developed in this framework and, although these systems have many limitations, they have been sufficiently effective to permit their use in robotics control systems (Nishihara, 1984).

From the point of view of biological systems, studies of the feasibility of such schemes (do they do what is claimed?) have run ahead of studies of their applicability (do biological systems actually work like this?). To some degree, this was inevitable for historical and practical reasons: The models have complicated properties, which need full-time attention to sort out. On the other hand, there are some close analogies between the construction of models and the design of experiments. Both deal in particularities (a specific computer program; a set of stimuli and responses), but they attempt to press home general points. Both make the often reasonable, but sometimes disastrous, assumption that small variation in particularities will not affect general conclusions. Often experiments do not fall neatly into the "hypothesis-testing" view of science and, like many modeling exercises, they are constructed so as to illustrate a general approach to a problem. So it would seem that one of the most useful functions of experimental investigations in parallel with modeling is that, as well as establishing factual points, experiments will enforce a critical appraisal of which fea-

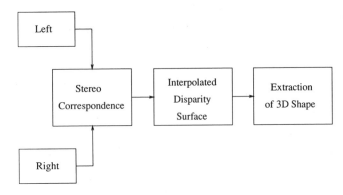

Fig. 22.1
Outline of a processing scheme for the use of stereo vision in extracting information about 3D shape. The general form was suggested by Marr and collaborators at MIT in the late 1970s, but many people have subsequently adapted this framework for their own use.

tures of models are central to their approach and which features simply reflect a consequence of choosing to implement a model in a particular way.

We have carried out a set of experimental investigations in order to understand human stereo vision in more detail and to evaluate the effectiveness of the computational approach for formulating empirical questions about biological visual systems. The three main areas of experimental investigation are: (1) the detection and registration of stereo disparities; (2) the combination of local disparity measures into a smooth surface; and (3) the use of stereo disparity and other cues to extract 3D shape information.

Orientation-specific Masking in Stereo Vision

One open question about stereo vision is the similarity in the shapes of spatial bandpass channels thought to underlie contrast detection (see Watson, 1983; Wilson, 1983) and the shapes of those involved in the detection of stereo disparity. Are the channels involved in stereo detection—particularly detection of fine-grain disparities in random-dot patterns—orientation selective? Mayhew and Frisby (1978) suggested that they are not, because with stereo targets (made from random noise filtered to retain only a limited band of spatial frequencies and orientations) they found that masking noise was equally effective in destroying stereo regardless of its orientation content.

Such a conclusion would provide strong grounds for arguing that the visual channels involved in spatial con-

trast detection are unlike those involved in depth identification. This conclusion would also generate some degree of anomaly with neurophysiological evidence, which suggests that most binocular cells in V1 are selective for orientation, especially in the cat (Hubel & Wiesel, 1962). Although there is evidence for binocular cells in primate V1 with essentially no orientation preference at all (Hawken & Parker, 1984), such cells seem to be relatively poor in the spatial localization of luminance contrast targets (Parker & Hawken, 1985) and it is difficult to see how good stereo performance could be built out of poor localization performance. Moreover, most binocular cells in the primate show an orientation preference, even if they do have a weaker response at orientations orthogonal to the best response (Hawken & Parker, 1984; Livingstone & Hubel, 1984).

The substantial aspects of the Mayhew and Frisby (1978) study are:

• Random-dot stereograms were filtered to exclude all components outside two orthogonal orientation bands (each $\pm 10°$ bandwidth and centered at $0°$ and $90°$ or $\pm 45°$).

• Masking noise filtered in the same way was added to one eye so that either the orientations of the test stereogram and mask were aligned or they differed by $45°$.

• Over a range of relative contrasts of test and mask, there was no difference in the subjective quality of stereopsis for masks aligned with the test stereogram or differing in orientation by $45°$.

Experimental Procedure

In our experiments, a sequence of 8-bit Gaussian random integers was used to generate Julesz-type stereograms (mean luminance = 110 cd m^{-2}; angular size = 1.67°) with a central square patch (angular size = 0.42°) of either crossed or uncrossed disparity, 4 min arc. The random sequence was produced by a method based on the Box-Müller method, implemented as part of the HIPS software package (Landy, Cohen & Sperling, 1984). The images were represented by 256 graylevels corresponding to the 8-bit random integers and were viewed on a Manitron VLR2044 display monitor (P4 phosphor). In high-contrast images, the patch appeared as a raised square in depth above the background or as a sunken square in depth behind the background. These stereo images were filtered in the 2D Fourier domain, using filters with the following form of pass-band in spatial frequency and orientation:

$$F(f, \theta) = \exp\left[-\frac{1}{2}\left(\frac{f - f_{peak}}{\omega f_{peak}}\right)^2\right]$$

$$\times \exp\left[-\frac{1}{2}\left(\frac{\theta - \theta_{peak}}{\beta}\right)^2\right]. \qquad (1)$$

The parameters were chosen to select spatial frequencies centered around 7.5 cycles/degree with bandwidth, ω, set to 0.2. The orientation bandwidth, β, was 20°. The left and right halves were filtered with either $\theta_{peak} = 0°$ (vertical) or $\theta_{peak} = 90°$ (horizontal). The selection of these parameters was motivated by the following considerations: a desire to stay as closely as possible to the parameter values used by Mayhew and Frisby (1978), and the need to explore a range of masking interactions over orientations from 0° to 90°. The filtered stereo pairs formed the signal target for depth identification by the observers. The task of the observer was to make a forced-choice decision as to whether the square was in front of or behind the background.

Sets of masks were generated by filtering additional samples of random noise with $\theta_{peak} = 0°, 30°, 45°, 60°$, and 90°. Different masks of the same θ_{peak} were added independently to the left and right halves of the signal stereo pairs; the masks always had the same contrast in the left and right eyes. All targets and masks had the same bandwidth, so contrast was defined in terms of root mean square (r.m.s.) values. Contrast was calculated separately for each sample of filtered noise. The contrast of the stereo signal target (-27dB re unity contrast, about 4 times detection threshold) was held constant and the frequency of correctly identifying the disparity (either "in front of" or "behind") was measured for different levels of mask contrast in a forced-choice procedure.

The probability of correctly identifying the depth is plotted for observer JSM in figure 22.2A as a function of the *amplitude ratio* of the signal and mask contrasts, for the case where the signal stereo pair was filtered with $\theta_{peak} = 0°$ (vertical) and for three orientations of mask (0°, 45°, 90°). Figure 22.2B shows for two observers a summary of the values of signal/noise ratio for 75 percent correct identification for five orientations of masking noise. It can be seen that performance steadily improves as the angle between signal and mask increases. Figure 22.2C shows the same procedure for a test orientation θ equal to 90° and the same improvement can be seen as the difference in orientations increases.

Discussion

Figure 22.2 shows an orientation-dependent component in the masking of stereo depth identification. Where the test and mask patterns differ in orientation by 90°, the test pattern is more readily visible by a factor of about 10 dB, compared to the condition where test and mask orientations were aligned. These data are contrary to the conclusions reached by Mayhew and Frisby (1978), but it is more difficult to determine if these quantitative results are incompatible with the demonstration stereograms presented in their paper. The main difference is the use of a forced-choice detection procedure in this study, as opposed to subjective reports concerning the quality of stereopsis. No direct feedback was given to the observers during the trials, but it is interesting to note that, by the end of the many trials of observations, neither observer found the original Mayhew and Frisby demonstrations convincing.

The demonstration offered by Mayhew and Frisby (1978) is a comparison between masks that are aligned with the test patterns and those that are rotated by 45°. Our data suggest that this should have led to about a 5 dB difference in the detectability of the test pattern. There was also a significant elevation of stereo identification thresholds by masking patterns that are at 90° to the test pattern, an effect which Mansfield (in preparation) has characterized in more detail. It is therefore possible that casual inspection of the Mayhew and Frisby figures may not suffice to reveal the orientation-dependent component in the effectiveness of their masks.

A further point is that both the test patterns and masks used by Mayhew and Frisby (1978) were two-component patterns, containing a pair of orientations orthogonal to each other. This approach restricts to $\pm 45°$ the range of orientation differences that can be explored. Mayhew and Frisby (1978) mentioned that they found stereo judgments to be more difficult with one-component patterns, but this was not a problem for our observers. This is probably because the orientation bandwidth of our stimuli was broader, being 20° rather than 10° as for Mayhew and Frisby (1978). For simple detection, there is a difference in the efficacy of one- and two-component sinewave grating masks (Derrington & Henning, 1989). The

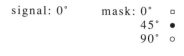

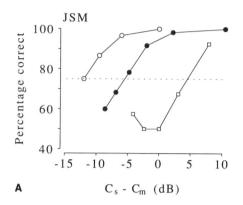

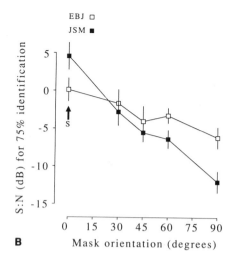

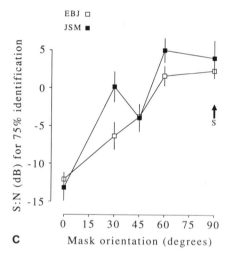

Fig. 22.2

(A) Psychometric functions for the detection of depth information as a function of contrast in spatially filtered random-dot targets in the presence of masking noise (see text for details of spectral characteristics of masks and filters). The abscissa shows the difference in dB between the contrast of the signal target (itself held constant at −27 dB *re* unity contrast) and the contrast of the masking noise. The ordinate shows the percentage of correct decisions in a forced-choice task, where the observer had to say whether a central square region in the stereogram was in front of or behind the surrounding region. The target stereogram was filtered to leave information only in a band of orientations about the vertical; different symbols indicate psychometric functions for the detection of stereo depth in the presence of different orientations of masking noise, ranging from 0° (vertical—same as stereo target) to 90° (horizontal—orthogonal to stereo target). The dashed horizontal line shows the criterion level of 75 percent correct. (B) The masking effect of added noise on depth identification as a function of the orientation of the noise pattern. The ordinate shows the ratio of target contrast to mask contrast expressed in dB for a performance of 75 percent correct, derived from forced-choice data as illustrated in (A). The orientation of the signal target was vertical, 0°, the abscissa shows the orientation of the added masking noise. The masking noise is much less effective when its orientation differs from that of the signal target. Different symbols are for two observers. (C) Same as (B), except that the target stereogram was filtered to leave only horizontal orientations.

data in figure 22.2 were gathered with one-component test patterns and masks, so it is possible that the using two-component tests and masks may broaden the bandwidth of masking, as appears to be the case for contrast detection (Derrington & Henning, 1989).

It may also be suggested that the extended nature of forced-choice testing procedure leads in itself to a change in the type of mechanism used for stereo detection, from

nonoriented to orientation selective (Bülthoff, Frisby, personal communication). Little can be said about this without more data, but asymptotically stable responses are usually sought before any psychophysical measurements are undertaken. Certainly, if a comparison with other masking experiments is required, then the subjects should be made thoroughly familiar with the task before formal data collection is begun.

The real issue at stake is whether the orientation dependence of masking of stereo detection is significantly different from that found for masking of simple monocular contrast detection. Phillips and Wilson (1984) measured the masking effect of cosine gratings of different orientations on the detectability of stimuli whose luminance profile had a sixth derivative of a Gaussian cross-section. Although their results indicate the existence of orientation-specific masking for contrast detection and can be processed to yield convincing estimates of channel bandwidths, it is clear that masking remains a complex and uncertain paradigm for investigating the properties of visual channels, as illustrated by the results of Derrington and Henning (1989), who show masking effects on contrast detection by orientation components as far as 67.5° from the test target. Perhaps the most positive point that can be made at this stage is that the Frisby and Mayhew (1978) result can no longer be taken as a firm indication of the contribution of nonoriented mechanisms to stereopsis. Equally, neither do the present results prove that stereo processing occurs exclusively through orientation-selective stereo channels.

Disparity Pooling

A number of psychophysical and computational studies point to the existence of processes concerned with combining local information from individual disparity-detecting elements into a globally consistent interpretation. A simple random-dot stereogram is readily seen as a continuous, smooth surface in depth, with all the individual dots belonging to this surface. Even with a very low spatial density of dots, the perception of continuity persists. This subjective impression of continuity is in accord with other psychophysical observations implying the construction of global organization from local ones and with computational proposals that there may be a stage of interpolation within the disparity field, *after* stereo correspondences have been established (Grimson, 1982; Terzopoulos, 1988).

It is worth reflecting on the motivations for the computational proposals for surface interpolation (e.g., Grimson, 1982). Crudely characterized, the need to smooth the disparity field arose because of (1) the noisiness of the edge features as found by the Laplacian of a Gaussian ($\nabla^2 G$) edge-finder and (2) the scarcity of suitable edge-features for stereo matching, especially in many natural scenes. Attempts to help with the noise problem by increasing the space constant of the Gaussian smoothing filter used in the edge-finder only served to make even more sparse the distribution of suitable edges within the image. The natural framework for recovering a continuous function from a sparse distribution of matched edges is that of interpolation.

Whatever the form of the process that smooths the disparity field, one may expect that the disparity values of spatially adjacent points will interact with one another. Mitchison and Westheimer (1984) and Westheimer (1986) have demonstrated this kind of effect with isolated line elements. In these experiments, we attempted to study disparity interactions using random dot targets. Stereograms were created in which two distinctly different disparity values were essentially superposed within the same spatial region. A more extensive account of the results of this section has recently appeared in full form (Parker & Yang, 1989).

Stimuli and Methods

The technique used to construct the stereograms was originally devised by Schumer (1979). In a simple stereogram depicting a planar patch of frontoparallel surface, all the dots in the patch are displaced horizontally by the same distance. By contrast, in those studied here, different displacements were applied to alternate rows of dots within the patch. Thus the odd-numbered rows might be shifted by one disparity (d_1), while the even-numbered rows might be shifted by a different disparity (d_2). Such a target will be called a mixed disparity target, with a difference between the component disparities: $\Delta d = d_1 - d_2$. The "averaged disparity" of such a region is a depth plane defined as $(d_1 + d_2)/2$ and regions where $d_1 = d_2$ are termed "normal." In figure 22.3, the left and right eye patterns are shown, with arrows indicating the correspondences between the rows. This diagram is only schematic, because the actual rows of elements in test patterns used in the experiments were 2 pixels in height (28 sec arc) and not 1 pixel as shown for the sake of illustration in figure 22.3.

The left and right images of a random-dot stereogram were generated on a CRT display (the monochrome graphics console of a SUN 3/160M workstation). The images were brought into alignment at the viewing distance (4.34 m) by first-surface mirrors. Each pixel subtended 14.25 sec arc, and the whole stereogram subtended approximately 1.4°. Two horizontal bars (approximately 0.7° wide by 0.27° high) were defined in the stereogram in depth planes different from the background. The bars were located above and below the fixation point, which was presented before and after each trial, approximately 1 sec in duration. The task of the observer was to say which of

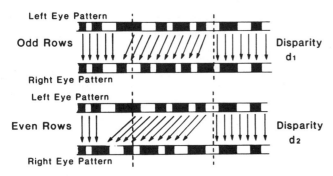

Fig. 22.3
Method of constructing random dot stereograms to test for disparity averaging. Alternative rows of dots in the stereo image are assigned different disparities, d_1 and d_2. Under some conditions, the disparities fuse together to form a single region with a depth value, $(d_1 + d_2)/2$. (Reprinted with permission from *Vision Research*, 29, Parker & Yang, Spatial properties of a stereo disparity pooling process, copyright 1989, Pergamon Press PLC.)

the two bars was nearer. Typically, the upper bar was a test target containing mixed disparities and the lower bar was one of a set of normal comparison targets, each containing just one disparity. This set of normal targets (five or seven in number) was arranged to span the point at which the lower and upper bars were expected to have subjectively equal depth. At least 200 trials of this forced choice procedure were carried out for each test target. A cumulative Gaussian curve was fitted to the psychometric function and the mean of the Gaussian (50 percent point on the psychometric function) was taken as the point of subjective equality, subsequently called the "matching" or "apparent" disparity. The standard deviation of the cumulative Gaussian (describing the slope of the psychometric function) was taken as a measure of stereo acuity with this configuration.

Results

Figure 22.4A indicates the arrangement of test and comparison targets during the psychophysical trials and figure 22.4B shows a sample psychometric function generated by observer YY. It can be seen that the disparity value of the comparison stimulus corresponding to $p = 0.5$ agrees well with the calculated mean disparity of the test target, $(d_1 + d_2)/2$. Moreover, the steepness of the psychometric function demonstrates that the test stimulus is not ambiguous, with one value of perceived depth on some trials and a different one on others. In fact, over a reasonable range of combinations of disparities in the test target,

stereo acuity is relatively close to that for "normal" test targets (Parker & Yang, 1989).

The phenomenon of disparity averaging, in the form illustrated in figure 22.4B, occurs only for a restricted set of combinations of disparities, d_1 and d_2. Within these limits, observers report the subjective impression of a single surface, almost smooth in appearance though not identical with a normal test target. As the disparity difference between the components increases, this single surface starts to break up into a "noisy" surface with many individual points at different disparities. At large differences, two surfaces can be seen; the nearer of these is, in some sense or other, transparent (Schumer, 1979; Tyler, 1983).

A simple prediction based on linear pooling of component disparities is that the depth plane perceived by the observer should lie at the calculated mean disparity of the target, $(d_1 + d_2)/2$, (e.g., Mitchison & Westheimer, 1984). How close to this simple expectation are our results, and for what ranges of test disparities does the expectation hold up? The stereo acuity of observers with normal test targets was used to set an objective criterion for deciding whether or not data were consistent with the prediction based on disparity averaging. The estimates of stereo acuity (10.5 sec arc for YY; 23 sec arc for DS) were obtained from the slope of the cumulative Gaussian describing the psychometric function with normal test targets. If the difference between the actual match and the predicted match fell within ± 1 j.n.d. of zero, then the combination of disparities in the test target was taken as consistent with the simple linear pooling prediction. Throughout the psychophysical judgments, observers were asked to respond to the nearest surface if there was any subjective ambiguity in the display. Probably as a consequence, as soon as the display takes on "thickened" appearance, the observer's matches are forced away from the match predicted on simple linear pooling.

Figure 22.5 shows the combinations of component disparities that support the linear pooling prediction with observers YY and DS. When the averaged disparity of the test target is offset from the fixation plane, a larger difference between the components can be tolerated. At the largest offsets from the fixation plane (greater than 300 sec arc), disparity averaging is again poor, possibly because one of the component disparities then falls outside the effective range of Panum's fusional area with these targets.

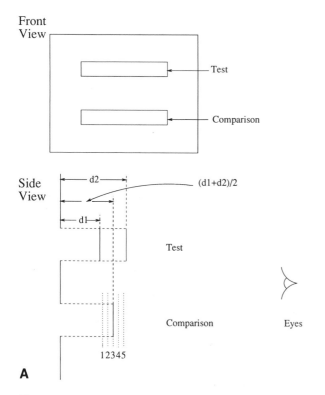

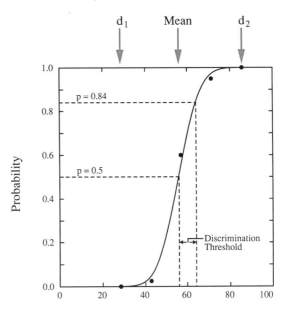

Psychometric Function

B Disparity of Comparison Stimulus (sec arc)

Fig. 22.4

(A) Relationship between test and match targets during measurements of disparity averaging. The observer was required to make judgments of the relative depths of the upper (test) target and the lower (comparison) target. The set of comparison targets was arranged to span the averaged depth of the test region, $(d_1 + d_2)/2$. (B) Psychometric function for depth judgments with a mixed disparity target. The data points indicate probability of reporting the comparison target as nearer than the test target as a function of the disparity of the comparison stimulus. The data are well described by the cumulative Gaussian function. (After a figure in Parker & Yang, 1989.)

What is the Site of Interpolation?

At least two hypotheses can be entertained for the averaging effect studied here. The first is that disparity signals are associated internally with each of the component disparities in the image; then there is a process of interpolation over those disparity values. The second is that, during the process of stereo matching, local features within the monocular images are extracted from a region covering several pixels (as a consequence of low-pass filtering of the image), thus effectively pooling together the information that could potentially define the component disparities as separate. Hence, disparity averaging could be a consequence of processing taking place either at a monocular stage or possibly actually at the point where stereo correspondence is established.

Several points suggest the second of these alternatives. Disparity averaging occurs only over a restricted range of test disparities and the pattern of results with changes in the combinations of disparities is not obviously related to the operation of a simple interpolation process. Quantitatively, the upper limit of averaging at the fixation plane is about 80 sec arc for the observer with good stereo acuity (YY); this agrees well with an upper limit of at most 22 cycles/degree for supporting stereo acuity determined by Westheimer and McKee (1980). In separate experiments with slanted and sinusoidally corrugated surfaces (Yang & Parker, 1988), we have been able to investigate the significance of potentially important factors such as spatial extent of the target, disparity gradient, and total range of disparities within the mixed disparity target. The actual shape of the surface itself is relatively unimportant in determining the occurrence of disparity averaging, whereas the actual range of disparities within the target is important. This suggests that with these targets disparity pooling is determined primarily by the local interactions between point disparities and does not involve the use of higher order derivatives of the disparity field.

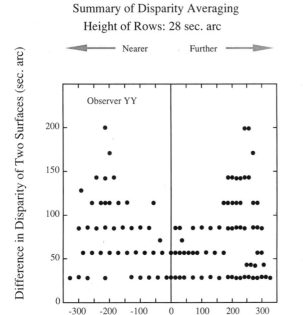

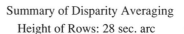

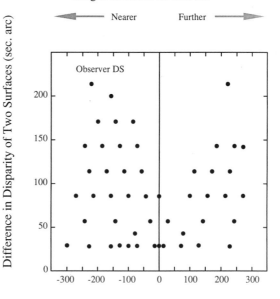

Summary of Disparity Averaging
Height of Rows: 28 sec. arc

◄— Nearer   Further —►

Observer YY

Difference in Disparity of Two Surfaces (sec. arc)

Averaged Disparity of Two Surfaces (sec. arc)

Summary of Disparity Averaging
Height of Rows: 28 sec. arc

◄— Nearer   Further —►

Observer DS

Difference in Disparity of Two Surfaces (sec. arc)

Averaged Disparity of Two Surfaces (sec. arc)

Fig. 22.5

Summary of conditions supporting disparity averaging in random-dot figures. Each point shows a combination of averaged disparity in the target, $(d_1 + d_2)/2$, plotted on the abscissa, and difference between the component disparities, $\Delta d = d_1 - d_2$, plotted on the ordinate. Each point illustrated here supports the perceptual phenomenon of disparity averaging. Close to the zero disparity plane, only small differences ($\Delta d \approx 80$ sec arc) can be tolerated, but at nonzero disparities larger differences are successfully fused together ($\Delta d \approx 200$ sec arc). (Reprinted with permission from *Vision Research*, 29, Parker & Yang, Spatial properties of a stereo disparity pooling process, copyright 1989, Pergamon Press PLC.)

Disparity Gradient Limits and The Ordering Constraint

A variation on the stimulus patterns used in the last section provides some insight into how candidate matches in stereo processing might be selected. Often in a pair of images, there is a large number of low-level features that contribute to matching up the left and right images of the stereo pair and, therefore, there are many opportunities for establishing correspondences that are locally feasible but globally false. Accordingly, machine-based visual systems make assumptions about the configuration of objects and surfaces in the natural world, and these assumptions yield a number of constraints that can be applied to eliminate inappropriate correspondences.

One of the most common assumptions is that 3D surfaces are opaque, as well as locally continuous and smooth. Abrupt discontinuities are tolerable, provided they do not occur "too often." This has led to the formulation of a number of different constraints, which differ in detail but have a common purpose. Essentially, they attempt to eliminate candidate matches between pairs of points where the nearer would occlude the latter (corresponding to one object lying behind another in 3D). On the other hand, they permit (or even positively encourage) candidate matches that would yield similar disparity values for pairs of points that are near each other in the visual field, because this would correspond geometrically to a smooth surface in 3D space. The effect of this can be seen in figure 22.6: Candidate matches corresponding to points *P* and *A* would be mutually exclusive outcomes, whereas candidate matches to *P* and *B* would be mutually acceptable, or even mutually reinforcing. The embodiment of this general principle in a computational model dates back at least to the Marr/Poggio Mark-1 stereo algorithm (Marr & Poggio, 1976) and before (Dev, 1975), and it has continued to appear as a significant element in computational modeling (see chapter 21).

Baker (1982) developed a formulation termed the *ordering constraint*, whose basis is the observation that the projection of points *P* and *B* has the same order in left and

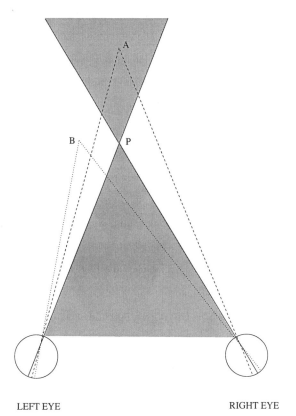

Fig. 22.6
The geometry of stereo correspondence is regard to the ordering constraint and the "forbidden" zone. The interocular separation is greatly exaggerated with respect to typical viewing distances. The observer is looking at point P. Point A is in the "forbidden" zone: From left to right on the retinae, the order of projections is P_L, A_L in the left eye and A_R, P_R in the right eye. By contrast, the ordering of projections for points P and B is the same in the two eyes. This geometrical relationship has been used to eliminate potential stereo matches within stereo algorithms—matches to P and A would not be allowed to coexist, whereas P and B would be allowed. Simultaneous matches to P and A would also violate the disparity gradient limit.

right images (the projection of B is to the right of P in both images), whereas the projection of points P and A is in reverse order. Baker developed an algorithm for machine-based stereo matching applying this principle along epipolar lines in the images. Thus the ordering constraint implies a forbidden zone (shaded area in figure 22.6) around each possible stereo match. The boundaries of the zone correspond to the classic Panum's limiting case, where one feature in one eye would be required to match simultaneously to two spatially separated features in the other eye.

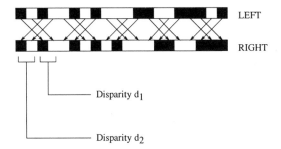

Fig. 22.7
The method of constructing stereograms to test the ordering constraint at local spatial scales. The procedure is similar to that in figure 22.3, except that columns of dot-pairs are interchanged so as to give individual columns different disparity values, d_1 and d_2. This interchange of colums necessarily means that the local order of features along a horizontal line (see figure 22.6) is interchanged in the left and right eyes, and so the ordering constraint for those features is violated.

A forbidden zone of dimensions similar to the region depicted in figure 22.6 is implied by matching schemes that exploit a limit based on *disparity gradient*—for present purposes, the disparity gradient can be expressed as the derivative of horizontal disparity with respect to cyclopean visual angle. In accord with the conclusions of Burt and Julesz (1980) about human vision, these matching schemes reject any pairs of matches that imply disparity gradients higher than a criterion value (typically, 1 or 2, for example, Pollard, Mayhew & Frisby, 1985). *Any match that violates the ordering constraint would also exceed the commonly accepted limits on the disparity gradient.* Moreover, Trivedi and Lloyd (1985) showed that disparity gradients of less than 2 are always produced, if the disparity field is consistent with viewing a continuous, opaque 3D surface.

Experimental Strategy and Results

Both the phenomenon of transparency in random-dot stereograms and of stereopsis in Panum's limiting case create problems for the above schemes (Braddick, 1978). Here we used random-dot stereograms in which we embedded many pairs of points that violated the ordering constraint (and thereby the disparity gradient limit). In figure 22.7, the rows of dots represent single rows from the 2D random-dot pattern. Within the *test* region, vertical columns of dot-pairs were interchanged according to the illustrated scheme. Thus, pixel-pairs with labels A_L, B_L, C_L, D_L,..., in the left image were ordered as B_R, A_R,

Width of Columns: 28 sec. arc
Summary of Disparity Averaging

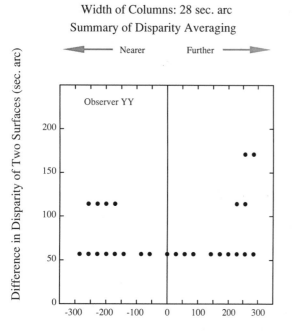

Width of Columns: 28 sec. arc
Summary of Disparity Averaging

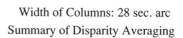

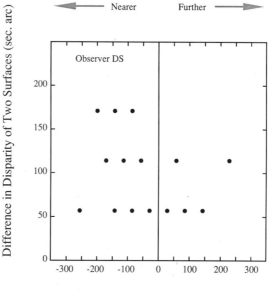

Fig. 22.8

Summary of conditions where stereopsis is achieved with local violations of the ordering constraint. Each point shows a combination of averaged disparity in the target, $(d_1 + d_2)/2$, plotted on the abscissa, and difference between the component disparities, $\Delta d = d_1 - d_2$, plotted on the ordinate. Each point illustrated here supports the perceptual phenomenon of disparity averaging using the same criterion that was applied to the results in figure 22.5. The points are more sparsely spaced than those in figure 22.5, owing to the geometrical constraints on the selection of different disparity combinations. The range over which the component disparities are assimilated into a single depth value, $(d_1 + d_2)/2$ is possibly a little more restricted than in figure 22.5, but the overall pattern of results is broadly similar.

D_R, C_R, ..., in the right image. The interchange of columns of dot-pairs together with any overall disparity applied to both columns resulted in test regions having two component disparities (d_1 and d_2) embedded within it. There is, of course, a strong similarity between this stimulus and those studied in the previous section.

As previously, the observers made judgments of relative depth between a comparison region, which contained only one disparity, and the test region. From the results discussed earlier (see Disparity Pooling), if the test region contains two disparities defined in different *rows* of dots, then the two disparities are sometimes integrated into a single plane, whose depth is estimated to be at the aver-

age of d_1 and d_2 (*disparity averaging*). When there is a large difference between d_1 and d_2, two surfaces are seen, the nearer of the two being transparent or lacy. The same set of subjective phenomena are observed with these targets where *columns* of dots are interchanged.

Both disparity averaging and transparency were observed with the stimuli studied here, which involved an interchange of columns and therefore a violation of the ordering constraint. We used the same quantitative criteria as applied before for deciding whether disparity averaging was occurring. Figure 22.8 summarizes results from two observers. Each point represents a combination of disparities d_1, d_2 that successfully supported disparity averaging. The two disparities are reexpressed as the average disparity $[(d_1 + d_2)/2]$ on the abscissa and the disparity difference $[\Delta d = d_1 - d_2]$ on the ordinate. It should be noted that the reason for the sparseness of points is that feasible combinations of d_1 and d_2 are limited by the geometry of construction of the random-dot figures. Also, the quantitative criterion for disparity averaging is probably rather strict. The overall range of disparities that support pooling seems much the same under these conditions as those discussed earlier, where rows of dots received different disparity values.

Transparency

The existence of transparency with some configurations seems to conflict with one of the constraints on matching employed by Marr and Poggio (1976) and others. At first, transparency seems to suggest that two matches may be permitted along a single cyclopean line of sight, thus breaking the *uniqueness* constraint. Braddick (1978) noted this complication and mentioned also the problems raised by Panum's limiting case, a stimulus configuration in which the right eye sees one vertical line and the left eye sees two vertical lines slightly separated. This configuration gives the impression of stereo depth, as if the single bar in the right eye can simultaneously match up with both bars in the left eye. Braddick (1978) also created a random-dot equivalent of this configuration. In the case of the stimulus targets studied in this section and the previous, the subjective appearance of transparency is difficult to interpret unambiguously. Certainly, the subjective appearance by itself is not a "knockdown" argument against the uniqueness constraint, especially when that constraint is cast in the form of a local disparity gradient around each potential match (Prazdny, 1985). The reason is that an alternative interpretation of the reported appearance is that the observer sees the nearer surface as "lacy" (Pollard, Mayhew & Frisby, 1985), in the sense that it is an opaque surface with holes in it. The stereo matches defining the rear surface could be established locally through the holes.

The feasibility of such a scheme has been established by the simulations of Pollard, Mayhew, and Frisby (1985) and Prazdny (1985). However, there are problems with the range of test targets used for evaluating these computational models, so the general applicability of their schemes is not secure. Their test patterns consisted of relatively sparse random-dot stereograms and there would be ample opportunity for isolated stereo matches to co-exist for both front and rear planes. The problem is that the sparseness of the dots isolates individual dots sufficiently to allow the formation of enough local matches that do not violate the disparity gradient limit. It is therefore uncertain how well these algorithms would cope with the more densely packed random dot patterns used in this work.

The Effects of Spatial Filtering

The disparity pooling observed with interchange of columns in this section seems to be generally similar to that involving the interchange of rows described in the section Disparity Pooling. In the case of stimuli involving interchange of columns, one may observe qualitatively, that, while the manipulations of disparity upset short-range ordering of stereo matches, longer-range ordering is still preserved and is still subject to the ordering constraint. In principle, this longer-range ordering could be made manifest by low-pass filtering of the image and the next section explores this possibility using a cross-correlation matching model.

Properties of A Cross-correlation Model

To illustrate the general effects of early monocular filtering on disparity pooling, suppose, somewhat unrealistically, that stereopsis is modeled as a stage of low-pass filtering of the image followed by an area-based correlation between the two images. In what follows, the description of graylevels in the images will be by means of contrast values and will set aside the overall mean luminance (d.c. level) of the image. Thus some authors will refer to the following calculation as forming a covariance sum rather than a correlation, although usage differs (Bracewell, 1986).

It is simplest to deal with the correlation as if it were a 1D correlation function along corresponding horizontal lines in the left and right eye images. Note that the cross-correlation function of the left and right portions of the random-dot stereogram is a unit impulse function centered at the disparity of the region (assuming the stimulus is truly random and infinite in extent). The cross-correlation of the filtered version of the stereogram is the unit impulse function convolved with the shape of the filter itself (see Bracewell, 1986, for a discussion of these mathematical properties). Thus, if we model the filter by a single Gaussian, the cross-correlation function of the mixed disparity target consists of two Gaussian functions, whose peaks are separated by the difference ($\Delta d = d_1 - d_2$) in the component disparities.

The two Gaussian functions arise either from the pooling of adjacent horizontal rows (see Disparity Pooling) or they reflect the pattern of disparities embedded within alternate columns (see Disparity Gradient Limits). The task faced by the visual system is to segregate these two Gaussian functions. At small separations, the two Gaussian functions result in a single function whose peak is

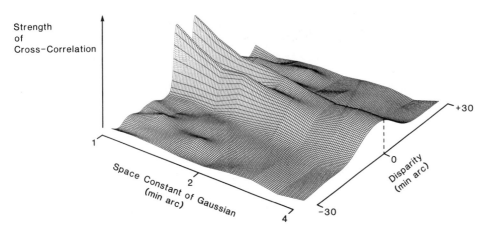

Strength of Cross-Correlation

Space Constant of Gaussian (min arc)

Disparity (min arc)

Fig. 22.9

Scale-space diagram of correlation model of stereo matching. The left and right 1D images that were input to the model consisted of randomly black (-1) or white ($+1$) dots organized to incorporate two component disparities, d_1 and d_2, as illustrated in figure 22.7. The left and right images were filtered spatially with a Gaussian filter whose space constant ranged from 1 to 4 min arc. The resulting signals are cross-correlated without normalization. The figure shows a plot of disparity along the y-axis, the space constant of the Gaussian filter along the x-axis and the strength of the cross-correlation is indicated by the vertical z-axis. At small spatial scales (1 min arc), the component disparities create two peaks in the cross-correlogram at d_1 and d_2, but the smoothing effect of the Gaussian filter fuses these two peaks together at coarser spatial scales. The values of d_1 and d_2 are among the more extreme explored in the experiments, while the range of space constants for the Gaussian filters is thought to be typical for human foveal vision.

halfway between the peaks of the two components; this would correspond to disparity averaging. As separation increases, the individual peaks of the Gaussians are distinct; this would correspond to seeing two surfaces. The suggestion for disparity pooling is not restricted to this simplified schematic model. Almost any model with spatial filtering and stereo matching—for example, the sign correlation model of Nishihara (1984, 1989)—will show similar behavior.

A simple 1D model was constructed to illustrate this point. The prime purpose was to reveal the sorts of information present in the stereograms that could be exploited by the human visual system; the model is not intended as a serious contender to account for human stereo vision. The model was applied to the stereograms studied in the section on disparity gradient limits, which had violations of the ordering constraint owing to the interchange of columns, but the same principles will apply

to the stereograms from the section on disparity pooling, where individual rows were interchanged.

Single corresponding rows of dots from the left and right stereo images were each convolved in the space domain with a single Gaussian function. The resulting left and right eye signals were cross-correlated. This calculation was carried out for a set of Gaussian filters with space constants ranging from 1 min arc to 4 min arc—a realistic choice for human foveal vision. The resulting set of correlation functions is represented in figure 22.9: The y-axis represents disparity (ranging from -30 min arc to $+30$ min arc), the x-axis represents the space constant of the Gaussian filter (from 1 min arc to 4 min arc on a logarithmic scale) and the z-axis represents different strengths of the cross-correlation product. The value of the cross-correlation product has not been normalized, because the form of the cross-correlation function is the only point of interest in this demonstration. At small scales, the two peaks in the cross-correlation are clearly seen, while at coarser scales, the two peaks merge into one. The implication of the greater range of disparity averaging at disparities away from the fixation plane would be that such disparities are processed through coarser scales of filter.

Are the ranges of interactions predicted by this kind of model sufficient to account for the disparity averaging phenomena? Certainly, the parameters used for the simulation illustrated in figure 22.9 were conservatively chosen: the disparity difference (Δd) was one of the largest tested (460 sec arc) and the peaks of the two correlation functions are fused at scales of Gaussian filter coarser than about 2 min arc space constant. Hence, the disparity pooling effects studied experimentally in this work could easily be accommodated by a simple model based on spatial filtering. With a further modification, the model could, in principle, predict the depth repulsion effects studied by Westheimer (1986) and Westheimer and Levi (1987). Suppose, quite reasonably, that the spatial monocular filters applied to the left and right images are bandpass in shape ather than lowpass. The consequence in the cross-correlation diagrams would be to replace the Gaussian peaks with peaks surrounded by valleys of *anticorrelation*. Consider a pair of such peak and valley functions that are initially superimposed but then are drawn apart gradually, simulating a steady change in Δd. As the peaks separate and interact with the valleys, there will be a limited region of interaction in which an effective repulsion of the peaks takes place. It remains to determine for certain whether these interactions in the cross-correlation diagram are sufficiently large to account for the experimentally observed sizes of disparity interactions.

3D Shape Judgments

A crucial aspect of the $2\frac{1}{2}$D sketch was that the visual system should be able to make some useful judgments about true 3D shape based on the information within the $2\frac{1}{2}$D sketch. Marr and Nishihara (1978) suggested volumetric representations based on generalized cylinders for the next stage. Earlier Koenderink and van Doorn (1976) had noted some of the invariant properties of stereo disparity fields and later work explored the computational properties of a variety of representations (Besl & Jain, 1986; Brady, Ponce, Yuille & Asada, 1985). In all of this work, the assumption has been that, in a heavily textured image, stereo will offer a moderately robust route to extracting 3D shape information from visual scenes. How well can human observers use stereo information in a shape judgment task?

The experiments presented here arose from a chance observation during some studies of the curvature discrimination capabilities of human observers (Johnston & Parker, 1987a,b, 1988) with surfaces defined by stereo depth. The stimuli for that study were 3D half-cylinders with the axis of symmetry lying in the horizontal meridian of the observer's visual field. It was noted that, even though the experimenter had arranged the geometrical distribution of disparities within the target to correspond exactly with a truly solid shape of exact hemicircular

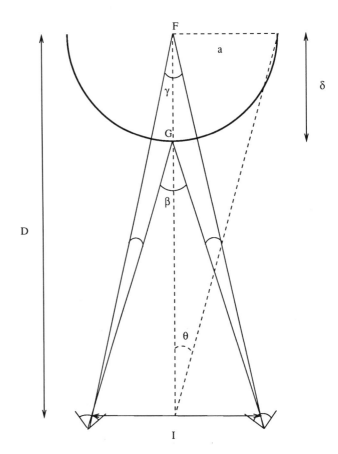

Fig. 22.10

Illustration of the geometrical relationships between angular measures (visual angle and stereo disparity) and distance measures (lateral extent and depth) when an observer is viewing a segment of cylindrical surface with symmetric convergence in the midline. The relationship between lateral extent (a) and visual angle (θ) scales with $1/D$, where D is the absolute viewing distance, while the relationship between depth (δ, which equals a for a circle) and stereo disparity (μ) scales with $1/D^2$. In detail, using small angle approximations, $\theta = a/D$ and $\mu = \beta - \gamma = I/(D - \delta) - I/D \approx I\delta/D^2$.

cross-section, the figures had a distorted shape and appeared hemielliptical in cross-section.

It seemed likely that the source of the distortion was an inappropriate estimate of absolute viewing distance by the observer. Figure 22.10 illustrates the point that, for shapes of circular cross-section viewed symmetrically in the midline, the stereo disparities and true depth are related as the inverse square of viewing distance, while the visual angle and true width or height are linearly related as the inverse of viewing distance—accepting the usual small angle approximations for trigonometry. Thus, if the observer uses the wrong estimate of viewing distance and the observer treats these artificial targets with the same rules that apply to the natural world, shape distortions should arise because disparity and visual angle scale differently with viewing distance.

The insight gained by considering estimates of absolute viewing distance has some interesting consequences for the notion of the $2\frac{1}{2}$D sketch. If we refer back to the sources of information that might contribute to the $2\frac{1}{2}$D sketch, for example in the table presented by Marr (1982, page 276), it may be seen that some kinds of information would need scaling with an estimate of viewing distance (stereo disparity and structure from motion), whereas others would not (surface orientation in the simple Lambertian shading model). Thus, before the visual system could begin to combine information about a single 3D object from different sources, it would be necessary to get such information into equivalent formats.

Experimental Method

In these experiments, we have investigated the effect of changes in absolute viewing distance on a 3-D shape judgment task. The task was constructed with the following points in mind:

• It should be obvious what the observer has to do and easy for her or him to do it.

• Ideally, the task should not rely on depth probes presented over the target since they might interact with the test shapes.

• Cross-modal judgments such as reaching or pointing with the hand are notoriously biased and error-prone.

• The use of external, visual reference lines or other configurations, whose spatial extent should be adjusted to match the depth dimension in the test shape, is also unsatisfactory since such visual targets are subject to a whole set of visual incongruencies of their own—the classical, visual illusions.

• In the last case, a further problem is the possible interaction of apparent size with estimates of viewing distance: Unless the visual reference target is located perceptually at the same distance as the test target—and this would be hard to prove—there can be no confidence in the size estimates derived from it.

Accordingly, a novel visual shape judgment was devised (Johnston, 1988, 1989), which we have termed the apparently circular cylinder (ACC). The main advantage of the

task is that it deals with judgments about the intrinsic configuration of a single target. The observer is presented with a perceptually solid 3D hemicylinder, which may have the cross-sectional form of (1) an ellipse whose major axis is the depth dimension, (2) a circle, or (3) an ellipse whose minor axis is the depth dimension. The task of the observer is to make a forced-choice judgment as to whether the cylindrical shape is perceptually overelongated or flattened in the depth dimension. The 50 percent point (point of subjective equality) in these forced-choice judgments corresponds to the target that is perceptually circular in form. The cylindrical shapes were generated as random dot stereograms, with a sparse density of dots to avoid complications from occlusions. Each cylinder was aligned along the horizontal meridian of the observer and extended in length equally either side of the vertical midline, so that no cues derived from seeing a 2D elliptical disk forming the base of the cylinder were available to observers—from this vantage point, the bases of the cylinder would always be occluded by the sides.

The detailed method of constructing the stereograms was as follows. A single random dot pattern of black and white dots was created on a 500 by 500 pixel grid with a 37.5 percent density of white dots. The average luminance of such a pattern on the display screen (SUN 3/50M workstation) was 7.2 cd m^{-2} and each pixel was approximately 0.03 by 0.03 cm on the screen (corresponding to visual angles of 28.9 sec arc, 57.8 sec arc, and 115.6 sec arc at the three viewing distances used—214 cm, 107 cm, and 53.5 cm, respectively). The original pattern was copied to make a left and right eye pair and horizontal disparities were introduced between the two by adjusting the position of individual dots to depict a cylinder for stereo viewing. The disparity (μ) to be introduced was calculated using the small angle approximation for midline viewing ($\mu = I\delta/(D(D - \delta))$; see figure 22.10) and was applied by incorporating half the required amount in opposite directions to corresponding horizontal rows in each of the two eyes' images. In true physical spatial dimensions, every cylinder was 8 cm in horizontal extent.

The absolute fixation distance was set for the observer by means of the viewing arrangement illustrated in figure 22.11. The left and right portions of the stereogram were presented to the observer using half-silvered mirrors. Through the mirrors, both left and right eyes could view a single physical fixation marker, consisting of a black outline square and diagonal cross. The fixation square had

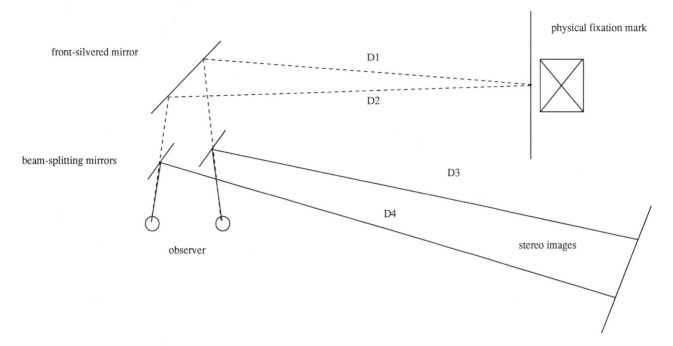

front-silvered mirror

physical fixation mark

D1

D2

beam-splitting mirrors

D3

D4

observer

stereo images

Fig. 22.11
Diagram of the viewing arrangements during the apparently circular cylinder (ACC) task. The observer viewed a single physical fixation marker through a pair of beam-splitting mirrors. The left and right halves of the stereo pair displayed on the CRT monitor were each reflected from one of the beam-splitting mirrors. The mirrors were carefully aligned to bring the CRT images and the physical fixation marker into precise correspondence before any data were collected.

the same angular, spatial extent as the stereograms themselves and, before any trials were carried out at a particular viewing distance, a test image on the CRT screen and the physical fixation marker had to be carefully aligned for left and right eyes independently. To facilitate this, the half-silvered mirrors were mounted on high-precision Ealing optical mountings, which could be positioned in azimuth and elevation to about 1 min arc accuracy. The experimenter created left and right eyes' copies of the fixation target on the single CRT screen, which was placed at the same optical distance as the real physical fixation mark, and then the half-silvered mirrors were rotated accurately into alignment. This procedure ensured the 3D congruence of the stereo targets and the physical fixation marker. The physical fixation marker was present continuously during all observations and the CRT fixation markers appeared between every trial, thus allowing regular monitoring by the subjects of their ocular alignment.

The test shapes for the observers were specified in terms of their notional, true 3D depth coordinates; thus the specification for a cylindrical shape of circular cross-section is given as the radius of the circle in *centimeters.* Suppose that a truly solid object having a circular cross-section is viewed by an observer who misestimates the absolute viewing distance or range of the shape. If the observer applies the incorrect viewing distance in conjunction with a correct registration of the angular stereo disparities, then the transformed shape will be usually elliptical in form, but, at one particular viewing distance, the transformed shape is itself circular as well. As a consequence, two parameters, describing the minor and major axes of the ellipse, will be needed to specify the test shapes.

The basic form of results from a single test session is shown in figure 22.12. The left-hand side shows a diagrammatic example of a set of test targets, which vary in depth b relative to vertical extent $2a$, and the right-hand side shows the forced-choice judgments of circularity, expressed as the probability of saying $b/a > 1$ as a function of the value of b, expressed in *centimeters.* In this case, the subject experienced a considerable distortion in perceived shape and the value of b is considerably smaller than the value of a at the point of subjective equality. We wished to explore these judgments over a range of test shapes and absolute viewing distances. To some extent,

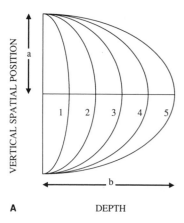

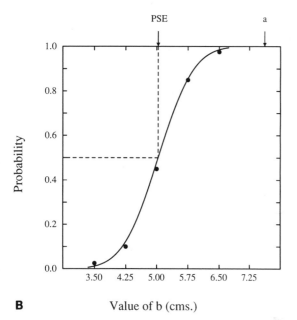

A

VERTICAL SPATIAL POSITION

a

DEPTH

b

B

Value of b (cms.)

Probability

PSE

a

Fig. 22.12

Illustration of the forced-choice judgments of ellipticity of the 3D cylindrical shape. (A) Diagram of a set of test targets that differ in elongation in depth (b) relative to lateral extent (a). (B) A set of forced-choice judgments that are adequately described by a cumulative Gaussian function and that indicate that the observer's perception of 3D shape was considerably distorted. The 50 percent point (5.07 cm) from the psychometric function was used as a measure of which physical shape appeared circular in cross-section to the observer (JSM). The shape had a lateral extent given by $a = 7.5$ cm, so at this viewing distance (53.5 cm) the shape was distorted by about 30 percent in linear dimensions.

the final choice was something of a compromise, since trivial factors such as spatial size of the display screen, the desire to limit the overall range of disparities within the target, and the geometry of the viewing system inevitably placed some constraints on our choice. Five test cylinders were used with a (half the vertical spatial extent) set to 2.5, 3.75, 5.0, 6.25, and 7.5 cm; these were tested at three viewing distances, 53.5, 107, and 214 cm.

A summary of the results for two observers is shown in figure 22.13. This plots the value of b for which the cylinder is perceptually circular in form against the value of a, which corresponds to half the vertical spatial extent of the cylinder. If the observers' choices had corresponded exactly to physical dimensions, then the matches should all be described by the dashed line (of slope $+1$) shown on the graphs. It can be seen that there is systematic variation in slope with viewing distance. At far viewing distances, a cylinder that is physically circular appears flattened in depth to observers, so they have to add more disparity than might be expected to make the cylinder appear circular. Conversely, at near viewing distances, a cylinder that is physically circular appears overextended in depth, so observers add less disparity than might be expected. At intermediate viewing distances (about 100 cm), matches are close to veridical.

In more detail, it may be seen that these results are consistent with a systematic misestimation of viewing distance by human observers. If observers underestimate viewing distance, then their matches should be linearly proportional to the actual physical dimensions of the target, but the constant of proportionality should be greater than 1. Conversely, overestimating viewing distance leads to a linear relationship with proportionality less than 1. These simple linear transformations describe the data quite well and are consistent with estimating targets actually placed at 214 cm as being only about 110 cm away, while targets actually placed at 53.5 cm are treated as if they were 75 cm away.

Proportionate Depth Perception

This pattern of perceptual misestimation of viewing distance is, of course, echoed in the studies on the apparent frontoparallel plane (AFPP) horopter and other measures of visual space perception in 3D viewing (Foley, 1980). The adherence of the data to the linear relationship described above is an example of what von Kries (see note

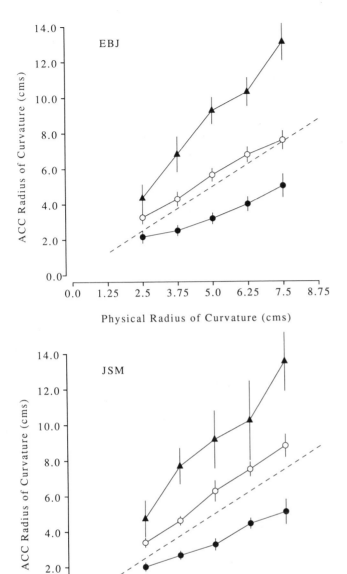

Fig. 22.13

Values of physical depth plotted in *centimeters b* vs. vertical spatial extent *a* for horizontally aligned cylinders that appear circular in form to the observer (apparently circular cylinders—ACC). The different symbols for the data points indicate the observers' judgments at the three viewing distances (*filled circles*, 53.5 cm; *open circles*, 107 cm; *triangles*, 214 cm). The dotted line of slope +1 indicates where judgments should lie at all three viewing distances, if the observer were able to scale the pattern of stereo disparities and angular subtenses accurately for absolute viewing distance (range).

9 to section 30 in Helmholtz, 1962/1925/1910) termed *proportionate depth perception*. According to this principle, the geometric relationships between all the visual angles, including stereo disparities, within the visual scene will be preserved, but the figure as a whole will be interpreted with a mistaken estimate of absolute viewing distance or range.

For example, the AFPP task requires the observer to adjust the distances of five or seven vertical rods placed at equal horizontal intervals apart, until the the rods appear to lie in a plane perpendicular to the observers primary cyclopean line of sight. The selected shape of the AFPP horopter is physically a convex curved surface (apex towards the observer) at far viewing distances, planar at intermediate viewing distances and concave at near viewing distances. Foley (1980) applied the concept of proportionate depth perception to such data and demonstrated that a single "correction factor," namely the *effective viewing distance*, would account for all the data collected at one physical viewing distance. Such a transformation also applies to the present data.

Hence, proportionate depth perception does not apply just to the layout of visual space, but also to the shape of 3D objects within it. This point was clearly appreciated by von Kries (see Helmholtz, 1962), who mentions two examples. In the first, Heine arranged three vertical rods to form a triangular prism. The observer's task was to adjust the rods until the prism was equiangular (60°). Heine reports the same pattern of perceptual misestimation for this task as we found for the ACC task. In the second example, Elschnig mentions that solid spheres appear distorted in shape. Of course, in these earlier studies, multiple cues for depth and 3D shape would be present within the stimuli themselves, rather than purely stereo as in the figures studied here. Without computer control of the stimuli, it would be difficult to dissect the contribution of these different cues. However, those earlier results did encourage the notion that it might be worth exploring more complex stimulus patterns with the ACC task.

Stereo, Texture, and Shading

Accordingly, a new form of cylindrical shape was devised, in which stereo, texture gradient cues, and luminance shading cues were all present. The stimuli were constructed by mapping a texture onto a cylindrical surface and then using a ray-tracing procedure to determine two perspective projections, which corresponded to the left and right eyes' viewpoints for stereo viewing (see Bülthoff and Mallot (1988) and chapter 20 for a discussion of the general principles behind this approach). The choice of texture was somewhat arbitrary, but eventually a black and white checkerboard was selected because it would provide strong vertical and horizontal contours in the final images and because observers would be familiar with the canonical form of the texture. The cylinder was illuminated with a single light source located above the observer's head. The reasons for this location were (1) it was undesirable in the first instance to use a position in which the light source would create visible shadows from the bounding rim of the cylinder and (2) it would have been unnatural to have the light source at a location where the observer's own body should have fallen as a shadow on the scene. The cylindrical surface was assumed to have a purely Lambertian reflectance characteristic without specularities and, as there were no other objects in the scene, the effects of mutual illumination (Forsyth & Zisserman, 1989a, b) were ignored. The albedo of the black squares was fixed at 0.1 and of the white squares was 1.0, and an ambient, diffuse illumination equivalent to about 10 percent of the directed light source was added. In the final images, the luminance was about 110 cd m^{-2} and the maximum contrast in the image was locally as large as 0.8.

The ray-tracing procedure was carried out with reversed light paths and initiated from each pixel location in the final images, so as to reduce aliasing effects. A photograph of an example of the final stereo pairs is shown in figure 22.14, but the reader should be warned that this is not exactly to scale and includes some geometric distortion due to the photographic process. The particular interest of these images is that the luminance shading, and possibly also the texture gradient information, could provide the observer with cues to surface orientation that do not depend on the absolute viewing distance. The ability to exploit knowledge of the surface orientation over the cylinder would be an alternative strategy for an observer in solving the ACC task, without an explicit computation of the depth dimension and comparison with the vertical spatial extent. The results of the ACC judgments are shown in figure 22.15 for two observers. The overall pattern of behavior is similar to that for the case of stereo alone, although the judgments are closer to the true

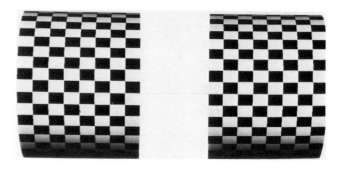

Fig. 22.14
Appearance of the cylinders used to investigate the combination of different cues to 3D shape (stereo, texture, and shading). The photograph is not accurately to scale, so that the pattern of cues in this example does not necessarily correspond in exact geometry to the binocular viewing of a real physical object. By contrast, in the experimental set-up, this condition was fulfilled as accurately as possible.

physical expectations. The variability of the observer's responses (derived from the slope of the psychometric functions) is lower than for the pure stereo case, and it should be emphasized that the sensitivity of observers to *changes* in 3D shape is excellent, even though they misestimate shape in absolute terms. Yet again, this is an example of a task where the human visual system has good relative sensitivity, but much poorer absolute sensitivity.

Recovery of Viewing Distance

When observers are given these shape judgment tasks, it seems that they scale the disparity relationships within the figure in a way that indicates they are sensitive to viewing distance as a parameter. The internal estimates of viewing distance used by the observer are related to the physical viewing distance, but are only partially correct. What sources of information about absolute viewing distance are present within the experimental set-up? The use of the physical fixation marker ensures that strong signals are available for the classical cues of convergence of the eyes and accommodative effort associated with focussing the lens of the eye. With close attention to the geometric alignment of the stereo images and the true physical fixation marker, the pattern of vertical disparities can be made to correspond exactly to the viewing of a real 3D object. A critical test of the rôle of purely visual cues in specifying the absolute viewing distance can then be made (Cumming, Johnston & Parker, 1991).

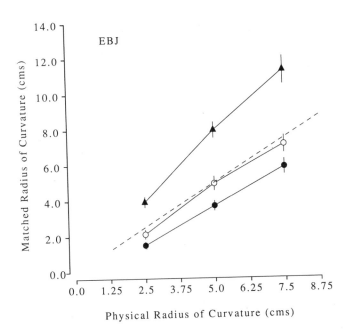

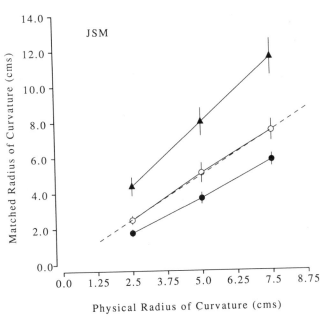

Fig. 22.15
Similar to figure 22.13, but for the case where the shapes had texture and shading cues as well as stereo. The different symbols for the data points indicate the observers' judgments at the three viewing distances (*filled circles*, 53.5 cm; *open circles*, 107 cm; *triangles*, 214 cm).

Recently, Bishop (1989) has reviewed the literature on depth constancy and concluded that there was a reasonable case for its existence and that constancy could, in principle, be achieved through processing of vertical disparity information. However, most of the experimental studies that he quotes are flawed because they rely on measurement methods of the sort that we rejected before devising the ACC task. Bishop (1989), like Mayhew and Longuet-Higgins (1982), attributes a role to vertical disparities in recovering the absolute viewing distance of the target. Unfortunately, when vertical disparities are directly manipulated, observers do not seem very sensitive to such changes (Westheimer, 1984). The inferred sensitivity to vertical disparities from measurements of the induced effect is rather better (Mayhew & Longuet-Higgins, 1982). Also, in chapter 20 Bülthoff suggests that vertical disparities may be important in processing specular reflections, when these are present. We are investigating the role of vertical disparities further by manipulating them directly as a parameter in the ACC task (Cumming, Johnston & Parker, 1991) and by exploring a range of eccentric gaze angles, a condition that gives rise to much larger vertical disparities.

Finally, Koenderink and van Doorn (1976) predated the work on vertical disparities with a more general treatment based on a vector field description of binocular disparity. They argue that by using the deformation component of this vector field it is possible to recover on a ratio scale the absolute distances between the observer and various points on the surface of an object up to an overall scale constant, a conclusion that is remarkably similar to our experimental results. However, their theory predicts that the most veridical recovery of 3D shape should take place for the smallest cylinders (highest curvature) at the furthest viewing distance. As yet in our data, there is no interrelationship between curvature of the shapes and viewing distance. Shape perception corresponds most accurately with physical reality at intermediate viewing distances, not the furthest viewing distances.

Representations for Shape and Surfaces

It is inconceivable that a single experiment should reject an idea as complex and as general as the $2\frac{1}{2}$D sketch. Yet, taken together, these experiments raise some difficulties about the suitability of the $2\frac{1}{2}$D sketch in our present understanding of it. The two main roles of an intermediate level representation should be to draw together efficiently the information derived from early visual processing and to present that information in a convenient format for later processing stages. How does the current notion of the $2\frac{1}{2}$D sketch stand up to these criteria and the experimental evidence presented above?

Interpolation

The experimental work presented in the sections on disparity pooling and disparity gradient limits suggests that in human stereo vision much of the effective interpolation may be carried out by early filtering stages that occur prior to a stage such as the $2\frac{1}{2}$D sketch. Regardless of the source of information (stereo, motion, texture, shading, contour), filtering through multiple spatial frequency channels (or at multiple spatial scales) will provide some effective smoothing of the visual inputs to later stages. The significant question is whether the smoothing provided by early visual filtering is sufficient in quantitative terms to account for the behavior of the system as a whole. For the random-dot stereo targets examined in this work, the effects of the early processes do seem to be sufficient, but it is an open question how far this can be generalized, even to other stereo targets, such as simple line and dot figures. In addition, more information is needed about the nature of the spatial filtering that is applied prior to stereo combination: even straightforward issues such as the orientation selectivity of the filters (see earlier section on orientation specific masking in stereo) are hard to settle convincingly. A further assumption in the present work is that interpolation is a process that would be automatically applied over the whole scene. There are hardly any experimental data or modeling efforts that have investigated the possibility of a more "intelligent" interpolation process that is driven only by significant geometric features within the images—such features might be points of high curvature on contours, or occlusion boundaries as signaled at trijunctions in the graylevel image. The work of Collett (1985) and Buckley, Frisby, and Mayhew (1989) are significant exceptions.

Assimilation of Information from Different Sources

As well as smoothing and interpolation, another important role of the $2\frac{1}{2}$D sketch might be to bring together information from different visual cues within the scene.

Alternatively, separate processes might extract "shape from X" into a set of intrinsic images (Barrow & Tenenbaum, 1978), but the multiple sources of information would be used for cross-checking and verification. For example, in scenes with many smooth surfaces (e.g., manmade objects), depth or shape from stereo can be weak, because there are very few surface features to drive stereo matching. Our experiments on 3D shape (see 3D Shape Judgments) emphasize that the various "shape from X" processes do not offer information to a $2\frac{1}{2}$D sketch in formats that are easily compared with each other. For example, the relationship between surface orientation and stereo disparities (in angular terms) is complex and depends on absolute viewing distance or range. Marr's table of information (Marr, 1982, p. 276) that might contribute to the $2\frac{1}{2}$D sketch sets aside this problem by explicitly assuming orthographic projections for stereo and implicitly assuming a constant vergence angle. But we have seen that the problem is not easily evaded, since the necessity of considering perspective projections and the need to know eye position lead straight into the question of assessing 3D shape, a function for the sake of which the $2\frac{1}{2}$D sketch supposedly exists.

The apparent unity of single sources of visual information, as exemplified by the phrase "shape from X," may also be partly to blame for this confusion. In the case of stereo information, one could list not only the classical point disparities, but also local differences in orientation (Blakemore, Fiorentini & Maffei, 1972; Koenderink & van Doorn, 1976) and spatial frequency (Blakemore, 1970), local differences in curvature (Rogers & Cagenello, 1989), and a host of local differential forms of the disparity field (Koenderink & van Doorn, 1976). Each of these stereo cues can provide subtly different information about the local geometry of the disparity field and each cue should relate to other general image features (Koenderink & van Doorn, 1986) according to precise geometric principles. Thus, schemes for combining sources of information into a $2\frac{1}{2}$D sketch based on simple statistical combination of intrinsic images (Poggio, Gamble & Little, 1988) set aside the potential that has been offered as a consequence of recognizing the richness and subtlety of visual information in natural scenes. On the other hand, it is arguable that this potential has yet to show its worth!

The key improvement would be to insist that when information is integrated into something like the $2\frac{1}{2}$D sketch, the representation should incorporate a form of "label" or "tag" stating how the component pieces of evidence were acquired and what the quality of the evidence is. For example, the second Marr/Poggio stereo algorithm (Marr & Poggio, 1979) suggests the use of stereo matches derived from filtering at coarse spatial scales to guide the assignment of matches derived from filtering at finer spatial scales; this scheme must use knowledge about which spatial scale of filter is providing the evidence under evaluation. Thus the later stages can access information about the scale of the filter through which visual information has arrived. The same organizational feature may allow the system to exploit computational regularities such as the ordering constraint (see earlier section on disparity gradient limits) more effectively.

Distributed Representation for Depth

The suggestion that even just "depth from stereo" could be represented in several ways (e.g., disparity and its gradient and curvature) raises the obvious possibility that the representation for depth may be distributed over the responses of many neurons rather than being collected together into a single exclusive assertion about what is happening along a single cyclopean line of sight. The phenomenon of transparency is often cited as arguing for a distributed representation for depth. Although we have noted some weaknesses with this argument, it is undeniable that the explanation we have offered for disparity pooling would be naturally captured by a distributed representation. More strongly, the existence of stereo in Panum's limiting case (Braddick, 1978; Westheimer, 1986) also suggests a distributed representation.

Dynamics of Shape Perception

Perhaps the deepest weakness of the $2\frac{1}{2}$D sketch is its static and single view of the world. Of course, it is reasonable that if one starts by asking what can be computed about shape from one snapshot of the world (or two snapshots in the case of stereo or motion), then one would probably choose something like a $2\frac{1}{2}$D sketch. However, what this hides is the fact that much of shape perception is dynamic, both in terms of the integration of information from multiple viewpoints and in terms of the selection of new viewpoints to explore. Purely by way of illustration, suppose that a professional mechanic were given the job of deciding which of two straight, solid metal rods was circular in cross-section and which was

elliptical. The task is analogous to the shape-judgment task discussed in the section on 3D Shape Judgments, yet naturally the strategy would be to inspect the two rods end on, not from the side. Clearly, for humans some views of an object are easier to cope with than others—whether this means that those viewpoints are more informative is still an open question. Hence, between the leap from a viewer-centered coordinate frame ($2\frac{1}{2}$D sketch) to an object-centered coordinate frame (true 3D shape), there is an essential component of understanding what will happen to the $2\frac{1}{2}$D sketch under a movement of the viewpoint and an essential insight in appreciating that the behavior of certain features in the $2\frac{1}{2}$D sketch under motion of the viewpoint will give good information about 3D structure without the need for explicit object recognition (Koenderink & van Doorn, 1980).

Shape of the Future?

The directions that this area of work will follow over the next few years have two recognizable strands. First, there is a drive to increased realism in visual stimuli. To a large extent this is a technological impetus, which will permit experimenters to introduce realism into their visual stimuli in a controlled fashion. "Controlled realism" will require the continued improvement of models of image formation through understanding of the physics of natural images. Second, there is a need to understand the interaction of visual sensing with visually guided movements. Eye movements may be a useful model system because they are moderately well understood on the motor output side and because they are a sufficiently complex system for controlled motions of the sensor to take place. Underpinning these approaches will be the continued development of psychophysical procedures for the investigation of higher levels of visual processing.

Acknowledgments

This research was supported by the Science and Engineering Research Council (GR/D/64193) and by the The Wellcome Trust. Some of the work used the HIPS package from New York University (see Landy, Cohen & Sperling, 1984).

References

Baker, H. H. (1982). *Depth from edge and intensity based stereo.* Stanford University, California: Report No. STAN-CS-82-930.

Barrow, H. & Tenenbaum, J. M. (1978). Recovering intrinsic scene characteristics from images. In A. R. Hanson & E. M. Riseman (Eds.), *Computer vision systems.* Orlando, FL: Academic Press.

Besl, P. J. & Jain, R. C. (1986). Invariant surface characteristics for 3D object recognition in range images. *Computer Vision, Graphics and Image Processing, 33,* 33–80.

Bishop, P. O. (1989). Vertical disparity, egocentric distance and stereoscopic depth constancy: a new interpretation. *Proceedings of the Royal Society of London B, 237,* 445–469.

Blakemore, C. (1970). A new kind of stereoscopic vision. *Vision Research, 10,* 1181–1189.

Blakemore, C., Fiorentini, A. & Maffei, L. (1972). A second neural mechanism of binocular depth discrimination. *Journal of Physiology, London, 226,* 725–749.

Bracewell, R. N. (1986). *The Fourier transform and its applications* (2nd ed.). New York: McGraw-Hill.

Braddick, O. J. (1978). Multiple matching in stereopis. Unpublished.

Brady, M., Ponce, J., Yuille, A. & Asada, H. (1985). Describing surfaces. In H. Hanafusa & H. Inoue (Eds.), *Proceedings of the 2nd International Symposium on Robotics Research* (pp. 5–16). Cambridge, MA: MIT Press.

Buckley, D, Frisby, J. P. & Mayhew, J. E. W. (1989). Integration of stereo and texture cues in the formation of discontinuities during three-dimensional surface interpolation. *Perception, 18,* 563–588.

Bülthoff, H. H. & Mallot, H. A. (1988). Integration of depth modules: Stereo and shading. *Journal of the Optical Society of America A, 5,* 1749–1758.

Burt, P. & Julesz, B, (1980). A disparity gradient limit for binocular fusion. *Science, 208,* 615–617.

Collett, T. S. (1985). Extrapolating and interpolating surfaces in depth. *Proceedings of the Royal Society of London B, 224,* 43–56.

Cumming, B. G., Johnston, E. B. & Parker, A. J. Vertical disparities and the perception of three-dimensional shape. *Nature, 349,* 411–413.

Derrington, A. M. & Henning, G. B. (1989). Some observations on the masking effects of two-dimensional stimuli. *Vision Research, 29,* 241–246.

Dev, P. (1975). Perception of depth surfaces in random-dot stereograms: A neural model. *International Journal of Man-Machine Studies, 7,* 511–528.

Foley, J. M. (1980). Binocular distance perception. *Psychological Review, 87,* 411–434.

Forsyth D. & Zisserman A. (1989a). Mutual illumination. *Proceedings of Conference on Computer Vision and Pattern Recognition (CVPR89),* San Diego.

Forsyth D. & Zisserman A. (1989b). Shape from shading in the light of mutual illumination. *Proceedings of the Alvey Vision Conference (AVC89),* Reading. Also to appear in *Image and Vision Computing.*

Grimson, W. E. L. (1982). A computational theory of visual surface interpolation. *Philosophical Transactions of the Royal Society of London B, 298,* 395–427.

Hawken, M. J. & Parker, A. J. (1984). Contrast sensitivity and orientation selectivity in lamina IV of the striate cortex of Old-World monkeys. *Experimental Brain Research, 54,* 367–373.

Helmholtz, H. von (1962/1925/1910). *Treatise on Physiological Optics* Volume III, translated from the 3rd edition (1910) of *Handbuch der Physiologischen Optik* by Southall, J. P. C. (1925). Republished (1962) by Dover Publications Inc., New York.

Horn, B. K. P. (1986). *Robot vision.* Cambridge, MA: MIT Press.

Hubel, D. H. & Wiesel, T. N. (1962). Receptive fields, binocular interaction and functional architecture in the cat's visual cortex. *Journal of Physiology, London, 160,* 106–154.

Johnston, E. B. (1988). Systematic distortions of shape from stereo. Supplement to *Investigative Ophthalmology and Visual Science, 29,* 399.

Johnston, E. B. (1989). Human perception of three-dimensional shape. Unpublished D. Phil. thesis, University of Oxford.

Johnston, E. & Parker, A. J. (1987a). Surface curvature as a descriptor of three dimensional shape. Supplement to *Investigative Ophthalmology and Visual Science, 28,* 294.

Johnston, E. B. & Parker, A. J. (1987b). Shape discrimination based on curvature acuity. *Perception, 16,* 234.

Johnston, E. B. & Parker, A. J. (1988). Measures of surface shape from disparity fields. *Perception, 17,* 365–366.

Koenderink, J. J. & van Doorn, A. J. (1976). Geometry of binocular vision and a model for stereopsis. *Biological Cybernetics, 21,* 29–35.

Koenderink, J. J. & van Doorn, A. J. (1980). Photometric invariants related to solid shape. *Optica Acta, 27,* 981–986.

Koenderink, J. J. & van Doorn, A. J. (1986). Dynamic shape. *Biological Cybernetics, 53,* 383–396.

Landy, M. S., Cohen, Y. & Sperling, G. (1984). HIPS: Image processing under UNIX. Software and applications. *Behavior Research Methods, Instruments, & Computers, 16,* 199–216.

Livingstone, M. S. & Hubel, D. H. (1984). Anatomy and physiology of a color system in the primate visual cortex. *Journal of Neuroscience, 4,* 309–356.

Marr, D. (1982). *Vision.* San Francisco: W. H. Freeman.

Marr, D. & Nishihara, H. K. (1978). Representation and recognition of the spatial organization of three-dimensional shapes. *Proceedings of the Royal Society of London B, 200,* 269–294.

Marr, D. & Poggio, T. (1976). Cooperative computation of stereo disparity. *Science, 194,* 283–287.

Marr, D. & Poggio, T. (1979). A computational theory of human stereo vision. *Proceedings of the Royal Society of London B, 204,* 301–328.

Mayhew, J. E. W. & Frisby, J. P. (1978). Stereopsis masking in humans is not orientationally tuned. *Perception, 7,* 431–436.

Mayhew, J. E. W. & Longuet-Higgins, H. C. (1982). A computational model of binocular depth perception. *Nature, London, 297,* 376–378.

Mitchison, G. & Westheimer, G. (1984). The perception of depth in simple figures. *Vision Research, 24,* 1063–1073.

Nishihara, H. K. (1984). Practical real-time imaging stereo matcher. *Optical Engineering, 23,* 536–545.

Nishihara, H. K. (1989). Tests of a sign correlation model for binocular stereo. (ARVO abstract). *Investigative Ophthalmology and Visual Science, 30, (Supplement),* 389.

Parker, A. J. & Hawken, M. J. (1985). Capabilites of monkey cortical cells in spatial resolution tasks. *Journal of the Optical Society of America A, 2,* 1101–1114.

Parker, A. J. & Yang, Y. (1989). Spatial properties of a stereo disparity pooling process. *Vision Research, 29,* 1525–1538.

Phillips, G. C. & Wilson, H. R. (1984). Orientation bandwidths of spatial mechanisms measured by masking. *Journal of the Optical Society of America A, 1,* 226–232.

Poggio, T., Gamble, E. B. & Little, J. J. (1988). Parallel integration of vision modules. *Science, 242,* 436–440.

Pollard, S. B., Mayhew, J. E. W. & Frisby, J. P. (1985). PMF: A stereo correspondence algorithm using a disparity gradient limit. *Perception, 14,* 449–470.

Prazdny, K. (1985). Detection of binocular disparities. *Biological Cybernetics, 52,* 93–99.

Rogers, B. & Cagenello, R. (1989). Disparity curvature and the perception of three-dimensional surfaces *Nature, London, 339,* 135–137.

Schumer, R. A. (1979). *Mechanisms in human stereopsis.* Ph.D. Thesis, Stanford University, Palo Alto, California.

Terzopoulos, D. (1988). The computation of visible-surface representations. *Proceedings of the IEEE: Pattern Analysis and Machine Intelligence, 10,* 417–438.

Trivedi, H. & Lloyd, S. A. (1985). The role of disparity gradient in stereo vision. *Perception, 14,* 685–690.

Tyler, C. W. (1983). Sensory Processing of Binocular Disparity. In C. M. Schor & K. J. Ciuffreda (Eds.), *Vergence eye movements: Basic and clinical aspects* (pp. 199–295). Boston, MA: Butterworth.

Watson, A. B. (1983). Detection and recognition of simple spatial forms. In O. J. Braddick & A. C. Sleigh (Eds.), *Physical and biological processing of images* (pp. 100–114). New York: Springer-Verlag.

Westheimer, G. (1984). Sensitivity for vertical retinal image differences. *Nature, 307,* 632–634.

Westheimer, G. (1986). Spatial interactions in the domain of disparity signals in human stereoscopic vision. *Journal of Physiology, 370,* 619–629.

Westheimer, G. & Levi, D. (1987). Depth attraction and repulsion of disparate foveal stimuli. *Vision Research, 27,* 1361–1368.

Westheimer, G. & McKee, S. P. (1980). Stereoscopic acuity with defocused and spatially filtered retinal images. *Journal of the Optical Society of America, 70,* 772–778.

Wilson, H. R. (1983). Psychophysical evidence for spatial channels. In O. J. Braddick & A. C. Sleigh (Eds.), *Physical and biological processing of images* (pp. 88–99). New York: Springer-Verlag.

Yang, Y. & Parker, A. J. (1988). Averaging of stereo disparity in sinusoidally-corrugated surfaces. Supplement to *Investigative Ophthalmology and Visual Science, 29,* 410.

Author Index

Abramov, I., 80
Adelson, E. H., 16–17, 46, 57, 66, 109–110, 120–122, 128, 169, 213, 216, 229, 232–233, 236–242, 254, 259–260, 275, 277–278, 285
Aguilar, M., 66
Ahn, S. J., 177
Ahnelt, P. K., 23
Ahuja, N., 333, 335, 353
Ahumada, A. J., Jr., 23, 31–32, 44, 101, 109, 120, 122, 138, 147, 153, 232, 234
Aitsebaomo, A. P., 156, 161
Albers, J., 176
Albrecht, D. G., 11, 84, 101–102, 104–105, 125, 129–130, 155, 255, 257, 285
Albright, T. D., 238–239, 241, 312, 354
Aliomonos, J., 303, 307
Allebach, J. P., 26
Amari, S., 32
Amthor, F. R., 241
Anastasio, T. J., 340
Andersen, R. A., 232, 248
Andrews, B. W., 125, 234
Andrews, D. P., 161
Anstis, S. M., 231–240, 248
Arend, L. E., 177, 210
Arnold, R. D., 315, 344
Arsenin, V. Y., 243
Asada, H., 371
Ayache, N., 336

Bajcsy, R., 307
Baker, C. L., Jr., 241
Baker, H. H., 337, 341, 366–367
Ballard, D. H., 236, 345
Banks, M. S., 32, 100, 147
Barlow, H. B., 12, 32, 109, 147
Barnard, S. T., 321, 328, 335–337, 378
Barrow, H. G., 205, 210, 307
Battaile, B., 203
Bauer, R., 92
Baylor, D. A., 58–60, 63–64, 66, 173
Beck, J., 3, 205, 210, 213, 261, 273–279, 281, 283, 286–287, 316
Bennett, J. M., 188
Bennett, P. J., 100, 147
Benzschawel, T., 177

Bergen, J. R., 3, 16–17, 46, 109–111, 120–122, 128, 130, 169, 229, 232–233, 237, 239, 241–242, 254–255, 257, 260, 273, 275, 277–278, 287, 291, 297
Bernard, G. D., 52
Berns, R. S., 177
Bertero, M., 243
Besag, J., 219
Besl, P. J., 371
Beverley, K. I., 241
Biederman, I., 210
Billings, S. A., 333–334
Binford, T. O., 205, 315, 341, 344
Birch, D. G., 57–65
Birch, E. E., 58
Birdsall, T. G., 148–149
Bishop, P. O., 101, 110, 125, 127, 377
Bisti, S., 232, 234
Bitmead, R. R., 29
Blackwell, K. T., 177
Blake, A., 205, 211, 306, 312, 314–315, 319, 327, 337, 339, 353
Blakemore, C., 86, 340, 378
Blakeslee, B., 105
Blasdel, G. G., 91
Blinn, J. F., 188, 191
Blom, J., 32
Bonds, A. B., 120, 130, 259, 285
Boring, E. G., 171
Bouman, M. A., 163
Bovik, A. C., 273, 275, 277
Bowen, J. B., 337, 340, 352–353
Bowmaker, J., 72
Bowne, J. F., 164
Boycott, B. B., 72, 84, 89, 159, 166
Boynton, R. M., 65, 173
Bracewell, R. N., 96, 195, 204, 295, 369
Braddick, O. J., 367, 369, 379
Brady, M., 333, 336, 348, 371
Brainard, D. H., 172–175, 179–183, 199
Brelstaff, G. J., 315
Brent, R. P., 257
Brewer, W. L., 171
Brill, M. H., 172
Brindley, G. S., 174
Brint, A. T., 336
Brodatz, P., 261
Brookes, A., 307, 319
Brooks, R. A., 333
Brown, C. M., 210, 345
Brown, C. R., 345
Brown, K. J., 58
Bruch, T. A., 66
Bruno, N., 324
Buchsbaum, G., 172, 176–177
Buckley, D., 310, 337, 354, 378

Bullier, J., 241
Bülthoff, H. H., 169, 177, 205, 210–212, 216, 237, 240, 242, 306–308, 310–311, 313–314, 316, 319–321, 323–325, 327, 335, 337, 339, 344, 354, 362, 376
Burbeck, C. A., 153, 157, 167
Burnham, R. W., 171, 176
Burr, D. C., 16, 109–110, 120, 150, 285
Burt, P. J., 255, 257, 342–344, 367
Byram, G. M., 35

Cabral, B., 188, 192
Caelli, T. M., 254, 273, 277, 293
Cagenello, R., 378
Campbell, F. W., 28, 35, 38, 46, 85, 87–88, 119, 164
Canny, J., 341–342, 349, 351–352
Carmignoto, L., 232, 234
Cass, P. F., 35
Chalupa, L., 232
Chen, B., 50
Chen, D. S., 26
Chen, S. E., 203
Cheney, F. E., 35
Chou, P. B., 210
Chubb, C., 273–274, 277–278
Cicerone, C. M., 72
Citron, M. C., 114, 128, 232, 237, 241
Clark, J., 321, 324, 328
Clark, M., 273, 275, 277
Cobbs, W. H., 59, 64, 66
Coggins, J. M., 273
Cohen, D. S., 240
Cohen, M. F., 203
Cohen, Y., 360
Cohn, T. E., 147, 149
Coletta, N. J., 22, 35–38, 44–45, 52–54, 72
Collett, T. S., 354, 378
Collier, R., 44
Connolly, M., 84, 91
Conte, M., 273, 287
Cook, R. L., 188, 190–191, 196–197, 205
Coombs, G. H., 100
Cooper, G. F., 85, 119
Cornsweet, T. N., 172
Cowan, W. B., 199
Cowey, A., 42, 84, 89–90
Creutzfeldt, O., 129–130
Cronin, T. W., 11
Cumming, B. G., 376–377
Cunitz, R. J., 159–166
Cunningham, M. J., 28
Cunningham, R. B., 105
Curcio, C. A., 23, 36–38, 42, 53, 89–90, 102, 105, 158
Cutting, J. E., 307, 324
Cynader, M., 17

Daniel, P. M., 166
Daugman, J. G., 101, 121, 233–234, 273, 275
Davila, K. D., 23
DaVinci, L., 4–5
Davis, E. T., 232, 237
Daw, N. W., 177
Dawis, S., 85, 111
Dean, A. F., 129, 150
Dean, P., 340
DeAngelis, G., 17
de Faller, J. M., 58
Delman, S., 210
DeMonasterio, F. M., 71–72
DePriest, D. D., 285
Derrington, A. M., 46, 75–76, 78–80, 84–85, 88, 92, 96, 100, 285, 361–363
Dev, P., 321–322, 341, 366
DeValois, K. K., 3, 285
DeValois, R. L., 3, 11, 84, 101–102, 153, 155, 239, 255, 257
DeYoe, E. A., 32
Disbrow, D. T., 58
Dobbins, A., 17, 216
Dosher, B. A., 324
Dow, B. M., 92
Dowling, J. E., 72
Drew, M. S., 184
Duchon, J., 243
D'Zmura, M., 172, 184, 205

Egelhaaf, M., 242
Elfar, S. D., 239
Emerson, R. C., 16, 110, 114, 128, 232, 237, 241
Enroth-Cugell, C., 22, 57, 69, 73, 84–85, 96, 112, 119, 123, 259, 285
Epstein, L. I., 340
Eskin, T. A., 106
Evans, B. M., 171, 176

Fahle, M., 232, 323, 327, 344
Fairchild, M. D., 177
Farrar, S., 105
Farrell, J. E., 44
Faverjon, B., 336
Feldman, J. A., 236
Feller, W., 298
Ferrera, V. P., 242, 259
Field, D. J., 85, 104, 275
Finkelstein, M. A., 57, 285
Fiorentini, A., 127–128, 234, 378
Fischler, M. A., 335, 337
Fish, G. E., 57–58, 64
Flannery, B. P., 192, 204, 285
Fleet, D. J., 232, 240
Fogel, I., 273, 275, 277–278
Foley, J. M., 155–156, 374–375

Forsyth, D., 376
Fox, W. C., 148–149
Freeman, R. D., 17, 105, 110, 113, 116, 129–130, 150, 259, 285
French, A. S., 160
Frisby, J. P., 260, 262, 306, 310, 313, 315–316, 321, 332–341, 344–348, 350–354, 360–363, 366–367, 369, 378
Fukada, Y., 242
Funt, B. V., 184
Furuya, M., 212, 216

Gabor, D., 121, 233
Gaddum, J. H., 241
Gallego, A., 72
Galli, L., 232, 234
Gamble, E. B., 210, 219, 248, 378
Gaska, J. P., 17
Geiger, D., 321–323
Geisler, W. S., 23, 40, 100–101, 147, 217, 273, 275, 277
Gelade, G., 4
Gelatt, C. D., 322
Gelb, A., 322
Gelb, D. J., 153, 155, 163–165, 167
Gel'Fand, I. M., 192
Geman, D., 219, 222, 224, 321, 327
Geman, S., 219, 222, 224, 321, 327
Gennert, M. A., 313, 321, 323, 328
Gerstein, G. L., 110
Gervais, M. J., 254
Giblin, P., 315
Gibson, J. J., 5
Gilbert, C. D., 150
Gilchrist, A. L., 210
Gillam, B., 339
Ginsberg, I. W., 188–189
Girosi, F., 241, 321–322
Gizzi, M. S., 238–239, 241
Goetz, K. G., 36
Golden, R., 219
Goldstein, R., 210
Gonzalez, R. C., 266
Goral, C. M., 203
Gordon, J., 80
Gorzynski, M. E., 177
Gouras, P., 71
Graham, M., 354
Graham, N. V. S., 3, 12, 130, 135, 137, 140, 143, 147, 273–279, 281, 283, 286–287, 291, 297
Granit, R., 58
Granlund, G. H., 16–17
Green, D. G., 35, 39, 46, 87–88
Green, D. M., 29, 138, 148
Greenberg, D. P., 203
Greenstein, V., 57, 64
Gregory, R. L., 326

Grimson, W. E. L., 312, 321, 337, 348, 353, 363
Grosof, D. H., 239
Grossberg, S., 210, 277–278, 286
Grossmann, A., 241
Grünert, U., 71, 84, 89, 159, 166
Grzywacz, N. M., 120, 122, 232, 234–244, 247–249, 316, 321, 328
Gubisch, R. W., 28, 87–88

Hagins, W. A., 58–60, 63–64, 66
Hall, J. L., 137
Hamilton, D. B., 101, 104–105, 125, 129–130, 285
Hammond, P., 232, 237
Harris, C., 336
Harvey, L. O., 254
Hauske, G., 156
Hawken, M. J., 84–89, 96, 100–101, 103, 155, 360
Hayhoe, M. M., 66, 72
Haynes, S. M., 307
Healey, G., 205
Heeger, D. J., 105, 120, 232, 234, 236–237, 259–260, 278, 285–286
Heeley, D. W., 165–167
Helson, H., 171, 176
Hendrickson, A. E., 23, 36–38, 42, 53, 89–90, 102, 105
Henning, G. B., 361–363
Henry, G. H., 110
Hepler, N., 255–257
Herman, M., 159, 166
Herman, W. K., 58
Hess, R. F., 100
Heynen, H. G. M., 58
Hicks, T. P., 100
Hikosaka, D., 242
Hildreth, E. C., 237, 240, 242–244, 246–248, 312–313, 316
Hirsch, J., 25, 28, 42, 102, 105, 158, 163, 165–167
Ho, J., 184
Hobson, E. W., 192
Hochstein, S., 16, 110, 112, 234, 278
Hochstrasser, U. W., 298
Hodgkin, A. L., 59, 63–64
Hoff, M. E., 27
Hoff, W., 333, 335, 353
Hoffman, K. 192
Holub, R. A., 231–232, 235, 237, 241
Hood, D. C., 57–65, 285
Hopkins, J. M., 72
Horn, B. K. P., 4, 187–189, 203, 209–210, 242–243, 246–247, 307, 359
Houde, J., 91
Hsia, J. J., 188–189
Hubel, D. H., 3, 14, 75, 77, 84–85, 110, 115, 119, 255, 360
Humphrey, A. L., 110
Hungerford, T. W., 182
Hunt, R. W. G., 171, 176–177
Hunter, R. S., 191
Hurlbert, A. C., 177

Hurvich, L. M., 171, 177
Hutchinson, J., 248
Hylton, R., 25, 28, 163, 165–167

Ikeda, H., 231–232, 237
Ikeuchi, K., 307
Ishihara, S., 178
Iverson, G., 273
Iverson, L., 216
Ivry, R., 213, 273–274, 287
Iwai, E., 242

Jaarsma, D., 149
Jacobsen, A., 210
Jacobson, L. D., 17
Jain, A. K., 273
Jain, R. C., 307, 371
Jameson, D., 171, 177
Jeffers, V. B., 171, 176
Jepson, A. D., 232, 240
Jerri, A. J., 26
Johnston, E. B., 335–336, 371–372, 376–377
Jones, D. G., 333–334
Jones, J. P., 101, 115, 125, 241
Jones, R. C., 147
Judd, D. B., 171–172, 176, 180
Jukes, J., 164
Julesz, B., 3, 254–255, 261, 273, 306, 316, 333, 336–337, 341–344, 348, 360, 367

Kajiya, J. T., 201, 203
Kalina, R. E., 23, 36–38, 42, 53, 89–90
Kanade, T., 184, 205
Kanizsa, G., 214, 216
Kaplan, E., 84–85, 96, 100, 111
Kass, M. H., 214, 344, 353–354
Kender, J. R., 307
Kennedy, H., 241
Kersten, D., 210, 212, 216–217
Kim, C. B. Y., 163, 165
King-Smith, P. E., 137
Kirkpatrick, S., 322
Klein, S. A., 114, 128, 153, 156–158, 161, 166–167, 232, 237, 273
Klinker, G. J., 184, 205
Knight, B. W., 144
Knowles, G., 307, 312
Knutsson, H., 16
Koch, C., 219, 236–237, 248, 312, 341
Koenderink, J. J., 7, 9, 17, 32, 307, 315, 339, 353, 371, 377–379
Koffka, K., 231
Köhler, W., 32
Kohonen, T., 25, 32
Kolb, H., 23, 72
Kraft, T. W., 173
Krauskopf, J., 72, 75–76, 79–80, 147

Kröger-Paulus, A., 72
Krol, J. D., 347
Kulikowski, J. J., 101, 125, 127, 137
Kunze, R., 192

Lamb, T. D., 59, 63–64
Land, E. H., 172, 177, 209–210
Landy, M. S., 130, 257, 260, 273–275, 277–278, 287–291, 297, 303, 307, 324, 360
Lange-Malecki, B., 177
Laplace, P. S., 192
Lasley, D. J., 149
Lawergren, B., 339
Lee, B. B., 100
Lee, H., 172, 177, 184
Legendre, A. M., 192, 298
Legge, G. E., 155–156
Lennie, P., 46, 72, 75–76, 78–80, 84–85, 88, 92, 96, 100, 104, 129, 172, 184, 205, 285
LeVay, S., 91
Levi, D. M., 153, 155–158, 161, 166–167, 371
Levick, W. R., 109
Levine, M. D., 4
Li, C., 129–130
Lieberman, L., 307
Limperis, T., 188–189
Linsker, R., 32
Little, J. J., 210, 219, 237, 240, 242, 313, 316, 327, 378
Livingstone, M. S., 14, 360
Lloyd, S. A., 345, 367
Longuet-Higgins, H. C., 307, 315, 338–339, 377
Lubin, J., 286
Lund, J. S., 91–92, 103
Luo, J., 248

MacAdam, D. L., 176, 180
McCann, J. J., 172, 177
McCourt, M. E., 105
McCrane, E. P., 72
McFarlane, D. K., 154–156
Mach, E., 210, 216
McKee, S. P., 156–157, 177, 231, 239, 241, 365
McLaren, K., 172
McLauchlan, P., 333, 337, 353
McLean, J., 115–116, 125, 232
MacLeod, D. I. A., 41, 57, 66, 72, 177, 285
MacRobert, T. M., 192
Maddess, T., 105
Maffei, L., 110, 125, 127–129, 150, 153, 155, 232, 234, 285, 378
Magnenat-Thalmann, N., 212
Makous, W., 41, 50
Malik, J., 120, 273, 287
Mallat, S. G., 241
Mallot, H. A. 205, 210, 306–308, 310–311, 314, 320, 324–325, 335, 337, 340, 376

Maloney, L. T., 11, 22–23, 29, 31, 170, 172, 176, 219, 303, 324
Mansfield, J. S., 335–336, 361
Marcelja, S., 85, 101
Marchiafava, P. L., 241
Mariani, A., 72, 77
Marmarelis, P., 114–115
Marmarelis, V., 114–115
Marr, D., 4, 32, 211, 241–244, 303, 306, 312, 316, 321–322, 327, 333, 335, 337, 340–342, 345, 348–351, 354, 359, 366, 369, 371–372, 378–379
Marrocco, R. T., 72
Marroquin, J. L., 217
Marshall, N. J., 11
Mattsson, L., 188
Maunsell, J. H. R., 92, 104, 129, 166, 232, 285
Max, N., 188, 192
Mayer, M. J., 163, 165
Mayhew, J. E. W., 260, 262, 306, 310, 313, 315–316, 332–341, 344–346, 348, 350–354, 360–361, 363, 367, 369, 377–378
Mead, C., 248
Meister, M., 66
Merigan, W. H., 106
Metelli, F., 212–213
Metropolis, N., 322
Millard, R. T., 307
Miller, M. I., 219
Miller, W. H., 42, 52, 158
Mingolla, E., 205, 277–278, 286, 307, 309, 320
Minlos, R. A., 192
Mitchison, G., 363–364
Mollon, J., 72
Moravec, H. P., 336
Moreland, J. D., 80
Morgan, M. J., 153, 156–157, 166–167
Morlet, J., 241
Morley, J. W., 86
Morrone, M. C., 16, 109–110, 120, 125, 150, 285
Morton-Gibson, M., 231–232, 235, 237, 241
Mostafavi, H., 254
Movshon, J. A., 16, 101, 110–113, 120, 125, 127–128, 150, 155, 231–232, 236–242
Mulligan, J. B., 23, 31–32
Mullins, W. W., 137
Mumford, D., 327

Nachmias, J., 137–138, 148–149, 155–156, 164, 286
Nakatani, K., 66
Nakayama, K., 109, 212–213, 232, 239, 241–242, 247–248
Näsänen, R., 160
Nayar, S. K., 205
Neisser, U., 3
Nerger, J. L., 72
Newhall, S. M., 171, 176
Newsome, W. T., 92, 166, 232, 238–239, 241
Nickerson, D., 174

Nicodemus, F. E., 188–189
Nielsen, K. R. K., 138, 140, 153
Nishihara, H. K., 359, 370, 371
Nolte, L. W., 149
Nothdurft, H. C., 263, 273, 277
Nunn, B. J., 58–60, 64, 66

Oakley, J. P., 28
Ogle, K. N., 343
Ohzawa, I., 17, 110, 113, 116, 129–130, 259, 285
Olzak, L., 3
Orban, G. A., 241
Østerberg, G., 23, 42

Packer, O., 23, 36–38, 42, 53, 89–90, 102, 105
Palmer, L. A., 85, 101, 115–116, 125, 232, 241
Papoulis, A., 96–99
Parisi, G., 321
Parker, A. J., 84–85, 87–89, 96, 100–101, 103, 155, 335–336, 351, 360, 363–366, 371, 376–377
Paulus, W., 72
Pavel, M., 23, 31
Pearson, D. E., 44
Peek, S. A., 339
Peli, E., 279
Pelli, D. G., 103, 138, 141, 143–144, 147–150
Penn, R. D., 58–60, 63–64, 66
Pentland, A. P., 120, 187, 307
Perona, P., 120, 273, 287
Perry, V. H., 42, 72–73, 84, 89–90, 285
Peterson, W. W., 148–149
Petrov, A. P., 339
Pettigrew, J. D., 340
Pflug, R., 23
Phillips, G. C., 154–156, 231, 244–245, 255, 305, 362
Phong, B. T., 188, 191, 195, 305, 309–311, 320, 325
Pirchio, M., 125
Plummer, D. J., 210
Poggio, G. F., 14, 312, 333, 337, 354
Poggio, T., 14, 210, 219, 232, 234, 237, 240–244, 248, 306, 312–313, 316, 321–322, 327, 333, 335, 337, 341–342, 345, 348–349, 353–354, 366, 369, 378–379
Pointer, J. S., 100
Poirson, A. B., 173
Pokorny, J., 3, 72, 173
Polit, A., 254
Pollard, S. B., 313, 315, 321, 333, 336–337, 340–347, 350–354, 366–367, 369
Pollen, D. A., 125, 234
Ponce, J., 371
Porrill, J., 332, 336–341, 344–346, 350–353
Powell, M. J. D., 257
Prazdny, K., 213, 274, 306–307, 343–344, 348, 369
Press, W. H., 192, 204, 285

Pridmore, T. P., 337, 340, 352–353
Pugh, E. N., Jr., 59, 64, 66

Quick, R. F., 137, 285

Ramachandran, V. S., 216, 231, 248
Ramoa, A. S., 150
Ratliff, F., 237
Raugh, M. R., 29, 32
Reck, J., 232, 237
Reeves, A., 147, 177
Regan, D., 157, 166–167, 241, 333, 353–354
Reichardt, W. E., 109, 232, 242
Reichart, T. A., 137
Reid, R. C., 109, 111–115, 117, 125, 127–128, 131, 241
Relkin, E. M., 150
Richards, W. A., ix, 161–162, 166, 212–213, 254
Richmond, J. C., 188–189
Ritter, H., 32
Robinson, D. A., 340
Robson, J. G., 69, 73, 84–85, 96, 112, 119–120, 137, 140, 163–164, 259, 278, 285, 293
Rodieck, R. W., 73, 85
Rodman, H. R., 238–239, 241
Rogers, B. J., 339, 353–354, 378
Rogowitz, B., 177
Röhrenbeck, J., 72, 84, 89, 159, 166
Ronner, S., 234
Rose, A., 147
Rosenbluth, A., 322
Rosenfeld, A., 274
Ross, J., 16, 109, 120
Roth, B., 340
Rovamo, J., 153, 155, 160
Roysam, B., 219
Rubenstein, R. S., 275
Rygol, M., 345

Sachs, M. B., 137
Sagi, D., 273, 275, 277–278
Saito, H., 242
Sakitt, B., 66
Sakrison, D. J., 254
Saleh, B. E. A., 39
Samy, C. N., 102, 105
Sanderson, A. C., 205
Sandini, G., 125
Sanger, T. D., 17, 120
Sansbury, R. V., 148, 155–156
Saul, A. B., 110
Saye, A., 336
Schein, S. J., 72, 84, 89
Schlögl, R. W., 242
Schnapf, J. L., 57–60, 64, 66, 173, 285

Schor, C. M., 333, 348, 353
Schulten, K., 32
Schulze, E., 340
Schumer, R. A., 363–364
Schunck, B. G., 242–243, 246–247
Schweitzer-Tong, D. E., 85, 96
Sclar, G., 72, 104, 110, 113, 116, 129–130, 259, 285
Scott, A. B., 332
Sekuler, R., 231, 244–245
Shadlen, M., 150
Shafer, S. A., 172, 184, 205
Shah, J., 328
Shapiro, Z., 192
Shapley, R. M., 22, 57, 72, 84–85, 96, 100, 109, 111–115, 117, 123, 125, 127–128, 131, 172, 234, 241, 259, 285
Shepard, R. N., 179
Shevell, S. K., 72
Shimojo, S., 212–213
Shulman, D., 303, 354
Siegel, R. M., 232, 248
Silverman, G. H., 212–213, 232, 239, 242, 247–248
Silverman, M. S., 239
Sjoberg, R. W., 188–189
Skottun, B. C., 150
Sloan, K. R., 23, 36–38, 42, 53, 89–90
Smith, J. A., 232, 242–243, 248
Smith, K., 219
Smith, R. A., 35
Smith, V. C., 3, 72, 173
Sneyd, J., 59, 66
Snyder, A. W., 32, 92, 160
Sondhi, M. M., 123, 137
Soodak, R. E., 85, 109, 111–114, 117, 127–128, 131
Sparrow, E. M., 191
Spekreijse, H., 285
Sperling, G., 109, 122–123, 273, 278, 324, 341, 360
Sperling, H. G., 72
Sperry, R. W., 32
Spitzer, H., 16, 110, 278
Springmeyer, R., 188, 192
Stavenga, D. G., 160
Steinman, R. M., 159, 166
Stephens, M., 336
Stevens, K. A., 307, 319
Stiles, W. S., 66, 179, 181, 199
Stone, G. O., 27
Storjohann, K., 340
Stromeyer, C. F., 255
Sutter, A. K., 273–279, 281, 283, 286–287
Sutter, E., 114–115
Swain, M. J., 307, 312
Swanson, W. H., 159
Swarztrauber, P. N., 192, 194

Swets, J. A., 29, 138, 148
Szeliski, R. S., 203

Tadmor, Y., 120, 125–126
Talman, J. D., 192, 202
Tamura, T., 66
Tanaka, K., 242
Tanner, W. P., Jr., 138, 148–149
Taylor, T. H., 177
Teller, A., 322
Teller, E., 322
Tenenbaum, J. M., 205, 210, 307, 378
Terras, A., 192
Terzopoulos, D., 210, 214, 224, 353–354, 363
Teukolsky, S. A., 192, 204, 285
Thacker, N., 336–337, 340
Thalmann, D., 212
Thibos, L. N., 35
Thomas, J. P., 3
Thompson, B. J., 44
Thompson, I. D., 16, 100, 112, 120, 125, 127–128, 155
Thompson, R. J., 165
Thompson, W. B., 336
Thorell, L. G., 11, 84, 101–102, 155, 255, 257
Tiana, C. L. M., 36–38, 54
Tikhonov, A. N., 243
Timberlake, G. T., 159, 166
Todd, J. T., 205, 307, 309, 320
Todorović, D., 210
Toet, A., 32
Tolhurst, D. J., 16, 85, 101, 110–113, 120, 125–128, 150, 155, 231–232, 237
Tominaga, S., 172, 205
Tootell, R. B., 285
Torrance, K. E., 188, 190–191, 196–197, 203, 205
Torre, V., 219, 241, 243, 312, 341
Tranchina, D., 59, 66, 85, 111
Treisman, A., 4
Trivedi, H. P., 336–337, 345, 367
Troy, J. B., 96, 100–101
Tsai, R. A., 337, 342
Turner, M. R., 120, 273, 275, 277
Tyler, C. W., 156, 241, 273, 332–333, 343, 353, 364

Udding, J. T., 219
Ullman, S., 209, 231, 236, 241–242, 307

Valberg, A., 177
Valeton, J. M., 66
van den Berg, T. J. T. P., 285
van Doorn, A. J., 7, 9, 17, 315, 353, 371, 377–379
van Essen, D. C., 32, 84, 91–92, 166
van Norren, D., 58, 285
van Santen, J. P. H., 109, 122

Varner, F. D., 177
Vaughn, W. J., 114, 128, 232, 237
Vautin, R. G., 92
Vecchi, M. P., 322
Vergnet, R. L., 336
Verri, A., 241
Vetterling, W. T., 192, 204, 285
Victor, J. D., 114–115, 259, 273, 277, 287
Vidyasagar, T. R., 100
Vimal, R. L. P., 72
Virsu, V., 160
von der Malsburg, C., 32
von Gavel, L., 36
von Helmholtz, H., 169, 171, 190, 332–333, 339, 374–375
Vorhees, H., 244

Walker, J. S., 192
Wallace, J. R., 203
Walraven, J., 57, 66, 177, 285
Walraven, P. L., 163
Walsh, D. J., 35
Wandell, B. A., 140, 170, 172–176, 180–181, 183, 199, 205, 219
Warren, M., 171, 176
Wässle, H., 72, 84, 89, 159, 166
Watson, A. B., 3, 32, 44, 85, 96, 98, 100–101, 104–105, 109,
     120, 122, 138–139, 147–148, 153, 163–164, 232, 234, 255, 257,
     275, 360
Watt, R. J., 153, 156–157, 161, 167
Wegman, M., 323, 327
Weinshall, D., 313, 347
Weiss, L. E., 205
Welch, L., 231, 241
West, G., 172
Westheimer, G., 154, 156–157, 159, 339, 363–365, 371, 377, 379
Whitten, D. N., 65
Whitteridge, D., 166
Widrow, B., 27
Wiesel, T. N., 75, 77, 84–85, 110, 115, 119, 150, 255, 360
Williams, D. R., 22, 35–38, 41–42, 44–46, 50, 52–54, 72
Williams, D. W., 231, 244–245
Willshaw, D. J., 32
Wilson, H. R., 153–157, 159–167, 242, 254–255, 259, 360, 362
Wintz, P., 266
Witkin, A. P., 205, 212–214, 244, 307, 353–354
Wood, I., 348
Woolfson, M. M., 172
Wright, M. J., 231–232, 237
Wurst, S., 324
Wyszecki, G. W., 171, 176, 179, 180–181, 199

Yang, T., 323
Yang, Y., 335–336, 363–366
Yap, Y. L., 157–158, 166
Yau, K.-W., 66
Yellott, J. I., Jr., 21, 23, 31–32, 42–43, 273

Young, R. A., 10–11, 72
Yuille, A. L., 203, 221, 231–232, 234–240, 242–244, 247–249, 306,
     316, 321–324, 328, 371
Yukio, M., 242
Yund, E. W., 255, 257

Zheng, Y., 333–334
Zisserman, A., 306, 312, 315, 337, 353, 376
Zucker, S. W., 17, 216

Subject Index

Acuity
  grating, 159
  hyperacuity, 32, 154, 156, 160–161
  stereo. *See* Stereopsis, stereo acuity
  vernier, 18, 154–156, 159–160
Adaptation
  chromatic, 171, 176–177
  light, 22, 64–66, 123, 285
  spatial frequency, 154
Aliasing, 13
  spatial, 21, 32, 35–55, 161, 340, 376
  temporal, 37
Aperture problem. *See* Motion, aperture problem
A-wave. *See* Electroretinogram, a-wave

Back-pocket model. *See* Texture, back-pocket model
Bandwidth. *See* Linear filtering
Bayesian analysis, 217–219, 226, 320–324, 327–328
Beta. *See* Psychometric function, slope
Binocular stereopsis. *See* Stereopsis
Bipolar cell, 72, 77
Blue-yellow cell. *See* Color, opponency
B-wave. *See* Electroretinogram, b-wave

Channel, 136, 138, 143–144, 147, 153–157, 161–163, 254–255,
      273–279, 282–287, 335–336, 360, 363
Clique, 220
Color
  appearance, 38, 171–184
  assimilation, 176
  constancy, 169, 171, 176, 183
  opponency, 12–14, 69, 71–81
  simultaneous color contrast, 171, 176
Complex cell, 16, 119, 124–125, 128, 255, 278
Compressive nonlinearity. *See* Nonlinearity, compressive
Computer graphics, 169, 191, 316, 325, 375–376
Cone
  aperture, 39, 41, 49–50
  density, 23, 73, 83–84, 89–90, 158
  mosaic, 35–36, 39, 41–43, 50, 54, 70–72, 79, 87–92, 158–160
  ratio (R : G), 72, 79
  spectral sensitivity, 72, 173–174
Contrast, 148–150, 213–214, 277–278, 293
  gain, 96, 98–99
  gain control. *See* Nonlinearity, contrast gain control
  independence, 154, 164, 167

Contrast (cont.)
  response, 128–131
  reversal, 112–113, 127–128
  sensitivity, 83, 85–89, 95–106
Cooperativity. See Cue integration; Motion, cooperativity
Correspondence. See Stereopsis, correspondence
Cortex. See Visual cortex
Cortical magnification. See Visual cortex, cortical magnification
Counterphase. See Contrast, reversal
Cross-correlation, 115, 139, 264–268, 313, 333, 369–371
CSF. See Contrast, sensitivity
Cue integration, 209–210, 224–226
  depth, 206, 303, 305–312, 319–324, 354, 375–379
  transparency, 214
Curvature discrimination. See Discrimination, curvature

d', 148–150
Dark adaptation. See Adaptation, light
Decision, 40, 46–48, 138, 148–150, 264–265, 297
Delta rule, 27–30
Depth. See Shape
Detection, 135–136, 138, 147
Differential invariant, 339, 371
Direction selectivity, 109–117, 231–233, 237, 241
Directional derivative, 8–10, 257
Directional index, 112–113, 127–128
Discrimination, 135
  curvature, 161–162, 371
  displacement, 18
  motion, 36, 38, 40, 48–50, 231
  orientation, 36–38, 40
  spatial frequency, 154, 163–166
  spatial pattern, 23, 153, 155–158, 166, 253, 264–269
  temporal order, 18
  wavelength, 18
Disparity. See Stereopsis, disparity
DOG. See Gaussians, difference of

Edge, 6–7, 10, 14, 335
Edge detection, 210, 216, 248, 266, 297, 341–342, 352
Efficiency, 147
Electroretinogram
  a-wave, 57–58, 61–66
  b-wave, 57–58, 62
End-stopping, 17
Energy measure. See Motion; Stereopsis; Texture
Epipolar constraint. See Stereopsis, epipolar constraint
Equiluminance. See Isoluminance
ERG. See Electroretinogram
Eye movement, 22, 29, 54, 159

Fourier analysis, 295–296
  spatial, 42–43, 84–87, 126, 273
  spatiotemporal, 40–41, 44, 96, 116, 234

spherical, 188–205
Fovea, 11, 21, 23, 25, 35, 42, 52, 72, 75, 87, 89–90, 100, 105
Frequency doubling, 110, 128
Fundamental. See Cone, spectral sensitivity

Gabor function
  spatial, 85, 101, 104, 121, 126, 263, 275
  spatiotemporal, 122, 128, 233–234, 241
Gain. See Contrast, gain
Gain control. See Nonlinearity, contrast gain control
Ganglion cell, 71, 72, 79, 84–85, 159
Gaussians, difference of, 73–74, 85–86, 88–89, 100
  with separation, 85–89
Gibbs distribution, 219, 222, 224, 226, 321
Gloss. See Reflectance, specular

Highlight. See Reflectance, specular
Horizontal cell, 72
Horopter. See Stereopsis, horopter
Hyperacuity. See Acuity, hyperacuity

Ideal observer, 40, 148, 217–218, 226
Identification. See Discrimination
Impulse response
  spatial, 121, 125–126
  spatiotemporal, 96, 110–111, 122
  temporal, 12, 58
Induced effect. See Stereopsis, induced effect
Inhibition, 125, 150, 154, 276
  cross-frequency, 124, 285
  cross-orientation, 110, 120, 124, 285
  shunting, 125, 241
Integration. See Cue integration
Interference fringe, 35, 38
Interpolation, 25–32, 313–314, 321, 323–324, 353, 365, 378
Isoluminance, 253

Kernel, 114–117

Lambertian reflectance. See Reflectance, Lambertian
Laplacian operator, 9, 12, 192, 243, 306, 312–313, 363
Lateral geniculate nucleus, 73, 83–89, 100–106, 111, 119
Legendre polynomial, 192–194, 298
LGN. See Lateral geniculate nucleus
Light adaptation. See Adaptation, light
Lighting, 169
Lightness, 210, 287
Line element model, 139–141, 155–156
Line process, 219–221, 248, 321, 327–328
Linear filtering, 9–10, 39, 119–121, 188–190
  optical, 21, 28, 87–88
  orientation bandwidth, 257, 260, 275
  spatial, 155, 254–255, 275–276, 297–298, 335–336, 360–361, 369–370

spatial frequency bandwidth, 102, 104, 275
spatiotemporal, 100, 122, 232–235, 237
temporal, 12, 59

Macular pigment, 77–78
Magnocellular (M) stream, 69, 71, 84
Markov random field, 214, 219–221, 226
Masking, 154–155, 286, 335–336, 360–363
Mechanism. *See* Channel
Metamerism, 179, 183–184, 199, 205, 254
Micropattern, 253, 261
Modulation transfer function, 88, 96, 100–101, 121–122, 125–126, 188
Mondrian, 210, 225–226
Motion
    aperture problem, 235–236, 239, 241, 247–248
    capture, 248
    cooperativity, 231, 244–246
    discontinuity, 231, 240, 242, 248
    energy, 16, 110, 120–121, 123, 130, 229, 232–242, 277
    opponency, 46–47
    parallax, 14
    reversal, 35–36, 45, 48–50, 52
    structure-from-motion. *See* Shape, from motion
    velocity, 231–249
MRF. *See* Markov random field
M-sequence, 114–117
MT. *See* Visual cortex, MT
MTF. *See* Modulation transfer function
Multiple cues. *See* Cue integration

Neural network model, 23–32, 339–340
Noise, 96–101, 147–150, 265–266
Nonlinearity, 113, 148–149, 155–156, 161, 166, 269, 274, 282–285, 297–300
    compressive, 65, 213, 334
    contrast gain control, 116–117, 123–125, 130, 259–260, 285–287
    rectification, 112, 120, 122–123, 126–127, 130–131, 278–279, 283
    saturation, 59, 63–64, 66, 129
Normalization. *See* Nonlinearity, contrast gain control
Nyquist frequency, 21, 33, 36, 38, 42–43, 45–46, 48, 50–51, 87

Occlusion, 210, 212, 307, 340, 378
Opponency. *See* Color, Motion; Orientation
Ordering constraint. *See* Stereopsis, ordering constraint
Orientation, 260–261
    opponency, 47–48, 52, 258–259, 287
    reversal, 35–37, 45–46, 52–53
    selectivity, 85, 153, 160, 255, 257

Panum's fusional area, 343, 364
Panum's limiting case, 347, 367, 369, 379
Parvocellular (P) stream, 69, 71–81, 84, 100, 104–106
Phase, spatiotemporal response, 112–113, 127, 131

Phong reflectance. *See* Reflectance, Phong
Photoisomerization, 58–59
Photoreceptor. *See* Cone; Rod
Plaid, 236, 238–239
Plenoptic function, 1, 4–14, 17, 169, 229–230
Point spread function, 28, 195
Primary visual cortex. *See* Visual cortex, V1
Probability summation, 138, 140, 147, 149
Psychometric function, 148, 155
    slope, 138–139, 141–144
Pyramid, Gaussian/Laplacian, 255–258, 275

Quadrature, 16, 111, 120–121, 234–235, 258

Receptive field, 10, 96, 297
    ganglion cell, 73–74, 78
    lateral geniculate nucleus, 11, 73–74, 78, 83–92, 100
    model, 84–87, 121–122, 138, 154–155, 275, 281
    V1, 11, 83–92, 119, 125
Rectification. *See* Nonlinearity, rectification
Red-green cell. *See* Color, opponency
Reflectance, 169, 210, 217
    function, 172, 187–192, 195–206
    Lambertian, 187, 305, 308–310, 312, 320, 325, 372
    Phong, 191, 195, 309–311, 320, 325
    specular, 187–188, 205–206, 211, 305–306, 313–319, 325
Representation, 307–309, 320, 332–333, 377–379
Retina, 71–72, 241
Retinal disease, 57, 64–66
Rod, 58–66, 173

Saccade. *See* Eye movement
Sampling, 11–12, 21
    disordered, 23, 26, 35, 38, 42, 52, 54, 72, 105, 154, 158–161, 164–166
    hexagonal, 41–42, 72, 79, 87
    regular, 26–29, 33
    wavelength, 11, 38
Saturation. *See* Nonlinearity, saturation
Sensitivity. *See* Contrast, sensitivity
Sensor. *See* Channel
Separability, 100–101, 110–112, 115, 117
Shadow, 205, 210–212, 221
Shading. *See* Reflectance; Shape, from shading
Shape, 303. *See also* Cue integration; Stereopsis
    from contour, 206
    from highlight, 306, 311–319
    from motion, 209, 226
    from shading, 187, 206, 209, 305–314, 319–320, 375–377
    from texture, 305, 308, 310–312, 318, 375–377
Signal detection theory, 97–98, 138, 148–150
Simple cell, 109–117, 124–128, 155, 255, 278
Simulated annealing, 224, 322
Spectral power distribution, 169, 171–174, 176, 205

Specularity. *See* Reflectance, specular
Spherical harmonic. *See* Fourier analysis, spherical
Stereopsis, 214–215, 226, 306, 309–310, 312–323, 327–328, 359–379
  correspondence, 13, 212, 331–354
  disparity, 13, 18, 206, 313, 316–317, 321–323, 327, 363–366
    gradient, 323, 342–347, 366–370
    vertical, 315, 318, 332, 337–339, 354, 377
  energy, 16
  epipolar constraint, 315–316, 327, 337–338, 340, 342, 347
  horopter, 331–332, 374–375
  induced effect, 339, 377
  ordering constraint, 341, 346, 349, 366–370
  stereo acuity, 364–365
Striate cortex. *See* Visual cortex, V1
Subthreshold summation, 138–144, 154
Subunit, 16, 119, 128
Superposition, 119–121
Surface
  property, 169, 307–308, 316
  reflectance. *See* Reflectance

Template matching, 138–144
Texture
  back-pocket model, 274, 276, 297–298
  energy, 16, 120, 229, 255–256, 258–263, 276–277
  segregation, 229, 253–270, 273–288, 293–294, 297–300
  shape-from-texture. *See* Shape, from texture
Transducer function. *See* Nonlinearity
Transparency, 210–226, 240, 248, 323, 348, 369
Trichromacy, 38, 172–173

Uncertainty
  observer, 138, 140–144, 149–150
  sampling, 158–161, 164–166
Undersampling. *See* Aliasing

V1. *See* Visual cortex, V1
Vector magnitude model. *See* Line element model
Velocity. *See* Motion, velocity
Vernier acuity. *See* Acuity, vernier
Visual cortex
  cortical magnification, 92, 159
  MT, 237–242
  V1, 83–92, 100–105, 110–117, 119–120, 278

Wavelength, 5, 172–174
Weber's law, 157–158, 164–165
Window of visibility, 39, 44–46, 50–51